Principles of Psych
Assessment

This book highlights the principles of psychological assessment to help researchers and clinicians better develop, evaluate, administer, score, integrate, and interpret psychological assessments. It discusses psychometrics (reliability and validity), the assessment of various psychological domains (behavior, personality, intellectual functioning), various measurement methods (e.g., questionnaires, observations, interviews, biopsychological assessments, performance-based assessments), and emerging analytical frameworks to evaluate and improve assessment including: generalizability theory, structural equation modeling, item response theory, and signal detection theory. It also discusses ethics, test bias, and cultural and individual diversity.

Key Features

- Gives analysis examples using free software
- Helps readers apply principles to research and practice
- Provides text, analysis code/syntax, R output, figures, and interpretations integrated to guide readers
- Uses the freely available petersenlab package for R

Principles of Psychological Assessment: With Applied Examples in R is intended for use by graduate students, faculty, researchers, and practicing psychologists.

Dr. Isaac T. Petersen is assistant professor at the University of Iowa. He completed his Bachelor of Arts in psychology and French at the University of Texas, his PhD in psychology at Indiana University, and his clinical psychology internship from Western Psychiatric Hospital at the University of Pittsburgh Medical Center.

Dr. Petersen is a licensed clinical psychologist with expertise in developmental psychopathology. His clinical expertise is in training parents how to deal with difficult children. He is interested in how children develop individual differences in adjustment, including behavior problems as well as competencies, so that more effective intervention and prevention approaches can be developed and implemented. He is particularly interested in the development of externalizing behavior problems (e.g., ADHD, conduct problems, and aggression) and underlying self-regulation difficulties. Dr. Petersen's primary interests include how children develop self-regulation as a function of bio-psycho-social processes including brain functioning, genetics, parenting, temperament, language, and sleep, and how self-regulation influences adjustment. A special emphasis of his work examines neural processes underlying the development of self-regulation and externalizing problems, using electroencephalography (EEG) and event-related potentials (ERPs). He uses longitudinal designs, advanced quantitative methods, and multiple levels of analysis, including bio-psycho-social processes, to elucidate mechanisms in the development of externalizing problems. His work considers multiple levels of analysis simultaneously, in interaction, and over lengthy spans of development in ways that identify people's change in behavior problems over time while accounting for the changing manifestation of behavior problems across development (heterotypic continuity).

Chapman & Hall/CRC
Statistics in the Social and Behavioral Sciences Series

Series Editors
Jeff Gill, Steven Heeringa, Wim J. van der Linden, Tom Snijders

Recently Published Titles

Big Data and Social Science: Data Science Methods and Tools for Research and Practice, Second Edition
Ian Foster, Rayid Ghani, Ron S. Jarmin, Frauke Kreuter and Julia Lane

Understanding Elections through Statistics: Polling, Prediction, and Testing
Ole J. Forsberg

Analyzing Spatial Models of Choice and Judgment, Second Edition
David A. Armstrong II, Ryan Bakker, Royce Carroll, Christopher Hare, Keith T. Poole and Howard Rosenthal

Introduction to R for Social Scientists: A Tidy Programming Approach
Ryan Kennedy and Philip Waggoner

Linear Regression Models: Applications in R
John P. Hoffman

Mixed-Mode Surveys: Design and Analysis
Jan van den Brakel, Bart Buelens, Madelon Cremers, Annemieke Luiten, Vivian Meertens, Barry Schouten and Rachel Vis-Visschers

Applied Regularization Methods for the Social Sciences
Holmes Finch

An Introduction to the Rasch Model with Examples in R
Rudolf Debelak, Carolin Stobl and Matthew D. Zeigenfuse

Regression Analysis in R: A Comprehensive View for the Social Sciences
Jocelyn H. Bolin

Intensive Longitudinal Analysis of Human Processes
Kathleen M. Gates, Sy-Min Chow, and Peter C. M. Molenaar

Applied Regression Modeling: Bayesian and Frequentist Analysis of Categorical and Limited Response Variables with R and Stan
Jun Xu

The Psychometrics of Standard Setting: Connecting Policy and Test Scores
Mark Reckase

Crime Mapping and Spatial Data Analysis using R
Juanjo Medina and Reka Solymosi

Computational Aspects of Psychometric Methods: With R
Patricia Martinková and Adéla Hladká

Principles of Psychological Assessment
With Applied Examples in R
Isaac T. Petersen

For more information about this series, please visit: https://www.routledge.com/Chapman--Hall CRC-Statistics-in-the-Social-and-Behavioral-Sciences/book-series/CHSTSOBESCI

Principles of Psychological Assessment

With Applied Examples in R

Isaac T. Petersen

CRC Press
Taylor & Francis Group
Boca Raton London New York

CRC Press is an imprint of the
Taylor & Francis Group, an **informa** business
A CHAPMAN & HALL BOOK

First edition published 2024
by CRC Press
2385 Executive Center Drive, Suite 320, Boca Raton, FL 33431, U.S.A.

and by CRC Press
4 Park Square, Milton Park, Abingdon, Oxon, OX14 4RN

CRC Press is an imprint of Taylor & Francis Group, LLC

Library of Congress Cataloging-in-Publication Data

Names: Petersen, Isaac T., author.
Title: Principles of Psychological Assessment : with Applied Examples in R/ Isaac T. Petersen.
Description: First edition. | Boca Raton : CRC Press, 2024. | Series: Statistics in the social and behavioral sciences series | Includes bibliographical references and index. | Summary: "The book highlights the principles of psychological assessment to help researchers and clinicians better develop, evaluate, administer, score, integrate, and interpret psychological assessments. It discusses psychometrics (reliability and validity), the assessment of various psychological domains (behavior, personality, intellectual functioning), various measurement methods (e.g., questionnaires, observations, interviews, biopsychological assessments, performance-based assessments), and emerging analytical frameworks to evaluate and improve assessment including: generalizability theory, structural equation modeling, item response theory, and signal detection theory. It also discusses ethics, test bias, and cultural and individual diversity"-- Provided by publisher.
Identifiers: LCCN 2023039827 (print) | LCCN 2023039828 (ebook) |
ISBN 9781032411347 (pbk) |
ISBN 9781032413068 (hbk) | ISBN 9781003357421 (ebk)
Subjects: LCSH: Psychodiagnostics--Data processing. | Mental illness--Diagnosis--Methodology. | R (Computer program language)
Classification: LCC RC469 .P48 2024 (print) | LCC RC469 (ebook) | DDC 616.89/075--dc23/eng/20240102
LC record available at https://lccn.loc.gov/2023039827
LC ebook record available at https://lccn.loc.gov/2023039828

ISBN: 978-1-032-41306-8 (hbk)
ISBN: 978-1-032-41134-7 (pbk)
ISBN: 978-1-003-35742-1 (ebk)

DOI: 10.1201/9781003357421

Typeset in Latin Modern font
by KnowledgeWorks Global Ltd.

Publisher's note: This book has been prepared from camera-ready copy provided by the authors.

To our daughter, Maisie.

Contents

List of Figures

List of Tables

Acknowledgments

This book was supported by a grant from the University of Iowa Libraries.

This book would not be possible without the help of others. Much of the content of this book was inspired by Richard Viken's course in psychological assessment that I took as a graduate student. I thank W. Joel Schneider who provided several examples that were adapted for this book. I thank Danielle Szabreath, Samar Haddad, and Michele Dumont for help in copyediting. I acknowledge my wife, Alyssa Varner[1], who helped design several of the graphics used in this book, in addition to all of her support throughout the process.

[1] https://alyssajovarner.com

Introduction

About This Book

First, let us discuss what this book is *not*. This book is not a guide on how to assess each psychological construct or disorder. This book is also not a comparative summary of the psychometrics of different measures. There already exist many resources that summarize and compare the reliability and validity of measures in psychology (Buros Center for Testing, 2021). Instead, this book is about the *principles* of psychological assessment.

This book was originally written for a graduate-level course on psychological assessment. The chapters provide an overview of topics that each could have its own class and textbook, such as structural equation modeling, item response theory, generalizability theory, factor analysis, prediction, cognitive assessment, psychophysiological assessment, etc. The book gives readers an overview of the breadth of the field of assessment and various assessment approaches. As a consequence, the book does not cover any one assessment device or method in great depth.

The goal of this book is to help researchers and clinicians learn to think critically about assessments so they can better develop, evaluate, administer, score, integrate, and interpret psychological assessments. Learning important principles of assessment will put you in a better position to learn any assessment device and to develop better ones. This book applies a scientific perspective to the principles of psychological assessment. The assessments used in a given situation—whether in research or practice—should be supported by the strongest available science, or they should be used cautiously while undergoing development and study. In addition to discussing principles, however, analysis scripts in the software `R` (R Core Team, 2022) are also provided, so that you are able to apply the principles discussed in this book. Analysis exercises for each chapter are freely available in the online version of the book: https://isaactpetersen.github.io/Principles-Psychological-Assessment/

Why R?

`R` is free, open source, open platform, and widely used. Unlike proprietary software used for data analysis, `R` is not a black box. You can examine the code for any function or computation you perform. You can even modify and improve these functions by changing the code, and you can create your own functions. `R` also has advanced capabilities for data wrangling and has many packages available for advanced statistical analysis and graphing. In addition, there are strong resources available for creating your analyses in `R` so they are reproducible by others (Gandrud, 2020).

About the Author

Regarding my background, I am a licensed clinical psychologist. My research examines how children develop behavior problems. I am also a trained clinician, and I supervise training clinicians in assessment and therapy, particularly assessment and treatment of children's disruptive behavior. Given my expertise, many of the examples in the book deal with topics in clinical psychology, but many of the assessment principles discussed are relevant to all areas of psychology—and science more broadly—and are often overlooked in research and practice. As a clinical scientist, my perspective is that the scientific epistemology is the strongest approach to knowledge and that assessment should be guided first and foremost by the epistemology of science, regardless of whether one is doing research or practice.

What Is Assessment?

Assessment is the gathering of information about a person, group, setting, or context. In psychological assessment, we are interested in gathering information about people's psychological functioning, including their thoughts, emotions, and behaviors. Psychological assessment can also consider biological and physiological processes that are linked to people's thoughts, emotions, and behaviors. Many assessment approaches can be used to assess people's thoughts, emotions, and behaviors, including self-report questionnaires, questionnaires reported by others (e.g., spouse, parent, teacher, or friend), interviews, observations, biopsychological assessments (e.g., cortisol, heart rate, brain imaging), performance-based assessments, archival approaches (e.g., chart review), and combinations of these.

Why Should We Care About Assessment (and Science)?

In research, assessments are conducted to advance knowledge, such as improved prediction or understanding. For example, in my research, I use assessments to understand what processes influence children's development of disruptive behavior. In society, assessments are conducted to improve decision-making. For instance, assessments are conducted to determine whether to hire a job candidate or promote an employee. In a clinical context, assessments are conducted to improve treatment and the client's outcomes. As an example, assessments are conducted to determine which treatment would be most effective for a person suffering from depression. Assessments can be valuable to understanding current functioning as well as making predictions. To best answer these questions and address these goals, we need to have confidence that our devices yield accurate answers for these purposes for the assessed individuals. Science is crucial for knowing how much (or how little) confidence we have in a given assessment for a given purpose and population. Effective treatment often depends on accurate assessment. Thus, knowing how to conduct and critically evaluate science will make you more effective at selecting, administering, and interpreting assessments.

Decisions resulting from assessments can have important life-altering consequences. High-stakes decisions based on assessments include decisions about whether a person is hospitalized, whether a child is removed from their abusive home, whether a person is deemed competent to stand trial, whether a prisoner is released on parole, and whether an applicant is admitted to graduate school. These important assessment-related decisions should be made using the best available science.

The problem is that there has been a proliferation of pseudo-science in assessment and treatment. There are widely used psychological assessments and treatments that we know are inaccurate, do not work, or in some cases, that we know to be harmful. Lists of harmful psychological treatments (e.g., Lilienfeld, 2007) and inaccurate assessments (e.g., Hunsley et al., 2015) have been published, but these treatments and assessments are still used by professional providers to this day. Practice using such techniques violates the aphorism, "First, do no harm." This would be inconceivable for other applied sciences, such as chemistry, engineering, and medicine. For instance, the prescription of a particular medication for a particular purpose requires approval by the U.S. Food and Drug Administration (FDA). Psychological assessments and treatments do not have the same level of oversight.

The gap between what we know based on science and what is implemented in practice (the science–practice gap) motivated McFall's (1991) "Manifesto for a Science of Clinical Psychology," which he later expanded (McFall, 2000). The Manifesto has one cardinal principle and four corollaries:

> Cardinal Principle: Scientific clinical psychology is the only legitimate and acceptable form of clinical psychology.
>
> First Corollary: Psychological services should not be administered to the public (except under strict experimental control) until they have satisfied these four minimal criteria:
>
> 1. The exact nature of the service must be described clearly.
> 2. The claimed benefits of the service must be stated explicitly.
> 3. These claimed benefits must be validated scientifically.
> 4. Possible negative side effects that might outweigh any benefits must be ruled out empirically.
>
> Second Corollary: The primary and overriding objective of doctoral training programs in clinical psychology must be to produce the most competent clinical scientists possible.
>
> Third Corollary: A scientific epistemology differentiates science from pseudo-science.
>
> Fourth Corollary: The most caring and humane psychological services are those that have been shown empirically to be the most effective, efficient, and safe.

The Manifesto orients you to the scientific perspective from which we will be examining psychological assessment techniques in this book.

Assessment and the Replication Crisis in Science

Assessment is also crucial to advancing knowledge in research, as summarized in the maxim, "What we know depends on how we know it." Findings from studies boil down to the methods that were used to obtain them—thus, everything we know comes down to methods.

Many domains of science, particularly social science, have struggled with a replication crisis, such that a large proportion of findings fail to replicate when independent investigators attempt to replicate the original findings (Duncan et al., 2014; Freese & Peterson, 2017; Larson & Carbine, 2017; Lilienfeld, 2017; Open Science Collaboration, 2015; Shrout & Rodgers, 2018; Tackett, Brandes, King, et al., 2019). There is considerable speculation on what factors account for the replication crisis. For instance, one possible factor is the researcher degrees of freedom, which are unacknowledged choices in how researchers prepare, analyze, and report their data that can lead to detecting significance in the absence of real effects (Loken & Gelman, 2017). This is similar to Gelman & Loken (2013)'s description of research as the garden of forking paths, where different decisions along the way can lead to different outcomes (see Figure 1). A second possibility for the replication crisis is that some replication studies have had limited statistical power (e.g., insufficiently large sample sizes). A third possibility may be that there is publication bias such that researchers tend to publish only significant findings, which is known as the file-drawer effect. A fourth possibility is that researchers may engage in ethically questionable research practices, such as multiple testing and selective reporting.

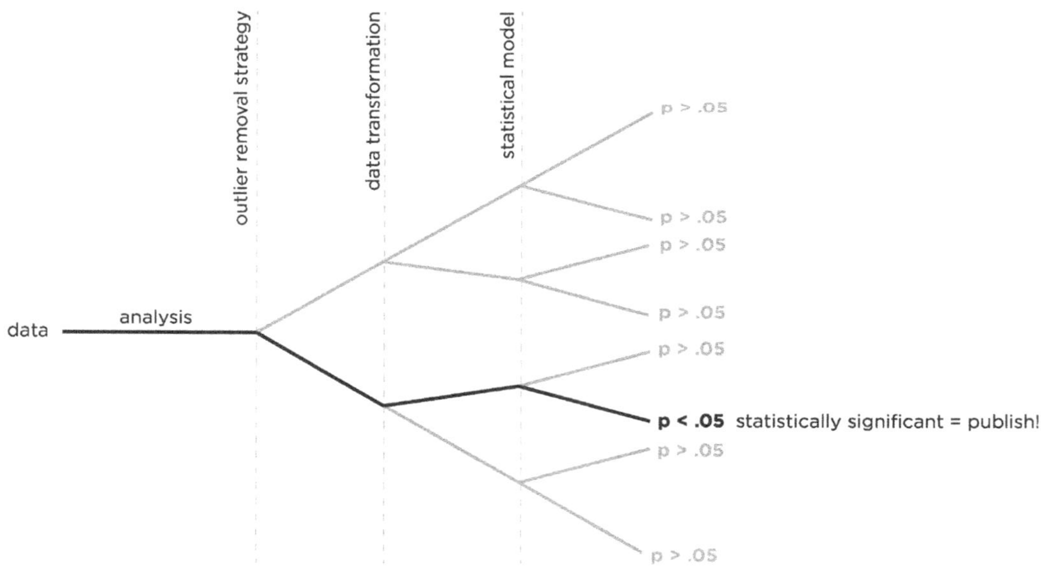

FIGURE 1 Garden of Forking Paths. (Adapted from https://www.si.umich.edu/about-umsi/news/ditch-stale-pdf-making-research-papers-interactive-and-more-transparent [archived at https://perma.cc/R2V9-CP3F].)

However, difficulties with replication could exist even if researchers have the best of intentions, engage in ethical research practices, and are transparent about all of the methods they used and decisions they made. The replication crisis could owe, in part, to noisy (imprecise and inaccurate) measures. The field has paid insufficient attention to measurement unreliability as a key culprit in the replication crisis. As Loken & Gelman (2017) demonstrated, when measures are less noisy, measurement error weakens the association between the measures. But when using noisy measures and selecting what to publish based on statistical significance, measurement error can make the association appear stronger than it is. This is what Loken & Gelman (2017) describe as the *statistical significance filter*: In a study with noisy measures and a small or moderate sample size, statistically significant estimates are likely to have a stronger effect size than the actual effect size—the "true" underlying effects could be small or nonexistent. The statistical significance filter exists because, with a small sample size, the effect size will need to be larger in order to detect it as statistically significant due to larger standard errors. That is, when researchers publish a statistically significant effect with a small or moderate sample size and noisy measures, the effect size will necessarily be large enough to detect it (and likely larger than the true effect). However, the effect of noise (measurement error) diminishes as the sample size increases. So, the goal should be to use less noisy measures with larger sample sizes. And, as discussed in Chapter 13 on ethical considerations in psychological assessment, the use of pre-registration could be useful to control researcher degrees of freedom.

The lack of replicability of findings has the potential to negatively impact the people we study through misinformed assessment, treatment, and policy decisions. Therefore, it is crucial to use assessments with strong psychometric properties and/or to develop better assessments. Psychometrics refer to the reliability and validity of measures. These concepts are described in greater detail in Chapters 3 and 4, but for now, think about reliability as *consistency* of measurement and validity as *accuracy* of measurement.

Science Versus Pseudo-Science in Assessment

Science is the best system of epistemology we have to pursue truth. Science is a process, not a set of facts. It helps us overcome blind spots. The system is revisionary and self-correcting. Science is the epistemology that is the least susceptible to error due to authority, belief, intuition, bias, preference, etc. Clients are in a vulnerable position and deserve to receive services consistent with the strongest available evidence. By providing a client a service, you are implicitly making a claim and prediction. As a psychologist, you are claiming to have expert knowledge and competence. You are making a prediction that the client will improve because of your services. Ethically, you should be making these predictions based on science and a risk-benefit analysis. It is also important to make sure the client knows when services are unproven so they can provide fully informed consent. Otherwise, because of your position as a psychologist, they may believe that you are using an evidence-based approach when you are not.

We will be examining psychological assessment from a scientific perspective. Here are characteristics of science that distinguish it from pseudo-science:

1. Risky hypotheses are posed that are falsifiable. The hypotheses can be shown to be wrong.
2. Findings can be replicated independently by different research groups and different methods. Evidence converges across studies and methods.
3. Potential alternative explanations for findings are specified and examined empirically (with data).
4. Steps are taken to guard against the undue influence of personal beliefs and biases.
5. The strength of claims reflects the strength of evidence. Findings and the ability to make judgments or predictions are not overstated. For instance, it is important to present the degree of uncertainty from assessments with error bars or confidence intervals.

6. Scientifically supported measurement strategies are used based on their psychometrics, including reliability and validity.

Science does not progress without advances in measurement, including

- more efficient measurement (see Chapters 8 and 20)
- more precise measurement (i.e., reliability; see Chapter 3)
- more accurate measurement (i.e., validity; see Chapter 4)
- more sophisticated modeling (see Chapter 23)
- more sophisticated biopsychological (e.g., cognitive neuroscience) techniques, as opposed to self-report and neuropsychological techniques (see Chapter 19)
- considerations of cultural and individual diversity (see Chapter 24)
- ethical considerations (see Chapter 13)

These considerations serve as the focus of this book.

Prerequisites

Applied examples in `R` are provided throughout the book. Each chapter that has `R` examples has a section on "Getting Started," which provides the code to load relevant libraries, load data files, simulate data, add missing data (for realism), perform calculations, and more. The data files used for the examples are available on the Open Science Framework (OSF): https://osf.io/3pwza.

Most of the `R` packages used in this book can be installed from the Comprehensive R Archive Network (CRAN) using the following command:

```
install.packages("INSERT_PACKAGE_NAME_HERE")
```

Several of the packages are hosted on GitHub repositories, including `uroc` (Gneiting & Walz, 2021), `dmacs` (Dueber, 2019), and `petersenlab` (Petersen, 2024).

You can install the `uroc` and `dmacs` packages using the following code:

```
install.packages("remotes")
remotes::install_github("evwalz/uroc")
remotes::install_github("ddueber/dmacs")
```

Many of the `R` functions used in this book are available from the `petersenlab` package (Petersen, 2024): https://github.com/DevPsyLab/petersenlab. You can install the `petersenlab` package (Petersen, 2024) using the following code:

```
install.packages("remotes")
remotes::install_github("DevPsyLab/petersenlab")
```

The code that generates this book is located on GitHub: https://github.com/isaactpetersen/Principles-Psychological-Assessment.

1

Scores and Scales

Assessments yield information. The information is encoded in scores or in other types of data. It is important to consider the different types of data because the types of data restrict what options are available to analyze the data.

1.1 Getting Started

1.1.1 Load Libraries

First, we load the `R` packages used for this chapter:

```
library("petersenlab")
library("MOTE")
library("here")
library("tidyverse")
library("tinytex")
library("knitr")
library("kableExtra")
library("rmarkdown")
library("bookdown")
```

1.1.2 Prepare Data

1.1.2.1 Simulate Data

For this example, we simulate data below.

```
set.seed(52242)

rawData <- rnorm(
  n = 1000,
  mean = 200,
  sd = 30)

scores <- data.frame(
  rawData = rawData,
  rawDataNoMissing = rawData)
```

1.1.2.2 Add Missing Data

Adding missing data to dataframes helps make examples more realistic to real-life data and helps you get in the habit of programming to account for missing data.

```
scores$rawData[c(5,10)] <- NA
```

1.2 Data Types

There are four general data types: nominal, ordinal, interval, and ratio. Depending on the use of the variable, the data could fall into more than one category. The type of data influences what kinds of data analysis you can do. For instance, parametric statistical analysis (e.g., *t* test, analysis of variance [ANOVA], and linear regression) assumes that data are interval or ratio.

1.2.1 Nominal

Nominal data are distinct categories. They are categorical and unordered. Nominal data make no quantitative claims. Nominal data represent things that we can name (e.g., cat and dog). Nominal data can be represented with numbers. For example, zip codes are nominal. Numbers that represent a participant's sex, race, or ethnicity are also nominal. Categorical data are often dummy-coded into binary (i.e., dichotomous) variables, which represent nominal data. Higher numbers of nominal data do not reflect higher (or lower) levels of the construct because the numbers represent categories that do not have an order.

1.2.2 Ordinal

Ordinal data are ordered categories: they have a name and an order. They make no claim about the conceptual distance between the ranks, only that higher values represent higher (or lower) levels of the construct. For example, ranks following a race are ordinal—that is, the person with rank 1 finished before the person with rank 2, who finished before the person with rank 3 ($1 > 2 > 3 > 4$). Ordinal data make a limited claim because the conceptual distance between adjacent numbers is not the same. For instance, the person who finished the race first might have finished 10 minutes before the second-place finisher; whereas the third-place finisher might have finished 1 second after the second-place finisher.

That is, just because the numbers have the same *mathematical* distance does not mean that they represent the same *conceptual* distance on the construct. For example, if the respondent is asked how many drinks they had in the past day, and the options are $0 = 0$ drinks; $1 =$ 1–2 drinks; $2 = 3$ or more drinks, the scale is ordinal. Even though the numbers have the same mathematical distance (1, 2, 3), they do not represent the same conceptual distance. Most data in psychology are ordinal data even though they are often treated as if they were interval data.

1.2.3 Interval

Interval data are ordered and have meaningful distances (i.e., equal spacing between intervals). You can sum interval data (e.g., 2 is 2 away from 4), but you cannot multiply interval data

($2 \times 2 \neq 4$). Examples of interval data are temperatures in Fahrenheit and Celsius—100 degrees Fahrenheit is not twice as hot as 50 degrees Fahrenheit. A person's number of years of education is interval, whereas educational attainment (e.g., high school degree, college degree, graduate degree) is only ordinal. Although much data in psychology involve numbers that have the same mathematical distance between intervals, the intervals likely do not represent the same conceptual distance. For example, the difference in severity of two people who have two symptoms and four symptoms of depression, respectively, may not be the same difference in depression severity as two people who have four symptoms and six symptoms, respectively.

1.2.4 Ratio

Ratio data are ordered, have meaningful distances, and have a true (absolute) zero that represents absence of the construct. With ratio data, multiplicative relationships are true. An example of ratio data is temperature in Kelvin—100 degrees Kelvin is twice as hot as 50 degrees Kelvin. There is a dream of having ratio scales in psychology, but we still do not have a true zero with psychological constructs—what does total absence of depression mean (apart from a dead person)?

1.3 Score Transformation

There are a number of score transformations, depending on the goal. Some score transformations (e.g., log transform) seek to make data more normally distributed to meet assumptions of particular analysis approaches. Score transformations alter the original (raw) data. If you change the data, it can change the results. Score transformations are not neutral.

1.3.1 Raw Scores

Raw scores are the original data, or they may be aggregations (e.g., sums or means) of multiple items. Raw scores are the purest because they are closest to the original operation (e.g., behavior). A disadvantage of raw scores is that they are scale dependent, and therefore they may not be comparable across different measures with different scales. An example histogram of raw scores is in Figure 1.1.

1.3.2 Norm-Referenced Scores

Norm-referenced scores are scores that are referenced to some norm. A norm is a standard of comparison. For instance, you may be interested in how well a participant performed relative to other children of the same sex, age, grade, or ethnicity. However, interpretation of norm-referenced scores depends on the measure and on the normative sample. A person's norm-referenced score can vary widely depending on which norms are used. Which reference group should you use? Age? Sex? Age and sex? Grade? Ethnicity? The optimal reference group depends on the purpose of the assessment. Pros and cons of group-based norms are discussed in Section 15.5.2.2.2.

A standard normal distribution on various norm-referenced scales is depicted in Figure 1.2, as adapted from Bandalos (2018).

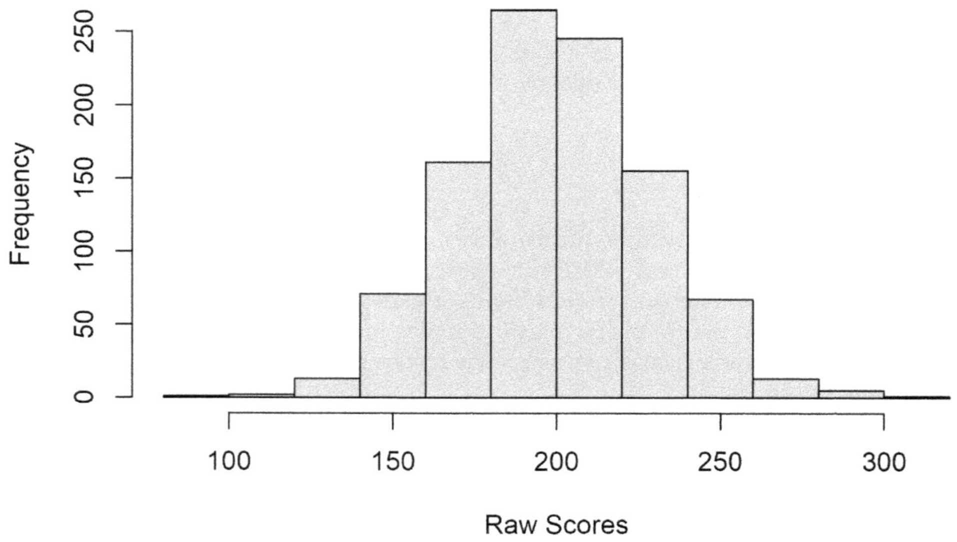

FIGURE 1.1 Histogram of Raw Scores.

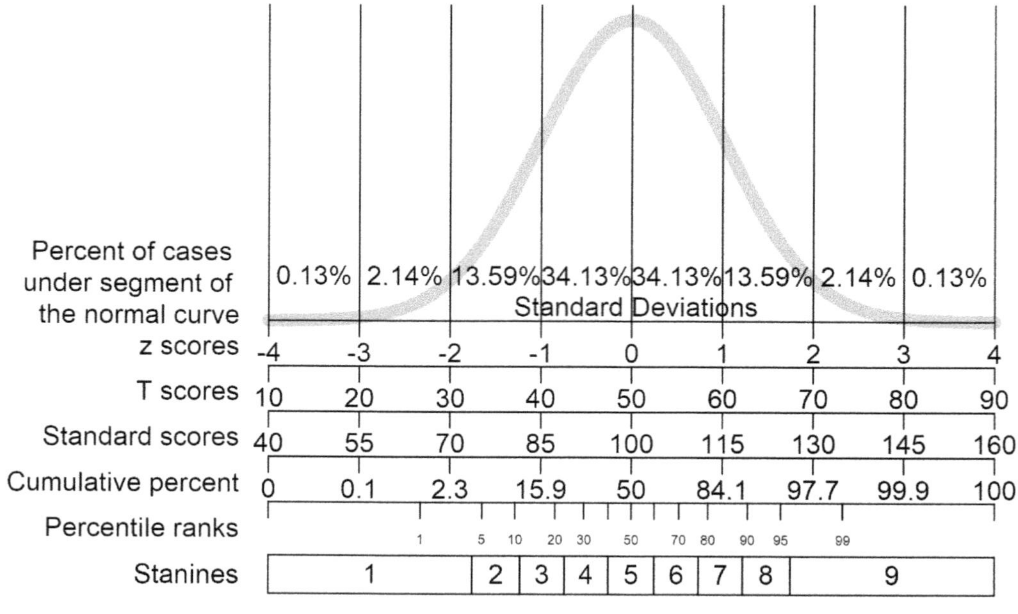

FIGURE 1.2 Various Norm-Referenced Scales.

1.3.2.1 Percentile Ranks

A percentile rank reflects what percent of people a person scored higher than, in a given group (i.e., norm). Percentile ranks are frequently used for tests of intellectual/cognitive ability, academic achievement, academic aptitude, and grant funding. They seem like interval data, but they are not intervals because the conceptual spacing between the numbers is not equal. The difference in ability for two people who scored at the 99th and 98th percentile, respectively, is not the same as the difference in ability for two people who scored at the 49th and 50th percentile, respectively. Percentile ranks are only judged against a baseline; there is no subtraction.

Percentile ranks have unusual effects. There are lots of people in the middle of a distribution, so a very small difference in raw scores gets expanded out in percentiles. For instance, a raw score of 20 may have a percentile rank of 50, but a raw score of 24 may have a percentile rank of 68. However, a larger raw score change at the ends of the distribution may have a smaller percentile change. For example, a raw score of 120 may have a percentile rank of 97, whereas a raw score of 140 may have a percentile rank of 99. Thus, percentile ranks stretch out differences for some people but constrict differences for others.

Here is an example of how to calculate percentile ranks using the `dplyr` package from the `tidyverse` (Wickham et al., 2019; Wickham, 2021):

```
scores$percentileRank <-
  percent_rank(scores$rawDataNoMissing) * 100
```

A histogram of percentile rank scores is in Figure 1.3.

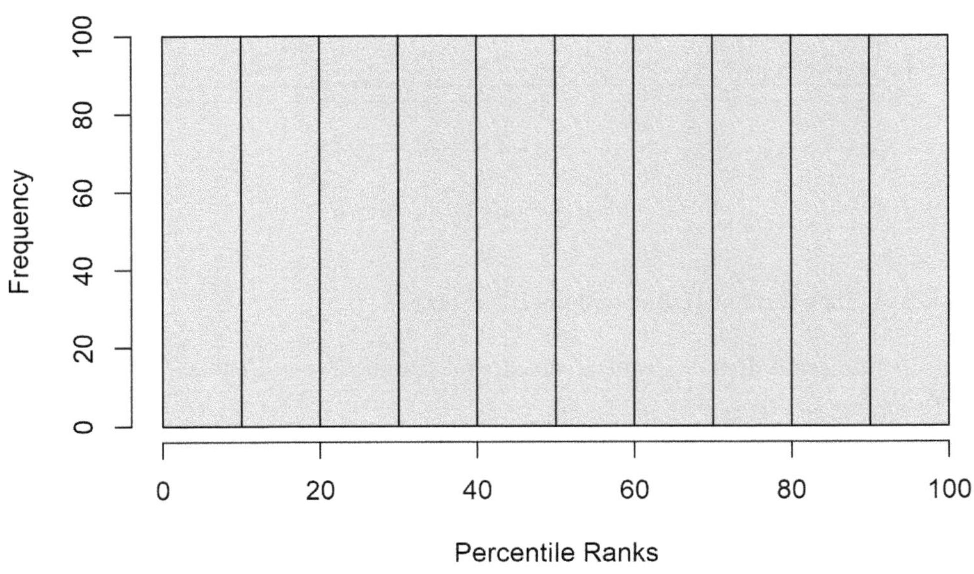

FIGURE 1.3 Histogram of Percentile Ranks.

1.3.2.2 Deviation (Standardized) Scores

Deviation or standardized scores are the transformation of raw scores to a normal distribution using some norm. The norm could be a comparison group, or it could be the sample itself. With deviation scores, you have similar challenges as with percentile ranks, including which reference group to use, but there are additional challenges. Deviation scores are more informative when the scores are normally distributed compared to when the scores are skewed. If scores are skewed, it can lead to two z scores on the opposite side of the mean having different probabilities.

Many constructs we study in psychology are not normally distributed. For example, the frequency of hallucinations among people would show a positively skewed distribution with a truncation at zero, representing a floor effect—i.e., most people do not show hallucinations. For instance, consider a hypothetical distribution of hallucinations. It might follow a folded distribution, as depicted in Figure 1.4.

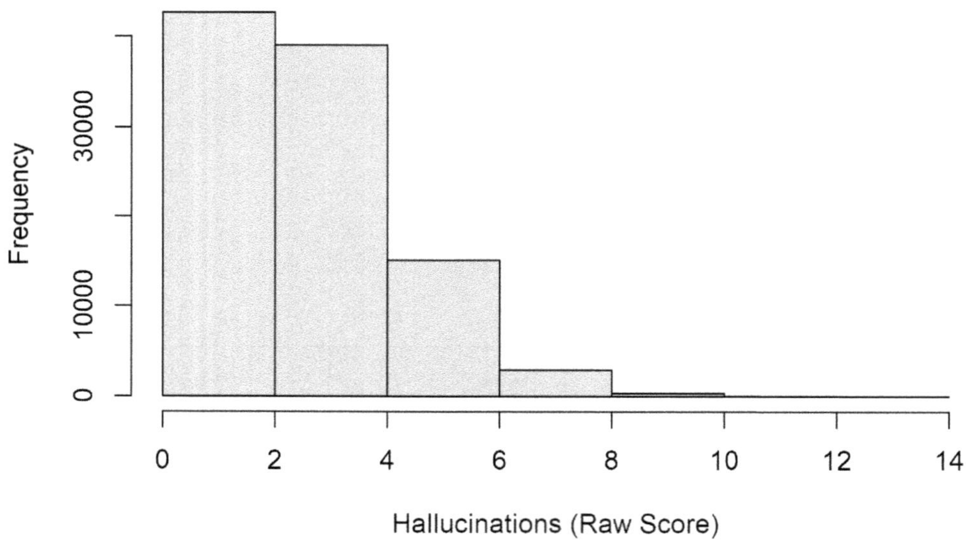

FIGURE 1.4 Histogram of Hallucinations (Raw Score).

Now consider the same distribution converted to a standardized (z) score, as depicted in Figure 1.5.

Thus, you can compute a deviation score, but it may not be meaningful if the data and underlying construct are not normally distributed.

1.3.2.2.1 z scores

The z score is the most common standardized score, and it can help put scores from different measures with different scales onto the same playing field. z scores have a mean of zero and a standard deviation of one. To get a z score that uses the sample as its own norm, subtract

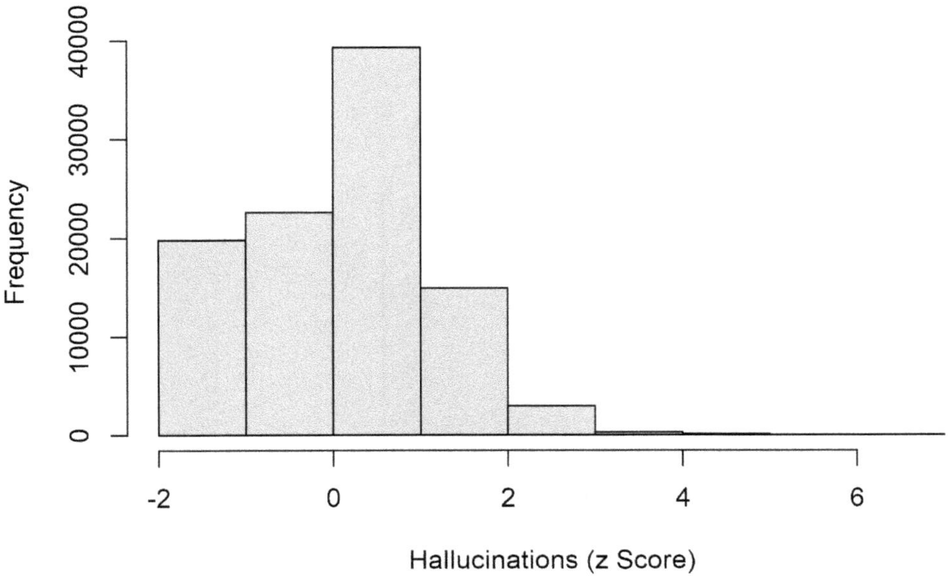

FIGURE 1.5 Histogram of Hallucinations (z Score).

the mean from all scores and divide by the standard deviation. Every z score represents how far that person's score is from the (normed) average, represented in standard deviation units. With a standard normal curve, 68% of scores fall within one standard deviation of the mean. 95% of scores fall within two standard deviations of the mean. 99.7% of scores fall within three standard deviations of the mean.

The area under a normal curve within one standard deviation of the mean is depicted in Figure 1.6 and is calculated below using the `pnorm()` function, which calculates the cumulative density function for a normal curve.

```
stdDeviations <- 1
pnorm(stdDeviations) - pnorm(stdDeviations * -1)
```

```
[1] 0.6827
```

The area under a normal curve within two standard deviations of the mean is depicted in Figure 1.7 and is calculated below:

```
stdDeviations <- 2
pnorm(stdDeviations) - pnorm(stdDeviations * -1)
```

```
[1] 0.9545
```

The area under a normal curve within three standard deviations of the mean is depicted in Figure 1.8 and is calculated below:

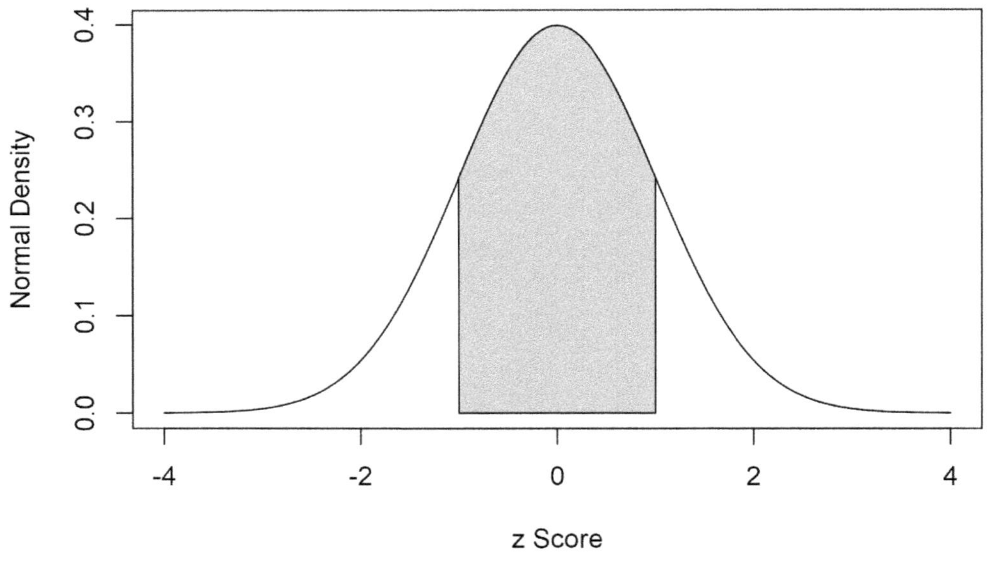

FIGURE 1.6 Density of Standard Normal Distribution. The gray region represents the area within one standard deviation of the mean.

```
stdDeviations <- 3
pnorm(stdDeviations) - pnorm(stdDeviations * -1)
```

```
[1] 0.9973
```

Alternatively, if you want to determine the z score associated with a particular percentile in a normal distribution, you can use the `qnorm()` function. For instance, the z score associated with the 37th percentile is:

```
qnorm(.37)
```

```
[1] -0.3319
```

z scores are calculated using Equation (1.1):

$$z = \frac{x - \mu}{\sigma} \tag{1.1}$$

where x is the observed score, μ is the mean observed score, and σ is the standard deviation of observed scores.

```
scores$zScore <- scale(scores$rawData)
```

An example histogram of z scores is in Figure 1.9.

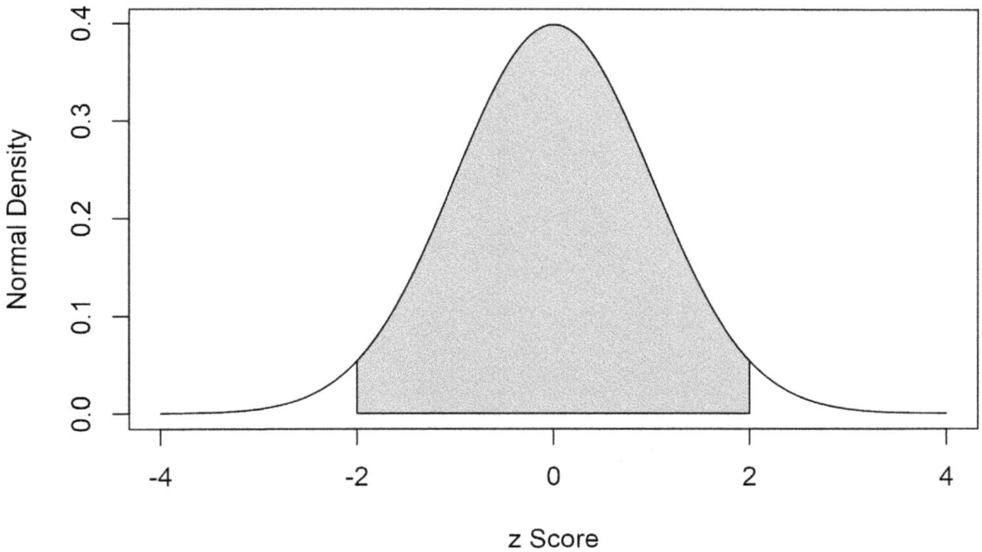

FIGURE 1.7 Density of Standard Normal Distribution. The gray region represents the area within two standard deviations of the mean.

1.3.2.2.2 T *scores*

T scores have a mean of 50 and a standard deviation of 10. T scores are frequently used with personality and symptom measures, where clinical cutoffs are often set at 70 (i.e., two standard deviations above the mean). For the Minnesota Multiphasic Personality Inventory (MMPI), you would examine peaks (elevations ≥ 70) and absences (≤ 30).

T scores are calculated using Equation (1.2):

$$T = 50 + 10z \tag{1.2}$$

where z are z scores.

```
scores$tScore <- 50 + 10*scale(scores$rawData)
```

An example histogram of T scores is in Figure 1.10.

1.3.2.2.3 Standard scores

Standard scores have a mean of 100 and a standard deviation of 15. Standard scores are frequently used for tests of intellectual ability, academic achievement, and cognitive ability. Intellectual disability is generally considered an I.Q. standard score less than 70 (two standard deviations below the mean), whereas giftedness is at 130 (two standard deviations above the mean).

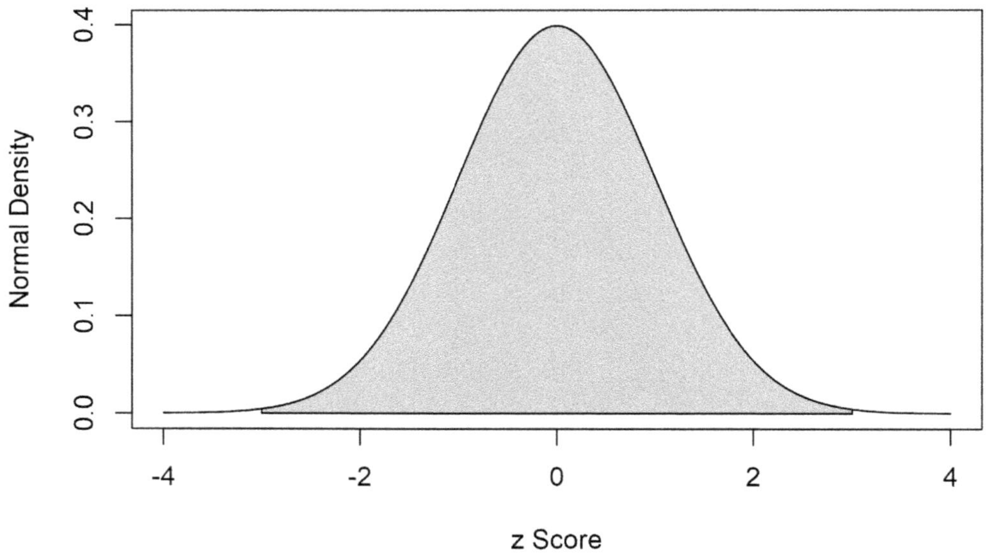

FIGURE 1.8 Density of Standard Normal Distribution. The gray region represents the area within three standard deviations of the mean.

Standard scores with a mean of 100 and standard deviation of 15 are calculated using Equation (1.3):

$$\text{standard score} = 100 + 15z \tag{1.3}$$

where z are z scores.

```
scores$standardScore <- 100 + 15*scale(scores$rawData)
```

An example histogram of standard scores is in Figure 1.11.

1.3.2.2.4 Scaled scores

Scaled scores are raw scores that have been converted to a standardized metric. The particular metric of the scaled score depends on the measure. On tests of intellectual or cognitive ability, scaled scores commonly have a mean of 10 and a standard deviation of 3.

Using this metric, scaled scores can be calculated using Equation (1.4):

$$\text{scale score} = 10 + 3z \tag{1.4}$$

where z are z scores.

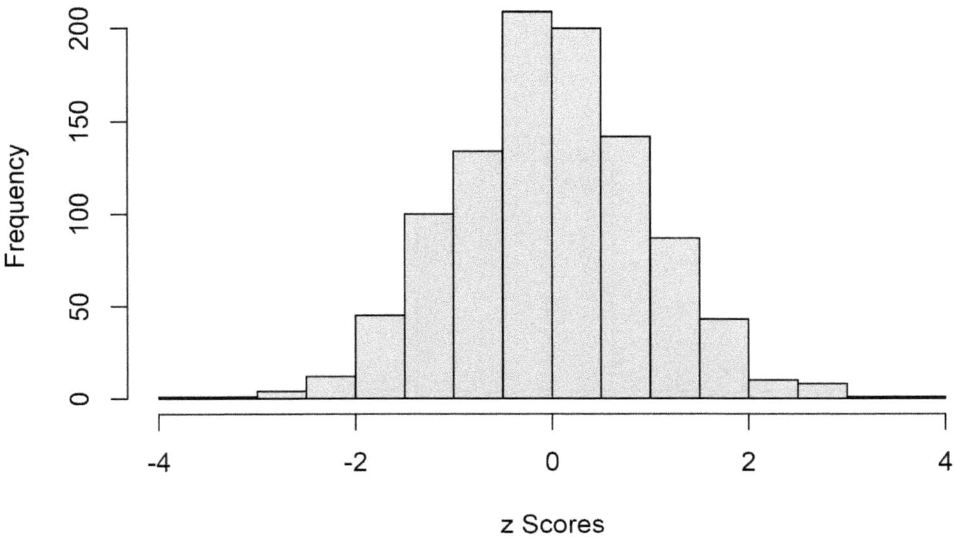

FIGURE 1.9 Histogram of z Scores.

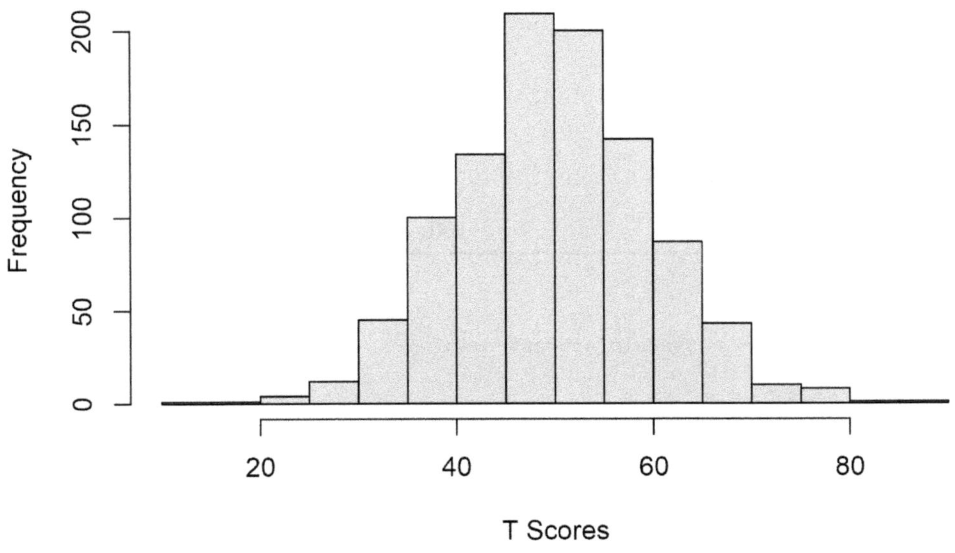

FIGURE 1.10 Histogram of T Scores.

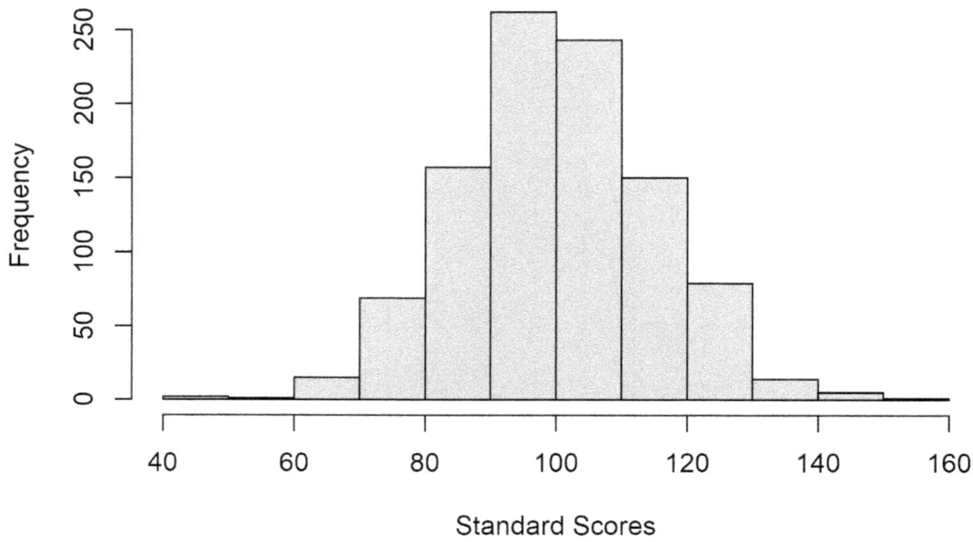

FIGURE 1.11 Histogram of Standard Scores.

TABLE 1.1 Calculating Stanine Scores

Stanine	Bracketed Percent	Cumulative Percent	z Score	Standard Score
1	4	4	below -1.75	below 74
2	7	11	-1.75 to -1.25	74 to 81
3	12	23	-1.25 to -0.75	81 to 89
4	17	40	-0.75 to -0.25	89 to 96
5	20	60	-0.25 to +0.25	96 to 104
6	17	77	+0.25 to +0.75	104 to 111
7	12	89	+0.75 to +1.25	111 to 119
8	7	96	+1.25 to +1.75	119 to 126
9	4	100	above +1.75	above 126

```
scores$scaledScore <- 10 + 3*scale(scores$rawData)
```

An example histogram of scaled scores is in Figure 1.12.

1.3.2.2.5 Stanine scores

Stanine scores (short for STANdard Nine) have a mean of 5 and a standard deviation of 2. The scores range from 1–9. Stanine scores are calculated using the bracketed proportions in Table 1.1. The lowest 4% receive a stanine score of 1, the next 7% receive a stanine score of 2, etc.

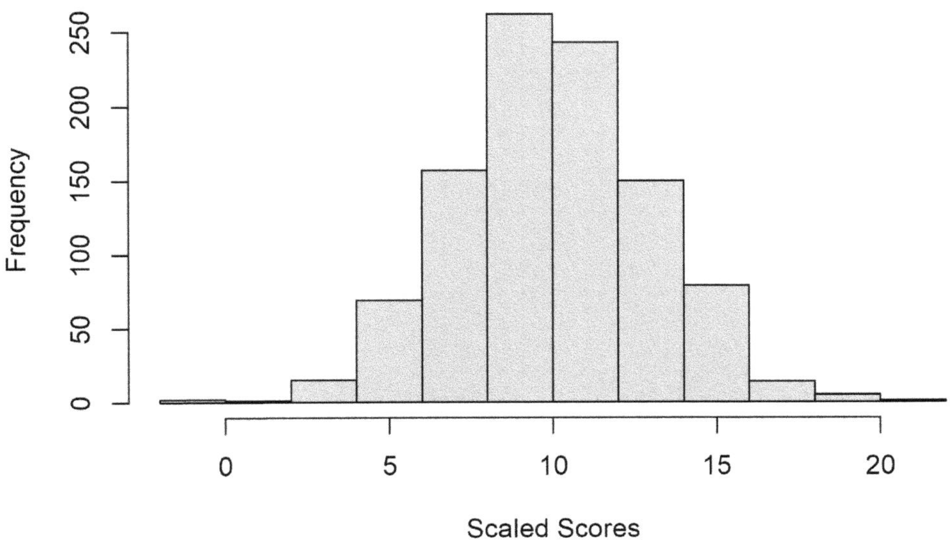

FIGURE 1.12 Histogram of Scaled Scores.

```
scores$stanineScore <- NA
scores$stanineScore[which(scores$percentileRank <= 4)] <- 1
scores$stanineScore[
  which(scores$percentileRank > 4 & scores$percentileRank <= 11)] <- 2
scores$stanineScore[
  which(scores$percentileRank > 11 & scores$percentileRank <= 23)] <- 3
scores$stanineScore[
  which(scores$percentileRank > 23 & scores$percentileRank <= 40)] <- 4
scores$stanineScore[
  which(scores$percentileRank > 40 & scores$percentileRank <= 60)] <- 5
scores$stanineScore[
  which(scores$percentileRank > 60 & scores$percentileRank <= 77)] <- 6
scores$stanineScore[
  which(scores$percentileRank > 77 & scores$percentileRank <= 89)] <- 7
scores$stanineScore[
  which(scores$percentileRank > 89 & scores$percentileRank <= 96)] <- 8
scores$stanineScore[which(scores$percentileRank > 96)] <- 9
```

A histogram of stanine scores is in Figure 1.13.

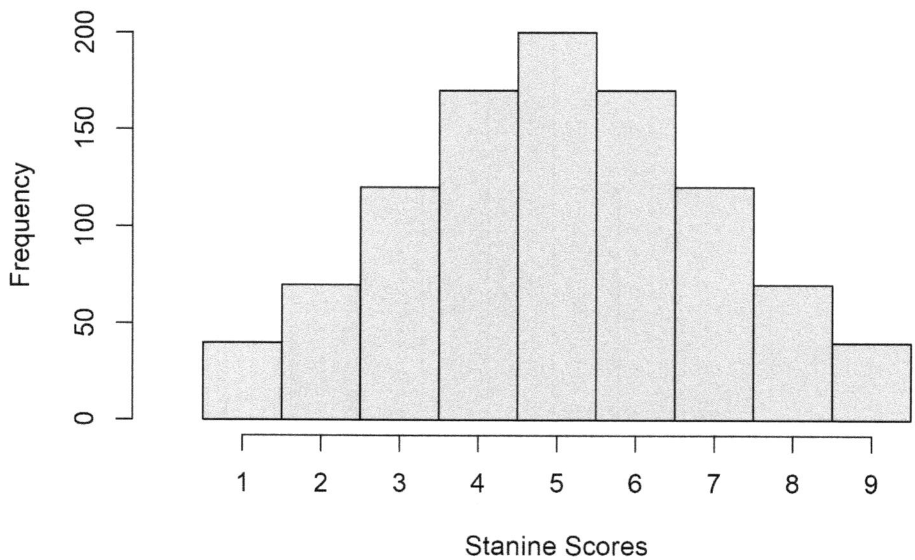

FIGURE 1.13 Histogram of Stanine Scores.

1.4 Conclusion

It is important to consider the types of data your data are because the types of data restrict what options are available to analyze the data. It is also important to consider whether the data were transformed because score transformations are not neutral—they can impact the results.

1.5 Suggested Readings

Childs et al. (2021): https://dzchilds.github.io/stats-for-bio/data-transformations.html (archived at https://perma.cc/3YEB-QW2V)

2

Constructs

2.1 Types of Constructs

A *construct* is a concept. A construct is generally considered a latent idea or phenomenon that is not directly observable. For example, depression could be considered a construct because we cannot directly measure someone's level of depression. Rather, we infer a person's level on the construct of depression by taking measurements of many indirect proxies that we think are *indicators* of the construct. An indicator is a measurement, and it could be thought of as a behavior or questionnaire item. Potential indicators of depression could include behaviors/items such as whether the person has low mood, low energy, sleep difficulties, loss of interest in formerly enjoyable activities, changes in weight or appetite, etc.

Because constructs are latent, unobservable phenomena, they are often estimated using latent variable models, as described in Section 2.5.

There are two main types of constructs: reflective constructs and formative constructs.

2.1.1 Reflective Construct

With a *reflective construct* (or reflective model), the construct is the cause of the measures, and the construct is reflected by the indicators, see Figure 2.1 (Bollen & Lennox, 1991).

An example of a reflective construct is extraversion; see Figure 2.2. We conceptualize extraversion as a latent concept that, although not directly observable, influences the measurements of indicators of extraversion, such as whether the person enjoys talking to strangers, goes to lots of parties, is energetic, and is happy. In a reflective model, the answers that people give on the items are thought to reflect a certain disposition—in this case, extraversion. None of these indicators, in isolation, is considered a direct measure of extraversion. Nevertheless, we feel that we can get a better estimate of the concept of extraversion by capturing the variance that covaries across these indicators, i.e., the common (systematic) variance among the indicators. Thus, the latent factor is estimated to reflect the common variance among the indicators. Because a reflective construct influences the indicators, the indicators are called *effect indicators*. What we observe, theoretically, are the effects of the underlying construct, which influences scores on each individual measure.

With a reflective construct, we would expect that the items would show strong internal consistency reliability. That is, we would expect that the indicators would all be correlated with each other, because all indicators are thought to be a reflection of the underlying construct. But in reality, there is often still residual correlation between items even after accounting for the latent factor.

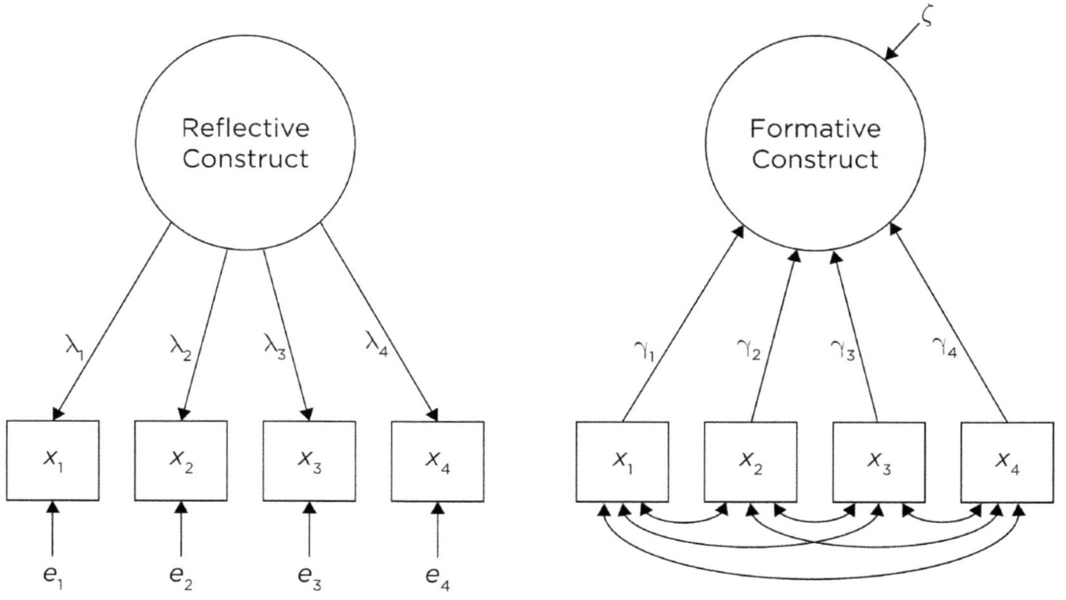

FIGURE 2.1 Reflective and Formative Constructs in Structural Equation Modeling.

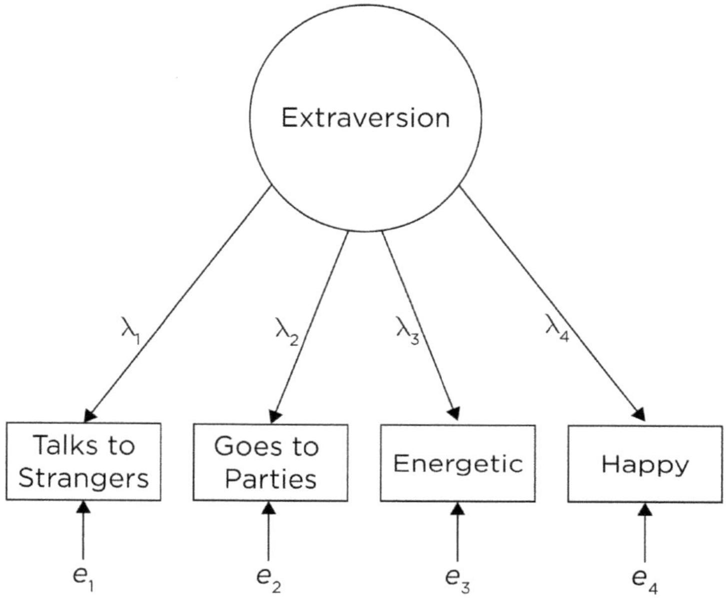

FIGURE 2.2 Extraversion as a Reflective Construct.

In a measurement model of a reflective construct (see Figure 2.1), the lambda (λ) values are called *factor loadings* that represent regression coefficients from observable indicators to latent variables. A factor loading is the relative weight that the item is given in the estimation of the latent factor, similar to the correlation between the construct and the measure. The stronger an item's factor loading on the construct, the more relative weight a given item has in the estimation of the latent factor. The epsilon (ϵ) term reflects measurement error. Structural equation modeling is an application of the same way we think about measurement according to classical test theory, but in a latent variable framework. According to classical test theory, the observed score is thought to be some combination of the true score and error (observed score = true score + error; $X = T + e$). Or, in a multiple regression framework: extraversion $= \lambda_1 \cdot$strangers$+\lambda_2 \cdot$parties$+\lambda_3 \cdot$happy$+$errors. That is, the true score influences the observed score on each measure. If a person's level on the construct (extraversion) changes, their score on each measure/indicator/item is expected to change (J. R. Edwards & Bagozzi, 2000).

2.1.2 Formative Construct

Formative constructs are the other fundamental way to understand the relation between a construct and a measure. With a *formative construct* (or formative model), the measures cause the construct; see Figure 2.1 (Bollen & Lennox, 1991). That is, the construct is created by the measures. Because the indicators influence the formative construct, the indicators are called *causal indicators*.

Examples of formative constructs include constructs such as socioeconomic status (SES), stress, and risk for cardiovascular disease. For instance, we may define SES such that it is the linear combination of a person's educational attainment, occupational prestige, and income, as in Figure 2.3. With a formative construct, if a person changes in their level on the construct, we might not expect that their scores on all of the measures/indicators/items would change (J. R. Edwards & Bagozzi, 2000). If a person's SES changes, you would not necessarily expect the person's score on all of these measures/items to change. For instance, if a person's SES increases from T1 to T2, you would not necessarily expect that their educational attainment increased; it could be instead that their occupational prestige or income increased.

In a structural equation model, the gamma (γ) values are regression coefficients from exogenous variables to endogenous variables. Endogenous variables are variables whose values are determined by the model (i.e., they are influenced by other variables), whereas exogenous variables are variables whose values are not determined by the model (i.e., they are not influenced by other variables). In a measurement model of a formative construct (see Figure 2.1), the gamma values reflect the relative weight that the item is given in the estimation of the latent factor, similar to the correlation between the construct and the measure. The stronger an item's factor loading on the construct, the more relative weight a given item has in the estimation of the latent factor.

With a formative construct, the disturbance term, zeta (ζ), represents the part of the construct that is not explained by the measures, i.e., the measurement error. However, the measures are thought (or at least assumed) to be error-free causes of the construct. The covariances between the indicators are permissive of item correlations, but unlike the reflective model, the formative model does not require that the items are correlated. In other words, for a formative model, it is not necessary that the items are correlated, even though the items could be correlated.

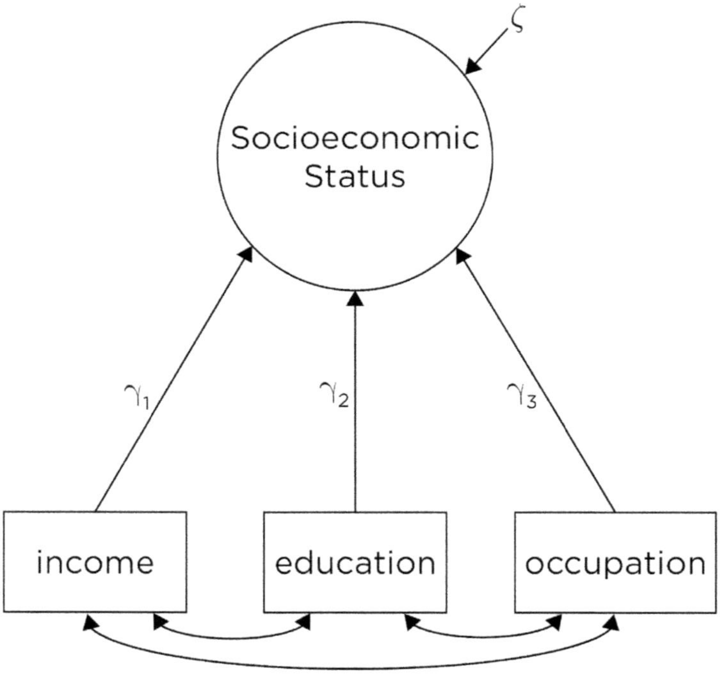

FIGURE 2.3 Socioeconomic Status as a Formative Construct.

A formative construct is determined by the measures, so if you change the measures, you change the construct. A formative model requires that you include all facets of the construct. This is not true in a reflective model because all items of a unidimensional reflective construct are interchangeable as long as the construct is unidimensional and the items are equally reliable because the construct influences the measure scores. With a reflective construct, all you need to do is find the items that reflect the underlying construct, and you could create parallel measures of the construct. This is impossible to do in a formative model.

Although formative conceptualizations of constructs may be useful in some cases, formative constructs can be controversial (J. R. Edwards, 2011; Hardin et al., 2011; Howell et al., 2007; Markus, 2018; Bollen & Bauldry, 2011; Bollen & Diamantopoulos, 2017; but see Bollen & Lennox, 1991; Diamantopoulos et al., 2008). It is important to think carefully about the construct of interest, as guided by theory, and how best to assess and estimate it.

2.2 Differences in Measurement Expectations

There are several differences in our measurement expectations based on the type of construct (formative or reflective) or indicator (causal or effect), as described by Bollen and Lennox (1991).

One difference we would expect between effect versus causal indicators is the actual correlations between the indicators. Causal indicators may not be correlated, whereas effect indicators must be correlated. So, when we are assessing internal consistency reliability of a measure, and we assume that higher correlations between items suggests higher internal consistency reliability, we are assuming that indicators of the construct have an effects relation to the construct. A scale assessing causal indicators would likely have very low internal consistency reliability.

A second difference we would expect between effect versus causal indicators is whether to use a sample or a census of indicators. The suggestions that we sample all facets of a construct when determining indicators is necessary only for causal indicators, for which a failure to assess a certain formative indicator changes the overall meaning of the construct. For effect indicators of a unidimensional construct, equally reliable measures are interchangeable.

A third difference we would expect between effect versus causal indicators is the optimal correlations between the indicators. For effect indicators, high correlations are desirable. For causal indicators, too high of a correlation between indicators is likely to introduce the problem of multicollinearity, so lower correlations are optimal. Multicollinearity is when two or more predictors are correlated such that their regression coefficients with the outcome variable (in this case, the factor loadings on the latent factor, i.e., λ) are erratic.

2.3 Practical Issues

There are important practical issues to consider with both reflective and formative models.

As described in Section 7.4 in the chapter on structural equation modeling, it is challenging to use formative constructs in a latent variable framework. In a structural equation modeling (SEM) framework, formative constructs must be used in the context of a model that allows some constraints. But one can easily estimate formative constructs outside of a SEM context, for example, with an average or weighted average composite, similar to principal component analysis. However, unlike latent variable approaches, linear composite approaches (e.g., mean or sum scores) do not account for measurement error. That is, linear composite approaches do not include a disturbance/error term. Therefore, a linear composite is not the same as a latent variable. If no disturbance term is included in a structural equation model, the model is equivalent to a linear composite approach (e.g., sum score, weighted average). Linear composite approaches are likely more defensible for formative constructs than for reflective constructs.

2.4 How to Estimate

To estimate a reflective construct, a latent variable modeling approach is necessary, such as structural equation modeling, factor analysis, or item response theory.

To estimate a formative construct, one may estimate an average or sum score across items (which gives each item equal weight), estimate a weighted average, use principal component analysis, use confirmatory composite analysis, or use structural equation modeling.

Thus, it is important to think about the nature of the construct before deciding how to estimate it. The nature of a construct is a theoretical question. Data alone cannot determine whether a construct is reflective or formative. Just because items are highly correlated does not mean that scientists think of the construct as reflective. By contrast, if items are not highly correlated, it suggests that a single unidimensional reflective construct may not adequately capture reality—the variance may be better captured by a formative or by multiple reflective constructs (i.e., a multidimensional model). In sum, although empiricism is relevant, theory is necessary to inform our understanding of the nature of constructs.

2.5 Latent Variable Modeling: IRT, SEM, and CFA

Item response theory (IRT), structural equation modeling (SEM), confirmatory composite analysis (CCA), and confirmatory factor analysis (CFA) are all approaches to latent variable modeling. CFA and IRT most commonly estimate reflective latent variables rather than formative latent variables. CCA estimates formative latent variables. SEM can estimate both reflective and formative latent variables. IRT is essentially a form of CFA with categorical, binary, or ordinal data. As we discuss in Chapter 7, SEM is CFA with regression paths that specify hypothesized causal relations between the latent variables (the structural component of the model).

2.6 Conclusion

It is important to think about the nature of a construct before deciding how to estimate it. For a formative construct, the indicators influence the construct, and a linear composite such as a weighted mean or sum score is justifiable. For a reflective construct, the construct influences the indicators, and it is more appropriate to estimate it with a reflective latent variable that reflects the common variance among the indicators using structural equation modeling, factor analysis, or item response theory.

2.7 Suggested Readings

Bollen & Lennox (1991); Bollen & Bauldry (2011); Bollen & Diamantopoulos (2017)

3

Reliability

3.1 Classical Test Theory

3.1.1 Overview

To understand the concept of reliability, it is helpful to understand *classical test theory* (CTT), which is also known as "true score theory." Classical test theory is one of various measurement theories, in addition to item response theory and generalizability theory. CTT has been the predominant measurement theory through the history of psychology. CTT is a theory of how test scores relate to a construct. A *construct* is the concept or characteristic that a measure is intended to assess.

Assume you take a measurement of the same object multiple times (i.e., repeated measure). For example, you assess the mass of the same rock multiple times. However, you obtain different estimates of the rock's mass each time. There are multiple possible explanations for this observation. One possible explanation could be that the rock is changing in its mass, which would be consistent with the idea proposed by the Greek philosopher Heraclitus that nothing is stable and the world is in flux. An alternative possibility, however, is that the rock is stable in its mass but the measurements are jittery—that is, they include error.

Based on the possibility that the rock is stable and that differences in scores across time reflect measurement error, CTT proposes the true score formula in Equation (3.1):

$$\begin{aligned} X &= T + e \\ \text{observed score} &= \text{true score} + \text{measurement error} \end{aligned} \tag{3.1}$$

X is the observed measurement or score, T is the classical (or psychometric) "true score," and e is the measurement error (i.e., error score).

This formula is depicted visually in the form of a path diagram in Figure 3.1.

It is important to distinguish between the classical true score and the Platonic true score. The *Platonic true score* is the truth, and it does not depend on measurement. The Platonic true score is an abstract notion because it is not directly observable and is based on Platonic ideals and theories of the construct and what a person's "true" level is on the construct. In CTT, we attempt to approximate the Platonic true score with the classical true score, (T). If we took infinite repeated observations (and the measurements had no carryover effect), the average score approaches the classical true score, T. That is, $\overline{X} = T$ as number of observations $\rightarrow \infty$. CTT attempts to partition variance into different sources. *Variance* is an index of scores' variability, i.e., the degree to which scores differ. Variance is defined as the average squared deviation from the mean, as in Equation (3.2):

$$\sigma^2_X = E[(X - \mu)^2] \tag{3.2}$$

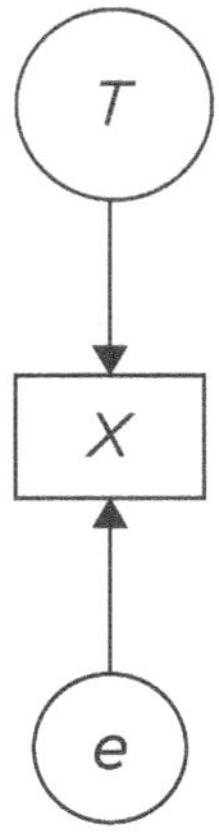

FIGURE 3.1 Classical Test Theory Formula in a Path Diagram.

According to CTT, any observed measurement includes both true score (construct) variance (σ^2_T) and error variance (σ^2_e). Given the true score formula ($X = T + e$), this means that their variance is as follows (see Equation (3.3)):

$$\begin{gathered}\sigma^2_X = \sigma^2_T + \sigma^2_e \\ \text{observed score variance} = \text{true score variance} + \text{error variance}\end{gathered} \tag{3.3}$$

Nevertheless, the *classical true score*, T, is the expected value and is not necessarily the same thing as the Platonic true score (Borsboom, 2003; Klein & Cleary, 1969) because the expected value would need to be entirely valid/accurate (i.e., it would need to be the construct score) for it to be the Platonic true score. The expected score could also be influenced by systematic sources of error such as other constructs, which would not fall into the error portion of the CTT formula because, as described below, CTT assumes that error is random (not systematic). The distinctions between construct score, (classical) true score, and observed score, in addition to validity, reliability, systematic error, and random error are depicted in Figure 3.2.

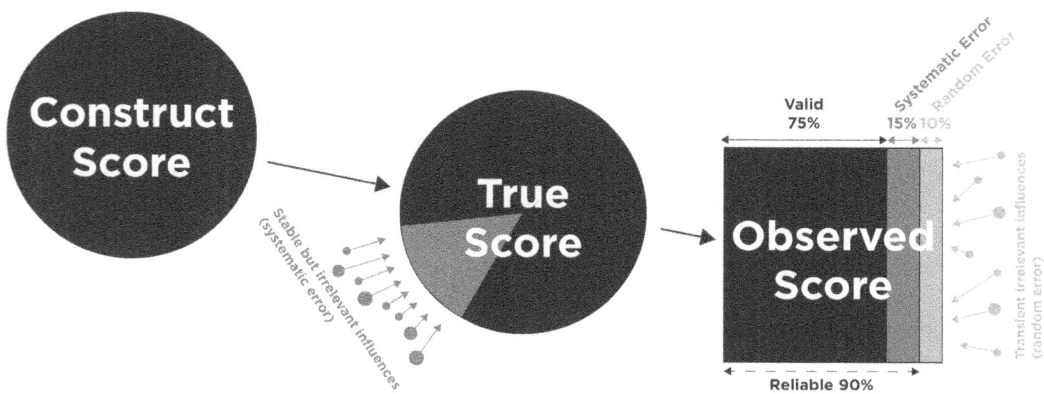

FIGURE 3.2 Distinctions Between Construct Score, True Score, and Observed Score, in Addition to Reliability, Validity, Systematic Error, and Random Error. (Adapted from W. Joel Schneider.)

The true score formula is theoretically useful, but it is not practically useful because it is an under-identified equation and we do not know the values of T or e based on knowing the observed score (X). For instance, if we obtain an observed score of 10, our formula is $10 = T + e$, and we do not know what the true score or error is. As a result, CTT makes several simplifying assumptions so we can estimate how stable (reliable) or noisy the measure is and what proportion of the observed score reflects true score versus measurement error.

1. $E(e) = 0$

   The first assumption of CTT is that the expected value of the error (i.e., error scores) is zero. Basically, the error component of the observed scores is expected to be random with a mean of zero. The likelihood that the observed score is an overestimate of T is assumed to be the same as the likelihood that the observed score is an underestimate of T. In other words, the distribution of error scores above T is assumed to be the same as the distribution of error scores below T. In reality, this assumption is likely false in many situations. For instance, social desirability bias is a systematic error where people rate themselves as better than they actually are; thus, social desirability results in biasing scores in a particular direction across respondents, so such an error would not be entirely random. But using the assumption that the expected value of e is zero also informs that the expected value of the observed score (X) equals the expected value of the true score (T), as in Equation (3.4):

$$\begin{aligned} E(X) &= E(T + e) \\ &= E(T) + E(e) \\ &= E(T) + 0 \\ &= E(T) \end{aligned} \tag{3.4}$$

2. $r_{T,e} = 0$

   The second assumption of CTT is that the correlation between T and e is zero—that is, people's true scores are uncorrelated with the error around their measurement (i.e., people's error scores). However, this assumption is likely false in many situations. For instance, one can imagine that, on a paper-and-pencil intelligence test, scores may have greater error for respondents with lower true scores and may have less error for respondents with higher true scores.

3. $r_{e_1,e_2} = 0$

   The third assumption of CTT is that the error is uncorrelated across time—that is, people's error scores at time 1 (e_1) are not associated with their error scores at time 2 (e_2). However, this assumption is also likely false in many situations. For example, if some people have a high social desirability bias at time 1, they are likely to also have a high social desirability bias at time 2. That is, the error around measurements of participants is likely to be related across time.

These three assumptions are implicit in the path analytic diagram in Figure 3.3, which depicts the CTT approach to understanding reliability of a measure across two time points.

In path analytic (and structural equation modeling) language, rectangles represent variables we observe, and circles represent latent (i.e., unobserved) variables. The observed scores at time 1 (X_1) and time 2 (X_2) are entities we observe, so they are represented by rectangles.

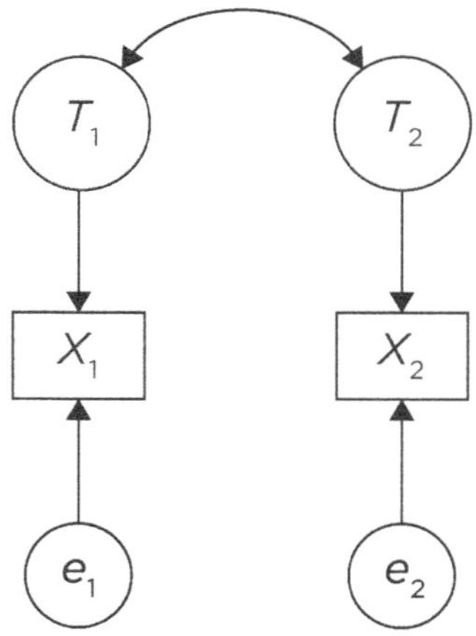

FIGURE 3.3 Reliability of a Measure Across Two Time Points, as Depicted in a Path Diagram.

We do not directly observe the true scores (T_1, T_2) and error scores (e_1, e_2), so they are considered latent entities and are represented by circles. Single-headed arrows indicate regression paths, where conceptually, one variable is thought to influence another variable. As the model depicts, the observed scores are thought to be influenced both by true scores and by error scores. We also expect the true scores at time 1 (T_1) and time 2 (T_2) to be correlated, so we have a covariance path, as indicated by a double-headed arrow. A *covariance* is an unstandardized index of the strength of association between two variables. Because a covariance is unstandardized, its scale depends on the scale of the variables. The covariance between two variables is the average product of their deviations from their respective means, as in Equation (3.5):

$$\sigma_{XY} = E[(X - \mu_X)(X - \mu_Y)] \tag{3.5}$$

The covariance of a variable with itself is equivalent to its variance, as in Equation (3.6):

$$\begin{aligned} \sigma_{XX} &= E[(X - \mu_X)(X - \mu_X)] \\ &= E[(X - \mu_X)^2] \\ &= \sigma^2_X \end{aligned} \tag{3.6}$$

By contrast, a *correlation* is a standardized index of the strength of association between two variables. Because a correlation is standardized (fixed between [-1,1]), its scale does not depend on the scales of the variables. In this figure, no other parameters (regressions, covariances, or means) are specified, so the following are implicit in the diagram:

- $E(e) = 0$
- $r_{T,e} = 0$
- $r_{e_1,e_2} = 0$

The factor loadings reflect the magnitude that the latent factor influences the observed variable. In this case, the true scores influence the observed scores with a magnitude of $\sqrt{r_{xx}}$, which is known as the *index of reliability*. The index of reliability is the theoretical estimate of the correlation between the true scores and the observed scores. This is depicted in Figure 3.4.

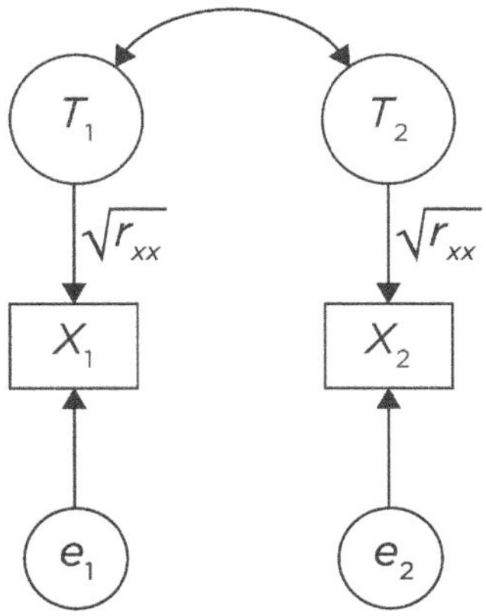

FIGURE 3.4 Reliability of a Measure Across Two Time Points, as Depicted in a Path Diagram; Includes the Index of Reliability.

We can use path tracing rules to estimate the reliability of the measure, where the reliability of the measure, i.e., the *coefficient of reliability* (r_{xx}), is estimated as the correlation between the observed score at time 1 (x_1) and the observed score at time 2 (x_2). According to path tracing rules (Pearl, 2013), the correlation between x_1 and x_2 is equal to the sum of the standardized coefficients of all the routes through which x_1 and x_2 are connected. The contribution of a given route to the correlation between x_1 and x_2 is equal to the product of all standardized coefficients on that route that link x_1 and x_2 that move in the following directions: (a) forward (e.g., T_1 to x_1) or (b) backward once and then forward (e.g., x_1 to T_1 to T_2 to x_2). Path tracing does not allow moving forward and then backward—that is, it does not allow retracing (e.g., e to x_1 to T_1) in the same route. It also does not allow passing more than one curved arrow (covariance path) or through the same variable twice in the same route. Once you know the contribution of each route to the correlation, you can calculate the total correlation between the two variables as the sum of the contribution of each route. Therefore, using one route, we can calculate the association between x_1 and x_2 as in Equation (3.7):

$$\begin{aligned} r_{x_1,x_2} &= \sqrt{r_{xx}} \times r_{T_1,T_2} \times \sqrt{r_{xx}} \\ &= r_{T_1,T_2} \times r_{xx} \\ &= \text{correlation of true scores across time} \times \text{reliability} \end{aligned} \tag{3.7}$$

When dealing with a stable construct, we would assume that the correlation between true scores across time is 1.0: $r_{T_1,T_2} = 1.0$, as depicted in Figure 3.5.

Then, to calculate the association between x_1 and x_2 of a stable construct, we can use path tracing rules as in Equation (3.8):

$$\begin{aligned} r_{x_1,x_2} &= \sqrt{r_{xx}} \times r_{T_1,T_2} \times \sqrt{r_{xx}} \\ &= \sqrt{r_{xx}} \times 1 \times \sqrt{r_{xx}} \\ &= r_{xx} \\ &= \text{coefficient of reliability} \end{aligned} \tag{3.8}$$

That is, for a stable construct (i.e., whose true scores are perfectly correlated across time; $r_{T_1,T_2} = 1.0$), we estimate reliability as the correlation between the observed scores at time

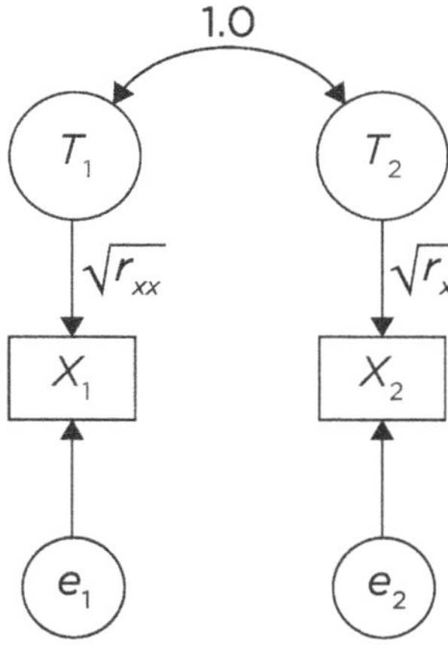

FIGURE 3.5 Reliability of a Measure of a Stable Construct Across Two Time Points, as Depicted in a Path Diagram.

1 (x_1) and the observed scores at time 2 (x_2). This is known as *test–retest reliability*. We therefore assume that the extent to which the correlation between x_1 and x_2 is less than one reflects measurement error (an unstable measure), rather than people's changes in their true score on the construct (an unstable construct).

As described above, the reliability coefficient (r_{xx}) is the association between a measure and itself over time or with another measure in the domain. By contrast, the *reliability index* (r_{xT}) is the correlation between observed scores on a measure and the true scores (Nunnally & Bernstein, 1994). The reliability index is the square root of the reliability coefficient, as in Equation (3.9).

$$\begin{aligned} r_{xT} &= \\ &= \sqrt{r_{xx}} \\ &= \text{index of reliability} \end{aligned} \tag{3.9}$$

3.1.2 Four CTT Measurement Models

There are four primary measurement models in CTT (J. M. Graham, 2006):

1. parallel
2. tau-equivalent
3. essentially tau-equivalent
4. congeneric

3.1.2.1 Parallel

The parallel measurement model is the most stringent measurement model for use in estimating reliability. In CTT, a measure is considered parallel if the true scores and error scores are equal across items. That is, the items must be unidimensional and assess the same construct, on the same scale, with the same degree of precision, and with the same amount of error (J. M. Graham, 2006). Items are expected to have the same strength of association (i.e., factor loading or discrimination) with the construct.

3.1.2.2 Tau-Equivalent

The tau (τ)-equivalent measurement model is the same as the parallel measurement model, except error scores are allowed to differ across items. That is, a measure is tau-equivalent if the items are unidimensional and assess the same construct, on the same scale, with the same degree of precision, but with possibly different amounts of error (J. M. Graham, 2006). In other words, true scores are equal across items but each item is allowed to have unique error scores. Items are expected to have the same strength of association with the construct. Variance that is unique to a specific item is assumed to be error variance.

3.1.2.3 Essentially Tau-Equivalent

The essentially tau (τ)-equivalent model is the same as the tau-equivalent measurement model, except items are allowed to differ in their precision. That is, a measure is essentially tau-equivalent if the items are unidimensional and assess the same construct, on the same scale, but with possibly different degrees of precision, and with possibly different amounts of error (J. M. Graham, 2006). The essentially tau-equivalent model allows item true scores to differ by a constant that is unique to each pair of variables. The magnitude of the constant reflects the degree of imprecision and influences the mean of the item scores but not its variance or covariances with other items. Items are expected to have the same strength of association with the construct.

3.1.2.4 Congeneric

The congeneric measurement model is the least restrictive measurement model. The congeneric measurement model is the same as the essentially tau (τ)-equivalent model, except items are allowed to differ in their scale. That is, a measure is congeneric if the items are unidimensional and assess the same construct, but possibly on a different scale, with possibly different degrees of precision, and with possibly different amounts of error (J. M. Graham, 2006). Items are not expected to have the same strength of association with the construct.

3.2 Measurement Error

Measurement error is the difference between the measured (observed) value and the true value. All measurements come with uncertainty and measurement error. Even a measure of something as simple as whether someone is dead has error.

There are two main types of measurement error: systematic (nonrandom) error and unsystematic (random) error. In addition, measurement error can be within-person, between-person, or both.

3.2.1 Systematic (Nonrandom) Error

An example of *systematic error* is depicted in Figure 3.6. Systematic error is error that influences consistently for a person or across the sample. An error is systematic if the error always occurs, with the same value, when using the measure in the same way and in the same case. An example of a systematic error is a measure that consistently assesses constructs other than the construct the measure was designed to assess. For instance, if a test written in English to assess math skills is administered in a nonnative English-speaking country, some portion of the scores will reflect variance attributable to English reading skills rather than the construct of interest (math skills). Other examples of systematic error include response styles or subjective, idiosyncratic judgments by a rater—for instance, if the rater's judgments are systematically harsh or lenient. A systematic error affects the average score (i.e., resulting in bias), which makes the group-level estimates less accurate and makes the measurements for an individual less accurate.

As depicted in Figure 3.6, systematic error does not affect the variability of the scores, but it does affect the mean of the scores, so the person-level mean and group-level mean are less accurate. In other words, a systematic error leads to a biased estimate of the average. However, multiple systematic errors may simultaneously coexist and can operate in the same direction (exacerbating the effects of bias) or in opposite directions (hiding the extent of bias).

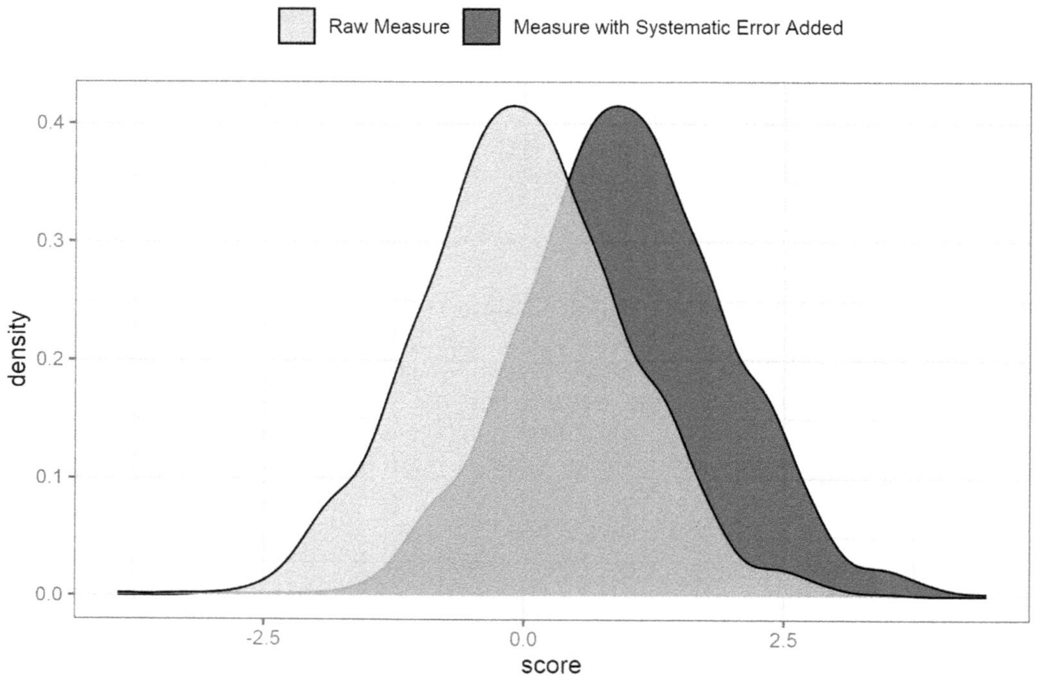

FIGURE 3.6 Systematic Error.

3.2.2 Unsystematic (Random) Error

An example of *unsystematic (random) error* is depicted in Figure 3.7. Random error occurs due to chance. For instance, a random error could arise from a participant being fatigued on a particular testing day or from a participant getting lucky in guessing the correct answer. Random error does not have consistent effects for a person or across the sample, and it may vary from one observation to another. Random error does not (systematically) affect the average, i.e., the group-level estimate—random error affects only the variability around the average (noise). However, random error makes measurements for an individual less accurate. A large number of observations of the same construct cancels out random error but does not cancel out systematic error.

As depicted in Figure 3.7, random error does not affect the mean of the scores, but it does increase the variability of the scores. In other words, the group-level mean is still accurate, but individuals' scores are less precise.

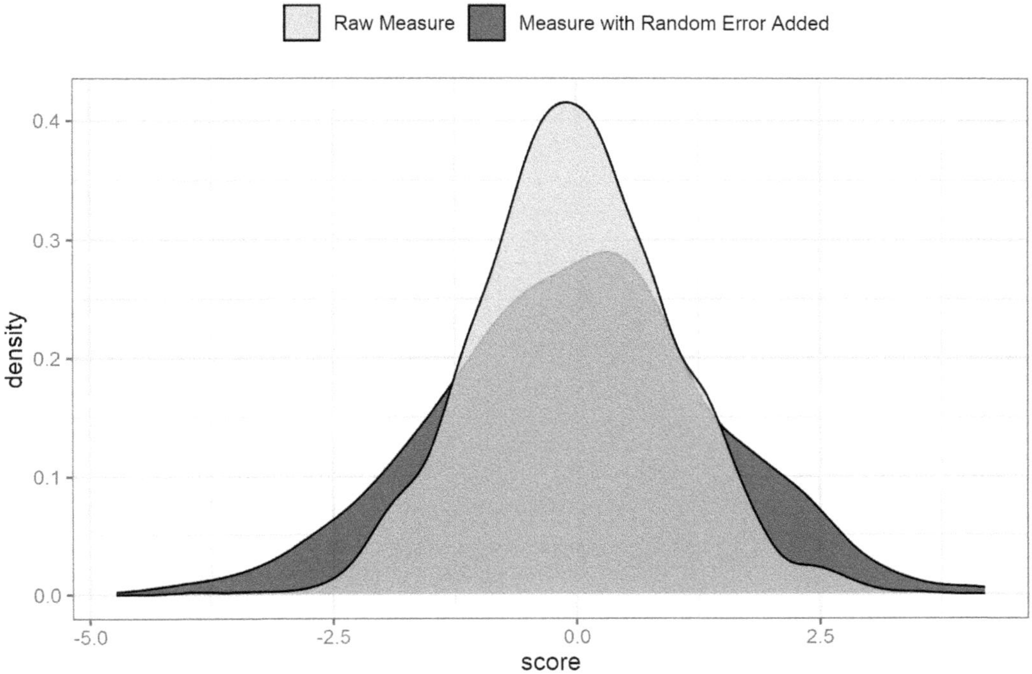

FIGURE 3.7 Random Error.

3.2.3 Within-Person Error

Consider two data columns, one column for participants' scores at time 1 and another column for participants' scores at time 2. Adding within-person error would mean adding noise (e) within the given row (or rows) for the relevant participant(s). Adding between-person error would mean adding noise (e) across the rows within the column.

Within-person error occurs within a particular person. For instance, you could add within-person error to a data set by adding error to the given row (or rows) for the relevant participant(s).

3.2.4 Between-Person Error

Between-person error occurs across the sample. You could add between-person random error to a variable by adding error across the rows, within a column.

3.2.5 Types of Measurement Error

There are four nonmutually exclusive types of measurement error: within-person random error, within-person systematic error, between-person random error, and between-person systematic error. The four types of measurement error are depicted in Figure 3.8, as adapted from Willett (2012).

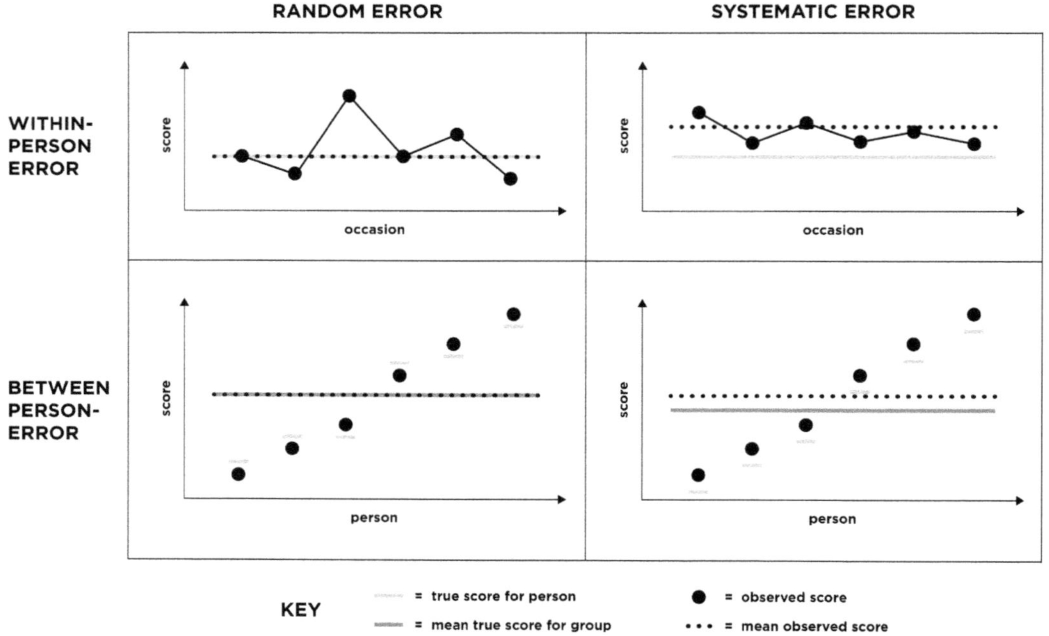

FIGURE 3.8 Types of Measurement Error.

3.2.5.1 Within-Person Random Error

Adding within-person random error would involve adding random noise (e) to the given row (or rows) for the relevant participant(s). This could reflect momentary fluctuations in the assessment for a specific person. When adding within-person random error, the person's and group's measurements show no bias, i.e., there is no consistent increase or decrease in the scores from time 1 to time 2 (at least with a sample size large enough to cancel out the random error, according to the law of large numbers). A person's average approximates their true score if many repeated measurements are taken. A group's average approximates the sample mean's true score, especially when averaging the repeated measures across time. The influence of within-person random error is depicted in Figure 3.9.

3.2.5.2 Within-Person Systematic Error

Adding within-person systematic error would involve adding systematic noise (e) (the same variance across columns) to the given row (or rows), reflecting the relevant participant(s). These are within-person effects that are consistent across time. For example, social desirability bias is high for some people and low for others. Another instance in which within-person systematic error could exist is when one or more people consistently misinterpret a particular question. Within-person systematic error increases person-level bias because the person's mean shows a greater difference from their true score. The influence of within-person systematic error is depicted in Figure 3.10.

	Participant	True Score	T1	T2	Influence	Person-Level			
						Bias at T1	Bias at T2	Mean of T1 and T2	Mean-Level Bias
	1	70	80	60	Add random error (+10 to T1, -10 to T2)	10	-10	70	0
	2	70	70	70		0	0	70	0
	3	80	80	80		0	0	80	0
	4	80	80	80		0	0	80	0
	5	90	90	90		0	0	90	0
	6	90	90	90		0	0	90	0
	7	100	100	100		0	0	100	0
	8	100	100	100		0	0	100	0
	9	110	110	110		0	0	110	0
	10	110	110	110		0	0	110	0
Group-Level	Mean	90	91	89		1	-1	90	0
	Variance	222.22	187.78	276.67				222.22	

FIGURE 3.9 Within-Person Random Error.

	Participant	True Score	T1	T2	Influence	Person-Level			
						Bias at T1	Bias at T2	Mean of T1 and T2	Mean-Level Bias
	1	70	80	80	Add systematic error (+10 to T1, +10 to T2)	10	10	80	10
	2	70	70	70		0	0	70	0
	3	80	80	80		0	0	80	0
	4	80	80	80		0	0	80	0
	5	90	90	90		0	0	90	0
	6	90	90	90		0	0	90	0
	7	100	100	100		0	0	100	0
	8	100	100	100		0	0	100	0
	9	110	110	110		0	0	110	0
	10	110	110	110		0	0	110	0
Group-Level	Mean	90	91	91		1	1	91	1
	Variance	222.22	187.78	187.78				187.78	

FIGURE 3.10 Within-Person Systematic Error.

3.2.5.3 Between-Person Random Error

Adding between-person random error at time 2 would involve adding random noise (e) across the rows, within the column.

Between-person random error would result in less accurate scores at the person level but would not result in bias at the group level. At a given timepoint, it results in overestimates of the person's true score for some people and underestimates for other people, i.e., there is no consistent pattern across the sample. Thus, the group average approximates the sample's mean true score (at least with a sample size large enough to cancel out the random error, according to the law of large numbers). In addition, the average of repeated measurements of the person's score would approximate the person's true score. However, the group's variance is inflated. The influence of between-person random error is depicted in Figure 3.11.

3.2.5.4 Between-Person Systematic Error

Adding between-person systematic error at time 2 would involve adding systematic noise (e) across the rows, within the column. Between-person systematic error results from within-person error that tends to be negative or positive across participants. For instance, this could reflect an influence with a shared effect across subjects. For example, social desirability leads to a positive group-level bias for rating their socially desirable attributes. Another example would be when a research assistant enters values wrong at time 2 (e.g., adding 10 to all participants' scores). Between-person systematic error increases bias because it results in a greater group mean difference from the group's mean true score. The influence of between-person systematic error is depicted in Figure 3.12.

						Person-Level			
	Participant	True Score	T1	T2	Influence	Bias at T1	Bias at T2	Mean of T1 and T2	Mean-Level Bias
	1	70	70	75	Add random error at T2 (5)	0	5	72.50	2.50
	2	70	70	65	Add random error at T2 (-5)	0	-5	67.50	-2.50
	3	80	80	83	Add random error at T2 (3)	0	3	81.50	1.50
	4	80	80	77	Add random error at T2 (-3)	0	-3	78.50	-1.50
	5	90	90	96	Add random error at T2 (6)	0	6	93	3
	6	90	90	84	Add random error at T2 (-6)	0	-6	87	-3
	7	100	100	110	Add random error at T2 (10)	0	10	105	5
	8	100	100	90	Add random error at T2 (-10)	0	-10	95	-5
	9	110	110	112	Add random error at T2 (2)	0	2	111	1
	10	110	110	108	Add random error at T2 (-2)	0	-2	109	-1
Group-Level	Mean	90	90	90		0	0	90	0
	Variance	222.22	222.22	260.89				231.89	

FIGURE 3.11 Between-Person Random Error.

						Person-Level			
	Participant	True Score	T1	T2	Influence	Bias at T1	Bias at T2	Mean of T1 and T2	Mean-Level Bias
	1	70	70	75	Add systematic error at T2 (5)	0	5	72.50	2.50
	2	70	70	75	Add systematic error at T2 (5)	0	5	72.50	2.50
	3	80	80	85	Add systematic error at T2 (5)	0	5	82.50	2.50
	4	80	80	85	Add systematic error at T2 (5)	0	5	82.50	2.50
	5	90	90	95	Add systematic error at T2 (5)	0	5	92.50	2.50
	6	90	90	95	Add systematic error at T2 (5)	0	5	92.50	2.50
	7	100	100	105	Add systematic error at T2 (5)	0	5	102.50	2.50
	8	100	100	105	Add systematic error at T2 (5)	0	5	102.50	2.50
	9	110	110	115	Add systematic error at T2 (5)	0	5	112.50	2.50
	10	110	110	115	Add systematic error at T2 (5)	0	5	112.50	2.50
Group-Level	Mean	90	90	95		0	5	92.50	2.50
	Variance	222.22	222.22	222.22				222.22	

FIGURE 3.12 Between-Person Systematic Error.

3.2.6 Summary

In sum, all types of measurement error (whether systematic or random) lead to less accurate scores for an individual. But different kinds of error have different implications. Systematic and random error have different effects on accuracy at the group-level. Systematic error leads to less accurate estimates at the group-level, whereas random error does not.

CTT assumes that all error is random. According to CTT, as the number of measurements approaches infinity, the mean of the measurements gets closer to the true score, because the random errors cancel each other out. With more measurements, we reduce our uncertainty and increase our precision. According to CTT, if we take many measurements and the average of the measurements is 10, we have some confidence that the true score (T) $\approx$ 10. In reality, however, error for a given measure likely includes both systematic and random error.

3.3 Overview of Reliability

The "Standards for Educational and Psychological Testing" set the standard for educational and psychological assessment and are jointly published by the American Educational Research Association, American Psychological Association, and National Council on Measurement in Education. According to the "Standards" (American Educational Research Association et al.,

2014, p. 33), reliability is the "consistency of the scores across instances of the testing procedure." In this book, we define reliability as how much repeatability, consistency, and precision the scores from a measure have.

Reliability (r_{xx}) has been defined mathematically as the proportion of observed score variance (σ^2_X) that is attributable to true score variance (σ^2_T), as in Equation (3.10):

$$\begin{aligned} r_{xx} &= \frac{\sigma^2_T}{\sigma^2_T + \sigma^2_e} \\ &= \frac{\sigma^2_T}{\sigma^2_X} \\ &= \frac{\text{true score variance}}{\text{observed score variance}} \end{aligned} \tag{3.10}$$

An alternative formulation is that reliability (r_{xx}) is the lack of error variance or the degree to which observed scores are correlated with true scores or uncorrelated with error scores. In CTT, reliability can be conceptualized in four primary ways, as depicted in Figure 3.13 (Furr, 2017).

Statistical basis of reliability in terms of...	Conceptual basis of reliability; Observed scores in relation to... **True Scores**	**Measurement Error**
Proportions of Variance	Ratio of true score variance to observed score variance: $r_{xx} = \frac{\sigma^2_T}{\sigma^2_X}$	Lack of error variance: $r_{xx} = 1 - \frac{\sigma^2_e}{\sigma^2_X}$
Correlations	Squared correlation between observed scores and true scores: $r_{xx} = r^2_{xT}$	Lack of correlation between observed scores and error scores: $r_{xx} = 1 - r^2_{xe}$

FIGURE 3.13 Four Different Ways of Conceptualizing Reliability.

However, we cannot *calculate* reliability because we cannot measure the true score component of an observation. Therefore, we *estimate* reliability (the coefficient of reliability) based on the relation between two observations of the same measure (for test–retest reliability) or using other various estimates of reliability.

The coefficient of reliability can depend on several factors. Reliability is inversely related to the amount of measurement error. The coefficient of reliability, like correlation, depends on the degree of spread (variability) of the scores. If the scores at one or both time points show restricted range, the scores will show a weaker association and coefficient of reliability, as shown in Figure 3.19. An ideal way to estimate the reliability of a measure would be to take a person and repeatedly measure them many times to get an estimate of their true score and each measurement's deviation from their true score, and to do this for many people. However, this is rarely done in practice. Instead of taking one person and repeatedly measuring them many times, we typically estimate reliability by taking many people and doing repeated measures twice. This is a shortcut to estimate reliability, but even this shorter approach is not often done. In short, researchers rarely estimate the test–retest reliability of the measures they use.

Reliability can also be related to the number of items in the measure. In general, the greater the number of items, the more reliable the measure (assuming the items assess the same construct) because we are averaging out random error.

We never see the true scores or the error scores, so we cannot compute reliability—we can only *estimate* it from the observed scores. This estimate of reliability gives a probabilistic answer of the reliability of the measure, rather than an absolute answer.

3.3.1 How Reliable Is Reliable Enough?

As described by Nunnally & Bernstein (1994), how reliable a measure should be depends on the proposed uses. If it is early in the research process, and the focus is on group-level inferences (e.g., associations or group differences), modest reliability (e.g., .70) may be sufficient and save time and money. Then, the researcher can see what the associations would be when disattenuated for unreliability, as described in Section 4.6 of the chapter on validity. If the disattenuated associations are promising, it may be worth increasing the reliability of the measure. Associations are only weakly attenuated above a reliability of .80, so achieving a reliability coefficient of .80 may be an appropriate target for basic research.

However, when making decisions about individual people from their score on a measure, reliability and precision are more important (than when making group-level inferences) because small differences in scores can lead to different decisions. Nunnally & Bernstein (1994) recommend that measures have at least a reliability of .90 and—when making important decisions about individual people—that measures preferably have a reliability of .95 or higher. Nevertheless, they also note that one should not switch to a less valid measure merely because it is more reliable.

3.3.2 Standard Error of Measurement

The estimate of reliability gives a general idea of the degree of uncertainty you have of a person's true score given their observed score. From this, we can estimate the standard error of measurement, which estimates the extent to which an observed score deviates from a true score. The standard error of measurement indicates the typical distance of the observed score from the true score. The formula for the standard error of measurement is in Equation (3.11):

$$\text{standard error of measurement (SEM)} = \sigma_x \sqrt{1 - r_{xx}} \tag{3.11}$$

where σ_x represents the standard deviation of scores. Thus, the standard error of measurement is directly related to the reliability of the measure. The higher the reliability, the lower the standard error of measurement. The standard error of measurement as a function of reliability of the measure and the standard deviation of scores is depicted in Figure 3.14.

The derivation of the SEM (from W. Joel Schneider) is in Equation (3.12):

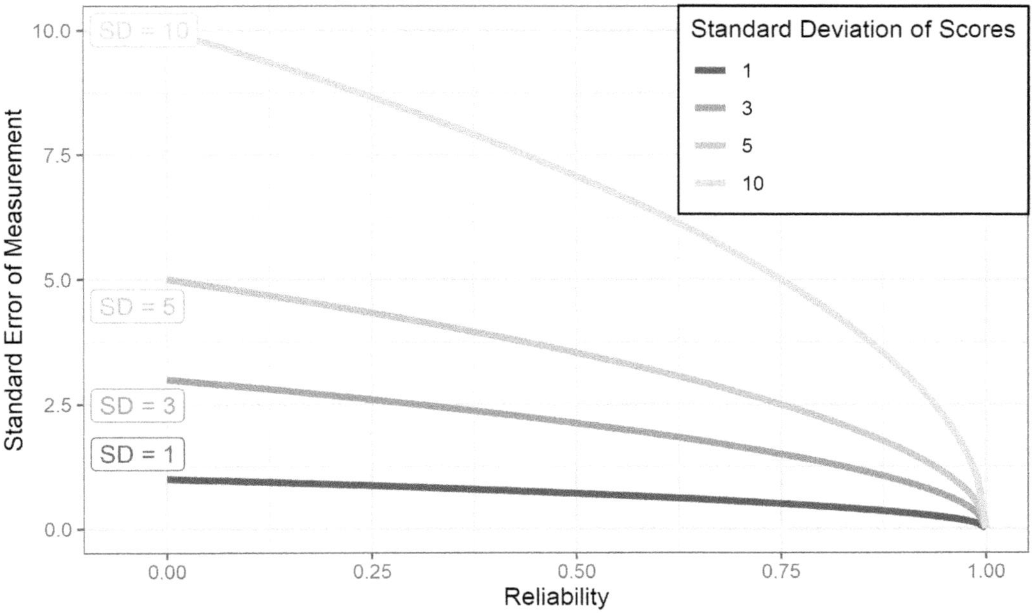

FIGURE 3.14 Standard Error of Measurement as a Function of Reliability.

$$
\begin{aligned}
\text{Remember, based on } X = T + e: &\quad \sigma^2_X = \sigma^2_T + \sigma^2_e \\
\text{Solve for } \sigma^2_T: &\quad \sigma^2_T = \sigma^2_X - \sigma^2_e \\
\text{Remember:} &\quad r_{xx} = \frac{\sigma^2_T}{\sigma^2_X} \\
\text{Substitute for } \sigma^2_T: &\quad = \frac{\sigma^2_X - \sigma^2_e}{\sigma^2_X} \\
\text{Multiply by } \sigma^2_X: &\quad \sigma^2_X \cdot r_{xx} = \sigma^2_X - \sigma^2_e \\
\text{Solve for } \sigma^2_e: &\quad \sigma^2_e = \sigma^2_X - \sigma^2_X \cdot r_{xx} \\
\text{Factor out } \sigma^2_X: &\quad \sigma^2_e = \sigma^2_X(1 - r_{xx}) \\
\text{Take the square root:} &\quad \sigma_e = \sigma_X\sqrt{1 - r_{xx}} \qquad (3.12)
\end{aligned}
$$

The SEM is equivalent to the standard deviation of measurement error (e) (Lek & Van De Schoot, 2018), as in Equation (3.13):

$$
\begin{aligned}
\text{standard error of measurement (SEM)} &= \sigma_x \sqrt{1 - r_{xx}} \\
&= \sqrt{\sigma_x^2}\sqrt{1 - r_{xx}} \\
&= \sqrt{\sigma_x^2(1 - r_{xx})} \\
&= \sqrt{\sigma_x^2 - \sigma_x^2 \cdot r_{xx}} \\
&= \sqrt{\sigma_x^2 - \sigma_x^2 \frac{\sigma_T^2}{\sigma_x^2}} \\
&= \sqrt{\sigma_x^2 - \sigma_T^2} \\
&= \sqrt{\sigma_e^2} \\
&= \sigma_e
\end{aligned}
\tag{3.13}
$$

Around 95% of scores would be expected to fall within ±2 SEMs of the true score (or, more precisely, within ±1.96 SEMs of the true score). In other words, 95% of the time, the true score is expected to fall within ±2 SEMs of the observed score. Given an observed score of $X = 15$ and SEM $= 2$, the 95% confidence interval of the true score is [11, 19]. So if a person gets a score of 15 on the measure, 95% of the time, their true score is expected to fall within 11–19. An empirical example of estimating the SEM is provided in Section 3.7.

Based on the preceding discussion, consider the characteristics of measures that make them more useful from a reliability perspective. A useful measure would show wide variation across people (individual differences), so we can more accurately estimate its reliability. And we would expect a useful measure to show consistency, stability, precision, and reliability of scores.

3.4 Getting Started

3.4.1 Load Libraries

```
library("petersenlab")
library("psych")
library("blandr")
library("MBESS")
library("lavaan")
library("semTools")
library("psychmeta")
library("irrCAC")
library("gtheory")
library("ggrepel")
library("performance")
library("MOTE")
library("here")
library("tidyverse")
library("tinytex")
library("knitr")
```

```
library("kableExtra")
library("rmarkdown")
library("bookdown")
```

3.4.2 Prepare Data

3.4.2.1 Simulate Data

```
sampleSize <- 100

set.seed(52242)

rater1continuous <- rnorm(n = sampleSize, mean = 50, sd = 10)
rater2continuous <- rater1continuous +
  rnorm(
    n = sampleSize,
    mean = 0,
    sd = 4)
rater3continuous <- rater2continuous +
  rnorm(
    n = sampleSize,
    mean = 0,
    sd = 8)

rater1categorical <- sample(
  c(0,1),
  size = sampleSize,
  replace = TRUE)
rater2categorical <- rater1categorical
rater3categorical <- rater1categorical

rater2categorical[
  sample(1:length(rater2categorical),
         size = 10,
         replace = FALSE)] <- 0
rater3categorical[
  sample(1:length(rater3categorical),
         size = 10,
         replace = FALSE)] <- 1

time1 <- rnorm(n = sampleSize, mean = 50, sd = 10)
time2 <- time1 + rnorm(n = sampleSize, mean = 0, sd = 4)
time3 <- time2 + rnorm(n = sampleSize, mean = 0, sd = 8)

item1 <- rnorm(n = sampleSize, mean = 50, sd = 10)
item2 <- item1 + rnorm(n = sampleSize, mean = 0, sd = 4)
item3 <- item2 + rnorm(n = sampleSize, mean = 0, sd = 8)
item4 <- item3 + rnorm(n = sampleSize, mean = 0, sd = 12)
```

```
Person <- as.factor(rep(1:6, each = 8))
Occasion <- Rater <-
  as.factor(rep(1:2, each = 4, times = 6))
Item <- as.factor(rep(1:4, times = 12))
Score <- c(
  9,9,7,4,9,8,5,5,9,8,4,6,
  6,5,3,3,8,8,6,2,8,7,3,2,
  9,8,6,3,9,6,6,2,10,9,8,7,
  8,8,9,7,6,4,5,1,3,2,3,2)
```

3.4.2.2 Add Missing Data

Adding missing data to dataframes helps make examples more realistic to real-life data and helps you get in the habit of programming to account for missing data.

```
rater1continuous[c(5,10)] <- NA
rater2continuous[c(10,15)] <- NA
rater3continuous[c(10)] <- NA

rater1categorical[c(5,10)] <- NA
rater2categorical[c(10,15)] <- NA
rater3categorical[c(10)] <- NA

time1[c(5,10)] <- NA
time2[c(10,15)] <- NA
time3[c(10)] <- NA

item1[c(5,10)] <- NA
item2[c(10,15)] <- NA
item3[c(10)] <- NA
item4[c(10)] <- NA
```

3.4.2.3 Combine Data into Dataframe

```
mydata <- data.frame(
  rater1continuous, rater2continuous, rater3continuous,
  rater1categorical, rater2categorical, rater3categorical,
  time1, time2, time3,
  item1, item2, item3, item4)

pio_cross_dat <- data.frame(Person, Item, Score, Occasion)
```

3.5 Types of Reliability

Reliability is not one thing. There are several types of reliability. In this book, we focus on test–retest, inter-rater, intra-rater, parallel-forms, and internal consistency reliability.

3.5.1 Test–Retest Reliability

Test–retest reliability is defined as the consistency of scores across time. Typically, this is based on a two-week retest interval. The intent of a two-week interval between the original testing and the retest is to provide adequate time to pass to reduce any carryover effects from the original testing while not allowing too much time to pass such that the person's level on the construct (i.e., true scores) would change. A carryover effect is an effect of the experimental condition that affects the participant's behavior at a later time. Examples of carryover effects resulting from repeated measurement can include fatigue, boredom, learning (practice effects), etc. Another potential issue is that measurement error can be correlated across the two measurements.

Test–retest reliability controls for transient error and random response error. If the construct is not stable across time (i.e., people's true scores change), test–retest reliability is not relevant because the CTT approach to estimating reliability assumes that the true scores are perfectly correlated across time (see Section 3.1).

The length of the optimal retest interval depends on the construct of interest. For a construct in which people's levels change rapidly, a shorter retest interval may be appropriate. But one should pay attention to ways to reduce potential carryover effects. By contrast, if the retest interval is too long, people's levels on the construct may change during that span. If people's levels on the construct change from test to retest, we can no longer assume that the true scores are perfectly correlated across time, which would violate CTT assumptions for estimating test–retest reliability of a measure. The longer the retest interval, the smaller the observed association between scores across time will tend to be. For weak associations obtained from a lengthy retest interval, it can be difficult to determine how much of this weak association reflects measurement unreliability versus people's change in their levels on the construct. Thus, when conducting studies to evaluate test–retest reliability, it is important to consider the length of the retest interval and ways to reduce carryover effects.

3.5.1.1 Coefficient of Stability (and Coefficient of Dependability)

The coefficient of stability is the most widely used index when reporting the test–retest reliability of a measure. It is estimated using a Pearson correlation of the scores at time 1 with the score at time 2. That is, the coefficient of stability assesses the stability of individual differences (i.e., rank-order stability). The Pearson correlation is called the coefficient of stability when the length of the retest interval (the delay between test and retest) is on the order of days or weeks. If the retest occurs almost at the same time as the original test (e.g., a 45-minute delay), the Pearson correlation is called the *coefficient of dependability* (Revelle & Condon, 2019).

We estimate the coefficient of stability below:

```
cor.test(x = mydata$time1, y = mydata$time2)
```

```
    Pearson's product-moment correlation

data:  mydata$time1 and mydata$time2
t = 25, df = 95, p-value <2e-16
alternative hypothesis: true correlation is not equal to 0
95 percent confidence interval:
 0.8994 0.9539
sample estimates:
   cor
0.9317

cor(mydata[,c("time1","time2","time3")],
    use = "pairwise.complete.obs")

      time1  time2  time3
time1 1.0000 0.9317 0.8291
time2 0.9317 1.0000 0.8426
time3 0.8291 0.8426 1.0000
```

The r value of .93 indicates a strong positive association. Figure 3.15 depicts a scatterplot of the time 1 scores on the x-axis and time 2 scores on the y-axis.

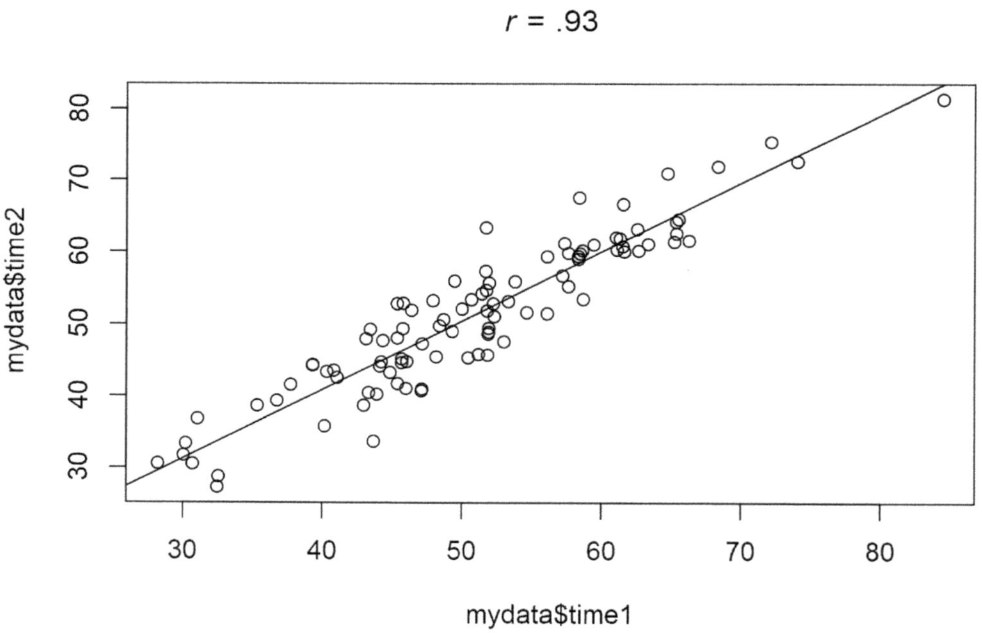

FIGURE 3.15 Test–Retest Reliability Scatterplot. The black line is the best-fitting linear line.

3.5.1.1.1 Considerations About the Correlation Coefficient

The correlation coefficient ranges from -1.0 to +1.0. The correlation coefficient (r) tells you two things: (1) the direction of the association (positive or negative) and (2) the magnitude of the association. If the correlation coefficient is positive, the association is positive. If the correlation coefficient is negative, the association is negative. If the association is positive, as X increases, Y increases (or conversely, as X decreases, Y decreases). If the association is negative, as X increases, Y decreases (or conversely, as X decreases, Y increases). The smaller the absolute value of the correlation coefficient (i.e., the closer the r value is to zero), the weaker the association and the flatter the slope of the best-fit line in a scatterplot. The larger the absolute value of the correlation coefficient (i.e., the closer the absolute value of the r value is to one), the stronger the association and the steeper the slope of the best-fit line in a scatterplot. See Figure 3.16 for a range of different correlation coefficients and what some example data may look like for each direction and strength of association.

Keep in mind that the Pearson correlation examines the strength of the *linear* association between two variables. If the association between two variables is nonlinear, the Pearson correlation provides the strength of the linear trend and may not provide a meaningful index of the strength of the association between the variables. For instance, Anscombe's quartet includes four sets of data that have nearly identical basic descriptive statistics (see Tables 3.1 and 3.2), including the same bivariate correlation, yet have very different distributions and whose association takes very different forms (see Figure 3.17).

TABLE 3.1 Anscombe's Quartet.

x1	y1	x2	y2	x3	y3	x4	y4
10	8.04	10	9.14	10	7.46	8	6.58
8	6.95	8	8.14	8	6.77	8	5.76
13	7.58	13	8.74	13	12.74	8	7.71
9	8.81	9	8.77	9	7.11	8	8.84
11	8.33	11	9.26	11	7.81	8	8.47
14	9.96	14	8.1	14	8.84	8	7.04
6	7.24	6	6.13	6	6.08	8	5.25
4	4.26	4	3.1	4	5.39	19	12.5
12	10.84	12	9.13	12	8.15	8	5.56
7	4.82	7	7.26	7	6.42	8	7.91
5	5.68	5	4.74	5	5.73	8	6.89

TABLE 3.2 Descriptive Statistics of Anscombe's Quartet.

Property	Value
Sample size	11
Mean of X	9.0
Mean of Y	~7.5
Variance of X	11.0
Variance of Y	~4.1
Equation of regression line	Y = 3 + 0.5X
Standard error of slope	0.118
One-sample t-statistic	4.24

Property	Value
Sum of squares of X	110.0
Regression sum of squares	27.50
Residual sum of squares of Y	13.75
Correlation coefficient	.816
Coefficient of determination	.67

As an index of correlation, the coefficient of stability (and dependability) has important weaknesses. It is a form of *relative* reliability rather than *absolute* reliability: It examines the consistency of scores across time relative to variation across people. Higher stability coefficients reflect greater stability of individual differences—not greater stability in people's absolute level on the measure. This is a major limitation. Figure 3.18 depicts two example data sets that show strong relative reliability (a strong coefficient of stability) but poor absolute reliability based on inconsistency in people's absolute level across time.

Another limitation of the coefficient of stability (and dependability) is that it is sensitive to outliers. Additionally, if there are little or no individual differences in scores on a given measure, the coefficient of stability will be low relative to the true reliability because correlation coefficients tend to be attenuated in the presence of a restricted range, and it may not be a useful index of reliability depending on the purpose. For more information see Section 23.3.4.3.2 on the reliability paradox in the chapter on cognitive assessment.

See Figure 3.19 for an example of how a correlation coefficient tends to be attenuated when the range of one or both of the variables has restriction of range. The figure depicts the correlation with and without restriction of range on x (i.e., x is restricted to values between 55 and 65).

The observed correlation became much weaker due to restriction of range. Thus, when developing measures, it is important to ensure there is adequate variability of scores (i.e., individual differences) and that scores are not truncated due to ceiling or floor effects. Moreover, when interpreting associations with truncated variability, it is important to keep in mind that the true association is likely to be even stronger than what was observed if the measures did not have restricted range.

To address these limitations of the coefficient of stability, it is important to consider additional indices of test–retest reliability, such as the coefficient of repeatability and bias that are depicted in Bland-Altman plots, as described later.

3.5.1.2 Coefficient of Agreement

The intraclass correlation (ICC) can be used to evaluate the extent of absolute agreement of scores within a person across time. ICC ranges from 0–1, with higher scores indicating greater agreement. ICC was estimated using the `psych` package (Revelle, 2022).

```
ICC(mydata[,c("time1","time2")], missing = FALSE)
```

```
Call: ICC(x = mydata[, c("time1", "time2")], missing = FALSE)

Intraclass correlation coefficients
                         type  ICC  F df1 df2       p lower bound
Single_raters_absolute   ICC1 0.93 28  99 100 1.1e-45        0.90
```

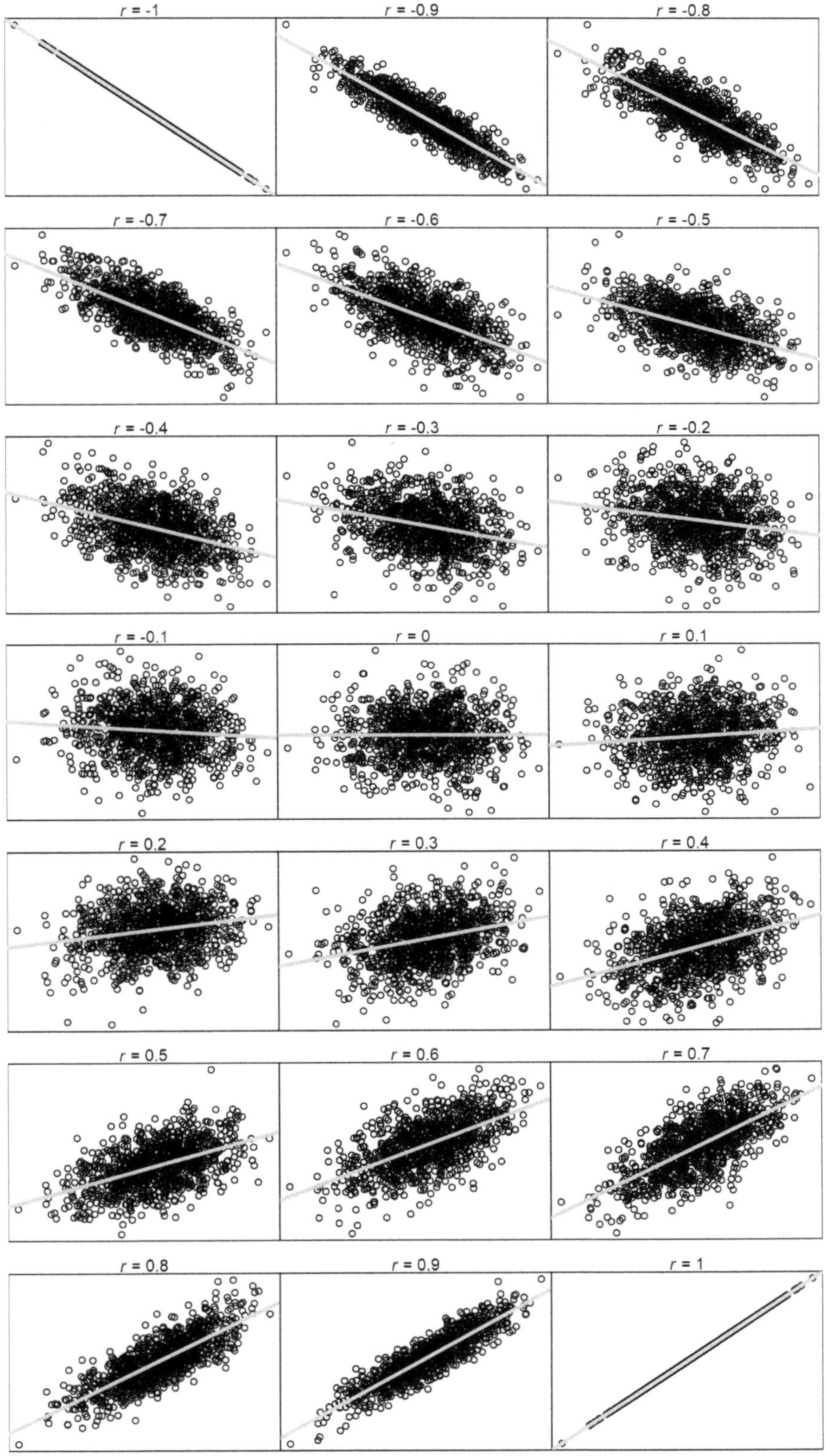

FIGURE 3.16 Correlation Coefficients.

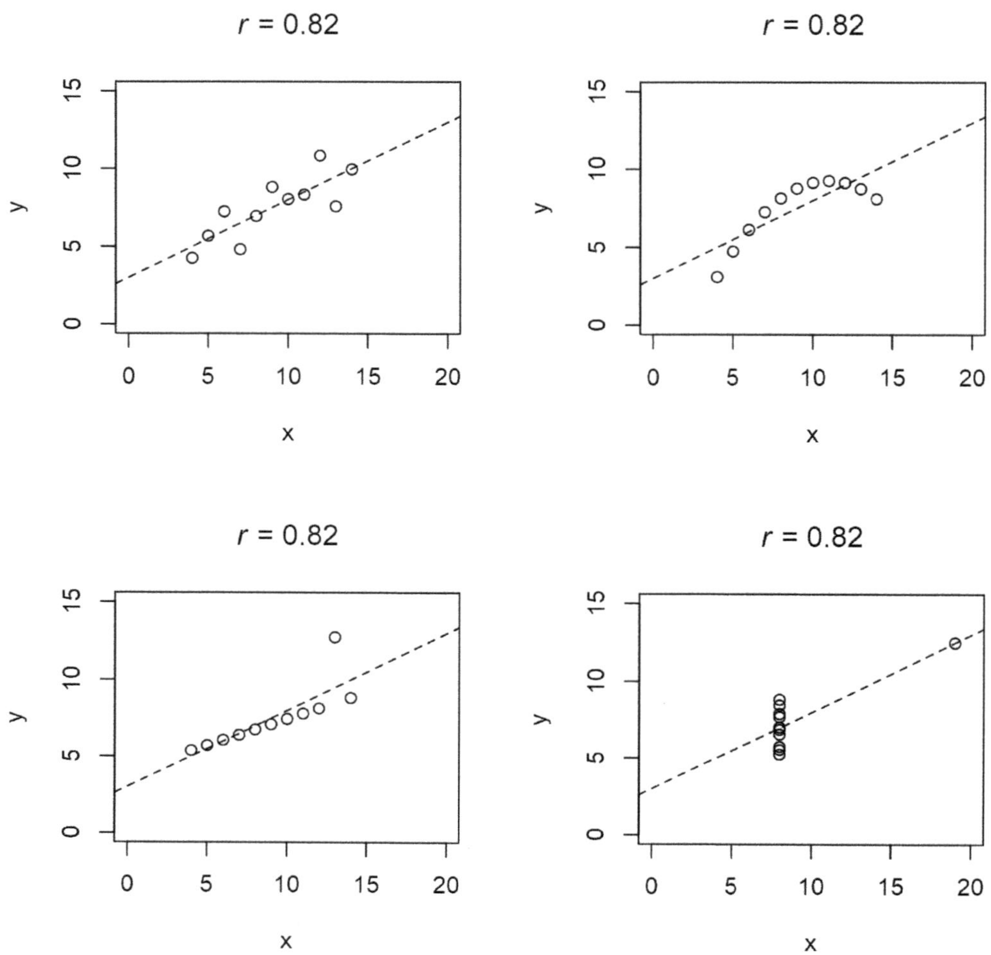

FIGURE 3.17 Anscombe's Quartet.

```
Single_random_raters      ICC2  0.93 28  99  99 2.6e-45         0.90
Single_fixed_raters       ICC3  0.93 28  99  99 2.6e-45         0.90
Average_raters_absolute  ICC1k 0.96 28  99 100 1.1e-45         0.95
Average_random_raters    ICC2k 0.96 28  99  99 2.6e-45         0.95
Average_fixed_raters     ICC3k 0.96 28  99  99 2.6e-45         0.95
                         upper bound
Single_raters_absolute         0.95
Single_random_raters           0.95
Single_fixed_raters            0.95
Average_raters_absolute        0.98
Average_random_raters          0.98
Average_fixed_raters           0.98

 Number of subjects = 100     Number of Judges =  2
```

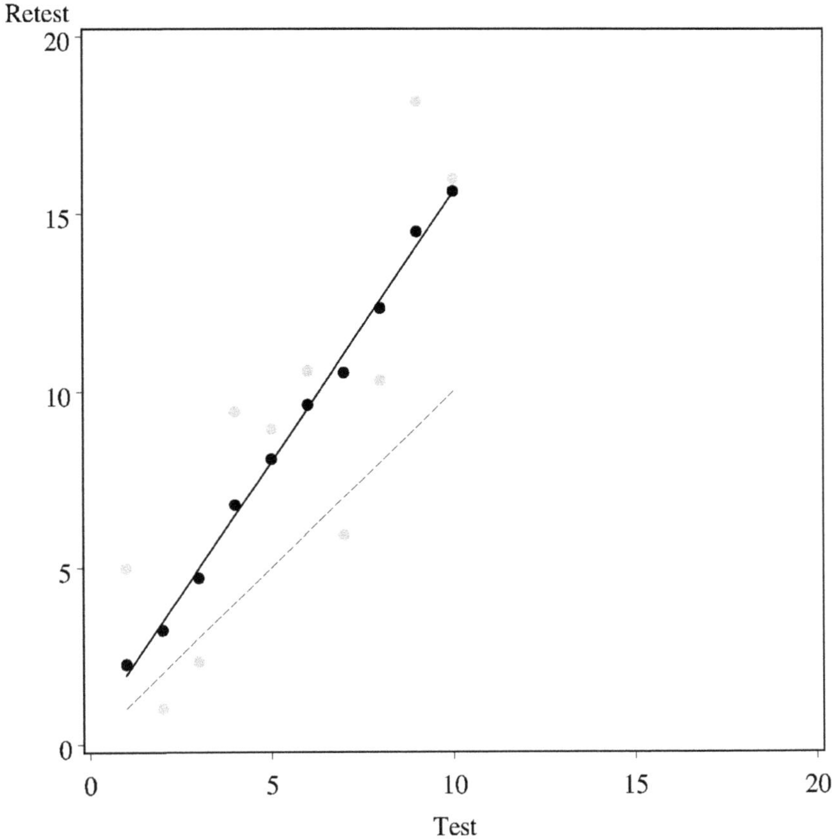

FIGURE 3.18 Hypothetical Data Demonstrating Good Relative Reliability Despite Poor Absolute Reliability. The figure depicts two fictional data sets (black and gray circles), which both exhibit a similar linear association. The line of best fit is the solid line in the graph and is the same for both data sets, but the black circles sit much closer to the line than the gray circles, leading to a much higher coefficient of stability ($r = .99$ and .84, respectively). However, neither sets of circles are on the line of complete agreement represented by the dashed line in the graph. If the circles fall on the line of complete agreement, it indicates that the measure's scores show consistency in absolute scores across time. Thus, although the measures show strong relative reliability, they show poor absolute reliability. (Figure reprinted from Vaz et al. (2013), figure 1, p. 3. Vaz, S., Falkmer, T., Passmore, A. E., Parsons, R., & Andreou, P. (2013). The case for using the repeatability coefficient when calculating test–retest reliability. *PLoS ONE*, *8*(9), e73990. https://doi.org/10.1371/journal.pone.0073990)

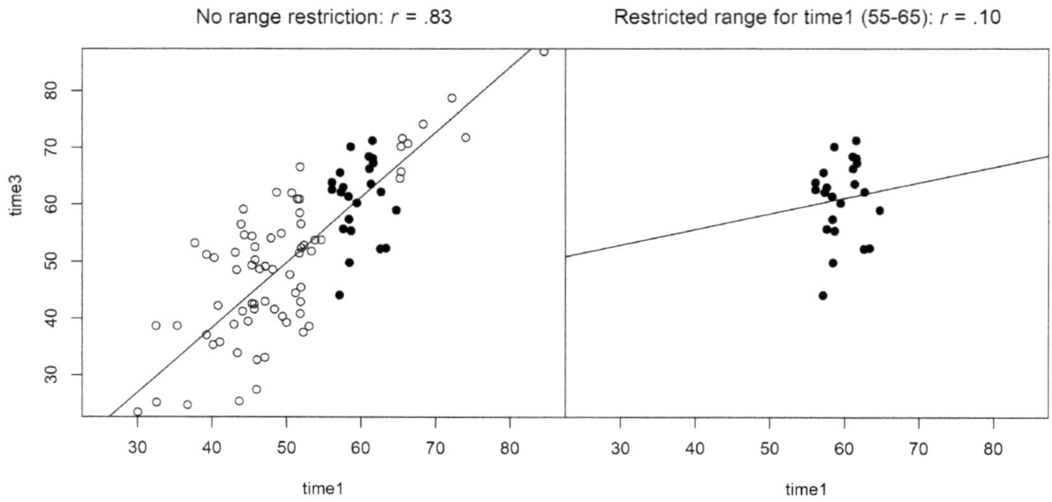

FIGURE 3.19 Example of Correlation With (Right Panel) and Without (Left Panel) Range Restriction. Filled black points represent the points in common across the two scatterplots.

```
See the help file for a discussion of the other 4 McGraw and Wong estimates,
```

There are various kinds of ICC coefficients. To read more about the various types of ICC coefficients, type the following command:

```
?ICC
```

3.5.1.3 Coefficient of Repeatability

The coefficient of repeatability (CR), also known as the "smallest real difference," is a form of *absolute* reliability. That is, it reflects the consistency of scores across time within a person. It is calculated as ~1.96 times the standard deviation of the mean differences between the two measurements (d_1 and d_2), as in Equation (3.14): https://www.medcalc.org/manual/bland-altman-plot.php (archived at https://perma.cc/MEH3-3TGN) (Bland & Altman, 1986, 1999). The CR is used for determining the lower and upper limits of agreement because it defines the range within which 95% of differences between the two measurement methods are expected to be.

The minimum possible coefficient of repeatability is zero, but there is no theoretical limit on the maximum possible coefficient of repeatability. The smaller the coefficient of repeatability (i.e., the closer to zero), the more consistent the scores are across time within a person. The coefficient of repeatability is tied to the units of the measure, so how small is considered "good" absolute reliability depends on the measure. In general, however, given the same units of measurement, a smaller coefficient of repeatability indicates stronger absolute test–retest reliability.

$$CR = 1.96 \times \sqrt{\frac{\sum(d_1 - d_2)^2}{n}} \tag{3.14}$$

The `petersenlab` package (Petersen, 2024) contains the `repeatability()` function that estimates the repeatability of a measure's scores and generates a Bland-Altman plot in Figure 3.20. The coefficient of repeatability is labeled `cr` in the output.

```
repeatability(
  measure1 = mydata$time1,
  measure2 = mydata$time2)
```

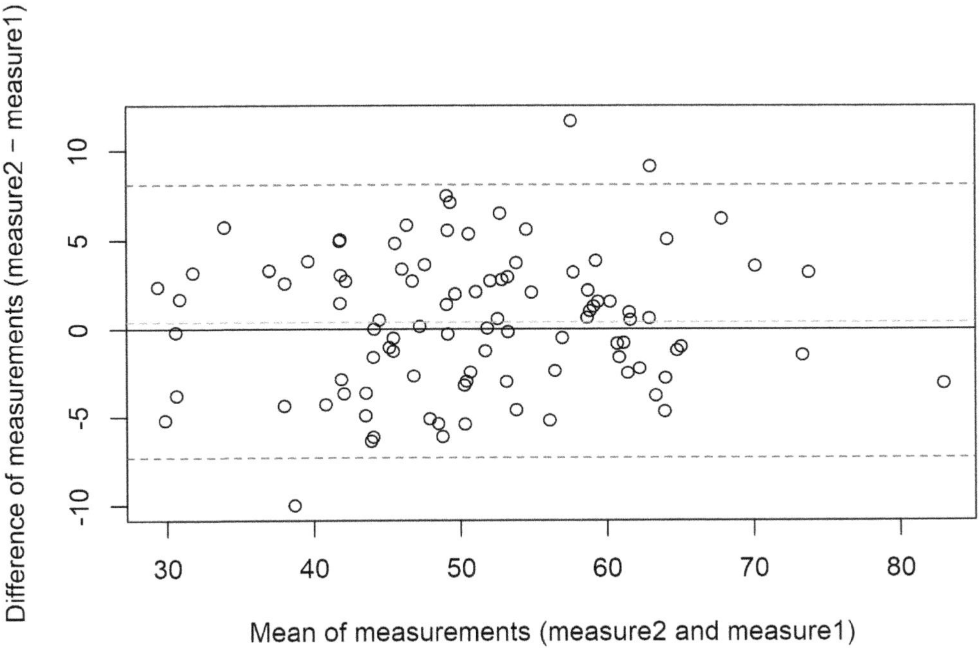

FIGURE 3.20 Bland-Altman Plot.

```
     cr   bias lowerLOA upperLOA
1 7.694 0.3956   -7.298     8.09
```

3.5.1.3.1 Bland-Altman Plot

The Bland-Altman plot can be useful for visualizing the degree of (in)consistency of people's absolute scores on a measure across two time points (Bland & Altman, 1986, 1999).

In a Bland-Altman plot, the x-axis represents the mean of a person's score across the two time points, and the y-axis represents the within-subject differences across time points. The horizontal line at $y = 0$ is called the line of identity. Points would fall on the line of identity if people's scores showed perfect consistency in their absolute level across time points (i.e., not relative level as in a cross-time correlation). Another line reflects the bias estimate (i.e., mean difference from the measure across the two points). The bias plus or minus the coefficient of repeatability is the upper or lower limit of agreement (LOA), respectively, as in Equations (3.15) and (3.16). The top dashed line reflects the upper LOA. The bottom dashed line reflects the lower LOA.

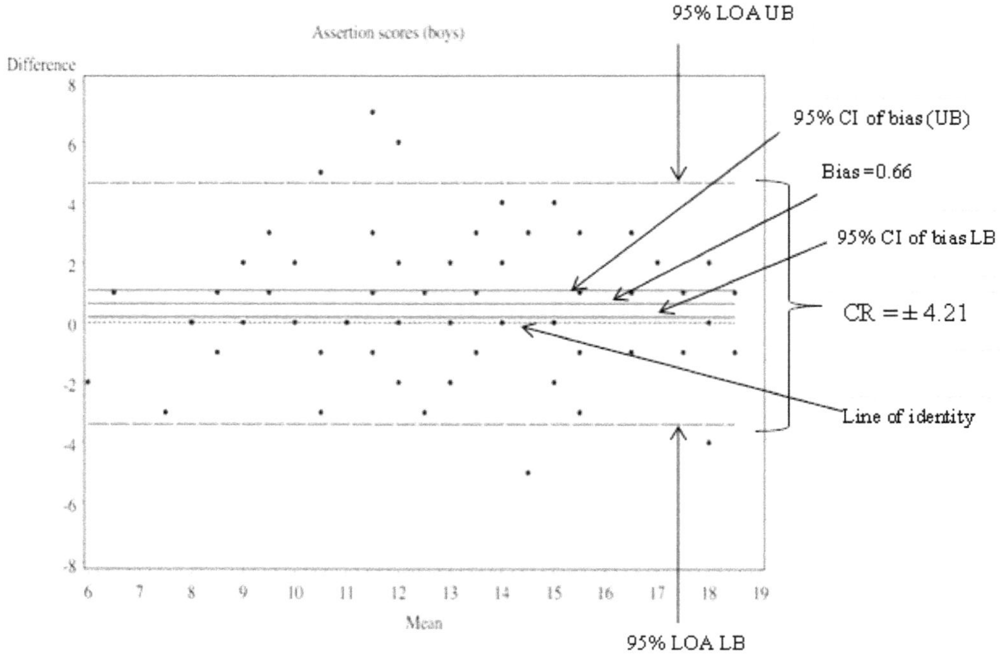

FIGURE 3.21 Example of a Bland-Altman Plot. (Figure reprinted from Vaz et al. (2013), figure 2, p. 4. Vaz, S., Falkmer, T., Passmore, A. E., Parsons, R., & Andreou, P. (2013). The case for using the repeatability coefficient when calculating test–retest reliability. *PLoS ONE*, *8*(9), e73990. https://doi.org/10.1371/journal.pone.0073990)

3.5.1.3.2 Bias

Bias is the degree of systematic measurement error. Bias is also called "mean error" in the context of assessing accuracy against a criterion (see Section 9.4.1.1.1). In a Bland-Altman plot, (test–retest) bias is estimated as the average of the within-subject differences between the two measurements. Estimated (test–retest) bias values that are closer to zero reflect stronger absolute test–retest reliability at the group-level. However, (estimated) bias values can still be close to zero while individuals show large differences because large positive and negative differences could cancel each other out. As a result, it is also important to examine other indices of test–retest reliability, including the coefficient of stability and the coefficient of repeatability.

The bias of 0.40 indicates that the scores at time 2 are somewhat larger, on average, than the scores at time 1.

3.5.1.3.3 95% Limits of Agreement

$$\text{Lower Limit of Agreement} = \text{Bias} - \text{Coefficient of Repeatability} \tag{3.15}$$

$$\text{Upper Limit of Agreement} = \text{Bias} + \text{Coefficient of Repeatability} \tag{3.16}$$

It is expected that the 95% limits of agreement (LOA) include 95% of differences between the two measurement methods (assuming the scores are normally distributed), based on how the coefficient of repeatability is calculated.

The limits of agreement indicate that 95% of scores at time 2 are expected to fall within $[-7.30, 8.09]$ of scores at time 1.

3.5.2 Inter-Rater Reliability

Inter-rater reliability is the consistency of scores across raters. For instance, two different raters may make a diagnostic decision for the same client, two different people may provide observational ratings of the same participant, or two different researchers may process psychophysiological data (e.g., electroencephalography, electrocardiography) from the same person. Consistency of scores can also be assessed within the same rater, which is known as *intra*-rater reliability and is described in Section 3.5.3. For assessing inter-rater reliability, intraclass correlation (ICC) is recommended for continuous data, such as ratings of a participant's mood. By contrast, Cohen's kappa (κ) is recommended for categorical variables, such as making a diagnostic decision whether to give someone a diagnosis of depression or not.

3.5.2.1 Continuous Data

Use intraclass correlation (ICC) for estimating inter-rater reliability of continuous data. ICC ranges from 0–1, with higher scores indicating greater agreement. ICC was estimated using the psych package (Revelle, 2022).

```
ICC(mydata[,c(
  "rater1continuous","rater2continuous","rater3continuous")],
  missing = FALSE)
```

```
Call: ICC(x = mydata[, c("rater1continuous", "rater2continuous", "rater3continuous")],
    missing = FALSE)

Intraclass correlation coefficients
                         type  ICC  F df1 df2       p lower bound
Single_raters_absolute   ICC1 0.81 14  99 200 2.7e-54        0.75
Single_random_raters     ICC2 0.81 14  99 198 6.4e-54        0.75
Single_fixed_raters      ICC3 0.81 14  99 198 6.4e-54        0.75
Average_raters_absolute ICC1k 0.93 14  99 200 2.7e-54        0.90
Average_random_raters   ICC2k 0.93 14  99 198 6.4e-54        0.90
Average_fixed_raters    ICC3k 0.93 14  99 198 6.4e-54        0.90
                        upper bound
Single_raters_absolute         0.86
Single_random_raters           0.86
Single_fixed_raters            0.86
Average_raters_absolute        0.95
Average_random_raters          0.95
Average_fixed_raters           0.95

 Number of subjects = 100     Number of Judges =  3
See the help file for a discussion of the other 4 McGraw and Wong estimates,
```

3.5.2.2 Categorical Data

For estimating the inter-rater reliability of categorical data, use Cohen's kappa (Bakeman & Goodman, 2020), Fleiss's kappa, the S index (Falotico & Quatto, 2010), or Gwet's AC1 statistic (Gwet, 2008; Gwet, 2021a, 2021b). Cohen's kappa was estimated using the `psych` package (Revelle, 2022). Fleiss's kappa and Gwet's AC1 statistic were estimated using the `irrCAC` package. These estimates of inter-rater reliability range from -1 to $+1$, with -1 indicating perfect disagreement, 0 indicating chance agreement, and 1 indicating perfect agreement. Larger, more positive scores indicate greater agreement.

```
cohen.kappa(mydata[,c(
  "rater1categorical","rater2categorical","rater3categorical")])
```

```
Cohen Kappa (below the diagonal) and Weighted Kappa (above the diagonal)
For confidence intervals and detail print with all=TRUE
                  rater1categorical rater2categorical rater3categorical
rater1categorical              1.00              0.86              0.90
rater2categorical              0.86              1.00              0.76
rater3categorical              0.90              0.76              1.00

Average Cohen kappa for all raters  0.84
Average weighted kappa for all raters  0.84
```

```
fleiss.kappa.raw(na.omit(mydata[,c(
  "rater1categorical","rater2categorical","rater3categorical")]))
```

```
$est
     coeff.name     pa     pe coeff.val coeff.se       conf.int p.value
1 Fleiss' Kappa 0.9175 0.5001     0.835  0.04483 (0.746,0.924)       0
      w.name
1 unweighted

$weights
     [,1] [,2]
[1,]    1    0
[2,]    0    1

$categories
[1] 0 1
```

```
gwet.ac1.raw(na.omit(mydata[,c(
  "rater1categorical","rater2categorical","rater3categorical")]))
```

```
$est
  coeff.name     pa     pe coeff.val coeff.se       conf.int p.value
1        AC1 0.9175 0.4999    0.8351  0.04479 (0.746,0.924)       0
      w.name
1 unweighted

$weights
```

```
     [,1] [,2]
[1,]    1    0
[2,]    0    1

$categories
[1] 0 1
```

3.5.3 Intra-Rater Reliability

Principles of intra-rater reliability are similar to principles of inter-rater reliability (described in Section 3.5.2), except the *same* rater provides ratings on two occasions, rather than using multiple raters.

3.5.4 Parallel- (or Alternate-) Forms Reliability

Parallel-forms reliability (also known as alternate-forms reliability) is the consistency of scores across two parallel forms. Parallel forms are two equivalent measures of the same construct that differ in content or format. The two measures can be administered in the same occasion, known as *immediate parallel-forms reliability*, or they can be administered separated by a delay, known as *delayed parallel-forms reliability*. Similar considerations of length of delay duration and ways to reduce carryover effects are relevant to parallel-forms reliability as they are to test–retest reliability.

Parallel-forms reliability is often estimated with the Pearson correlation, which is known as the *coefficient of equivalence*. The coefficient of equivalence is the consistency of scores across two parallel forms relative to variation across people. It is interpreted as the ratio of true score variance to observed score variance, consistent with the formal definition of reliability.

An example of parallel-forms reliability would be if we want to assess a participant twice with different measures of the same construct to avoid practice effects. This approach is often conducted in academic achievement testing, and it could involve retesting that is immediate or delayed. For instance, we could administer item set A at time 1 and item set B at time 2 for the same participant, to get rid of any possibility that the person's score differed across time because of improved performance that resulted merely from prior exposure to the same items. Many standardized academic achievement and aptitude tests have developed parallel forms, including the SAT, ACT, and GRE.

Parallel-forms reliability controls for specific error, i.e., error that is particular to a specific measure. However, parallel-forms reliability has the limitation that it assumes that the parallel forms are equivalent, such that it makes no difference which test you use. Two forms are considered equivalent when they assess the same construct, have the same mean and variance of scores, and have the same inter-correlations with external criteria. Technically, two instruments are only truly equivalent if they have the same true scores and variability of error scores, though this is difficult to establish empirically. Given these constraints, it can be difficult to assume that different forms are equivalent. Nevertheless, integrative data analysis and measurement harmonization may help make the assumption more tenable (Hussong et al., 2013, 2020). In general, parallel forms can be difficult to create and they can more than double the time it takes to develop a single measure, often with limited benefit, depending on the intended use.

3.5.5 Internal Consistency Reliability

Internal consistency reliability is the consistency of scores across items, that is, their inter-relatedness. Internal consistency is necessary, but insufficient, for establishing the homogeneity or unidimensionality of the measure, i.e., that the items on the measure assess the same construct.

There are many examples of internal consistency estimates, including Cronbach's coefficient alpha (α), Kuder-Richardson Formula 20 (which is a special case of Cronbach's alpha with dichotomous items), omega coefficients, average variance extracted, greatest lower bound, coefficient H, split-half reliability, average inter-item correlation, and average item–total correlation. In general, internal consistency ranges from 0–1, with higher scores indicating greater consistency. There is no magic cutoff for determining adequate internal consistency; however, values below .70 suggest that the items may not assess the same construct.

Internal consistency can be affected by many factors, such as

- wording of the item
- a participant's comprehension of the item, which could be impacted if using items with dated language or double negatives
- interpretation
- attention of the participant
- compliance of the participant

Although establishing internal consistency can help ensure that items in the measure are inter-related, you do not want to select items just based on internal consistency. If you did, you would end up with items that are too similar. For example, you could end up only with items that have similar item stems and are coded in the same direction. Therefore, selecting items solely based on internal consistency would likely not assess the breadth of the construct and would reflect strong method variance of the wording of the particular items. In other words, internal consistency can be *too* high. Internal consistency is helpful to a point, but you do not want items to be too homogeneous or redundant.

3.5.5.1 Average Inter-Item Correlation

One estimate of internal consistency is the average (mean or median) inter-item correlation.

```
interItemCorrelations <- cor(
  mydata[,c("item1","item2","item3","item4")],
  use = "pairwise.complete.obs")
diag(interItemCorrelations) <- NA
```

Here is the mean inter-item correlation for each item:

```
meanInterItemCorrelations <- colMeans(
  interItemCorrelations, na.rm = TRUE)
meanInterItemCorrelations
```

```
 item1  item2  item3  item4
0.7748 0.7787 0.7539 0.6595
```

Here is the mean inter-item correlation across all items:

```
psych::alpha(
  mydata[,c("item1","item2","item3","item4")])$total$average_r
```

```
[1] 0.7417
```

Here is the median inter-item correlation for each item:

```
medianInterItemCorrelations <- apply(
  interItemCorrelations, 2,
  function(x) median(x, na.rm = TRUE))
medianInterItemCorrelations
```

```
 item1  item2  item3  item4
0.7578 0.7792 0.7578 0.6317
```

Here is the median inter-item correlation across all items:

```
psych::alpha(mydata[,c(
  "item1","item2","item3","item4")])$total$median_r
```

```
[1] 0.7412
```

3.5.5.2 Average Item–Total Correlation

Another estimate of internal consistency is the average item–total correlation.

```
itemTotalCorrelations <- psych::alpha(
  mydata[,c("item1","item2","item3","item4")])$item.stats["raw.r"]

mean(itemTotalCorrelations$raw.r)
```

```
[1] 0.894
```

When examining the item–total correlation for a given item, it is preferable to exclude the item of interest from the total score, so that the item is associated with the total score that is calculated from the remaining items. This reduces the extent to which the association reflects that the item is associated with itself.

```
itemTotalCorrelationsDrop <- psych::alpha(
  mydata[,c("item1","item2","item3","item4")])$item.stats["r.drop"]

mean(itemTotalCorrelationsDrop$r.drop)
```

```
[1] 0.8053
```

3.5.5.3 Average Variance Extracted

The equivalent of the average item–total (squared) correlation when dealing with a reflective latent construct is the average variance extracted (AVE). AVE is estimated as the mean of the squared loadings of the indicators of a latent factor (i.e., the sum of the squared loadings divided by the number of indicators). When using unstandardized estimates, AVE is the item-variance weighted average of item reliabilities (Rönkkö & Cho, 2020). When using standardized estimates, AVE is the average indicator reliability (Rönkkö & Cho, 2020). AVE is equivalent to the communality of a latent factor. AVE was estimated using a confirmatory factor analysis model using the `lavaan` (Rosseel et al., 2022) and `semTools` (Jorgensen et al., 2021) packages.

```
latentFactorModel_syntax <- '
 latentFactor =~ item1 + item2 + item3 + item4
'

latentFactorModel_fit <- cfa(
  latentFactorModel_syntax,
  data = mydata,
  missing = "ML",
  estimator = "MLR",
  std.lv = TRUE)

AVE(latentFactorModel_fit)
```

```
latentFactor
        0.64
```

3.5.5.4 Split-Half Reliability

When estimating split-half reliability, we randomly take half of the items on the measure and relate scores on these items to the score on the other half of items. One challenge to split-half reliability is that, according to classical test theory, shorter tests tend to be less reliable than longer tests, so this would be an underestimate of the test's reliability. In general, the greater the number of items, the more reliable the test. To overcome this, the Spearman-Brown prediction (or prophecy) formula predicts the reliability of a test after changing the test length. Thus, the Spearman-Brown prediction formula accounts for the shorter test in predicting what the reliability of the full-length test would be when estimating split-half reliability.

The Spearman-Brown prediction formula is in Equation (3.17):

$$\text{predicted test reliability, } r_{xx} = \frac{n \cdot r_{xx'}}{1 + (n-1)r_{xx'}} \tag{3.17}$$

where $n =$ the number of tests combined (i.e., the ratio of the number of new items to the number of old items) and $r_{xx'} =$ the reliability of the original test.

So, according to Equation (3.18), doubling the length of a test whose reliability is .80 would be estimated to have a reliability of

$$\begin{aligned}\text{predicted test reliability, } r_{xx} &= \frac{2 \cdot .80}{1 + (2-1).80} \\ &= .89\end{aligned} \tag{3.18}$$

Another challenge to split-half reliability is that the reliability differs depending on which items go into which half.

One option is to calculate the split-half reliability of odd and even trials, while correcting for test length, as is performed with the `item_split_half()` function of the `performance` package (Lüdecke et al., 2021):

```
item_split_half(mydata[,c(
  "item1","item2","item3","item4")])
```

```
$splithalf
[1] 0.8734

$spearmanbrown
[1] 0.9324
```

Modern computational software allows for estimating the mean reliability estimate of all possible split-halves (Revelle & Condon, 2019), while correcting for test length, as seen below. Split-half reliability was estimated using the `psych` package (Revelle, 2022).

```
splitHalf(mydata[,c(
  "item1","item2","item3","item4")],
  brute = TRUE)
```

```
Split half reliabilities
Call: splitHalf(r = mydata[, c("item1", "item2", "item3", "item4")],
    brute = TRUE)

Maximum split half reliability (lambda 4) =  0.95
Guttman lambda 6                          =  0.93
Average split half reliability            =  0.92
Guttman lambda 3 (alpha)                  =  0.92
Guttman lambda 2                          =  0.92
Minimum split half reliability  (beta)    =  0.87
Average interitem r =  0.75  with median =  0.74
```

3.5.5.5 Cronbach's Alpha (Coefficient Alpha)

Cronbach's alpha (α), also known as coefficient alpha, is approximately equal to the mean reliability estimate of all split-halves, assuming that item standard deviations are equal. Alpha considers the inter-relatedness of a total set of items—giving us information about the extent to which each item in a set of items correlates with all other items. Alpha is the most commonly used estimate for internal consistency reliability, but it has many problems.

Cronbach's alpha assumes that the items are

- unidimensional: that there is one predominant dimension that explains the variance among the items
- essentially tau (τ) equivalent: that the items are equally related to the construct

Cronbach's alpha is affected by the

- number of items: The more items, the more inflated alpha is, even if correlations among the items are low.
- variance of the item scores: If the variances of item scores are low (e.g., dichotomous scores), alphas tend to be an underestimate of internal consistency reliability.

- violations of assumptions:
  - Cronbach's alpha assumes items are essentially tau equivalent—that the items are equally related to the construct. However, this is an unrealistic assumption.
  - Cronbach's alpha depends on the dimensionality of the scale: Alpha is only valid when the scale is unidimensional. If you use it with multidimensional scales, you know the extent to which items correlate with another but nothing about whether they are actually measuring the same constructs.

Cronbach's alpha is appropriate only in situations where a scale is unidimensional, where the items equally contribute to the scale, and you would like to determine whether its items are inter-related. However, Cronbach's alpha does not assess the dimensionality of the scale or any type of construct validity—it can only tell us how strongly the items hang together.

Cronbach's alpha (α) was estimated using the `psych` package (Revelle, 2022).

```
psych::alpha(mydata[,c(
  "item1","item2","item3","item4")])$total$raw_alpha
```

```
[1] 0.8924
```

However, because of the many weaknesses of Cronbach's alpha (Cortina, 1993; Dunn et al., 2014; Flora, 2020; Green & Yang, 2015; A. F. Hayes & Coutts, 2020; Kelley & Pornprasertmanit, 2016; McNeish, 2018; Peters, 2014; Raykov, 2001; Revelle & Condon, 2019; Sijtsma, 2008; but see Raykov & Marcoulides, 2019), current recommendations are to use coefficient omega (ω) instead, as described next.

3.5.5.6 Coefficient Omega (ω)

Current recommendations are to use McDonald's coefficient omega (ω) instead of Cronbach's alpha (α) for internal consistency reliability. Specifically, it is recommended to use omega total (ω_t) for continuous items that are unidimensional, omega hierarchical (ω_h) for continuous items that are multidimensional, and omega categorical (ω_C) for categorical items (i.e., items with fewer than five ordinal categories), with confidence intervals calculated from a bias-corrected bootstrap (Flora, 2020; Kelley & Pornprasertmanit, 2016).

3.5.5.6.1 Omega total (ω_t)

Omega total (ω_t) is the proportion of the total variance that is accounted for by the common factor (Flora, 2020). Omega total, like Cronbach's alpha, assumes that the items are unidimensional. Omega total (ω_t) was calculated using the `MBESS` package (Kelley, 2020). This code calculates a point estimate for omega total:

```
ci.reliability(
  mydata[,c("item1","item2","item3","item4")],
  type = "omega",
  interval.type = "none")$est
```

```
[1] 0.8761
```

3.5.5.6.2 Omega hierarchical (ω_h)

If the items are multidimensional and follow a bifactor structure, omega hierarchical (ω_h) is preferred over omega total. Omega hierarchical is the proportion of the total variance that is accounted for by the general factor in a set of multidimensional items (Flora, 2020). Use omega hierarchical for estimating internal consistency of continuous items that are multidimensional and that follow a bifactor structure. If the multidimensional items follow a higher-order structure, use omega higher-order [ω_{ho}; Flora (2020)].

Omega hierarchical was calculated using the `MBESS` package (Kelley, 2020).

```
ci.reliability(
  mydata[,c("item1","item2","item3","item4")],
  type = "hierarchical",
  interval.type = "none")$est
```

```
[1] 0.8453
```

3.5.5.6.3 *Omega categorical (ω_C)*

Use omega categorical (ω_C) for categorical items that are unidimensional. To handle categorical data, omega categorical is calculated using a polychoric correlation matrix instead of a Pearson correlation matrix. If the categorical items are multidimensional items and they follow a bifactor structure, use omega hierarchical categorical [$\omega_{h\text{-cat}}$; Flora (2020)]. If the categorical items are multidimensional and they follow a higher-order structure, use omega higher-order categorical [$\omega_{ho\text{-cat}}$; Flora (2020)].

Omega categorical was calculated using the `MBESS` package (Kelley, 2020).

```
ci.reliability(
  mydata[,c(
    "rater1categorical",
    "rater2categorical",
    "rater3categorical")],
  type = "categorical",
  interval.type = "none")$est
```

```
        [,1]   [,2]   [,3]
[1,] 1.0073 0.9852 0.9904
[2,] 0.9852 0.9636 0.9686
[3,] 0.9904 0.9686 0.9737
```

```
[1] 0.9601
```

3.5.6 Comparison

Even though the types of reliability described in Section 3.5 are all called "reliability," they are very different from each other. Test–retest reliability and inter-rater reliability tend to be lower than immediate parallel-forms reliability and internal consistency reliability because they involve administering measures at different times or with different raters. However, delayed parallel-forms reliability tends to be lower than test–retest reliability because it involves assessing the construct at a different time point *and* with different items. Thus, if we put the different types of reliability in order from low to high, they tend to be (but not always) arranged like this (Equation (3.19)):

$$\begin{aligned} &\text{delayed parallel-forms} < \\ &\text{test–retest, inter-rater} < \\ \text{immediate parallel-forms, internal consistency, intra-rater} \end{aligned} \tag{3.19}$$

3.5.7 Reliability of a Linear Composite Score

A linear composite score is a linear combination of variables, each of which has a given weight in the linear composite. Unit weights (i.e., weights of 1) would reflect an unweighted composite.

We first specify the variables used to generate the correlation matrix, and the reliability, standard deviation, and weight of each variable. We specify items 2 and 3 to have twice the weight as item 1 in the composite, and item 4 to have 1.5 times the weight as item 1 in the composite.

```
rxx <- c(0.70, 0.75, 0.80, 0.85) #reliability coefficients
rho <- cor(mydata[,c("item1","item2","item3","item4")],
           use = "pairwise.complete.obs")
sigma <- apply(
  mydata[,c("item1","item2","item3","item4")],
  2,
  function(x) sd(x, na.rm = TRUE)) #standard deviations
weights <- c(1, 2, 2, 1.5) #weights of each variable in the linear combination
```

Here is the reliability of an unweighted composite:

```
composite_rel_matrix(
  rel_vec = rxx,
  r_mat = rho,
  sd_vec = sigma)
```

```
[1] 0.9337
```

Here is the reliability of a weighted composite:

```
composite_rel_matrix(
  rel_vec = rxx,
  r_mat = rho,
  sd_vec = sigma,
  wt_vec = weights)
```

```
[1] 0.9317
```

3.5.8 Reliability of a Difference Score

Difference scores tend to be lower in reliability than the individual indices that compose the difference score. This is especially the case when the two indices are correlated. If the correlation between the indices is equal to the reliability of the indices, the reliability of the difference score will be zero (Revelle & Condon, 2019). If the correlation between the two indices is large, it requires a very high reliability for the difference score to show a strong reliability (Trafimow, 2015). To the extent that the two indices have unequal variances (e.g., if one index has a standard deviation that is four times the standard deviation of the second index), the reliabilities do not need to be quite as high for the difference score to be reliable (Trafimow, 2015).

The reliability of a difference score can be estimated using Equation (3.20) (Trafimow, 2015):

$$r_{x-y,x-y} = \frac{\sigma_x^2 r_{xx} + \sigma_y^2 r_{yy} - 2r_{xy}\sigma_x\sigma_y}{\sigma_x^2 + \sigma_y^2 - 2r_{xy}\sigma_x\sigma_y} \tag{3.20}$$

The `petersenlab` package (Petersen, 2024) contains the `reliabilityOfDifferenceScore()` function to estimate the reliability of a difference score:

```
reliabilityOfDifferenceScore(
  x = mydata$item1,
  y = mydata$item2,
  reliabilityX = .95,
  reliabilityY = .95)
```

```
[1] 0.2553
```

For instance, in this case, the reliability of the difference score is .26, even though the reliability of both indices is .95.

In Figures 3.22 and 3.23, the reliability of a difference score is depicted as a function of (a) the reliability of the indices that compose the difference score and (b) the correlation between them, assuming that both indices have equal variances.

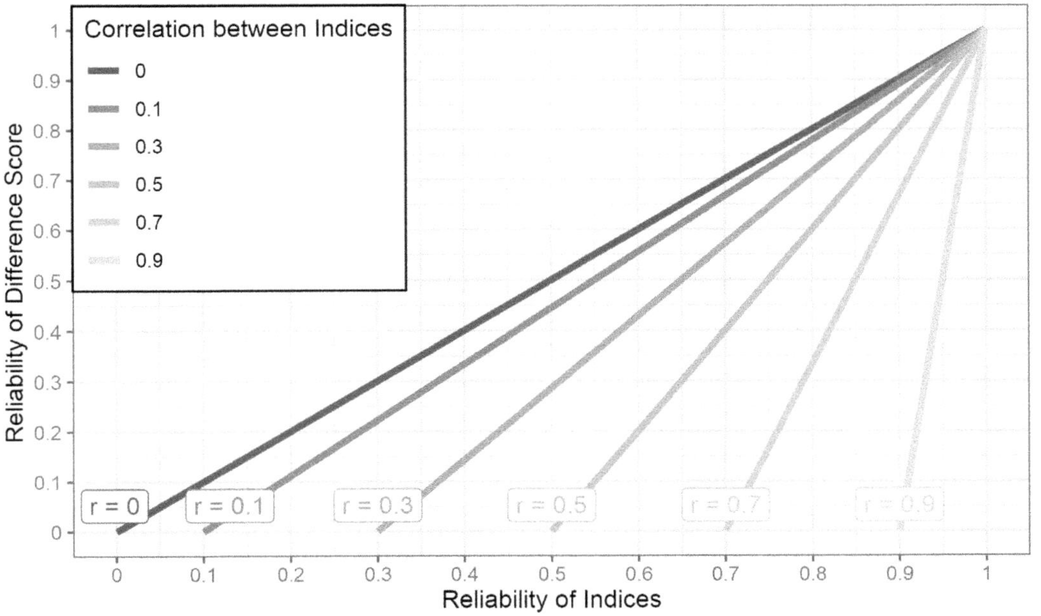

FIGURE 3.22 Reliability of Difference Score as a Function of Reliability of Indices and the Correlation Between Them.

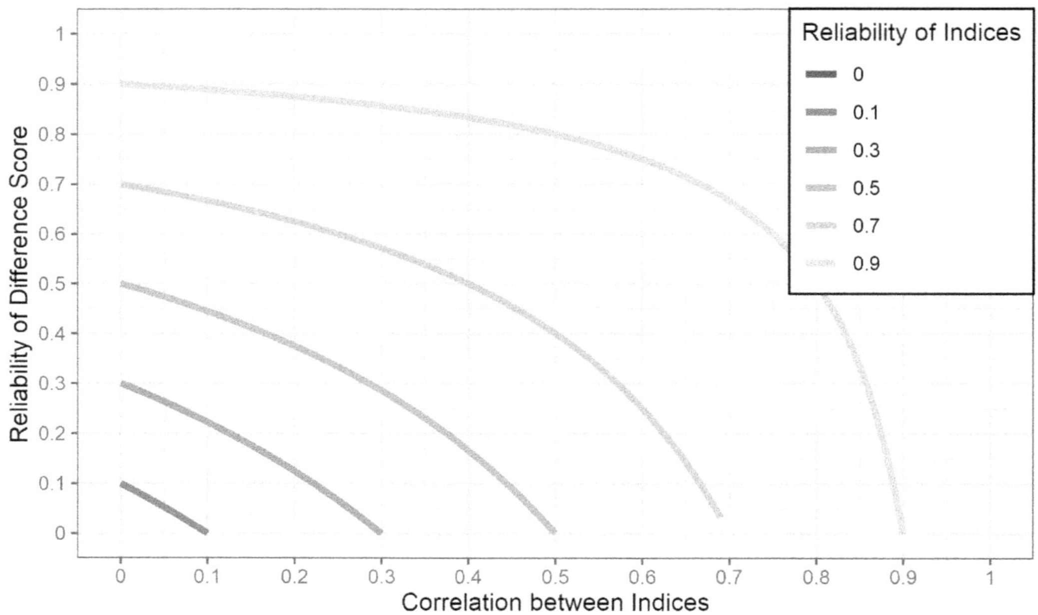

FIGURE 3.23 Reliability of Difference Score as a Function of Correlation Between Indices and Reliability of Indices.

3.6 Applied Examples

Although reliability is an important consideration for measures, stronger reliability is not always better. Reliability is not one thing; it is not monolithic. There are multiple aspects of reliability, and which aspects of reliability are most important depend on the construct of interest. That is, we want different kinds of reliability for measures of different constructs. In general, we want our measures to show strong inter-rater, intra-rater, immediate parallel-forms, and internal consistency reliability. However, we do not want internal consistency reliability to be too high so as to have redundant items that are correlated for reasons of shared method biases. Moreover, for some constructs (i.e., formative constructs such as stressful life events), we would not expect internal consistency reliability. And the extent to which our measures should show test–retest and delayed parallel-forms reliability depends on the stability of the construct and the time lag.

Consider the construct of reactive dysphoria. Assume that we assess people's reactive dysphoria with observations and several questionnaires today and one month from now. However, test–retest reliability is not meaningful because the phenomenon is not meant to be stable across time—it is supposed to be reactive to the situation, not a trait. Instead, we would expect that a strong measure of reactive dysphoria has high internal consistency reliability, a high coefficient of equivalence from immediate parallel-forms reliability, and high inter-/intra-rater reliability.

Consider the example of personality and intelligence. Personality is defined such that personality "traits" are thought to be stable across time and situation. Likewise, individual differences in intelligence are thought to be relatively stable in terms of individual differences across time (not in absolute level). Thus, strong measures of personality and intelligence should show high test–retest reliability, parallel-forms reliability, internal consistency reliability, and inter-/intra-rater reliability.

Just because one aspect of reliability is strong does not necessarily mean that other aspects of reliability will be strong. Measures of some constructs (e.g., depression) could be expected to show low test–retest reliability but high internal consistency reliability. You can also have measures that have low internal consistency reliability but that have high test–retest reliability (e.g., if our nonsensical measure averaged together z-scores of height and blood type).

Consider a questionnaire assessing people's extraversion. We would expect high stability of construct, and therefore a high coefficient of stability, but test and retest scores might not be equal. That is, the measures may show a somewhat lower repeatability coefficient because of random error—on a given day, the participant may be sick, stressed, or tired; they may have recently gotten into an argument; or they may be impacted by the season, the weather, or differences in the context (e.g., lab or online), just to name a few potential sources of random error.

3.7 Standard Error of Measurement

We presented and discussed the formula for estimating the standard error of measurement earlier in Equation (3.11).

The reliability of the measure was estimated here based on the test–retest reliability of the measure at T1 with the measure at T2.

```
reliabilityOfMeasure <- as.numeric(
  cor.test(
    x = mydata$time1,
    y = mydata$time2)$estimate)

sem <- sd(mydata$time1, na.rm = TRUE) * sqrt(1 - reliabilityOfMeasure)
sem
```

```
[1] 2.72
```

We can use the standard error of measurement to estimate the confidence interval around a person's score. A confidence interval indicates a range within which, with some degree of confidence (e.g., 95%), the person's true score is expected to be. For a 95% confidence interval, the true score is expected to fall within ± 1.96 SEMs of the observed score 95% of the time.

```
lower95CI <- mean(mydata$time1, na.rm = TRUE) - qnorm(.975)*sem
upper95CI <- mean(mydata$time1, na.rm = TRUE) + qnorm(.975)*sem

lower95CI
```

```
[1] 45.6
```

```
upper95CI
```

```
[1] 56.27
```

The 95% CI is [45.6, 56.27].

3.8 Influences of Measurement Error on Test–Retest Reliability

This section describes the influence of measurement error on reliability, specifically test–retest reliability. There are different types of measurement error, and each can have different impacts on reliability and, ultimately, your findings. As discussed in Section 3.2, a given error can be either systematic or random. In addition, error can be within-person, between-person, or both. However, error scores can include multiple errors simultaneously.

3.8.1 Add within-person random error

To add within-person random error, we added error that is randomly distributed around a mean of 0 and a standard deviation of 3 to all participants' scores at all time points. Adding within-person random error led to

- a weaker (lower) stability coefficient
- a weaker (higher) repeatability coefficient

3.8.2 Add within-person systematic error

To add within-person systematic error to all participants, we added error that is consistent across time for a given participant: pulled from a distribution with a mean of 5 and a standard deviation of 3. Adding within-person systematic error led to

- an artificially stronger (higher) stability coefficient
- no effect on the repeatability coefficient
- bias at the person level, but this bias would go undetected by the estimate of group-level bias in the Bland-Altman plot

3.8.3 Add between-person random error at T2

To add between-person random error, we added error that is randomly distributed around a mean of 0 and a standard deviation of 3 to all participants' scores at time 2 (see below). Adding between-person random error led to

- a weaker (lower) stability coefficient
- a weaker (higher) repeatability coefficient

3.8.4 Add between-person systematic error at T2

To add between-person systematic error, we added constant variance of 10 to all participants' scores at T2. Adding between-person systematic error led to

- no effect on the stability coefficient

- no effect on the repeatability coefficient
- bias at the person level and at the group level (detected by group-level estimate of bias in Bland-Altman plot)

3.8.5 Add constant variance of 10 to all participants at all time points

Adding constant variance (10) to all participants' scores at all time points led to

- no effect on the stability coefficient
- no effect on the repeatability coefficient
- bias at the person level and at the group level, but this bias would go undetected by the estimate of group-level bias in the Bland-Altman plot

3.8.6 Summary

To summarize the effects of measurement error, random error (both within- and between-person) results in (a) a worse (lower) stability coefficient because a smaller proportion of the observed score variance is attributable to true score variance, and (b) a worse (higher) repeatability coefficient because the standard deviation of the difference between the two measurements is greater. Neither type of random error leads to bias at the person or group level.

In terms of systematic error, all types of systematic error lead to increased bias, i.e., reduced accuracy for the person-level average and/or group-level average. Though multiple biases can coexist and can work in opposite directions, which can obscure bias even though it exists. In terms of within-person systematic error, it (a) artificially increases the stability coefficient, even though the measure is not actually more reliable, (b) has no effect on the repeatability coefficient because it is not changing the difference between the two measurements for a person, and (c) results in bias at the person level because the person's mean systematically differs from their true score.

In terms of between-person systematic error at time 2 (an example of adding constant variance to all participants), it (a) had no effect on the stability coefficient because the rank order of individual differences stays the same, (b) had no effect on the repeatability coefficient because the standard deviation of the difference between the two measurements is not changed, (c) resulted in bias at the person level and at the group level that would be detected in a Bland-Altman plot because the group-level average deviates from the group's average true score.

In sum, just because a measure has high estimates of test–retest reliability does not mean that the measure is actually reliable because systematic error does not reduce the stability and repeatability coefficients. Indeed, within-person systematic error actually (and artificially) *increases* the coefficient of stability. The coefficient of stability index of test–retest reliability is affected by the measure *and* variance across people, and it can be thrown off by outliers or by range restriction because the Pearson correlation strongly depends on these, as discussed in Section 3.5.1.1.1. And sample variation also has a strong influence, so it is important to cross-validate estimates of reliability in independent samples.

3.9 Effect of Measurement Error on Associations

As we describe in greater detail in the chapter on validity in Section 4.6, (random) measurement error weakens (or attenuates) the association between variables. The greater the random measurement error, the weaker the association.

3.9.1 Attenuation of True Test–Retest Reliability Due to Measurement Error

In the context of examining the association between test and retest (i.e., test–retest reliability), the estimate of the stability of the construct (i.e., true test–retest association) is attenuated to the extent that the measure is unreliable, as described in Equation (3.21):

$$
\begin{aligned}
r_{x_1 x_2} &= r_{x_{1_t} x_{2_t}} \sqrt{r_{xx} r_{xx}} \\
&= r_{x_{1_t} x_{2_t}} \sqrt{{r_{xx}}^2} \\
&= r_{x_{1_t} x_{2_t}} r_{xx} \\
\text{test–retest correlation of measure} &= (\text{true correlation of construct across two time points}) \\
&\quad \times (\text{reliability of measure})
\end{aligned}
\tag{3.21}
$$

Find the observed test–retest association if the true test–retest association (i.e., the stability of the construct) is .7 and the reliability of the measure is .9. The `petersenlab` package (Petersen, 2024) contains the `attenuationCorrelation()` function that estimates the observed association given the true association and the reliability of the predictor and criterion. When dealing with test–retest reliability, the predictor and criterion are the same, so we use the same reliability estimate for each:

```
trueAssociation <- 0.7
reliabilityOfMeasure <- 0.9

attenuationCorrelation(
  trueAssociation = trueAssociation,
  reliabilityOfPredictor = reliabilityOfMeasure,
  reliabilityOfCriterion = reliabilityOfMeasure)
```

```
[1] 0.63
```

3.9.2 Disattenuation of Observed Test–Retest Reliability Due to Measurement Error

Then, to disattenuate the observed test–retest reliability due to random measurement error, we can rearrange the terms in the formula above to estimate what the true stability of the construct is, according to Equation (3.22):

$$
\begin{aligned}
r_{x_{1_t} x_{2_t}} &= \frac{r_{x_1 x_2}}{r_{xx}} \\
\text{true correlation of construct across time points} &= \frac{\text{test–retest correlation of measure}}{\text{reliability of measure}}
\end{aligned}
\tag{3.22}
$$

Find the true correlation of the construct across two time points given an observed correlation if the observed reliability of the measure is .9. The `petersenlab` package (Petersen, 2024) contains the `disattenuationCorrelation()` function that estimates the observed association given the true association and the reliability of the predictor and criterion. When dealing with test–retest reliability, the predictor and criterion are the same, so we use the same reliability estimate for each:

```
observedAssociation <- as.numeric(cor.test(
  x = mydata$time2,
  y = mydata$time3)$estimate)

disattenuationCorrelation(
  observedAssociation = observedAssociation,
  reliabilityOfPredictor = reliabilityOfMeasure,
  reliabilityOfCriterion = reliabilityOfMeasure)
```

```
[1] 0.9362
```

The next section discusses method biases, including what they are, why they are important, and how to account for them.

3.10 Method Bias

3.10.1 What Method Biases Are and Why They Are Important

Method bias is the influence of measurement on a person's score that is not due to the person's level on the construct. Method bias is a form of systematic, nonrandom measurement error because it involves errors/biases that are shared/common to/correlated for two measures.

Method bias is problematic because it can bias estimates of a measure's reliability and validity, and its association with other measures/constructs. There is a biasing effect of assessing two or more constructs with the same method on estimates of the association between them—that is, some of the observed covariance may be due to the fact that they share the same method of measurement.

Although estimates vary widely from study to study, construct to construct, and measure to measure, estimates of method bias tend to be substantial. Meta-analyses suggest that around 20–40% of a given measure's variance reflects method variance (for a review, see Podsakoff et al., 2012). According to Podsakoff et al. (2012), response styles inflate the magnitude of observed correlations by 54% if there is a positive correlation between the constructs and a positive correlation between the response styles. Response styles inflate the magnitude of observed correlations by even more (67%) if there is a negative correlation between the constructs and a negative correlation between the response styles. Moreover, the method biases can also weaken the association between measures. If the direction of correlation between the constructs (e.g., positive) is incongruent with the direction of the correlation between the response styles (e.g., negative), the association between the measures is attenuated.

3.10.2 Types of Method Biases

There are many different types of method biases, including the effects of

- same source: Whether ratings or information comes from the same source can lead to systematic method variance.
- response styles (response biases): Response styles are systematic ways of responding to items or questions that are not due to the construct of interest. Different types of response styles can lead to systematic method variance across constructs. Examples of response styles include
  - acquiescence: the tendency to agree with items (both positively and negatively worded), regardless of content
  - disacquiescence: the tendency to disagree with items (both positively and negatively worded), regardless of content
  - extreme: the tendency to endorse items on the extremes (positive or negative) of the response scale, regardless of content
  - midpoint/central tendency: the tendency to endorse items on the middle scale category, regardless of content
  - noncontingent: the tendency to respond to items carelessly, randomly, or nonpurposefully
  - social desirability: the tendency to respond to items in a way that others will believe the respondent is better than they actually are. Social desirability includes multiple components, including self-deception and impression management. Impression management is the conscious effort to control the way people view oneself or the way one presents oneself.
- proximity: Items (of unrelated constructs) that are in closer proximity to one another in a measure are more likely to be correlated than items that are further apart. The associations of items assessing unrelated constructs are weakest when the pair of items are six or more items apart from each other. There is an exception for reversed items. For reversed items (e.g., reverse scored), the further apart the reversed item is placed from another item, the higher the negative correlation.
- item wording: Whether items are positively or negatively worded can influence the association between items (i.e., like-worded items go with like).
- item context: Manipulating the context of a measure can have an effect on the perceived association. You can observe a different association between constructs when you put the measure in a negative context versus in a positive context.
- item ambiguity: When respondents are less certain of how to accurately answer a question, it increases the likelihood that they will rely on response styles or succumb to the effect of context when responding, which biases scores.
- motivational factors: Researchers need to motivate participants to put in the cognitive effort to answer questions correctly, to decrease the likelihood that they will succumb to responding based on response style only. Also, researchers should decrease pressures for "optimal responding" on respondents. That is, researchers should attempt to reduce social desirability effects.
- the ability of the respondent: Respondents with low cognitive abilities, less education, more fatigue (after lots of questionnaires), less experience with the topic being assessed, and more uncertainty about how to respond are more likely to succumb to biasing factors.

3.10.3 Potential Remedies

There are numerous potential remedies to help reduce the effects of method bias, including

- obtain measures of the predictor and criterion from multiple or different sources
- create temporal, physical, and/or psychological separation between the predictor and criterion
- eliminate common scale properties; vary the scale types and anchor labels
- remove ambiguity in items—keep questions simple, (behaviorally) specific, and concise
- reduce social desirability in item wording
- provide anonymity to respondents
- for estimating the prevalence of a sensitive behavior, use the randomized response model (S. J. Clark & Desharnais, 1998), as described below
- provide incentives (e.g., compensation) to respondents
- reverse score some items to balance positively and negatively worded (i.e., reverse-scored) items
- separate items on the questionnaire to eliminate proximity effects
- maximize respondent motivation to give an accurate response
- develop a good cover story and clear instructions, with reminders as necessary
- match the measure difficulty to the respondent's ability; minimize frustration
- use confirmatory factor analysis or structural equation modeling, as described in Section 7.10.1
- use mixed models, as described below

3.10.3.1 Randomized Response Model

The randomized response model (S. J. Clark & Desharnais, 1998) is a technique to increase people's honesty in responding, especially around sensitive topics. The randomized response model sought to answer the question of how much information people withhold on surveys. It is no surprise that people lie on surveys, especially if the survey asks questions about sensitive topics, such as suicidality, criminal behavior (e.g., drug use), and child abuse or neglect. The randomized response model is based on the premise that respondents would give more honest answers if they could be certain that their survey answers would not reveal any sensitive information about themselves, and it is designed to reduce evasive-answer bias by guaranteeing privacy.

The randomized response model works by exploiting statistical probabilities. Consider a survey that asks respondents whether they have used various illegal drugs (e.g., "Have you used heroin?" or "Have you used cocaine?"). Each participant is given a coin. They are told to flip the coin before they answer each question. If the coin flip is "heads," they answer the question truthfully. If the coin flip is "tails," they answer the questions with a "yes" (i.e., the more sensitive answer) no matter what. That way, a yes could be due to the coin flip or could be the truth—so respondents feel as if they are divulging less.

Then, researchers can estimate the actual "no" rate by doubling the observed "no" rate for the sample. For instance, if 20% of people say they have never gambled and 80% say they have gambled, the actual "no" rate of gambling is 40%. That is, the actual gambling rate is 60%.

Findings using the randomized response model indicate that there are a lot of things that people are not sharing. The randomized response model is useful for estimating the true prevalence rate of sensitive behaviors. However, it is not great for individual differences research because you do not know whether any given individual truly engages in a behavior (because a "yes" response may have occurred merely because the coin flip was "heads").

Thus, the randomized response model is only helpful for knowing "true" overall rate of a given behavior in the sample.

3.10.3.2 Mixed Models

One approach to handle method biases is in mixed models, which are also called mixed-effects models, multilevel models, and hierarchical linear models (HLMs). Mixed models are similar to multiple regression in that they allow fitting a model that examines multiple predictor variables in relation to one outcome variable. One of the assumptions of multiple regression is that the data observations are independent from each other, as evidenced by the residuals being uncorrelated with each other. Mixed models are designed to handle nonindependent observations, that is, data that were collected from nonindependent units. Thus, mixed models can be fit to data that do not meet the nonindependence assumption of multiple regression.

Examples of data from nonindependent units include nested data, multiple membership data, and cross-classified data.

One example of nonindependent data is if your data are *nested*. When data are collected from multiple lower-level units (e.g., people) in an upper-level unit (e.g., married couple, family, classroom, school, neighborhood), the data from the lower-level units are considered nested within the upper-level unit. For example, multiple participants in your sample may come from the same classroom. Data from multiple people can be nested within the same family, classroom, school, etc. Longitudinal data can also be considered nested data, in which time points are nested within the participant (i.e., the same participant provides an observation across multiple time points). And if you have multiple informants of a child's behavior (e.g., parent-, teacher-, friend-, and self-report), the ratings could also be nested within the participant (i.e., there are ratings from multiple informants of the same child).

Another form of nonindependent data is when data involve *multiple membership*. Data involve multiple membership when the lower-level units belong to more than one upper-level unit simultaneously. As an example of multiple membership, children may have more than one teacher, and therefore, in a modeling sense, children "belong" to more than one teacher cluster.

Another form of nonindependent data is when data are *cross-classified* (also called crossed). Data are cross-classified when the lower-level units are classified by two or more upper-level units, but the upper-level units are not hierarchical or nested within one another. For instance, children may be nested within the crossing of schools and neighborhoods. That is, children are nested within schools, and children are also nested within neighborhoods; however, children attending the same school may not necessarily be from the same neighborhood. The data would still have a two-level hierarchy, but the data would be nested in specific school-neighborhood combinations. That is, children are nested within the cross-classification of schools and neighborhoods.

The general form of multiple regression is (see Equation (3.23)):

$$y = b_0 + b_1x + e \tag{3.23}$$

where b_0 is the intercept, e is the error term, and b_1 is the slope of the predictor, x, that states the relation between the predictor (x) and the outcome (y). However, the slope can exist at multiple levels when data are nested within groups or when time points are nested within people. For example, you can observe different associations of a predictor with an outcome at the between-individual level compared to the within-individual level. That is, the association between the predictor and outcome can differ when comparing across individuals versus when looking at the association between the predictor and outcome based on fluctuations within the individual. When the associations differ at multiple levels, this is known as *Simpson's paradox*. For an example of Simpson's paradox, see Figure 3.24 (R. Kievit et al., 2013). Thus, it is important to consider that the association between variables may differ at different levels (person level, group level, population level, etc.).

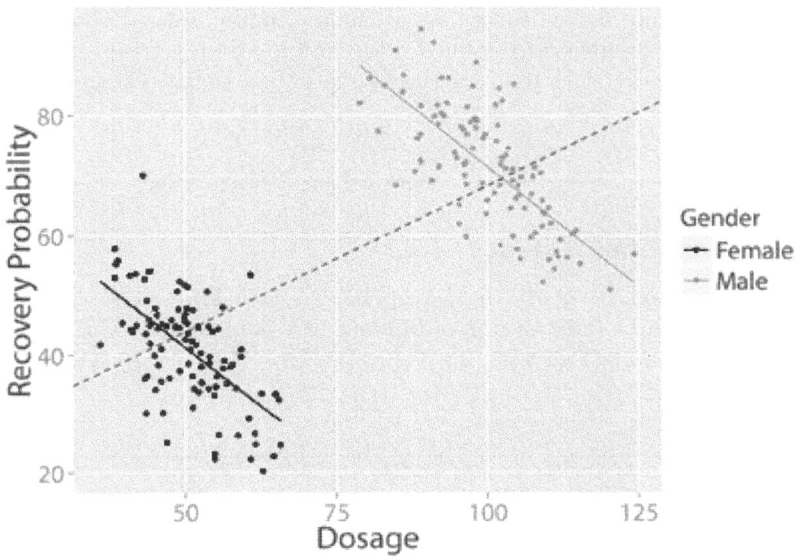

FIGURE 3.24 Example of Simpson's paradox, where the association between the predictor and outcome differs at different levels. In this case, the association between dosage and recovery probability is positive at the population-level (upper-level unit), but the association is negative among men and women separately (lower-level unit). (Figure reprinted from R. Kievit et al. (2013), figure 1, p. 2. Kievit, R., Frankenhuis, W., Waldorp, L., & Borsboom, D. (2013). Simpson's paradox in psychological science: a practical guide. *Frontiers in Psychology*, *4*(513). https://doi.org/10.3389/fpsyg.2013.00513)

To account for method biases in a mixed model, you could use scores from multiple measures and methods as the outcome variable. For instance, your mixed model could examine the association between income and optimism, where optimism is assessed by self-report, parent-report, and a performance-based measure. In the model, you could include, as a *fixed effect*, a factor that indicates the method of the measure, in addition to its interaction with income, to account for systematic ways in which the measurement method influences scores on the measures across the participants as a whole. You could also include a *random effect* of measurement method if you wanted to allow the effect of measurement method on the scores to differ from person to person.

3.11 Generalizability Theory

Up to this point, we have discussed reliability from the perspective of CTT. However, as we discussed, CTT makes several assumptions that are unrealistic (e.g., that all error is random). There are other measurement theories that conceptualize reliability differently than the way that CTT conceptualizes reliability. One such measurement theory is generalizability theory (Brennan, 1992), also known as G-theory and domain sampling theory. G-theory is described in detail in Chapter 5 on generalizability theory and is also discussed in the chapters on validity (Chapter 4, Section 4.7) and structural equation modeling (Chapter 7, Section 7.11).

3.12 Item Response Theory

In addition to CTT and G-theory, item response theory (IRT) is another measurement theory. IRT also estimates reliability in a different way compared to CTT, as described in Section 8.1.6. We discuss IRT in Chapter 8.

3.13 The Problem of Low Reliability

Using measures that have low reliability can lead to several problems, including

- over- or underestimation of the effects of interest. When sample sizes are large, measurement error tends to weaken effect sizes. However, when sample sizes are small to modest, measurement error can actually lead to overestimation of effect sizes as well as inaccurate estimates of the sign of the effect (positive or negative), due to the statistical significance filter (Loken & Gelman, 2017), as described in the section on "Assessment and the Replication Crisis" in the Introduction.
- reduced statistical power to detect the effects of interest
- failure to replicate findings
- invalid measurement for the proposed uses. As we described in the chapter on validity in Section 4.5, reliability constrains validity.

These concerns are especially important for individual differences research (e.g., correlational designs) or when making decisions about individual people based on their scores on measure. However, these concerns are also relevant for experimental designs.

3.14 Ways to Increase Reliability

Here are several potential ways to increase reliability of measurement:

1. Improve the clarity and homogeneity of items.
2. Use a structured response set and scoring system rather than unstructured ones.

3. Make sure participants know how to complete the task or items. For example, make sure they have appropriate instructions that are easily understood.
4. Adhere closely to the standardized procedures for administering and scoring a measure.
5. Make scoring rules as explicit as possible.
6. Train raters to some criterion of inter-rater reliability. Continue to monitor inter-rater reliability over time to reduce coder drift.
7. Use a more precise response scale. The smaller the number of response options, the greater the attenuation of a correlation due to measurement error (Rigdon, 2010).
8. Have a sample with a full range of variation in the items and measure.
9. If possible, do not use a difference score. This is discussed in greater detail in Section 3.5.8 and in Chapter 23 (Section 23.3.4.3.1) on cognitive assessment.
10. Remove items that reduce reliability. This may include items that have low variability because they are too easy or too difficult (i.e., items that show ceiling or floor effects), in addition to items that have a low item–total correlation.
11. Collect more information across people and time.
12. Aggregate: Add items, measures, observers, raters, and time points.
    a. Having more items that assess the same construct in the measure tends to increase reliability unless the additional items cause fatigue because the instrument is too long. Aggregation of like things reduces measurement error, because averaging together more items helps cancel out random error.
    b. Having multiple measures that assess the same construct can be beneficial, especially measures from different methods that do not share the same systematic errors (e.g., observation in addition to parent report).
    c. Items that aggregate a large amount of information tend to have strong predictive validity. In general, for predictive accuracy, it is often better to assess more things less well than to assess one thing extraordinarily well. Aggregation is a double-edged sword: It is your friend as a researcher, because of increased predictive utility, but it is your enemy as an interpreter because it is hard to interpret the theoretical meaning of predictive associations based on an aggregated variable because the measure is more general and nonspecific. If aggregation increases error, test–retest reliability will decrease. If error stays the same when aggregating, test–retest reliability will increase.
13. Use a latent variable approach to aggregate the multiple items, measures, observers, raters, or time points. Latent variable approaches include structural equation modeling and item response theory. Estimating a latent variable allows identifying the variance that is common to all of the measures (i.e., a better approximate of true score variance), and it discards variance that is not shared by all measures (i.e., error variance). Thus, latent variables have the potential to get purer estimates of the constructs by reducing measurement error.

3.15 Conclusion

Reliability is how much repeatability, consistency, and precision a measure's scores have. Reliability is not one thing. There are multiple aspects of reliability, and the extent to which a given aspect of reliability is important depends on the construct of interest. In general, we want our measures to show strong inter-rater, intra-rater, immediate parallel-forms, and internal consistency reliability. However, the extent to which our measures should show test–retest and delayed parallel-forms reliability depends on the stability of the construct and the time lag. Moreover, although we want our measures to show strong internal consistency reliability, the internal consistency reliability of a measure can be *too* high, and for some constructs (i.e., formative constructs), internal consistency would not be expected. In addition, reliability is not a characteristic that resides in a test. The reliability of a measure's scores reflects an interaction of the properties of the test with the population for whom it is designed and the sample, situation, and context in which it is administered. Thus, when reporting reliability in papers, it is important to adequately describe the aspects of reliability that have been considered and the population, sample, and context in which the measure is assessed. However, it is not enough for measures to be consistent or reliable; our interpretation of the measures' scores should also be accurate, meaningful, and useful for the intended uses. In other words, our interpretation of the measures' scores should be valid for the intended uses. In the next chapter (Chapter 4), we discuss validity of measurement.

3.16 Suggested Readings

For more information on inter-rater reliability, we suggest reading Gwet (2021a) and Gwet (2021b), for categorical and continuous ratings, respectively.

4

Validity

What we know depends on how we know it. – Anonymous

4.1 Overview

According to the *Standards for Educational and Psychological Testing* (American Educational Research Association et al., 2014, p. 11), measurement validity is "the degree to which evidence and theory support the interpretations of test scores for proposed uses of tests." We summarized reliability with three words: repeatability, consistency, and precision. A summary of validity in three words is accuracy, utility, and meaningfulness. Validity is tied to the *interpretation* of a measure's scores for the *proposed uses*, not (just) to the measure itself. The same set of scores can have different degrees of validity for different purposes. For instance, a measure's scores may have stronger validity for making a diagnostic decision than for making a prediction about future behavior. Thus, as *the Standards* indicate, it is incorrect to use the unqualified phrase "the validity of the measure" or "the measure is (in)valid," because these phrases do not specify which scores were used from the test, what the use is (e.g., predicting whether a person will succeed in a given job), and what interpretation was made of the test scores for this purpose.[1]

Below, we prepare the data to provide some validity-related examples throughout the rest of the chapter.

4.2 Getting Started

4.2.1 Load Libraries

```
library("petersenlab")
library("lavaan")
```

[1]For shorthand and to avoid repetition, we sometimes refer to the validity of the measure, but in such instances, we are actually referring to the validity of the interpretation of a measure's scores for a given use.

```
library("semPlot")
library("rockchalk")
library("semTools")
library("semPlot")
library("MASS")
library("psych")
library("simstandard")
library("DT")
library("MOTE")
library("here")
library("tidyverse")
library("tinytex")
library("knitr")
library("kableExtra")
library("rmarkdown")
library("bookdown")
```

4.2.2 Prepare Data

4.2.2.1 Simulate Data

```
sampleSize <- 1000

set.seed(52242)

means <- c(50, 100)
standardDeviations <- c(10, 15)

correlationMatrix <- matrix(.7, nrow = 2, ncol = 2)
diag(correlationMatrix) <- 1
rownames(correlationMatrix) <- colnames(correlationMatrix) <-
  c("predictor","criterion")

covarianceMatrix <- psych::cor2cov(
  correlationMatrix,
  sigma = standardDeviations)

mydataValidity <- as.data.frame(mvrnorm(
  n = sampleSize,
  mu = means,
  Sigma = covarianceMatrix,
  empirical = TRUE))

errorToAddToPredictor <- 3.20
errorToAddToCriterion <- 6.15

mydataValidity$predictorWithMeasurementErrorT1 <-
  mydataValidity$predictor +
```

```
  rnorm(n = sampleSize, mean = 0, sd = errorToAddToPredictor)

mydataValidity$predictorWithMeasurementErrorT2 <-
  mydataValidity$predictor +
  rnorm(n = sampleSize, mean = 0, sd = errorToAddToPredictor)

mydataValidity$criterionWithMeasurementErrorT1 <-
  mydataValidity$criterion +
  rnorm(n = sampleSize, mean = 0, sd = errorToAddToCriterion)

mydataValidity$criterionWithMeasurementErrorT2 <-
  mydataValidity$criterion +
  rnorm(n = sampleSize, mean = 0, sd = errorToAddToCriterion)

mydataValidity$oldpredictor <- mydataValidity$criterion +
  rnorm(n = sampleSize, mean = 0, sd = 7.5)

latentCorrelation <- .8
reliabilityPredictor <- .9
reliabilityCriterion <- .85

mydataValidity$predictorLatentSEM <- rnorm(sampleSize, 0 , 1)

mydataValidity$criterionLatentSEM <- latentCorrelation *
  mydataValidity$predictorLatentSEM + rnorm(
    sampleSize,
    0,
    sqrt(1 - latentCorrelation ^ 2))

mydataValidity$predictorObservedSEM <- reliabilityPredictor *
  mydataValidity$predictorLatentSEM + rnorm(
    sampleSize,
    0,
    sqrt(1 - reliabilityPredictor ^ 2))

mydataValidity$criterionObservedSEM <- reliabilityCriterion *
  mydataValidity$criterionLatentSEM + rnorm(
    sampleSize,
    0,
    sqrt(1 - reliabilityCriterion ^ 2))
```

4.2.2.2 Add Missing Data

Adding missing data to dataframes helps make examples more realistic to real-life data and helps you get in the habit of programming to account for missing data.

```
missingValuesPredictor <- sample(
  1:sampleSize,
  size = 50,
```

```
  replace = FALSE)
missingValuesCriterion <- sample(
  1:sampleSize,
  size = 50,
  replace = FALSE)

mydataValidity$predictor[
  missingValuesPredictor] <- NA
mydataValidity$predictorWithMeasurementErrorT1[
  missingValuesPredictor] <- NA
mydataValidity$predictorWithMeasurementErrorT2[
  missingValuesPredictor] <- NA
mydataValidity$predictorObservedSEM[
  missingValuesPredictor] <- NA

mydataValidity$criterion[
  missingValuesCriterion] <- NA
mydataValidity$criterionWithMeasurementErrorT1[
  missingValuesCriterion] <- NA
mydataValidity$criterionWithMeasurementErrorT2[
  missingValuesCriterion] <- NA
mydataValidity$criterionObservedSEM[
  missingValuesCriterion] <- NA

mydataValidity$oldpredictor[
  missingValuesPredictor] <- NA
```

4.3 Types of Validity

Like reliability, validity is not one thing. There are many types of validity. In this book, we discuss the following types of validity:

- face validity
- content validity
- criterion-related validity
- concurrent validity
- predictive validity
- construct validity
- convergent validity
- discriminant (divergent) validity
- incremental validity
- treatment utility of assessment
- discriminative validity
- elaborative validity
- consequential validity
- representational validity
- factorial (structural) validity

- ecological validity
- process-focused validity
- diagnostic validity
- social validity
- cultural validity
- internal validity
- external validity
- (statistical) conclusion validity

We arrange these types of validity into two broader categories: measurement validity and research design validity.

4.3.1 Measurement Validity

Aspects of *measurement validity* involve the validity of a particular measure, or more specifically, the validity of interpretations of scores from that measure for the proposed uses. Aspects of measurement validity include:

- face validity
- content validity
- criterion-related validity
- concurrent validity
- predictive validity
- construct validity
- convergent validity
- discriminant (divergent) validity
- incremental validity
- treatment utility of assessment
- discriminative validity
- elaborative validity
- consequential validity
- representational validity
- factorial (structural) validity
- ecological validity
- process-focused validity
- diagnostic validity
- social validity
- cultural validity

4.3.1.1 Face Validity

The interpretation of a measure's scores has *face validity* (for a given construct and a given use) if a typical person—a nonexpert—who looks at the content of each item will believe that the item belongs in the scale for this construct and for this use. The measure, and each item, looks "on its face" like it assesses the target construct. There are several advantages of a measure having face validity. First, outside groups will be less likely to be critical of the measure because it is intuitive. Second, use of a face valid measure is rarely objected to on ethical and bias charges for selling the measure to the public or clinicians. Third, face validity can be helpful for dissemination because more people may be receptive to it.

However, face validity also has important disadvantages. First, judgments of face validity are not based on theory. Second, face validity is based on subjective judgment, which can be inaccurate. Third, these subjective judgments are made by laypeople whose judgments may be inaccurate because of biases and lack of awareness of scientific knowledge. Fourth, a face valid measure may be too simple because anybody can understand the questions and what the questions are intended to assess, so (presumably) respondents can easily fake responses to achieve their goals. Faking of responses may be more of a concern in situations when there is an incentive for the respondent to achieve a particular outcome (e.g., be deemed competent to stand trial, be judged competent to obtain a job or custody of child, be judged to have a disorder to receive accommodations or disability benefits).

It is disputed whether having face validity is good or bad. Whether face validity is important to a given measure depends on the construct that is intended to be assessed, the context in which the assessment will occur, who will be paying for and/or administering the assessment, whether the respondents have incentives to achieve particular scores, and the goals of the assessment (i.e., how the assessment will be used). There is also controversy about whether face validity is a true form of validity; many researchers have argued that it is not a true psychometric form of validity, because the *appearance* of validity is not validity (Royal, 2016).

4.3.1.2 Content Validity

Content validity involves a judgment about whether or not the content (items) of the measure theoretically matches the construct that is intended to be assessed—that is, whether the operationalization accurately reflects the construct. Content validity is developed based on items generated and selected by experts of the construct and based on the subjective determination that the measure adequately assesses and covers the construct of interest. Content validity differs from face validity in that, for face validity, a *layperson* determines whether or not the measure seems to assess the construct of interest. By contrast, for content validity, an *expert* determines whether or not the measure adheres to the construct of interest.

For a measure to have content validity, its items should span the breadth of the construct. For instance, the construct of depression has many facets, such as sleep disturbances, weight/appetite changes, low mood, suicidality, etc., as depicted in Figure 4.1.

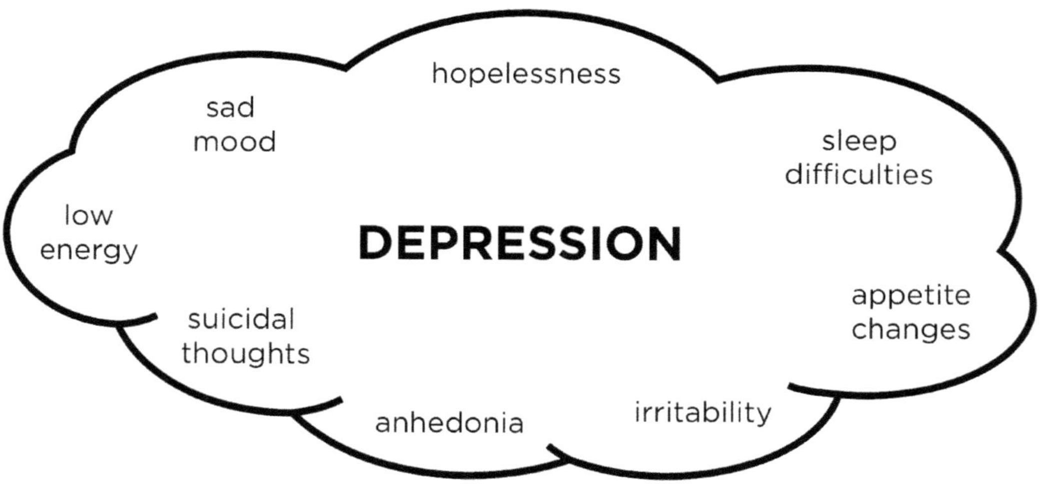

FIGURE 4.1 Content Facets of the Construct of Depression.

For a measure to have content validity, there should be no *gaps*—facets of the construct that are not assessed by the measure—and there should be no *intrusions*—facets of different constructs that are assessed by the measure. Consider the construct of depression. If theory states the construct includes various facets such as sadness, loss of interest in activities, sleep disturbances, lack of energy, weight/appetite change, and suicidal thoughts, then a content-valid measure should assess all of these facets. If the measure does not assess sleep disturbances (a gap), the measure would lack content validity. If the measure assessed facets of other constructs, such as impulsivity (an intrusion), the measure would lack content validity.

With content validity, it is important to consider the population of interest. The same construct may look different in different populations and may require different content to assess it. For instance, it is important to consider the cultural relativity of constructs. The content of a construct may depend on the culture, such as in the case of culture-bound syndromes. Culture-bound syndromes are syndromes that are limited to particular cultures. An example of a culture-bound syndrome among Korean women is *hwa-byung*, which is the feeling of an uncomfortable abdominal mass in response to emotional distress. Another important dimension to consider is development. Constructs can manifest differently at different points in development, known as heterotypic continuity, which is discussed in Section 22.8 of Chapter 22 on repeated assessments across time. When considering the different dimensions of your population, it can be helpful to remember the acronym *ADDRESSING*, which is described in Section 24.2.1 of Chapter 24 on cultural and individual diversity.

However, like face validity, content validity is based on subjective judgment, which can be inaccurate.

4.3.1.3 Criterion-Related Validity

Criterion-related validity examines whether a measure behaves the way it should given your theory of the construct. This is quantified by the correlation between a measure's scores and some (hopefully universally accepted) criterion we select. For instance, a criterion could be a diagnosis, a child's achievement in school, an employee's performance in a job, etc.

Below, we provide an example of criterion-related validity by examining the Pearson correlation between a predictor and a criterion.

```
cor.test(x = mydataValidity$predictor, y = mydataValidity$criterion)
```

```

	Pearson's product-moment correlation

data:  mydataValidity$predictor and mydataValidity$criterion
t = 30, df = 900, p-value <2e-16
alternative hypothesis: true correlation is not equal to 0
95 percent confidence interval:
 0.6738 0.7391
sample estimates:
   cor 
0.7079 
```

In this case, the estimate of criterion-related validity is $r = .71$. There are two types of criterion-related validity: concurrent validity and predictive validity.

4.3.1.3.1 Concurrent validity

Concurrent validity considers the *concurrent* association between the chosen measure and the criterion. That is, both the measure and the criterion are assessed at the same point in time. An example of concurrent validity would be examining self-report of court involvement in relation to current court records.

4.3.1.3.2 Predictive validity

Predictive validity considers the association between the chosen measure and the criterion at a *later* time point. An example of predictive validity would be examining the predictive association between children's scores on an academic achievement test in first grade and their eventual academic outcomes years later.

4.3.1.3.3 Empiricism and theory

Criterion-related validity arose out of a movement known as *radical operationalism.* Radical operationalism was a pushback against psychoanalysis. Psychoanalysis focused on grand theoretical accounts for how constructs relate. The goal of radical operationalism was to clarify concepts from a behavioristic perspective to allow predicting and changing behavior more successfully. An "operation" in radical operationalism refers to a fully described measurement.

Proponents of radical operationalism argued that all constructs in psychology that could not be operationally defined should be excluded from the field as "nonscientific." They asserted that operations should be well-defined enough to be able to replicate the findings. So, constructs had to be defined precisely according to this perspective, but how precisely? You could go on forever trying to more precisely describe a behavior in terms of its form, frequency, duration, intensity, situation, antecedents, consequences, biological substrates, etc. So, radical operationalists asserted that we should use theory of the construct to determine what is essential and what is not.

Radical operationalism was also related to *radical behavioralism*, which was espoused by B.F. Skinner. Skinner famously used a box (the "Skinner Box") to more directly control, describe, and assess behaviors. Skinner noted the major role that the environment played in influencing behavior. Skinner proposed a theory of implicit learning about a behavior or stimulus based on its consequences, known as operant conditioning. According to operant conditioning, something that increases the frequency of a given behavior is called a reinforcer (e.g., praise), and something that decreases the frequency of a behavior is called a punisher (e.g., loss of a privilege). Through this work, Skinner came to view everything an organism does (e.g., action, thought, feeling) as a behavior.

Related to these historical perspectives was a perspective known as *dustbowl empiricism.* Dustbowl empiricism focused on the empirical connections between things—how things were associated using data. It was a completely atheoretical perspective in which interpretation was entirely data driven. An example of dustbowl empiricism is the approach that was used to develop the first version of the Minnesota Multiphasic Personality Inventory (MMPI). The MMPI was developed using an approach known as empirical-criterion keying, where items were selected for the scale for no reason other than the items demonstrate an association with the criterion. That is, an item was selected if it showed a strong ability to discriminate (differentiate) between clinical and control groups. Using this method with hundreds of items (and thousands of inter-item correlations), the MMPI developed 10 clinical scales, which involved operational rules based on previously collected empirical evidence.

But what do you know with this abundance of correlations? You can use data reduction methods to reduce the many variables, based on their inter-correlations, down to a more parsimonious set of factors. But how do you name each factor, which is composed of many items? The developers originally numbered the MMPI clinical scales from 1 to 10. But numbered scales are not useful for other people, so the factors were eventually given labels (e.g., Paranoia). And if a client received an elevated score on a factor, many people would label the clients as ________ [the name of the factor], such as "paranoid." The MMPI is discussed in further detail in Chapter 17 on objective personality testing.

The idea of dustbowl empiricism was to develop a strong empirical base that would provide a strong foundation to help build up to a broad understanding that was integrated, coherent, and systematic. However, this process was unclear when there was only a table of correlations. Radical operationalists were opposed to content validity because it allows intrusion of our flawed thinking. According to operationalists, there are no experts. According to this perspective, the content does not matter; we just need enough data to bootstrap ourselves to a better understanding of the constructs.

Although the atheoretical approach can perform reasonably well, it can be improved by making better use of theory. An empirical result (e.g., a correlation) might not necessarily have a lot of meaning associated with it. As the maxim goes, correlation does not imply causation.

4.3.1.3.3.1 Correlation does not imply causation

Just because X is associated with Y does not mean that X causes Y. Consider that you find an association between variables X and Y, consistent with your hypothesis, as depicted in Figure 4.2.

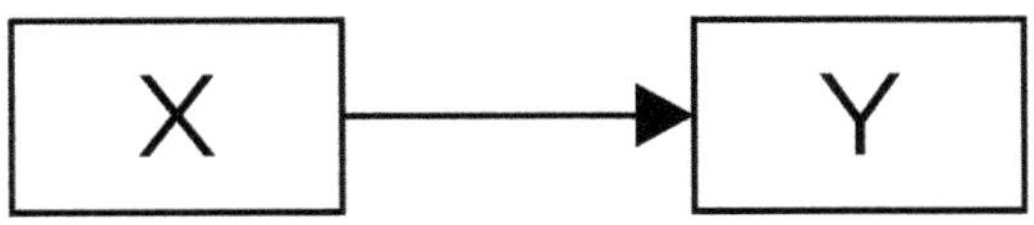

FIGURE 4.2 Hypothesized Causal Effect Based on an Observed Association Between X and Y, Such That X Causes Y.

There are three primary reasons that an observed association between X and Y does not necessarily mean that X causes Y. First, the association could reflect the opposite direction of effect, where Y actually causes X, as depicted in Figure 4.3.

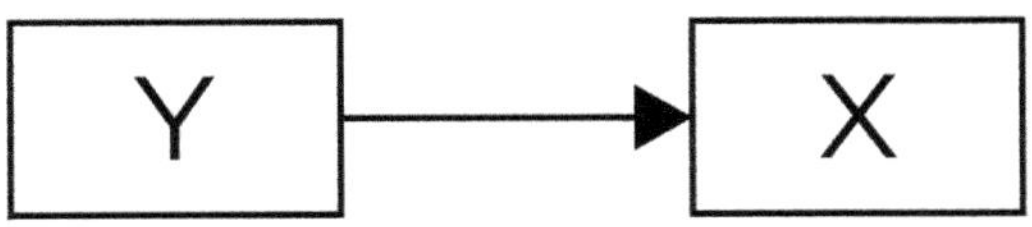

FIGURE 4.3 Reverse (Opposite) Direction of Effect from the Hypothesized Effect, Where Y Causes X.

Second, the association could reflect the influence of a third variable. If a third variable is a common cause of each and accounts for their association, it is a *confound.* An observed association between X and Y could reflect a confound—i.e., a cause (Z) that influences both X and Y, which explains why X and Y are correlated even though they are not causally related. A third variable confound that is a common cause of both X and Y is depicted in Figure 4.4.

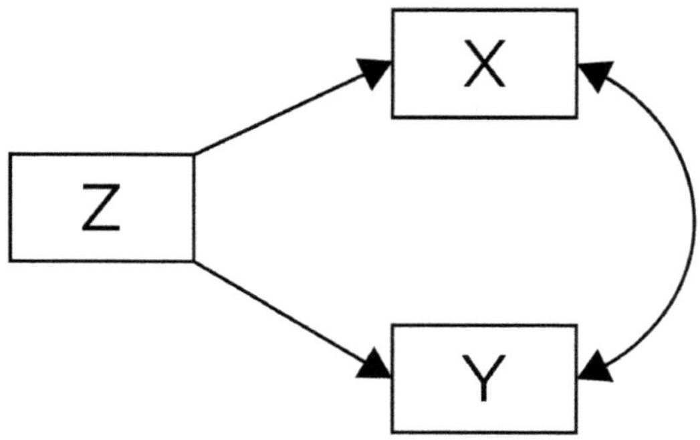

FIGURE 4.4 Confounded Association Between X and Y due to a Common Cause, Z.

Third, the association might be spurious. It might just reflect random variation (i.e., chance), and that when tested on an independent sample, what appeared as an association may not hold when testing whether the association generalizes.

However, even if the association between X and Y reflects a causal effect and that X causes Y, it does not necessarily mean that the effect is clinically actionable or useful. An association may reflect a static or unmodifiable predictor that is not practically useful as a treatment target.

4.3.1.3.3.2 Understanding the causal system

As Silver (2012) notes, "The numbers have no way of speaking for themselves. We speak for them. We imbue them with meaning" (p. 9). If we *understand* the variables in the system and how they influence each other, we can predict things more accurately than predicting for the sake of predicting. For instance, we have made great strides in the last decades when it comes to more accurate weather forecasts, including extreme weather events like hurricanes. These great strides have more to do with a better causal understanding of the weather system and the ability to conduct simulations of the atmosphere than merely because of big data (Silver, 2012). By contrast, other events are still incredibly difficult to predict, including earthquakes, in large part because we do not have a strong understanding of the system (and because we do not have ways of precisely measuring those causes because they occur at a depth below which we are realistically able to drill) (Silver, 2012).

4.3.1.3.3.3 Model over-fitting

Statistical models applied to big data (i.e., lots of variables and lots of samples) can *over-fit* the data, which means that the statistical model accounts for error variance (an overly specific prediction), which will not generalize to future samples. So, even though an over-fitting statistical model appears to be accurate, it is not actually that accurate—it will predict new data less accurately than how accurately it accounts for the data with which the model was built.

In Figure 4.5, the black line represents the true distribution of the data, and the gray line is an over-fitting model.

4.3.1.3.3.4 Criterion contamination

An important issue in predictive validity is the criterion problem—finding the right criterion. It is important to avoid *criterion contamination*, which is artificial commonality between

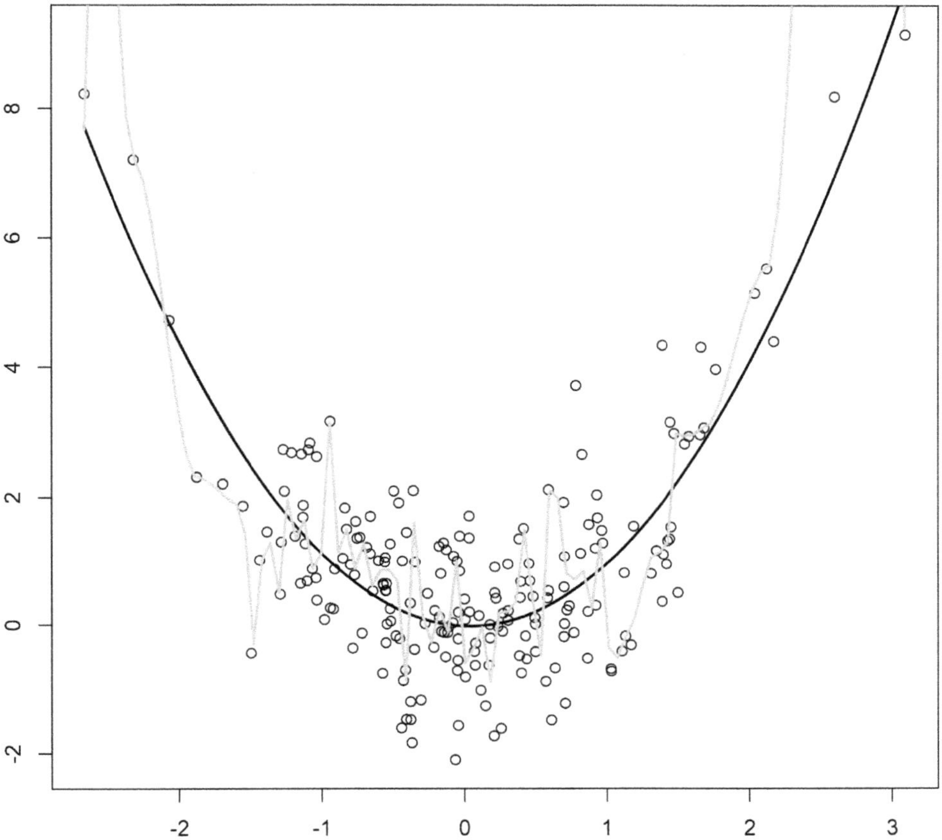

FIGURE 4.5 Over-fitting Model in Gray Relative to the True Distribution of the Data in Black.

the measure and the criterion. The criterion is not always a well-measured clear criterion to predict (like predicting death in the medical field). And you may not have access to a predictive criterion until a long time from now. So, what researchers often do is adopt intermediate assessments, which are not actually what they are interested in, but it is related to the criterion of interest, and it is in a window of time that allows for some meaningful prediction. For instance, intermediate graduate school markers of whether a graduate student will go on to have a successful career could include their grades in graduate school, whether they completed the dissertation, their performance in comprehensive/qualifying exams, etc. However, these intermediate assessments do not always indicate whether or not a student will go on to have a successful career (i.e., they are not always correlated with the real criterion of interest).

4.3.1.3.3.5 Using theory as a guide

So, empiricism is often not enough. It is important to use theory to guide selection of an intermediate criterion that will relate to the real criterion of interest. In psychology, even our long-term criteria are not well defined relative to other sciences. In clinical psychology, for example, we are often predicting a diagnosis, which is not that much more valid compared to our measure/predictor.

At the same time, in psychology, our theories of the causal processes that influence outcomes are not yet very strong. Indeed, we have misgivings calling them theories because they do not meet the traditional scientific standard for a theory. A scientific theory is an explanation of the natural world that is testable and falsifiable, and that has withstood rigorous scientific testing and scrutiny. In psychology, our "theories" are more like conceptual frameworks. And these conceptual frameworks are often vague, do not make specific predictions of effects *and* noneffects, and do not hold up consistently when rigorously tested. As described by Meehl (1978):

> I consider it unnecessary to persuade you that most so-called "theories" in the soft areas of psychology (clinical, counseling, social, personality, community, and school psychology) are scientifically unimpressive and technologically worthless ... Perhaps the easiest way to convince yourself is by scanning the literature of soft psychology over the last 30 years and noticing what happens to theories. Most of them suffer the fate that General MacArthur ascribed to old generals—They never die, they just slowly fade away. In the developed sciences, theories tend either to become widely accepted and built into the larger edifice of well-tested human knowledge or else they suffer destruction in the face of recalcitrant facts and are abandoned, perhaps regretfully as a "nice try." But in fields like personology and social psychology, this seems not to happen. There is a period of enthusiasm about a new theory, a period of attempted application to several fact domains, a period of disillusionment as the negative data come in, a growing bafflement about inconsistent and unreplicable empirical results, multiple resort to ad hoc excuses, and then finally people just sort of lose interest in the thing and pursue other endeavors. (pp. 806–807).

Even if we had strong theoretical understanding of the causal system that influences behavior, we would likely still have difficulty making accurate predictions because the field has largely relied on relatively crude instruments. According to one philosophical perspective known as LaPlace's demon, if we were able to know the exact conditions of everything in the universe, we would be able to know how the conditions would be in the future. This is an example of scientific determinism, where if you know the initial conditions, you also know the future. Other perspectives, such as quantum mechanics and chaos theory, would say that, even if we knew the initial conditions with 100% certainty, there would still be uncertainty in our understanding of the future. But assume, for a moment, that LaPlace's demon is true. The challenge in psychology is that we have a relatively poor understanding of the initial conditions of the universe. Thus, our predictions would necessarily be probabilistic, similar to weather forecasts. Despite having a strong understanding of how weather systems behave, we have imperfect understanding of the initial conditions (e.g., the position and movement of all molecules) (Silver, 2012).

4.3.1.3.3.6 Psychoanalysis versus empiricism

We can consider the difference between psychoanalysts and empiricists in cultural references. If we consider a scene from *The Hitchhiker's Guide to the Galaxy* where a man extrapolates a simulation of the universe from a single piece of cake, we find similarities to how psychoanalysts connect everything to everything else through grand theories. Psychoanalysts try to reconstruct the entire universe from a sparse bit of data with supposedly strong theoretical understanding (when, in reality, our theories are not so strong). Their "theories" make grand conceptual claims.

Let us contrast psychoanalysts with empiricists/radical operationalism. Figure 4.6 presents a depiction of empiricism. Empiricists evaluate how an observed predictor relates to an observed outcome. The rectangles in the figure represent entities that can be observed. For instance, an empiricist might examine the extent to which a person's blood pressure is related to the number of words they speak per minute.

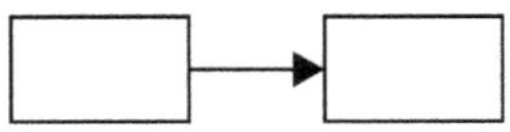

FIGURE 4.6 Conceptual Depiction of Empiricism.

Contrast the empirical approach with psychoanalysis, as depicted in Figure 4.7.

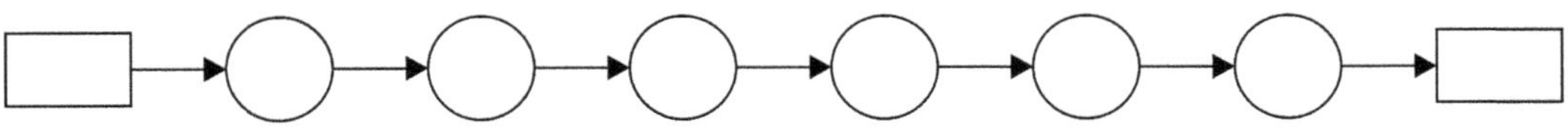

FIGURE 4.7 Conceptual Depiction of Psychoanalysis.

Circles represent unobserved, latent entities. For instance a psychoanalyst may make a conceptual claim that one observed variable influences another observed variable through a complex chain of intervening processes that are unobservable.

There is a classic and hilarious Monty Python video[2] that is an absurd example akin to radical operationalism taken to the extreme. In the video, the researchers make lots of measurements and predictions. The researchers identify interspecies differences in intelligence where humans show better performance on the English-based intelligence test (who got an IQ score of 100) than the penguins, who got an IQ score of 2. But the penguins did not speak English and were unable to provide answers to the English-based intelligence test. So, the researchers also assessed a group of non-English speaking humans as an attempt to control for language ability. They found that the penguins' scores were equal to the scores of the non-English speaking humans. They argued that, based on their smaller brain and equal IQ when controlling for language ability, that penguins are smarter than humans. However, the researchers clearly made mistakes about confounding variables. And inclusion of a control group of non-English speaking humans does not solve the problem of validity or bias; it just obscures the problem. In summary, radical operationalism provides rich lower-level information, but lacks the broader picture. So, it seems, that we need both theory *and* empiricism. Theory and empiricism can—and should—inform each other.

[2]https://osf.io/gc79d

4.3.1.4 Construct Validity

Construct validity is the extent to which a measure accurately assesses a target construct (Cronbach & Meehl, 1955). Construct validity is not quantified by a single index but rather consists of a "web of evidence" (the totality of evidence), which reflect the sum of inferences from multiple aspects of validity. That is, construct validity is the extent to which a measure assesses a target construct. Construct validity deals with the association between a measure and an unobservable criterion, i.e., a latent construct. By contrast, criterion-related validity deals with an observable criterion.

Construct validity encompasses all other types of measurement validity (e.g., content and criterion-related validity), in addition to

- scores on the measure show homogeneity—i.e., scores on the measure assess a single construct
- scores on the measure show theoretically expected developmental changes
- scores on the measure show theoretically expected group differences
- scores on the measure show theoretically expected intervention effects
- establishing the *nomological network* of a construct

4.3.1.4.1 Nomological network

A *nomological network* is the interlocking system of laws that constitute a theory. It describes how the concepts (constructs) of interest are causally linked, including their observable manifestations and the causal relations among and between them. An example of a nomological network is depicted in Figure 4.8.

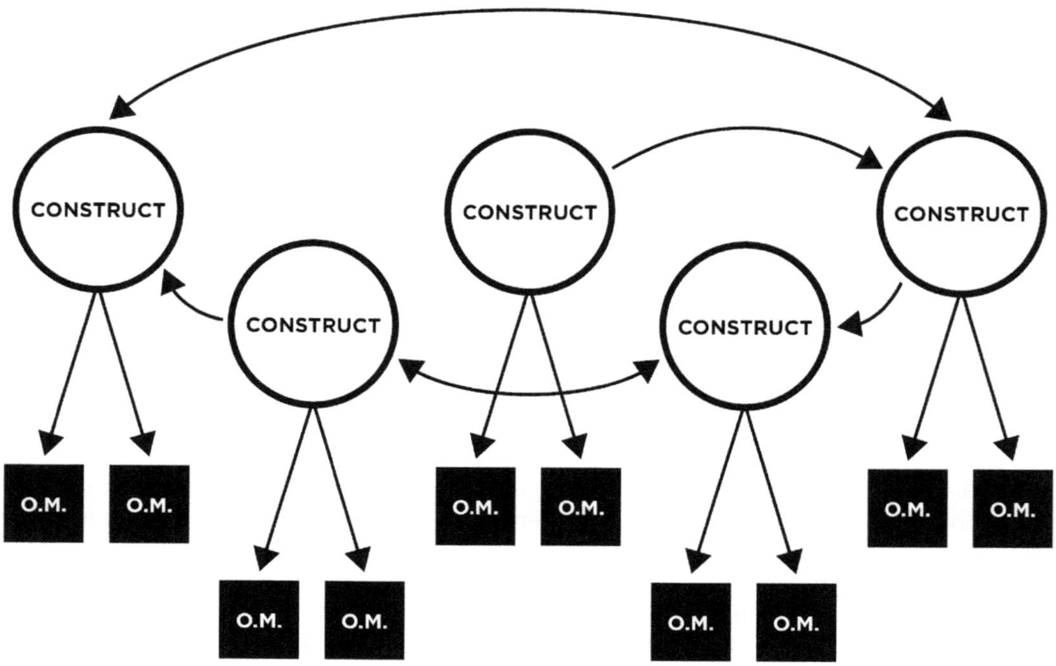

FIGURE 4.8 Example of a Nomological Network. O.M. = Observable Manifestation.

With construct validity, we can judge the quality of a measure by how well or how sensibly it fits in a nomological network. Latent constructs and observed measures improve each other step by step. But there is no established way to evaluate the process.

Historically, construct validity became a way for some researchers to skip out on other types of validity. People found a correlation between a measure's scores and some group membership and argued, therefore, that the measure has construct validity because there was a theoretically expected correlation between some measure and ________ (insert whatever measure). People started finding a correlation of a measure with other measures, asserting that it provides evidence of construct validity, and saying "that's my nomological network." But a theoretically expected association is not enough! For example, consider a measure of how quickly someone can count backward by seven. Performance is impaired in those with schizophrenia, anxiety (due to greater distractibility), and depression (due to concentration difficulties and cognitive slowing). Therefore, it is a low-quality claim that counting backward is part of the phenomenology of these disorders because it lacks differential deficit or discriminant validity (D. T. Campbell & Fiske, 1959). This is related to the "glop problem," which asserts that every bad thing is associated with every other bad thing—there is high comorbidity. Therefore, researchers needed some way to distinguish method variance from construct variance. This led to the development of the multitrait-multimethod matrix.

4.3.1.4.2 Multitrait-multimethod matrix (MTMM)

The *multitrait-multimethod matrix* (MTMM), as proposed by Campbell and Fiske (1959), is a concrete way to evaluate the validity of a measure. The MTMM allows you to split the variance of measures' scores into variance that is due to the method (i.e., method variance or method bias) and variance that is due to the construct (trait) of interest (i.e., construct variance). To create an MTMM, you need at least two methods and at least two constructs. For example, an MTMM could include self-report and observation of depression and introversion. You would then examine the correlations across combinations of construct and method.

For an example of an MTMM, see Figure 4.9. Several aspects of psychometrics can be evaluated with an MTMM, including reliability, convergent validity, and discriminant validity. The reliability diagonal of an MTMM is the correlation of a variable with itself, i.e., the test–retest reliability or monotrait-monomethod correlations. The reliability coefficients should be the highest values in the matrix because each measure should be more correlated with itself than with anything else.

A multitrait-multimethod matrix can be organized by method and then by construct or vice versa. An MTMM organized by method then by construct is depicted in Figure 4.10.

An MTMM organized by construct then by method is depicted in Figure 4.11.

4.3.1.4.2.1 Convergent validity

Convergent validity is the extent to which a measure is associated with other measures of the same target construct. In an MTMM, convergent validity evaluates whether measures targeting the same construct, but using different methods, converge upon the same construct. These are observed in the validity diagonals, also known as the convergent correlations or the monotrait-heteromethod correlations. For strong convergent validity, we would expect the values in the validity diagonals to be significant and high-ish.

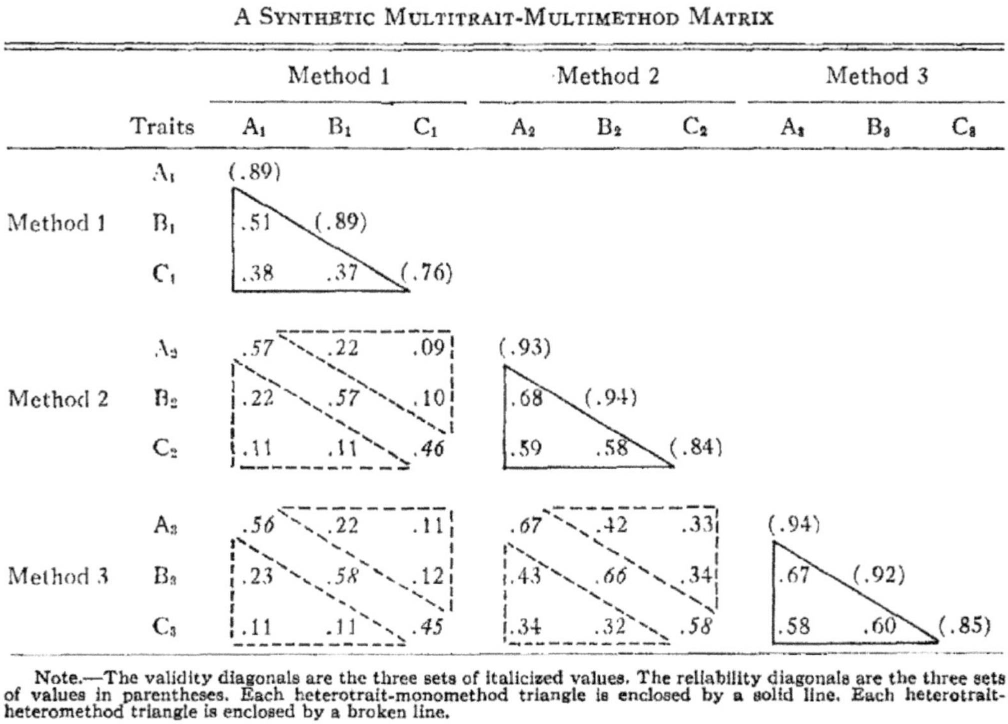

A SYNTHETIC MULTITRAIT-MULTIMETHOD MATRIX

		Method 1			Method 2			Method 3		
	Traits	A_1	B_1	C_1	A_2	B_2	C_2	A_3	B_3	C_3
Method 1	A_1	(.89)								
	B_1	.51	(.89)							
	C_1	.38	.37	(.76)						
Method 2	A_2	*.57*	.22	.09	(.93)					
	B_2	.22	*.57*	.10	.68	(.94)				
	C_2	.11	.11	*.46*	.59	.58	(.84)			
Method 3	A_3	*.56*	.22	.11	*.67*	.42	.33	(.94)		
	B_3	.23	*.58*	.12	.43	*.66*	.34	.67	(.92)	
	C_3	.11	.11	*.45*	.34	.32	*.58*	.58	.60	(.85)

Note.—The validity diagonals are the three sets of italicized values. The reliability diagonals are the three sets of values in parentheses. Each heterotrait-monomethod triangle is enclosed by a solid line. Each heterotrait-heteromethod triangle is enclosed by a broken line.

FIGURE 4.9 Multitrait-Multimethod Matrix. (Figure reprinted from Campbell, D. T., & Fiske, D. W. (1959). Convergent and discriminant validation by the multitrait-multimethod matrix. *Psychological Bulletin*, *56*, 81-105. https://doi.org/10.1037/h0046016. The content is in the public domain.)

4.3.1.4.2.2 Discriminant (divergent) validity

You can also evaluate the *discriminant validity*, also called divergent validity, of a measure in the context of an MTMM. Discriminant validity is the extent to which a measure is *not* associated (or less strongly associated) with measures of different constructs that are not theoretically expected to be related (compared to associations with measures of the same construct). In an MTMM, discriminant validity determines the extent to which a measure does not correlate with measures that share a method but assess different constructs. For strong discriminant validity, we would expect the discriminant correlations (heterotrait monomethod) to be low.

According to Campbell and Fiske (1959), discriminant validity of measures can be established when three criteria are met:

1. The convergent (monotrait-heteromethod) correlations are stronger than heterotrait-heteromethod correlations. This provides the weakest evidence for discriminant validity. That is, the convergent correlations are higher than the values in the same column or row in the same heteromethod block. This can be evaluated using the heterotrait-monotrait ratio (described below).
2. The convergent (monotrait-heteromethod) correlations are stronger than discriminant correlations (monomethod-heterotrait). This provides stronger evidence of discriminant validity.

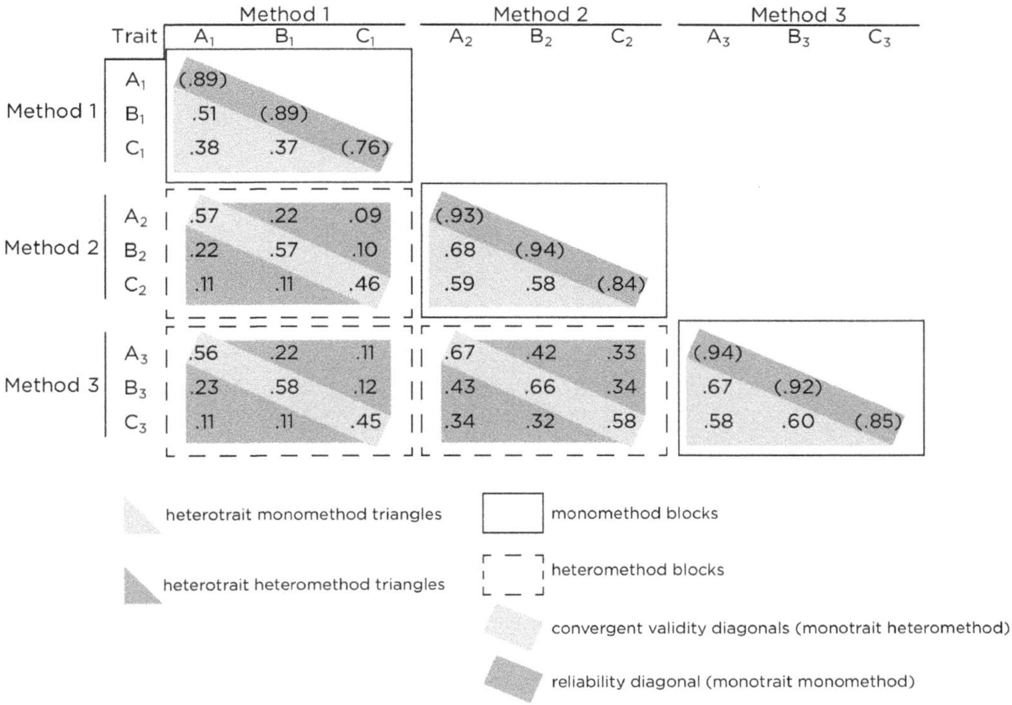

FIGURE 4.10 Multitrait-Multimethod Matrix Organized by Method Then by Construct.

3. The patterns of intercorrelations between constructs are the same, regardless of which measurement method is used. That is, the pattern of inter-trait associations is the same in all triangles. For example, if extraversion and anxiety are moderately correlated with each other but uncorrelated with achievement, we would expect this pattern of interrelations between constructs would hold, regardless of which method was used to assess the construct.

You can estimate a measure's degree of discriminant validity based on the *heterotrait-monotrait ratio* [HTMT; Henseler et al. (2015); Roemer et al. (2021)]. HTMT is the average of the heterotrait-heteromethod correlations (i.e., the correlations of measures from different measurement methods that assess different constructs), relative to the average of the monotrait-heteromethod correlations (i.e., the correlations of measures from different measurement methods that assess the same construct). As described here (http://www.henseler.com/htmt.html; archived at https://perma.cc/A9DU-WZWQ) based on evidence from Voorhees et al. (2016),

---

> If the HTMT is clearly smaller than one, discriminant validity can be regarded as established. In many practical situations, a threshold of 0.85 reliably distinguishes between those pairs of latent variables that are discriminant valid and those that are not.

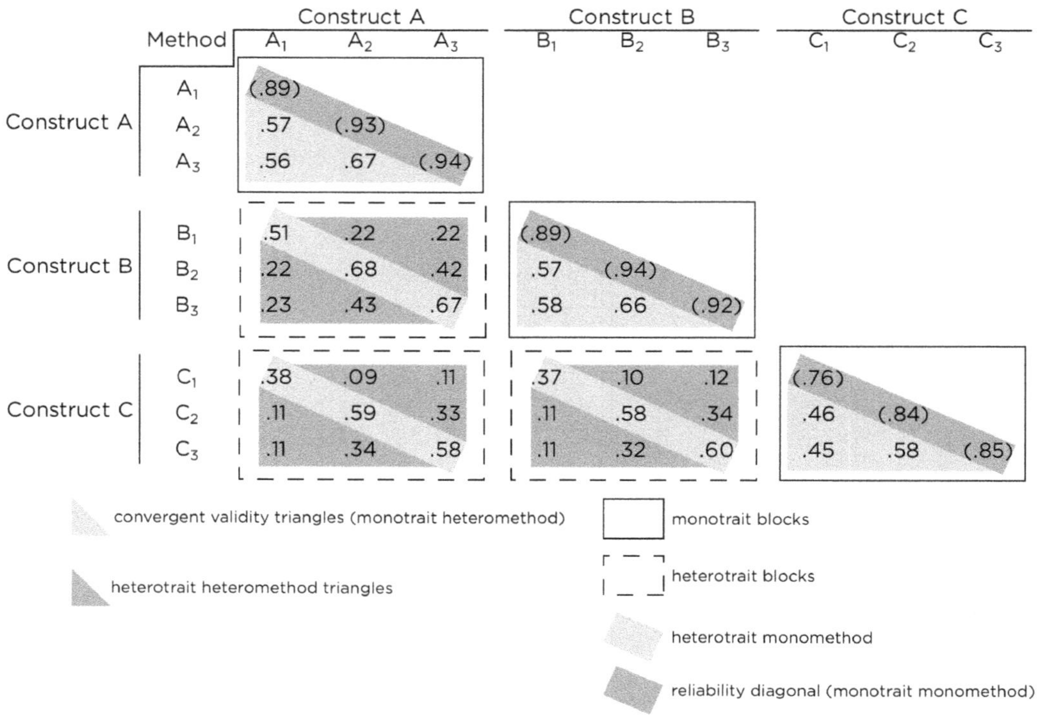

FIGURE 4.11 Multitrait-Multimethod Matrix Organized by Construct Then by Method.

The authors updated the HTMT to use the geometric mean of the correlations rather than the arithmetic mean of the correlations to relax the assumption of tau-equivalence (Roemer et al., 2021). They called the updated index HTMT2. HTMT2 was calculated below using the `semTools` package (Jorgensen et al., 2021). In this case, the HTMT values are less than .85, providing evidence of discriminant validity.

```
modelCFA <- '
  visual  =~ x1 + x2 + x3
  textual =~ x4 + x5 + x6
  speed   =~ x7 + x8 + x9
'

htmt(
  modelCFA,
  data = HolzingerSwineford1939,
  missing = "ml")
```

```
        visual textul speed
visual   1.000
textual  0.384  1.000
```

```
speed      0.387  0.280 1.000
```

Other indexes of discriminant validity include the CI_{CFA}(sys) (Rönkkö & Cho, 2020), χ^2(sys) (Rönkkö & Cho, 2020), and the Fornell-Larcker Ratio [FLR; Fornell & Larcker (1981)]. The FLR is based on the idea that a construct should be more strongly associated with its indicators than with other constructs, and is computed as the ratio of (a) the highest squared inter-correlation the construct has with other constructs to (b) the average variance extracted [AVE] by the construct. A criterion of FLR < 1 evaluates whether the AVE of a factor is greater than the highest squared inter-correlation between the factor and other factors in the model (Fornell & Larcker, 1981). Another index estimates the degree of correspondence of convergent and discriminant validity correlations with a priori hypotheses as an index of construct validity (Furr & Heuckeroth, 2019).

Using an MTMM, a researcher can learn a lot about the quality of a measure and build a nomological network. For instance, we can estimate the extent of method variance, or variance that is attributable to the measurement method rather than the construct of interest. Method variance is estimated by the difference between monomethod versus heteromethod blocks.

A poor example of an MTMM would be having two constructs such as height and depression and two methods such as Likert and true/false. This would be a poor MTMM for two reasons: (1) there are trivial differences in the methods, which would lead to obvious convergence, and (2) the differences between the constructs are not important—they are obviously discriminant. Using such an MTMM would find strong convergent associations because the methods are maximally similar and weak discriminant associations because the constructs are maximally different. It would be better to use maximally different measurement methods (e.g., self-report and performance-based measures) and to use constructs that are important to distinguish (e.g., depression and anxiey).

The paper by Campbell and Fiske (1959) that introduced the MTMM is one of the most widely cited papers in psychology of all time. *Psychological Bulletin* published a more recent paper by Fiske and Campbell (1992), entitled "Citations Do Not Solve Problems." They noted how their original paper was the most widely cited paper in the history of *Psychological Bulletin*, but they argued that nothing came of their paper. The MTMM matrices published today show little-to-no improvement compared to the ones they published in 1959. In part, this may be because we need better measures (i.e., a higher ratio of construct to method variance).

4.3.1.4.2.3 Multitrait-multimethod correlation matrix

This example is courtesy of W. Joel Schneider. First, we simulate data for an MTMM model using a fixed model with population parameters using the `simstandard` package (Schneider, 2021):

```
model_fixed <- '
 Verbal =~ .5*VO1 + .6*VO2 + .7*VO3 +
           .7*VW1 + .6*VW2 + .5*VW3 +
           .6*VM1 + .7*VM2 + .5*VM3
 Spatial =~ .7*SO1 + .7*SO2 + .6*SO3 +
            .6*SW1 + .7*SW2 + .5*SW3 +
            .7*SM1 + .5*SM2 + .7*SM3
 Quant =~ .5*QO1 + .7*QO2 + .5*QO3 +
```

TABLE 4.1 Multitrait-Multimethod Correlation Matrix.

	VO1	VO2	VO3	VW1	VW2	VW3	VM1	VM2	VM3	SO1	SO2	SO3	SW1	SW2	SW3	SM1	SM2	SM3	QO1	QO2	QO3	QW1	QW2	QW3	QM1	QM2	QM3
VO1	1.00																										
VO2	.50	1.00																									
VO3	.47	.57	1.00																								
VW1	.35	.43	.50	1.00																							
VW2	.30	.37	.43	.66	1.00																						
VW3	.27	.31	.37	.54	.43	1.00																					
VM1	.31	.37	.44	.43	.36	.33	1.00																				
VM2	.36	.42	.50	.50	.43	.37	.67	1.00																			
VM3	.25	.31	.35	.35	.30	.25	.46	.49	1.00																		
SO1	.36	.44	.43	.36	.30	.26	.30	.34	.24	1.00																	
SO2	.35	.44	.43	.35	.30	.26	.30	.34	.24	.58	1.00																
SO3	.42	.50	.45	.29	.26	.22	.25	.28	.22	.57	.57	1.00															
SW1	.20	.25	.29	.65	.50	.38	.26	.29	.21	.42	.43	.34	1.00														
SW2	.24	.29	.35	.65	.50	.42	.31	.35	.25	.49	.49	.41	.72	1.00													
SW3	.18	.22	.25	.54	.41	.33	.22	.25	.18	.35	.36	.30	.59	.61	1.00												
SM1	.25	.30	.36	.36	.31	.26	.54	.59	.39	.50	.50	.42	.43	.51	.36	1.00											
SM2	.18	.21	.26	.25	.21	.18	.46	.49	.32	.34	.34	.30	.29	.35	.26	.59	1.00										
SM3	.26	.31	.36	.36	.31	.27	.60	.64	.42	.50	.50	.42	.43	.50	.36	.79	.65	1.00									
QO1	.39	.47	.39	.22	.18	.16	.18	.22	.15	.35	.35	.44	.14	.17	.13	.17	.12	.18	1.00								
QO2	.32	.39	.39	.28	.25	.23	.25	.29	.21	.33	.33	.37	.19	.24	.17	.24	.17	.25	.53	1.00							
QO3	.30	.37	.33	.20	.17	.15	.18	.21	.15	.29	.29	.34	.13	.17	.12	.17	.12	.18	.49	.47	1.00						
QW1	.15	.19	.22	.45	.34	.28	.19	.21	.16	.18	.18	.15	.39	.38	.32	.18	.12	.18	.26	.35	.26	1.00					
QW2	.17	.20	.25	.49	.38	.31	.22	.25	.19	.21	.21	.17	.41	.42	.35	.23	.15	.22	.29	.41	.29	.46	1.00				
QW3	.19	.24	.29	.59	.45	.37	.25	.29	.20	.24	.25	.20	.50	.50	.43	.25	.16	.25	.34	.48	.35	.55	.61	1.00			
QM1	.14	.18	.22	.21	.18	.17	.39	.41	.27	.18	.17	.16	.14	.18	.14	.38	.32	.42	.25	.34	.24	.26	.30	.35	1.00		
QM2	.17	.21	.26	.25	.21	.20	.37	.40	.25	.20	.21	.17	.18	.20	.15	.36	.30	.39	.30	.42	.29	.30	.35	.41	.42	1.00	
QM3	.21	.25	.31	.31	.26	.24	.41	.45	.30	.24	.24	.21	.21	.26	.19	.39	.32	.43	.35	.49	.35	.35	.43	.49	.48	.50	1.00

```
           .5*QW1 + .6*QW2 + .7*QW3 +
           .5*QM1 + .6*QM2 + .7*QM3
  Oral =~ .4*VO1 + .5*VO2 + .3*VO3 +
          .3*SO1 + .3*SO2 + .5*SO3 +
          .6*QO1 + .3*QO2 + .4*QO3
  Written =~ .6*VW1 + .4*VW2 + .3*VW3 +
             .6*SW1 + .5*SW2 + .5*SW3 +
             .4*QW1 + .4*QW2 + .5*QW3
  Manipulative =~ .5*VM1 + .5*VM2 + .3*VM3 +
                  .5*SM1 + .5*SM2 + .6*SM3 +
                  .4*QM1 + .3*QM2 + .3*QM3
  Verbal ~~ .7*Spatial + .6*Quant
  Spatial ~~ .5*Quant
'

MTMM_data <- sim_standardized(
  model_fixed,
  n = 10000,
  observed = TRUE,
  latent = FALSE,
  errors = FALSE)
```

A multitrait-multimethod matrix correlation matrix is presented in Table 4.1.

4.3.1.4.2.4 Construct validity beyond Campbell and Fiske

There are a number of other approaches that can be helpful for establishing construct validity in ways that go beyond the approaches proposed by Campbell and Fiske (1959). One way is known as triangulation. Triangulation is conceptually depicted in Figure 4.12. Triangulation involves testing a hypothesis with multiple measures and/or methods to see if the findings are consistent—that is, whether the findings triangulate.

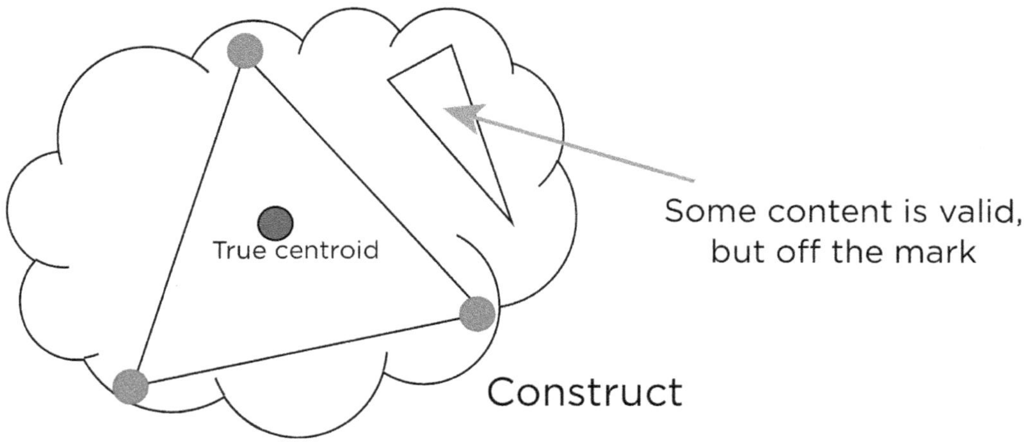

FIGURE 4.12 Using Triangulation to Arrive at a Closer Estimate of the Construct Using Multiple Measures and/or Methods.

A contemporary approach to multitrait-multimethod modeling uses confirmatory factor analysis, as described below.

4.3.1.4.2.5 MTMM in confirmatory factor analysis

Using modern modeling approaches, there are even more advanced ways of examining an MTMM. For instance, you can use structural equation modeling (SEM) or confirmatory factor analysis (CFA) to derive a latent variable of a construct from multiple methods to be free from method-related error variance to generate purer assessments of the construct to see how it relates to other constructs. For an example of an MTMM in confirmatory factor analysis, see Figure 4.13 and Section 6.4.2.12 in Chapter 6 on factor analysis.

4.3.1.5 Incremental Validity

Accuracy is not enough for a measure to be useful. Proposed by Sechrest (1963), measures should also be judged by the extent to which they provide an increment in predictive efficiency over the information otherwise easily and cheaply available. *Incremental validity* deals with the incremental value or utility over a measure beyond other sources of information. It must be demonstrated that the addition of a measure will produce better predictions than are made on the basis of information ordinarily available. It is not enough to show that the measure is better than chance, and the measure should not just be capitalizing on shared method variance with the criterion or on increased reliability of the measure. That is, the measure should explain truly unique variance—variance that was not explained before. Incremental validity demonstrates added value, unless the other measure is cheaper or less time-consuming. Incremental validity is a specific kind of criterion-related validity: significantly increased R^2 in hierarchical regression. The incremental validity of a measure can be evaluated by examining whether the measure explains significant unique variance in the criterion when accounting for other information, such as easily accessible information, traditionally available measures, or the current gold-standard measure. The extent of incremental validity of a measure can be quantified with the change in the coefficient of determination (ΔR^2) that compares (a) the model that includes the old predictor(s) to (b) the model that includes old predictors and the new predictor (measure).

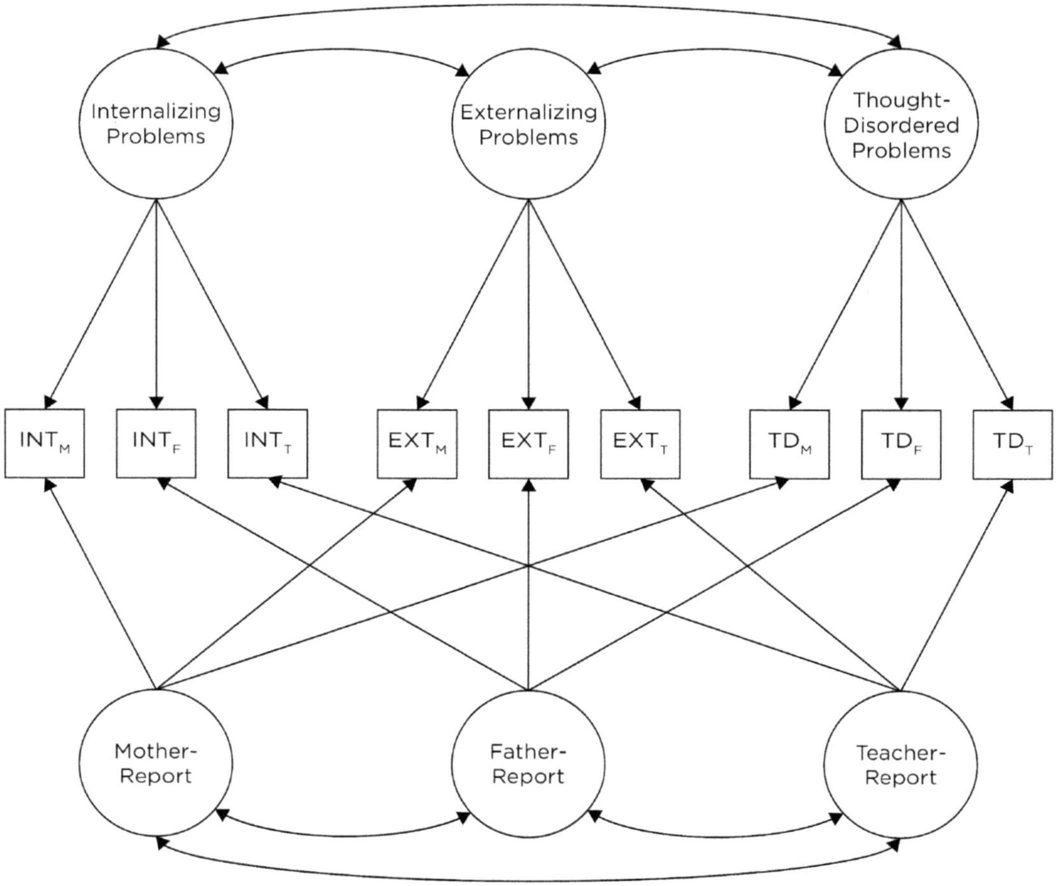

FIGURE 4.13 Multitrait-Multimethod Model in Confirmatory Factor Analysis with Three Constructs (Internalizing, Externalizing, and Thought-Disordered Problems) and Three Methods (Mother-, Father-, and Teacher-report).

```
model1 <- lm(
  criterion ~ oldpredictor,
  data = na.omit(mydataValidity))

model2 <- lm(
  criterion ~ oldpredictor + predictor,
  data = na.omit(mydataValidity))

model1Rsquare <- summary(model1)$r.squared
model2Rsquare <- summary(model2)$r.squared

deltaRsquare <- model2Rsquare - model1Rsquare

deltaRsquare
```

```
[1] 0.03628
```

```
anova(model1, model2)
```

```
Analysis of Variance Table

Model 1: criterion ~ oldpredictor
Model 2: criterion ~ oldpredictor + predictor
  Res.Df   RSS Df Sum of Sq   F Pr(>F)
1    900 44295
2    899 36886  1      7409 181 <2e-16 ***
---
Signif. codes:  0 '***' 0.001 '**' 0.01 '*' 0.05 '.' 0.1 ' ' 1
```

The predictor shows significant incremental validity above the old predictor in predicting the criterion. `Model 1` explains 78.31% of the variance ($R^2 = 0.78$), and `Model 2` explains 81.94% of the variance ($R^2 = 0.82$). Thus, the predictor explains only 3.63% additional variance in the criterion above the variance explained by the old predictor (ΔR^2).

4.3.1.6 Treatment Utility of Assessment

S. C. Hayes et al. (1987) argued that it is not enough for measures to be reliable and valid. The authors raised another important consideration for the validity of a measure: its treatment utility or usefulness. They asked the question: What goal do assessments accomplish in clinical psychology? In clinical psychology, the goal of assessment is to lead to better treatment outcomes. Therefore, the *treatment utility* of a measure is the extent to which a measure is shown to contribute to beneficial treatment outcomes. That is, if a clinician has the information/results from having administered this measure, do the clients have better outcomes? The treatment utility of assessment is a specific kind of criterion-related validity, with the idea that "all criteria are not created equal." And the criterion that is most important to optimize, from this perspective, when developing and selecting measures is a client's treatment outcomes.

S. C. Hayes et al. (1987) described different approaches to evaluating the extent to which a measure shows treatment utility. These are a priori group comparison approaches that examine whether a specific difference in the assessment approach relates to treatment outcome. They distinguished between (a) manipulated assessment and (b) manipulated use. Manipulated assessment and manipulated use are depicted in Figure 4.14.

In *manipulated assessment*, a single group of subjects is randomly divided into two subgroups, and either the collection or availability of assessment data is varied systematically. Therapists then design or implement treatment in accord with the data available. As an example, the measure of interest may be administered in one condition, and the standard measure may be administered in the other condition. Then the treatment outcomes would be compared across the two conditions. An advantage of manipulated assessment is that this type of design is more realistic than manipulated use. Making the assessment data available but not assigning a certain treatment based on the assessment outcomes better simulates a realistic clinical environment. Also, because the control group has no access to the data, it might serve as a stronger control. A disadvantage of manipulated assessment is that it depends on whether and how clinicians use the measure, which depends on how positively the measure was received by the clinicians.

In *manipulated use*, the same assessment information is available for all subjects, but the researcher manipulates the way in which the assessment information is used. For example,

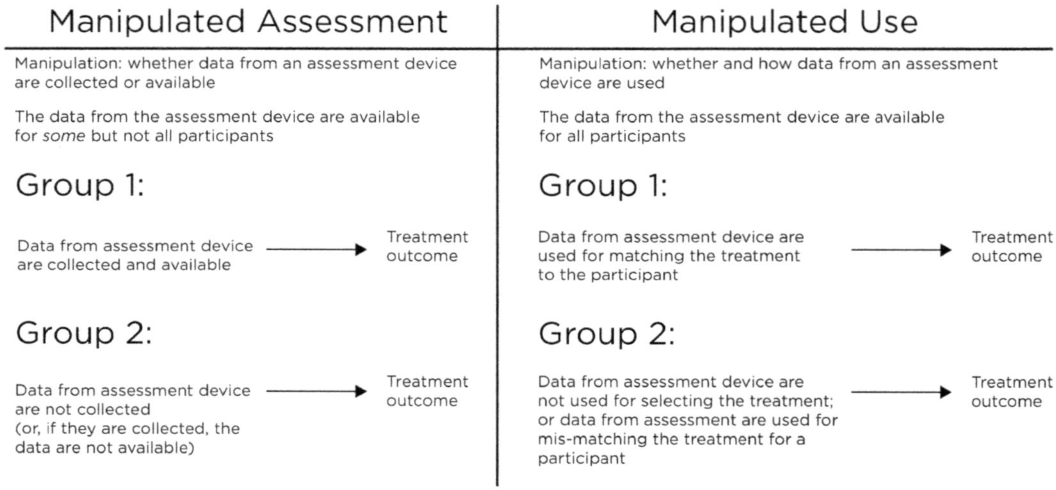

FIGURE 4.14 Research Designs That Evaluate the Treatment Utility of Assessment.

one group gets a treatment matched to assessment outcomes, and the other group gets a cross-matched treatment that does not target the problem identified by the assessment. So, in one group, the assessment information is used to match the treatment to the client based on their assessment results, whereas the other group receives a standard treatment regardless of their assessment results. An advantage of this design is that you can be certain that the treatment decisions are explicitly informed by the assessment results because the researcher ensures this, whereas the decision of how the assessment information is used is up to the clinician in manipulated assessment.

Relatively few measures show evidence of treatment utility of assessment. A review on the treatment utility of assessment is provided by Nelson-Gray (2003).

4.3.1.7 Discriminative Validity

Discriminative validity is the degree to which a measure accurately identifies persons placed into groups on the basis of another measure. Discriminative validity is not to be confused with discriminant (divergent) validity and discriminant analysis. A measure shows discriminant validity if it does not correlate with things that it would not be theoretically expected to correlate with. A measure shows discriminative validity, by contrast, if the measure is able to accurately differentiate things (e.g., two groups such as men and women). Discriminant analysis is a model that combines predictors to differentiate between multiple groups.

4.3.1.8 Elaborative Validity

Elaborative validity involves the extent to which a measure increases our theoretical understanding of the target construct or of neighboring constructs. It deals with a measure's meaningfulness. Elaborative validity is a type of incremental theoretical validity. It is a combination of criterion-related validity and construct validity that examines how much a given measure increases our understanding of a construct's nomological network. However, I am unaware of strong examples of measures that show strong elaborative validity in psychology.

4.3.1.9 Consequential Validity

Consequential validity is a form of validity that differs from evidential validity, or a test's potential to provide accurate, useful information based on research. Consequential validity takes a more macro-view and deals with the community, sociological, and public policy perspective. *Consequential validity* evaluates the consequences of our measures beyond the circumstances of their development, based on their impact. Measures can have positive, negative, or mixed effects on society. An example of consequential validity would be asking what the impacts of aptitude testing are on society—how aptitude testing affects society in the long run. Some would argue that, even in cases where the aptitude tests have some degree of evidential validity (i.e., they accurately assess to some degree what they tend to assess), they are consequentially invalid—that is, they have had a net negative effect on society and, due to their low value to society, are invalid. The tests themselves may be fine in terms of their accuracy, but consequential validity says that their validity depends on what we do with the test, i.e., how the test is used.

Another example of consequential validity is when the validity of a measure changes over time due to changes in people's or society's response, as depicted in Figure 4.15. Judgments and predictions can change the way society reacts and the way people behave so that the predictions become either more or less accurate. A prediction that becomes more accurate as a result of people's response to a prediction is a self-fulfilling prediction or prophecy. For instance, if school staff make a prediction that a child will be held back a grade, the teacher may not provide adequate opportunities for the child to learn, which may lead to the child being more likely to be held back.

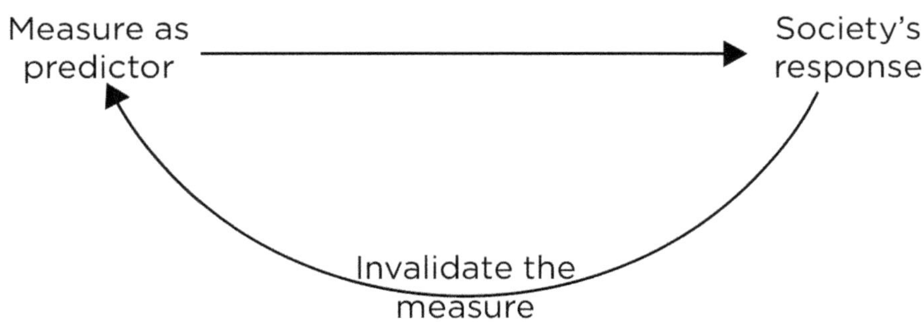

FIGURE 4.15 Invalidation of a Measure Due to Society's Response to the Use of the Measure.

A prediction that becomes less accurate as a result of people's response to a prediction is a self-canceling prediction. The most effective prediction about a flu outbreak might be one that leads people to safer behavior; therefore lowering flu rates, which does not correspond to the initial prediction (Silver, 2012). Society's response to a measure can invalidate the measure. For example, consider that an organization rates cities based on quality-of-life measures. If quality-of-life indices include the percent of solved cases by the city's police (i.e., the clearance rate), cities may try to improve their ratings of "quality-of-life" by increasing their clearance rate either by increasing the number of cases they mark as solved (such as by marking cases falsely as resolved) or by decreasing the number of cases (such as by investigating fewer cases). That is, cities may "game" the system based on the quality-of-life indices used by various organizations. In this case, the clearance rate becomes a less accurate measure of a city's quality of life.

Another example of a measure that becomes less valid due to society's response is the use of alumni donations as an indicator of the strength of a university that is used for generating university rankings. Such an indicator could lead schools to admit wealthier students who give the most donations, and students whose parents were alumni and provide lavish donations to the university. Yet another example could be standardized testing, where instructors may "teach to the test" such that better performance might not necessarily reflect better underlying competence.

4.3.1.10 Representational Validity

Representational validity examines the extent to which the items or content of a measure "flesh out" and mirror the true nature and mechanisms of the construct. There are many different types of validity, but many of them are overlapping and can be considered types of other forms of validity. For instance, representational validity is a type of elaborative validity and content validity.

4.3.1.11 Factorial (Structural) Validity

Factorial validity is examined in Section 6.1.4.2.2 on factor analysis. *Factorial validity* considers whether the factor structure of the measure(s) is consistent with the construct. According to factorial validity, if you claim that the measure is unidimensional with four items, factor analysis should support the unidimensionality. Thus, it involves testing empirically whether the measure has the same structure as would be expected based on theory. It is a type of construct validity.

4.3.1.12 Ecological Validity

Ecological validity examines the extent to which a measure provides scores that are indicative of the behavior of a person in the natural environment.

4.3.1.13 Process-Focused Validity

Process-focused validity attempts to get closer to the underlying mechanisms. *Process-focused validity* examines the degree to which respondents engage in a predictable set of psychological processes (which are specified a priori) when completing the measure (Bornstein, 2011; Furr, 2017). These psychological processes include effects of the instrument (e.g., observer versus third-party report versus projective test) as well as effects of the context (e.g., assessment setting, assessment instructions, affect state of the participant, etc.). To determine whether a test is valid in the process-focused technique, one experimentally manipulates variables that moderate the test score–criterion association—to better understand the underlying processes. The ideal outcome is a measure that both (1) has an adequate outcome (correlations where expected) as well as (2) adequate process validity—the psychological processes that one engages in are well hypothesized.

The idea of process-focused validity is that if a measure does not inform us about process or mechanisms, it is not worth doing. Process-focused validity is a type of elaborative validity and construct validity. For instance, consider the common finding that low socioeconomic status is associated with poorer outcomes. To make an impact, process-focused validity would argue that we need to know the mechanisms that underlie this association, and it involves how a measure helps us understand process.

4.3.1.14 Diagnostic Validity

Diagnostic validity is the extent to which the diagnostic category accurately captures the abnormal phenomenon of interest. It is a form of construct validity for diagnoses.

4.3.1.15 Social Validity

Social validity involves the extent to which the proposed procedures (assessment, intervention, etc.) will be well-liked and acceptable by those who receive and implement them.

4.3.1.16 Cultural Validity

Cultural validity refers to "the effectiveness of a measure or the accuracy of a clinical diagnosis to address the existence and importance of essential cultural factors" (Leong & Kalibatseva, 2016, p. 58). Essential cultural factors may include values, beliefs, experiences, communication patterns, and approaches to knowledge (epistemologies).

4.3.2 Research Design (Experimental) Validity

Aspects of *research design validity*, also called experimental validity, involve the validity of a research design for making various interpretations. Research design validity includes internal validity, external validity, and conclusion validity.

4.3.2.1 Internal Validity

Internal validity is the extent to which causal inference is justified from the research design. This encompasses multiple features including

- temporal precedence—does the (purported) cause occur before the (purported) effect?
- covariation of cause and effect—correlation is necessary (even if insufficient) for causality
- no plausible alternative explanations—such as third variables that could influence both variables and explain their covariation

There are number of potential threats to internal validity, which are important to consider when designing studies and interpreting findings. Examples of potential threats to internal validity include history, maturation, testing, instrumentation, regression, selection, experimental mortality, and an interaction of threats (Slack & Draugalis, 2001).

Research designs differ in the extent to which they show internal validity versus external validity. An experiment is a research design in which one or more variables (independent variables) are manipulated to observe how the manipulation influences the dependent variable. In an experiment, the researcher has greater control over the variables and attempts to hold everything else constant (e.g., by standardization and random assignment). In correlational designs, however, the researcher has less control over the variables. They may be able to statistically account for potential confounds using covariates or for the reverse direction of effect using longitudinal designs. Nevertheless, we can have greater confidence about whether a variable influences another variable in an experiment. Thus, experiments tend to have higher internal validity than correlational designs.

4.3.2.2 External Validity

External validity is the extent to which the findings can be generalized to the broader population and the real world. External validity is crucial to consider for studies that intend to make inferences to people outside of those who were assessed. For instance, norm-referenced assessments attempt to identify the distribution of scores for a given population from a sample within that population. The validity of the norms of a norm-referenced assessment are important to consider (Achenbach, 2001). The validity of norms and external validity, more broadly, can depend highly on how representative the sample is of the target population and how appropriate this population is to a given participant. Some measures are known to have poor norms, including the Exner Comprehensive System (Exner, 1974; Exner & Erdberg, 2005) for administering and scoring the Rorschach Inkblot Test, which has been known to over-pathologize (Wood, Teresa, et al., 2001; Wood, Nezworski, et al., 2001). The Rorschach is discussed in greater detail in Chapter 18.

4.3.2.2.1 Tradeoffs of internal validity and external validity

It is important to note that there is a tradeoff between internal and external validity—a single research design cannot have both high internal and high external validity. Some research designs are better suited for making causal inferences, whereas other designs tend to be better suited for making inferences that generalize to the real world. The research design that is best suited to making causal inferences is an experiment, where the researcher manipulates one variable (the independent variable) and holds all other variables constant to see how a change in the independent variable influences the outcome (dependent variable). Thus, experiments tend to have higher internal validity than other research designs. However, by manipulating one variable and holding everything else constant, the research takes place in a very standardized fashion that can become like studying a process in a vacuum. So, even if a process is theoretically causal in a vacuum, it may act very differently in the real world when it interacts with other processes.

Observational designs have greater capacity for external validity than experimental designs because people can be observed in their natural environments to see how variables are related in the real world. However, the greater external validity comes at a cost of lower internal validity. Observational designs are not well-positioned to make causal inferences because they have multiple threats to internal validity, including issues of temporal precedence in cross-sectional observational designs, and there are numerous potential third variables (i.e., confounds) that could act as a common cause of both the predictor and outcome variables. Thus, just because two variables are associated does not necessarily mean that they are causally related.

As the internal validity of a study's design increases, its external validity tends to decrease. The greater control we have over variables (and, therefore, have greater confidence about causal inferences), the lower the likelihood that the findings reflect what happens in the real world because it is studying things in a metaphorical vacuum. Because no single research design can have both high internal and external validity, scientific inquiry needs a combination of many different research designs so we can be more confident in our inferences—experimental designs for making causal inferences and observational designs for making inferences that are more likely to reflect the real world.

Case studies, because they have smaller sample sizes, tend to have lower external validity than both experimental and observational studies. Case studies also tend to have lower internal validity because they have less potential to control for threats to internal validity, such as potential confounds or temporal precedence. Nevertheless, case studies can still be useful for generating hypotheses that can then be tested empirically with a larger sample in experimental or observational studies.

4.3.2.3 (Statistical) Conclusion Validity

Conclusion validity, also called statistical conclusion validity, considers the extent to which conclusions are reasonable about the association among variables based on the data. That is, were the correct statistical analyses performed, and are the interpretations of the findings from those analyses correct?

4.3.3 Putting It All Together: An Organizational Framework

There are many types of measurement validity, but the central psychometric aspect of measurement validity is construct validity. That is, whether the measure accurately assesses the target construct is the most important consideration of measurement validity. As discussed earlier, construct validity includes the nomological network of the construct. Construct validity also subsumes other key types of measurement validity, including

- Convergent validity
- Discriminant (divergent) validity
- Criterion-related validity
  - Concurrent validity
  - Predictive validity
- Content validity

The organization of types of measurement validity that are subsumed by construct validity is depicted in Figure 4.16.

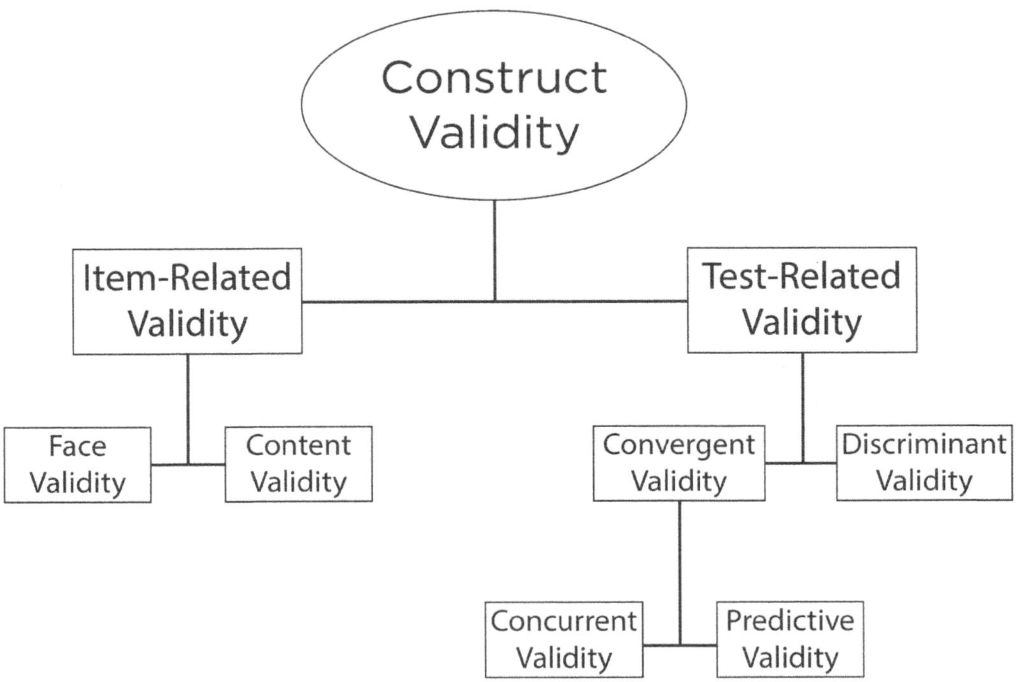

FIGURE 4.16 Organization of Types of Measurement Validity That are Subsumed by Construct Validity.

Moreover, many different types of reliability and validity can be viewed through the lens of construct validity:

- Internal consistency, which can be estimated as the coefficient of internal consistency, where the criterion for criterion-related validity is other items on the same measure
- Test–retest reliability, which can be estimated as the coefficient of stability, where the criterion for criterion-related validity is the same measure at another time point
- Parallel-forms reliability or convergent validity, which can be estimated as the coefficient of equivalence, where the criterion for criterion-related validity is the parallel form

4.4 Validity Is a Process, Not an Outcome

Validity (and validation) is a continual process, not an outcome. Validation is never complete. When evaluating the validity of a measure, we must ask: Validity for what and to what degree? We would not just say that a measure is or is not valid. We would express the strength of evidence on a measure's validity across the different types of validity for a particular purpose, with a particular population, in a particular context (consistent with generalizability theory).

4.5 Reliability Versus Validity

Reliability and validity are not the same thing. Reliability deals with consistency, whereas validity deals with accuracy. A measure can be consistent but not accurate (see Figure 4.17). That is, a measure can be reliable but not valid. However, a measure cannot be accurate if it is inconsistent; that is, a measure cannot be valid and unreliable.

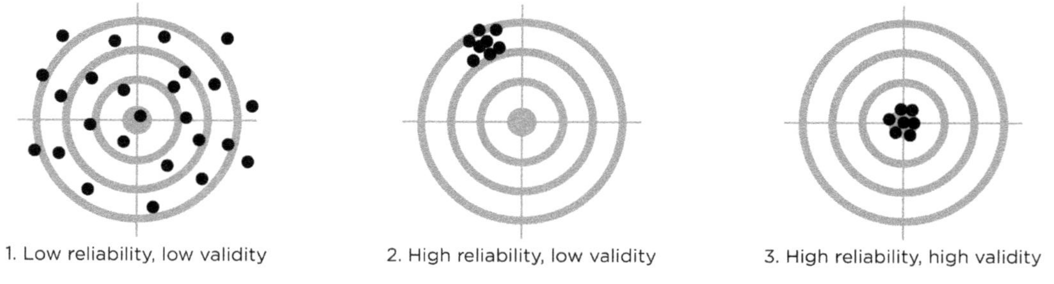

FIGURE 4.17 Traditional Depiction of Reliability (Consistency) Versus Validity (Accuracy).

The typical way of depicting the distinction between reliability and validity is in Figure 4.17, in which a measure can either have (a) low reliability and low validity, (b) high reliability and low validity, or (c) high reliability and high validity. However, it can be worth thinking about validity in terms of accuracy at the person level versus group level. When we distinguish between person- versus group-level accuracy, we can distinguish four general combinations of reliability and validity, as depicted in Figure 4.18: (a) low reliability, low accuracy at the person level, and low accuracy at the group level, (b) low reliability, low accuracy at the person level, and high accuracy at the group level, (c) high reliability, low accuracy at the person level, and low accuracy at the group level, and (d) high reliability, high accuracy at the person level, and high accuracy at the group level. However, as discussed before, reliability and validity are not binary states of low versus high—they exist to varying degrees.

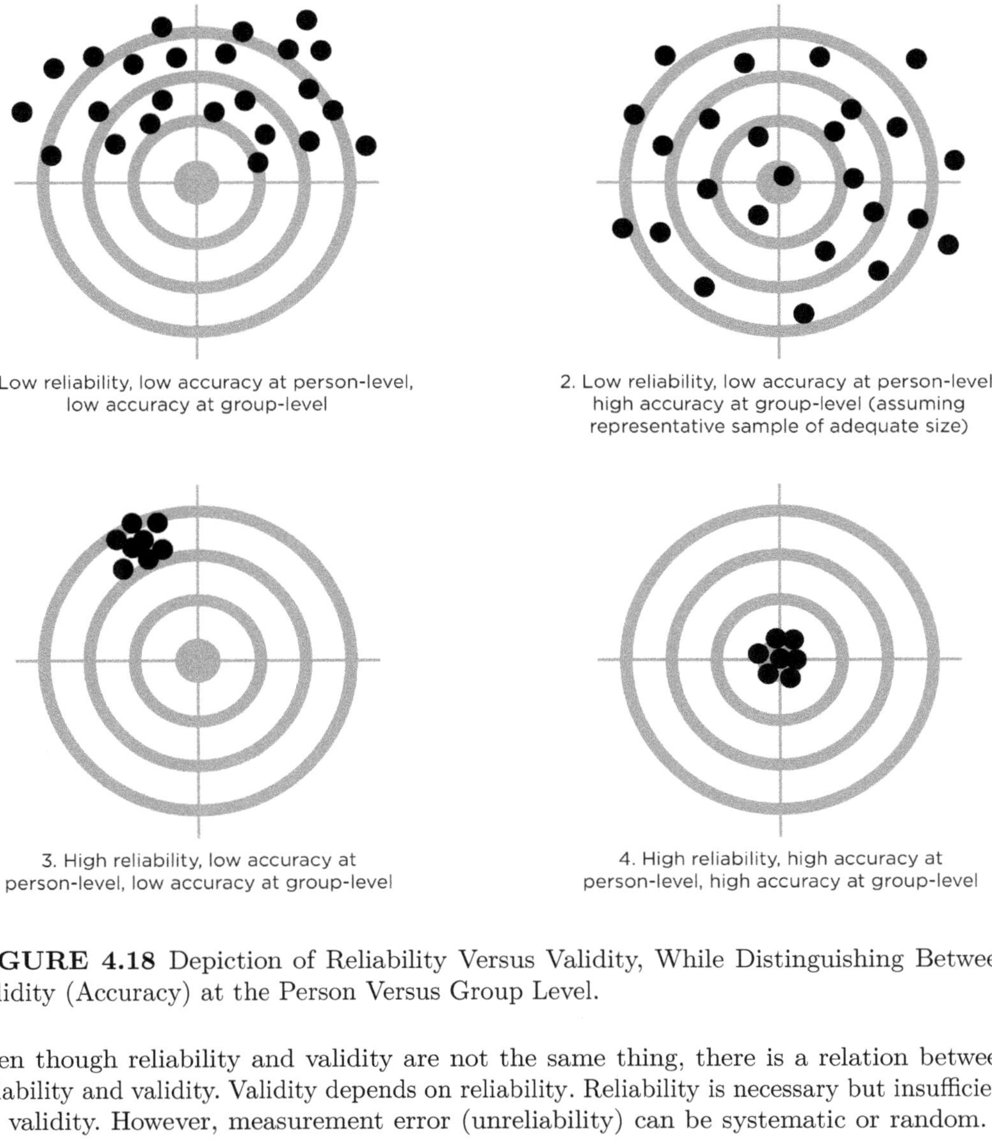

FIGURE 4.18 Depiction of Reliability Versus Validity, While Distinguishing Between Validity (Accuracy) at the Person Versus Group Level.

Even though reliability and validity are not the same thing, there is a relation between reliability and validity. Validity depends on reliability. Reliability is necessary but insufficient for validity. However, measurement error (unreliability) can be systematic or random. If measurement error is systematic, it reduces the validity of the measure. If measurement error is random, it reduces the precision of an individual's score on a measure, but the measure could still be a valid measure of the construct at the group level. However, random error would make it more difficult to make an accurate prediction for an individual person.

Reliability places the upper bound on validity because a measure can be no more valid than it is reliable. In other words, a measure should not correlate more highly with another variable than it correlates with itself. Therefore, the maximum validity coefficient is the square root of the product of the reliability of each measure, as in Equation (4.1):

$$\begin{aligned} r_{xy_{\max}} &= \sqrt{r_{xx}r_{yy}} \\ \text{maximum association between } x \text{ and } y &= \sqrt{\text{reliability of } x \text{ and } y} \end{aligned} \tag{4.1}$$

So, the maximum validity coefficient is based on the reliability of each measure. To the extent that one of the measures is unreliable, the validity coefficient will be attenuated relative to the true validity (i.e., the true strength of association of the constructs), as we describe below.

4.6 Effect of Measurement Error on Associations

Figure 4.19 depicts the classical test theory approach to understanding the validity of a measure, i.e., its association with another measure, which is the validity coefficient (r_{xy}).

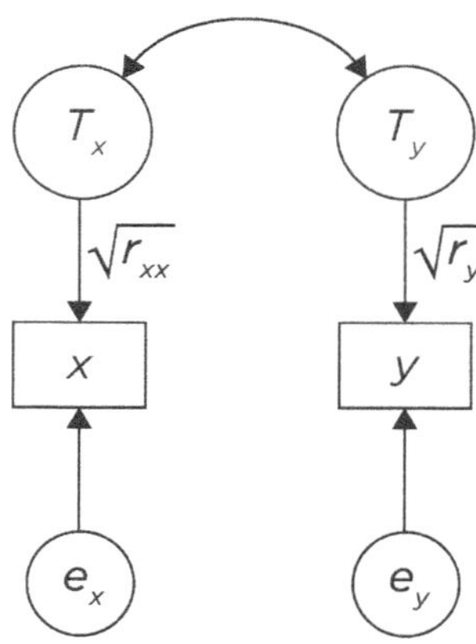

FIGURE 4.19 The Criterion-Related Validity of a Measure, i.e., Its Association with Another Measure, as Depicted in a Path Diagram.

As described above, (random) measurement error weakens (or attenuates) the association between variables (Goodwin & Leech, 2006; Schmidt & Hunter, 1996). The greater the random measurement error, the weaker the association. Thus, the correlation between x and y depends on both the true correlation of x and y ($r_{x_t y_t}$) and the reliabilities of x (r_{xx}) and y (r_{yy}). So, measurement error in x and y can reduce the observed correlation below the true correlation. This is known as the *attenuation formula* (Equation (4.2)):

$$\begin{aligned} r_{xy} &= r_{x_t y_t}\sqrt{r_{xx}r_{yy}} \\ \text{observed association between } x \text{ and } y &= (\text{true association of constructs}) \\ &\quad \times \sqrt{\text{reliability of } x \text{ and } y} \end{aligned} \tag{4.2}$$

The lower the reliability, the greater the attenuation of the validity coefficient relative to the true association between the constructs.

All of these r values (excluding the true correlation) are just estimates unless the sample size is infinite, so the observed association is an imperfect estimate. Hence, we need a correction for this attenuation (Schmidt & Hunter, 1996). This correction for the attenuation of an association due to measurement error (unreliability) is known as the disattenuation of a correlation, i.e., correction for the attenuation of an association due to measurement error to get a more accurate estimate of the true association between constructs. Rearranging the terms from the attenuation formula, the formula for disattenuation of a correlation (i.e., the *disattenuation formula*) is in Equation (4.3):

$$\begin{aligned} r_{x_t y_t} &= \frac{r_{xy}}{\sqrt{r_{xx} r_{yy}}} \\ \text{true association of constructs} &= \frac{\text{observed association between } x \text{ and } y}{\sqrt{\text{reliability of } x \text{ and } y}} \end{aligned} \tag{4.3}$$

All of this is implied in the path diagram (see Figure 4.19). The attenuation and disattenuation formulas are based on classical test theory, and therefore assume that all measurement error is random, that errors are uncorrelated, etc. Nevertheless, the attenuation formula can be informative for understanding how imperiled your research is when your measures have low reliability (i.e., when there is instability in the measure). Researchers recommend accounting for measurement reliability, to better estimate the association between constructs, either with the disattenuation formula (Schmidt & Hunter, 1996) or with structural equation modeling, as described in the next chapter.

4.6.1 Attenuation of True Correlation Due to Measurement Error

The attenuation formula is presented in Equation (4.2). We extend it to a specific example in Equation (4.4):

$$\begin{aligned} r_{xy} &= r_{x_t y_t} \sqrt{r_{xx} r_{yy}} \\ \text{observed correlation between } x \text{ and } y &= (\text{true association between construct } A \text{ and construct } B) \times \\ &\sqrt{\text{reliability of } x \times \text{reliability of } y} \end{aligned} \tag{4.4}$$

where $x =$ measure of construct A; $y =$ measure of construct B

Below is an example of how to find the observed correlation between the predictor and criterion if the true association between the constructs (i.e., correlation between true scores of constructs) is .70, the reliability of the predictor is .90, and the reliability of the criterion is .85. The `petersenlab` package (Petersen, 2024) contains the `attenuationCorrelation()` function that estimates the observed association given the true association and the reliability of the predictor and criterion:

```
attenuationCorrelation(
  trueAssociation = 0.7,
  reliabilityOfPredictor = 0.9,
  reliabilityOfCriterion = 0.85)
```

```
[1] 0.6122
```

The observed association ($r = .61$) is attenuated relative to the true association ($r = .70$).

4.6.2 Disattenuation of Observed Correlation Due to Measurement Error

The disattenuation formula is presented in Equation (4.3). We extend it to a specific example in Equation (4.5):

$$\begin{aligned} r_{x_t y_t} &= \frac{r_{xy}}{\sqrt{r_{xx} r_{yy}}} \\ \text{true association between construct } A \text{ and construct } B &= \frac{\text{observed correlation between } x \text{ and } y}{\sqrt{\text{reliability of } x \times \text{reliability of } y}} \end{aligned} \tag{4.5}$$

where $x =$ measure of construct A; $y =$ measure of construct B.

Find the true association between the construct assessed by the predictor and the construct assessed by the criterion given an observed association if the reliability of the predictor is .9, and the reliability of the criterion is .85: The `petersenlab` package (Petersen, 2024) contains the `disattenuationCorrelation()` function that estimates the observed association given the true association and the reliability of the predictor and criterion:

```
observedAssociation <- cor.test(
  x = mydataValidity$predictor,
  y = mydataValidity$criterion)$estimate

observedAssociation
```

```
   cor
0.7079
```

```
reliabilityOfPredictor <- 0.9
reliabilityOfCriterion <- 0.85

disattenuationCorrelation(
  observedAssociation = observedAssociation,
  reliabilityOfPredictor = reliabilityOfPredictor,
  reliabilityOfCriterion = reliabilityOfCriterion)
```

```
   cor
0.8094
```

The disattenuation of an observed correlation due to measurement error can be demonstrated using structural equation modeling. For instance, consider the following observed association:

```
cor(
  x = mydataValidity$predictorObservedSEM,
  y = mydataValidity$criterionObservedSEM,
  use = "pairwise.complete.obs")
```

```
[1] 0.6118
```

The observed association can be estimated in structural equation modeling in the `lavaan` package (Rosseel et al., 2022) using the following syntax:

TABLE 4.2 Parameter Estimates of Observed Association in Structural Equation Model.

lhs	op	rhs	est	se	z	pvalue	ci.lower	ci.upper	std.lv	std.all	std.nox
criterionObservedSEM		predictorObservedSEM	0.633	0.027	23.366	0.000	0.580	0.686	0.633	0.611	0.611
predictorObservedSEM		predictorObservedSEM	0.971	0.044	21.932	0.000	0.885	1.058	0.971	1.000	1.000
criterionObservedSEM		criterionObservedSEM	0.654	0.030	21.518	0.000	0.595	0.714	0.654	0.627	0.627
criterionObservedSEM	1		−0.012	0.027	−0.459	0.646	−0.064	0.040	−0.012	−0.012	−0.012
predictorObservedSEM	1		0.012	0.032	0.373	0.709	−0.050	0.074	0.012	0.012	0.012

```
observedSEM_syntax <- '
  criterionObservedSEM ~ predictorObservedSEM

  # Specify residual errors (measurement error)
  predictorObservedSEM ~~ predictorObservedSEM
  criterionObservedSEM ~~ criterionObservedSEM
'

observedSEM_fit <- sem(
  observedSEM_syntax,
  data = mydataValidity,
  missing = "ML")
```

Parameter estimates from the model are shown in Table 4.2.

Now consider when we account for the degree of unreliability of each measure. We can account for the (un)reliability of each measure by specifying the residual errors as 1 − reliability, as below:

```
disattenuationSEM_syntax <-
  paste(
    '
    # Factor loadings
    predictorLatent =~ 1*predictorObservedSEM
    criterionLatent =~ 1*criterionObservedSEM

    # Factor correlation
    criterionLatent ~ predictorLatent

    # Specify residual errors (measurement error)
    predictorObservedSEM ~~ (1 - ',
      reliabilityOfPredictor, ')*predictorObservedSEM
    criterionObservedSEM ~~ (1 - ',
      reliabilityOfCriterion, ')*criterionObservedSEM
    ',
    sep = "")

disattenuationSEM_fit <- sem(
  disattenuationSEM_syntax,
  data = mydataValidity,
  missing = "ML")
```

TABLE 4.3 Parameter Estimates of Disattenuated Association in Structural Equation Model.

lhs	op	rhs	est	se	z	pvalue	ci.lower	ci.upper	std.lv	std.all	std.nox
predictorLatent	=	predictorObservedSEM	1.000	0.000	NA	NA	1.000	1.000	0.933	0.947	0.947
criterionLatent	=	criterionObservedSEM	1.000	0.000	NA	NA	1.000	1.000	0.946	0.925	0.925
criterionLatent		predictorLatent	0.706	0.030	23.152	0.000	0.646	0.766	0.697	0.697	0.697
predictorObservedSEM		predictorObservedSEM	0.100	0.000	NA	NA	0.100	0.100	0.100	0.103	0.103
criterionObservedSEM		criterionObservedSEM	0.150	0.000	NA	NA	0.150	0.150	0.150	0.144	0.144
predictorLatent		predictorLatent	0.871	0.044	19.674	0.000	0.785	0.958	1.000	1.000	1.000
criterionLatent		criterionLatent	0.460	0.031	14.960	0.000	0.399	0.520	0.514	0.514	0.514
predictorObservedSEM	1		0.012	0.032	0.373	0.709	−0.050	0.074	0.012	0.012	0.012
criterionObservedSEM	1		−0.005	0.033	−0.143	0.887	−0.069	0.060	−0.005	−0.005	−0.005
predictorLatent	1		0.000	0.000	NA	NA	0.000	0.000	0.000	0.000	0.000
criterionLatent	1		0.000	0.000	NA	NA	0.000	0.000	0.000	0.000	0.000

Parameter estimates from the model are presented in Table 4.3.

The observed association ($\beta = 0.61$) becomes $\beta = 0.70$ when it is disattenuated for measurement error.

4.7 Generalizability Theory

Generalizability theory (G-theory) is discussed in greater detail in the chapter on reliability in Section 3.11 and in the chapter on generalizability theory. As a brief reminder, G-theory is a measurement theory that, unlike classical test theory, does not treat all measurement differences across time, rater, or situation as "error" but rather as a phenomenon of interest. G-theory can simultaneously consider multiple aspects of reliability and validity in the same model, something that classical test theory cannot achieve.

4.8 Ways to Increase Validity

Here are potential ways to increase the validity of the interpretation of a measure's scores for a particular purpose:

- Make sure the measure's scores are reliable. For potential ways to increase the reliability of measurement, see Section 3.14. But do not switch to a less valid measure or to items that are less valid merely because they are more reliable.
- Use multiple measures and multiple methods to remedy the effects of method bias.
- Design the measure with a particular population and purpose in mind. When describing the measure in papers or in public spheres, make it clear to others what the population and intended purposes are and what they are not.
- Make sure each item's scores are valid, based on theory and empiricism, for the particular population and purpose. For instance, the items should show content validity—the items should assess facets of the target construct for the target population as defined by experts, without item intrusions from other constructs. The items' scores should show convergent validity—the items' scores should be related to other measures of the construct, within the population of interest. The items' scores should show discriminant validity—the items'

scores should be more strongly related to measures that are intended to assess the same construct than they are to measures that are intended to assess other constructs.

- Obtain samples that are as representative of the population as possible, paying attention to including people who are traditionally under-represented in research (if such groups are part of the target population).
- Make sure that people in the population can understand, interpret, and respond to each item in a meaningful and comparable way.
- Make sure the measure and its items are not biased against any subgroup within the population of interest. Test bias is discussed in Chapter 15.
- Be careful to administer the measure to the population of interest under the conditions in which it is designed. If the measure must be administered to people from a different population or under different conditions from which it was designed, be careful to (a) note that the measure was not designed to be administered for these other populations or conditions, and (b) note that individuals' scores may not accurately reflect their level on the construct. If interpretations are made based on these scores, make them cautiously and say how the differences in population or condition may have influenced the scores.
- Continue to monitor the validity of the measure's scores for the given population and purpose. The validity of measures' scores can change over time for a number of reasons. Cohort effects can lead items to become obsolete over time. If people or organizations change their behavior in response to a measure, this can invalidate a measure's scores for the intended purpose, as described in Section 4.3.1.9 when discussing consequential validity.

4.9 Conclusion

Validity is how much accuracy, utility, and meaningfulness the interpretation of a measure's scores have for a particular purpose. Like reliability, validity is not one thing. There are multiple aspects of validity. Validity is also not a characteristic that resides in a test. The validity of a measure's scores reflect an interaction of the properties of the test with the population for whom it is designed and the sample and context in which it is administered. Thus, when reporting validity in papers, it is important to adequately describe the aspects of validity that have been considered and the population, sample, and context in which the measure is assessed.

4.10 Suggested Readings

Cronbach & Meehl (1955); L. A. Clark & Watson (2019)

5

Generalizability Theory

Up to this point, we have discussed reliability from the perspective of classical test theory (CTT). However, as we discussed, CTT makes several assumptions that are unrealistic. For example, CTT assumes that all error is random. In CTT, there is an assumption that there exists a true score that is an accurate measure of the trait under a *specific* set of conditions. There are other measurement theories that conceptualize reliability differently than the way that CTT conceptualizes reliability. One such measurement theory is generalizability theory (Brennan, 1992), also known as G-theory and domain sampling theory. G-theory is also discussed in the chapters on reliability (Chapter 3, Section 3.11), validity (Chapter 4, Section 4.7) and structural equation modeling (Chapter 7, Section 7.11).

5.1 Overview

G-theory is an alternative measurement theory to CTT that does not treat all measurement differences across time, rater, or situation as "error" but rather as a phenomenon of interest (Wiggins, 1973). G-theory is a measurement theory that is used to examine the extent to which scores are consistent across a specific set of conditions. In G-theory, the true score is conceived of as a person's *universe score*—the mean of all observations for a person over all conditions in the universe—this allows us to estimate and recognize the magnitude of multiple influences on test performance. These multiple influences on test performance are called *facets*.

5.1.1 The Universe of Generalizability

Instead of conceiving of all variability in a person's scores as error, G-theory argues that we should describe the details of the particular test situation (universe) that lead to a specific test score. The universe is described in terms of its facets:

- settings
- observers (e.g., amount of training they had)
- instruments (e.g., number of items in test)
- occasions (time points)
- attributes (i.e., what we are assessing; the purpose of test administration)

Measures with strong reliability show a high ratio of variance as a function of the person relative to the variance as a function of other facets or factors. To the extent that variance in scores is attributable to different settings, observers, instruments, occasions, attributes, or other facets, the reliability of the measure is weakened.

TABLE 5.1 Percent of Variance from Different Sources in Generalizability Theory Model with Three Facets: Person, Item, and Occasion (and Their Interactions). (Adapted from Webb et al. (2005), table 1, p. 2. Webb, N. M., & Shavelson, R. J. (2005). Generalizability theory: Overview. In B. S. Everitt & D. C. Howell (Eds.), *Encyclopedia of statistics in behavioral science* (Vol. 2, pp. 717–719). John Wiley & Sons, Ltd. https://doi.org/10.1002/0470013192.bsa703)

Source	Variance Accounted For (%)
Person (p)	30
Item (i)	5
Occasion (o)	3
p x i	25
p x o	5
i x o	2
p x i x o	10
residual	20

5.1.2 Universe Score

A person's universe score is the average of a person's scores across all conditions in the universe. According to G-theory, given the exact same conditions of all the facets in the universe, the exact same test score should be obtained. This is the universe score, which is analogous to the true score in CTT.

5.1.3 G-Theory Perspective on Reliability

G-theory asserts that the reliability of a test does not reside within the test itself; a test's reliability depends on the circumstances under which it is developed, administered, and interpreted. A person's test scores vary from testing to testing because of (many) variables in the testing situation. By assessing a person in multiple facets of the universe, this allows us to estimate and recognize the magnitude of multiple sources of measurement error. Such measurement error includes:

- day-to-day variation in performance (stability of the construct, test–retest reliability)
- variance in the item sampling (coefficient of internal consistency)
- variance due to both day-to-day and item sampling (coefficient of equivalence from parallel-forms reliability, or convergent validity, as discussed in Section 4.7)

In G-theory, all sources of measurement error (facets) are considered simultaneously—something CTT cannot achieve (Shavelson et al., 1989). This occurs through specifying many different variance facets in the estimation of the true score, rather than just one source of error variance as in CTT. This specification allows us to take into consideration variance due to occasion effects, item effects, and occasion × item effects (i.e., main effects of the facets in addition to their interaction), as in Table 5.1.

A score's usefulness largely depends on the extent to which it allows us to generalize accurately to behavior in a wider set of situations—i.e., a universe of generalization. The G-Theory equivalent of the CTT reliability coefficient of a measure is the generalizability coefficient or dependability coefficient.

5.1.4 G-Theory Perspective on Validity

G-theory can simultaneously consider multiple aspects of reliability and validity in the same model. For instance, internal consistency reliability, test–retest reliability, inter-rater reliability, parallel-forms reliability, and convergent validity (in the D. T. Campbell & Fiske, 1959 sense of the same construct assessed by a different method) can all be incorporated into a G-theory model.

For example, a G-theory model could assess each participant across the following facets:

- time: e.g., T1 and T2 (test–retest reliability)
- items: e.g., questions within the same instrument (internal consistency reliability) and questions across different instruments (parallel-forms reliability)
- rater: e.g., self-report and other-report (inter-rater reliability)
- method: e.g., questionnaire and observation (convergent validity)

Using such a G-theory model, we can determine the extent to which scores on a measure generalize to other conditions, measures, etc. Measures with strong convergent validity show a high ratio of variance as a function of the person relative to the variance as a function of measurement method. To the extent that variance in scores is attributable to different measurement methods, convergent validity is weakened.

An example data structure that could leverage G-theory to partition the variance in scores as a function of different facets (person, time, item, rater, method) and their interactions is in Table 5.2.

TABLE 5.2 Example Data Structure for Generalizability Theory with the Following Facets: Person, Time, Item, Rater, Method.

Person	Time	Item	Rater	Method	Score
1	1	"hits others"	1	questionnaire	10
1	1	"hits others"	1	observation	15
1	1	"hits others"	2	questionnaire	8
1	1	"hits others"	2	observation	13
1	1	"argues"	1	questionnaire	4
1	1	"argues"	1	observation	2
1	1	"argues"	2	questionnaire	5
1	1	"argues"	2	observation	7
1	2	"hits others"	1	questionnaire	8
1	2	"hits others"	1	observation	10
1	2	"hits others"	2	questionnaire	6
1	2	"hits others"	2	observation	7
1	2	"argues"	1	questionnaire	2
1	2	"argues"	1	observation	2
1	2	"argues"	2	questionnaire	4
1	2	"argues"	2	observation	6
2	1	"hits others"	1	questionnaire	5
...	...	...	...	...	...

In sum, G-theory can be a useful way of estimating the degree of reliability and validity of a measure's scores in the same model.

5.1.5 Generalizability Study

In G-theory, the goal is to conduct a generalizability study (G study) and a *decision study* (D study). A generalizability study examines the extent of variance in the scores that is attributable to various facets. The researcher must specify and define the universe (set of conditions) to which they would like to generalize their observations and in which they would like to study the reliability of the measure. For instance, it might involve randomly sampling from within that universe in terms of people, items, observers, conditions, timepoints, measurement methods, etc.

5.1.6 Decision Study

After conducting a generalizability study, one can then use the estimates of the extent of variance in scores that are attributable to various facets (estimated from the generalizability study) to conduct a decision study (D study). A decision study examines how generalizable scores from a particular test are if the test is administered in different situations. In G-theory, reliability is estimated with the *generalizability coefficient* and the *dependability coefficient*.

5.1.7 Analysis Approach

Traditionally, a generalizability theory approach would test the generalizability study and decision study using a factorial analysis of variance [ANOVA; Brennan (1992)], as exemplified in Section 5.2.4.1, (as opposed to simple ANOVA in CTT). However, ANOVA is limiting—it works best with balanced designs, such as with the same sample size in each condition/facet; but in most real-world applications, data are not equally balanced in each condition. So, it is better to fit G-theory models in a mixed model framework, as exemplified in Section 5.2.4.2.

5.1.8 Practical Challenges

G-theory is strong theoretically, but it has not been widely implemented. G-theory can be challenging because the researcher must specify, define, and assess the universe to which they would like to generalize their observations and to understand the reliability of the measure.

5.2 Getting Started

5.2.1 Load Libraries

```
library("petersenlab")
library("gtheory")
library("MOTE")
library("here")
library("tidyverse")
library("tinytex")
library("knitr")
library("kableExtra")
library("rmarkdown")
library("bookdown")
```

5.2.2 Prepare Data

5.2.2.1 Generate Data

```
set.seed(52242)

Person <- as.factor(rep(1:6, each = 8))
Occasion <- Rater <- as.factor(rep(1:2, each = 4, times = 6))
Item <- as.factor(rep(1:4, times = 12))
Score <- c(
  9,9,7,4,9,8,5,5,9,8,4,6,
  6,5,3,3,8,8,6,2,8,7,3,2,
  9,8,6,3,9,6,6,2,10,9,8,7,
  8,8,9,7,6,4,5,1,3,2,3,2)
```

5.2.2.2 Add Missing Data

Adding missing data to dataframes helps make examples more realistic to real-life data and helps you get in the habit of programming to account for missing data.

```
Score[30] <- NA
```

5.2.2.3 Combine Data into Dataframe

```
pio_cross_dat <- data.frame(Person, Item, Score, Occasion)
```

Below are examples implementing G-theory. The `pio_cross_dat` data file for these examples comes from the `gtheory` package (Moore, 2016). The examples are adapted from Huebner & Lucht (2019).

5.2.3 Universe Score for Each Person

Universe scores for each person are generated using the following syntax and are presented in Table 5.3.

```
universeScores <- pio_cross_dat %>%
  group_by(Person) %>%
  summarise(universeScore = mean(Score, na.rm = TRUE), .groups = "drop")
```

5.2.4 Generalizability (G) Study

Generalizability studies can be conducted in an ANOVA or mixed model framework. Below, we fit a generalizability study model in each framework. In these models, the item, person, and their interaction appear to be the three facets that account for the most variance in scores. Thus, when designing future studies, it would be important to assess and evaluate these facets.

TABLE 5.3 Participants' Universe Scores.

Person	Universe Score
1	7.000
2	5.500
3	5.500
4	6.143
5	8.250
6	3.250

5.2.4.1 ANOVA Framework

```
summary(aov(
  Score ~ Person*Item*Occasion,
  data = pio_cross_dat))
```

```
                     Df Sum Sq Mean Sq
Person                5  113.0    22.6
Item                  3  119.2    39.7
Occasion              1   14.2    14.2
Person:Item          15   35.6     2.4
Person:Occasion       5    6.6     1.3
Item:Occasion         3    2.3     0.8
Person:Item:Occasion 14   12.1     0.9
1 observation deleted due to missingness
```

5.2.4.2 Mixed Model Framework

The mixed model framework for estimating generalizability is described by Jiang (2018).

```
summary(lmer(
  Score ~ 1 + (1|Person) + (1|Item) + (1|Occasion) +
    (1|Person:Occasion) + (1|Person:Item) + (1|Occasion:Item),
  data = pio_cross_dat))
```

```
Linear mixed model fit by REML ['lmerMod']
Formula: Score ~ 1 + (1 | Person) + (1 | Item) + (1 | Occasion) + (1 |
    Person:Occasion) + (1 | Person:Item) + (1 | Occasion:Item)
   Data: pio_cross_dat

REML criterion at convergence: 174.7

Scaled residuals:
    Min      1Q  Median      3Q     Max
-1.3023 -0.6530 -0.0525  0.6356  1.3702

Random effects:
 Groups          Name        Variance Std.Dev.
 Person:Item     (Intercept) 0.78731  0.8873
 Person:Occasion (Intercept) 0.11728  0.3425
```

```
 Occasion:Item    (Intercept) 0.00157  0.0397
 Person           (Intercept) 2.47804  1.5742
 Item             (Intercept) 3.12380  1.7674
 Occasion         (Intercept) 0.53663  0.7326
 Residual                     0.83743  0.9151
Number of obs: 47, groups:
Person:Item, 24; Person:Occasion, 12; Occasion:Item, 8; Person, 6; Item, 4; Occasion, 2

Fixed effects:
            Estimate Std. Error t value
(Intercept)     5.96       1.23    4.83
```

```
PxIxO <- gstudy(
  data = pio_cross_dat,
  Score ~ (1|Person) + (1|Item) + (1|Occasion) + (1|Person:Item) +
    (1|Person:Occasion) + (1|Occasion:Item))

PxIxO
```

```
$components
           source      var percent n
1     Person:Item 0.787305    10.0 1
2 Person:Occasion 0.117284     1.5 1
3   Occasion:Item 0.001574     0.0 1
4          Person 2.478043    31.4 1
5            Item 3.123803    39.6 1
6        Occasion 0.536633     6.8 1
7        Residual 0.837426    10.6 1

attr(,"class")
[1] "gstudy" "list"
```

5.2.5 Decision (D) Study

The decision (D) study and generalizability (G) study, from which the generalizability and dependability coefficients can be estimated, were analyzed using the gtheory package (Moore, 2016).

```
decisionStudy <- dstudy(
  PxIxO,
  colname.objects = "Person",
  data = pio_cross_dat,
  colname.scores = "Score")
```

5.2.6 Generalizability Coefficient

The generalizability coefficient is analogous to the reliability coefficient in CTT. It divides the estimated person variance component (the universe score variance) by the estimated observed-score variance (with some adjustment for the number of observations). In other words, variance in a reliable measure should mostly be due to person variance rather than variance as a function of items, occasion, raters, methods, or other factors. The generalizability coefficient uses relative error variance, so it characterizes the similarity in the relative standing of individuals, similar to CTT-based estimates of relative reliability, such as Cronbach's alpha. Thus, the generalizability coefficient is an index of relative reliability. The generalizability coefficient ranges from 0–1, and higher scores reflect better reliability.

```
decisionStudy$generalizability
```

```
[1] 0.8731
```

5.2.7 Dependability Coefficient

The dependability coefficient is similar to the generalizability coefficient; however, it uses absolute error variance rather than relative error variance in the estimation. The dependability coefficient characterizes the absolute magnitude of differences across scores, not (just) the relative standing of individuals. Thus, the dependability coefficient is an index of absolute reliability. The dependability coefficient ranges from 0–1, and higher scores reflect better reliability.

```
decisionStudy$dependability
```

```
[1] 0.6374
```

5.3 Conclusion

G-theory provides an important reminder that reliability is not one thing. You cannot just say that a test "is reliable"; it is important to specify the facets across which the reliability and validity of a measure have been established (e.g., times, raters, items, groups, instruments). Generalizability theory can be a useful way of estimating multiple aspects of reliability and validity of measures in the same model.

5.4 Suggested Readings

Brennan (2001)

6

Factor Analysis and Principal Component Analysis

6.1 Overview

Factor analysis is a class of latent variable models that is designated to identify the structure of a measure or set of measures, and ideally, a construct or set of constructs. It aims to identify the optimal latent structure for a group of variables. Factor analysis encompasses two general types: confirmatory factor analysis and exploratory factor analysis. *Exploratory factor analysis* (EFA) is a latent variable modeling approach that is used when the researcher has no a priori hypotheses about how a set of variables is structured. EFA seeks to identify the empirically optimal-fitting model in ways that balance accuracy (i.e., variance accounted for) and parsimony (i.e., simplicity). *Confirmatory factor analysis* (CFA) is a latent variable modeling approach that is used when a researcher wants to evaluate how well a hypothesized model fits, and the model can be examined in comparison to alternative models. Using a CFA approach, the researcher can pit models representing two theoretical frameworks against each other to see which better accounts for the observed data.

Factor analysis is considered to be a "pure" data-driven method for identifying the structure of the data, but the "truth" that we get depends heavily on the decisions we make regarding the parameters of our factor analysis. The goal of factor analysis is to identify simple, parsimonious factors that underlie the "junk" (i.e., scores filled with measurement error) that we observe.

It used to take a long time to calculate a factor analysis because it was computed by hand. Now, it is fast to compute factor analysis with computers (e.g., often less than 30 ms). In the 1920s, Spearman developed factor analysis to understand the factor structure of intelligence. It was a long process—it took Spearman around one year to calculate the first factor analysis! Factor analysis takes a large dimension data set and simplifies it into a smaller set of factors that are thought to reflect underlying constructs. If you believe that nature is simple underneath, factor analysis gives nature a chance to display the simplicity that lives beneath the complexity on the surface. Spearman identified a single factor, g, that accounted for most of the covariation between the measures of intelligence.

Factor analysis involves observed (manifest) variables and unobserved (latent) factors. In a reflective model, it is assumed that the latent factor influences the manifest variables, and the latent factor therefore reflects the common (reliable) variance among the variables. A factor model potentially includes factor loadings, residuals (errors or disturbances), intercepts/means, covariances, and regression paths. A regression path indicates a hypothesis that one variable (or factor) influences another. The standardized regression coefficient represents the strength of association between the variables or factors. A factor loading is a regression path from a latent factor to an observed (manifest) variable. The standardized factor loading represents the strength of association between the variable and the latent factor. A residual is variance in a variable (or factor) that is unexplained by other variables or factors. An indicator's intercept is the expected value of the variable when the factor(s) (onto which it loads) is equal to zero. Covariances are the associations between variables (or factors).

In factor analysis, the relation between an indicator (X) and its underlying latent factor(s) (F) can be represented with a regression formula as in Equation (6.1):

$$\mathrm{X} = \lambda \cdot \mathrm{F} + \text{Item Intercept} + \text{Error Term} \tag{6.1}$$

where:

- X is the observed value of the indicator
- λ is the factor loading, indicating the strength of the association between the indicator and the latent factor(s)
- F is the person's value on the latent factor(s)
- Item Intercept represents the constant term that accounts for the expected value of the indicator when the latent factors are zero
- Error Term is the residual, indicating the extent of variance in the indicator that is not explained by the latent factor(s)

When the latent factors are uncorrelated, the (standardized) error term for an indicator is calculated as 1 minus the sum of squared standardized factor loadings for a given item (including cross-loadings).

Another class of factor analysis models are higher-order (or hierarchical) factor models and bifactor models. Guidelines in using higher-order factor and bifactor models are discussed by Markon (2019).

Factor analysis is a powerful technique to help identify the factor structure that underlies a measure or construct. As discussed in Section 6.1.4, however, there are many decisions to make in factor analysis, in addition to questions about which variables to use, how to scale the variables, etc. If the variables going into a factor analysis are not well assessed, factor analysis will not rescue the factor structure. In such situations, there is likely to be the problem of garbage in, garbage out. Factor analysis depends on the covariation among variables. Given the extensive method variance that measures have, factor analysis (and principal component analysis) tends to extract method factors. Method factors are factors that are related to the methods being assessed rather than the construct of interest. However, multitrait-multimethod approaches to factor analysis (such as in Section 6.4.2.12) help better partition the variance in variables that reflects method variance versus construct variance, to get more accurate estimates of constructs.

Floyd & Widaman (1995) provide an overview of factor analysis for the development of clinical assessments.

6.1.1 Example Factor Models from Correlation Matrices

Below, we provide some example factor models from various correlation matrices. Analytical examples of factor analysis are presented in Section 6.4.

Consider the example correlation matrix in Figure 6.1. Because all of the correlations are the same ($r = .60$), we expect there is approximately one factor for this pattern of data.

In a single-factor model fit to these data, the factor loadings are .77 and the residual error terms are .40, as depicted in Figure 6.2. The amount of common variance (R^2) that is

	v1	v2	v3	v4	v5	v6
v1	1					
v2	.6	1				
v3	.6	.6	1			
v4	.6	.6	.6	1		
v5	.6	.6	.6	.6	1	
v6	.6	.6	.6	.6	.6	1

FIGURE 6.1 Example Correlation Matrix 1.

accounted for by an indicator is estimated as the square of the standardized loading: $.60 = .77 \times .77$. The amount of error for an indicator is estimated as: error $= 1 -$ common variance, so in this case, the amount of error is: $.40 = 1 - .60$. The proportion of the total variance in indicators that is accounted for by the latent factor is the sum of the square of the standardized loadings divided by the number of indicators. That is, to calculate the proportion of the total variance in the variables that is accounted for by the latent factor, you would square the loadings, sum them up, and divide by the number of variables: $\frac{.77^2+.77^2+.77^2+.77^2+.77^2+.77^2}{6} = \frac{.60+.60+.60+.60+.60+.60}{6} = .60$. Thus, the latent factor accounts for 60% of the variance in the indicators. In this model, the latent factor explains the covariance among the variables. If the answer is simple, a small and parsimonious model should be able to obtain the answer.

Consider a different correlation matrix in Figure 6.3. There is no common variance (correlations between the variables are zero), so there is no reason to believe there is a common factor that influences all of the variables. Variables that are not correlated cannot be related by a third variable, such as a common factor, so a common factor is not the right model.

Consider another correlation matrix in Figure 6.4.

If you try to fit a single factor to this correlation matrix, it generates a factor model depicted in Figure 6.5. In this model, the first three variables have a factor loading of .77, but the remaining three variables have a factor loading of zero. This indicates that three remaining factors likely do not share a common factor with the first three variables.

Therefore, a one-factor model is probably not correct; instead, the structure of the data is probably best represented by a two-factor model, as depicted in Figure 6.6. In the model, Factor 1 explains why measures 1, 2, and 3 are correlated, whereas Factor 2 explains why measures 4, 5, and 6 are correlated. A two-factor model thus explains why measures 1, 2, and 3 are not correlated with measures 4, 5, and 6. In this model, each latent factor accounts for 60% of the variance in the indicators that load onto it: $\frac{.77^2+.77^2+.77^2}{3} = \frac{.60+.60+.60}{3} = .60$. Each latent factor accounts for 30% of the variance in all of the indicators: $\frac{.77^2+.77^2+.77^2+0^2+0^2+0^2}{6} = \frac{.60+.60+.60+0+0+0}{6} = .30$.

Consider another correlation matrix in Figure 6.7.

One way to model these data is depicted in Figure 6.8. In this model, the factor loadings are .77, the residual error terms are .40, and there is a covariance path of .50 for the association between Factor 1 and Factor 2. Going from the model to the correlation matrix is deterministic. If you know the model, you can calculate the correlation matrix. For instance,

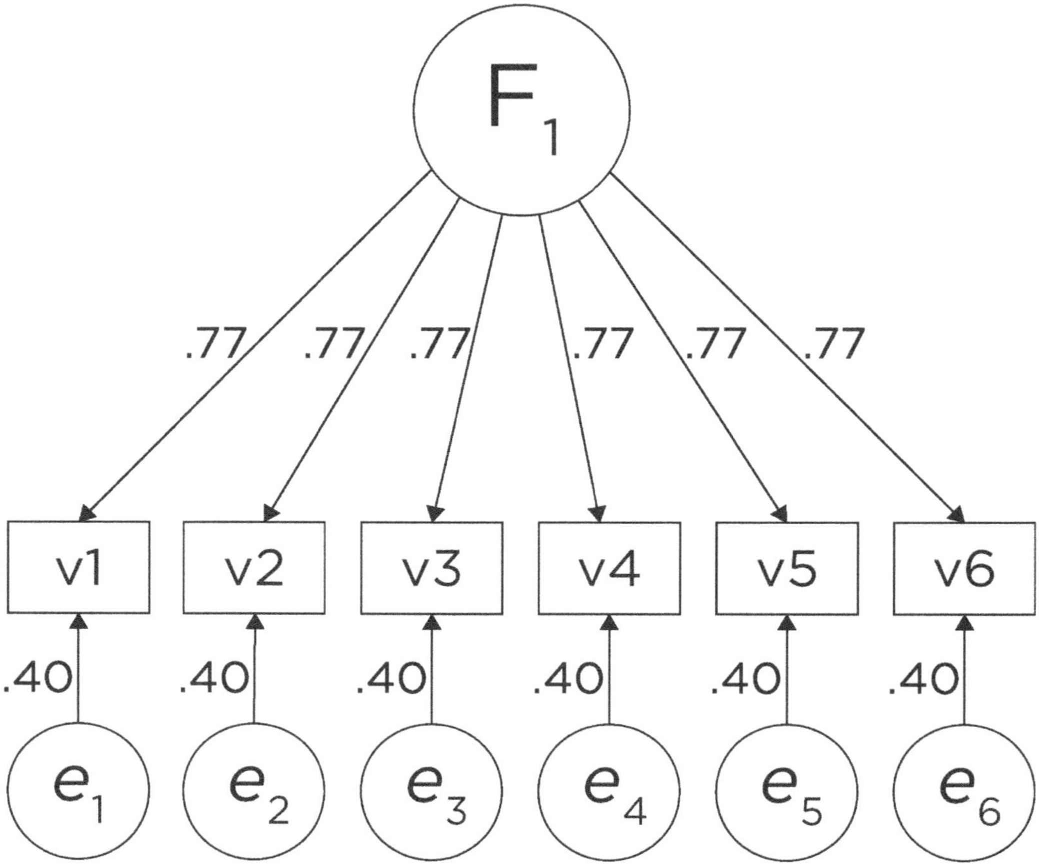

FIGURE 6.2 Example Confirmatory Factor Analysis Model: Unidimensional Model.

	v1	v2	v3	v4	v5	v6
v1	1					
v2	0	1				
v3	0	0	1			
v4	0	0	0	1		
v5	0	0	0	0	1	
v6	0	0	0	0	0	1

FIGURE 6.3 Example Correlation Matrix 2.

	v1	v2	v3	v4	v5	v6
v1	1					
v2	.6	1				
v3	.6	.6	1			
v4	0	0	0	1		
v5	0	0	0	.6	1	
v6	0	0	0	.6	.6	1

FIGURE 6.4 Example Correlation Matrix 3.

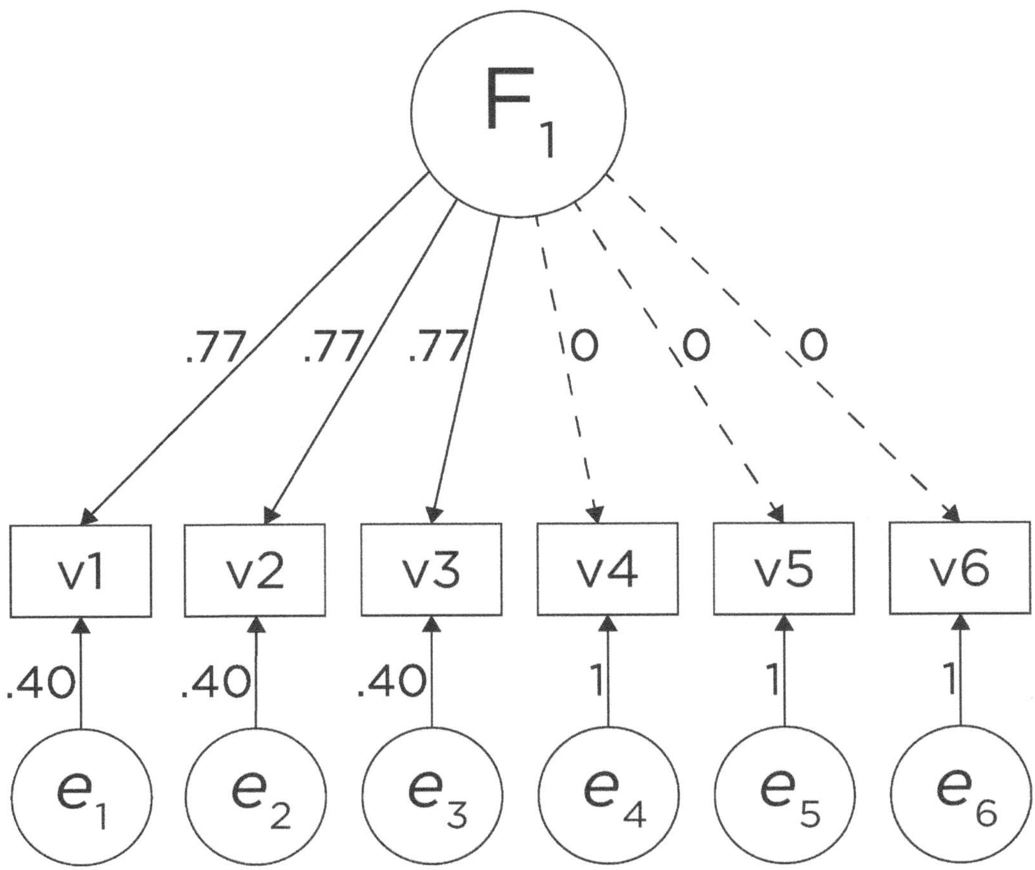

FIGURE 6.5 Example Confirmatory Factor Analysis Model: Multidimensional Model.

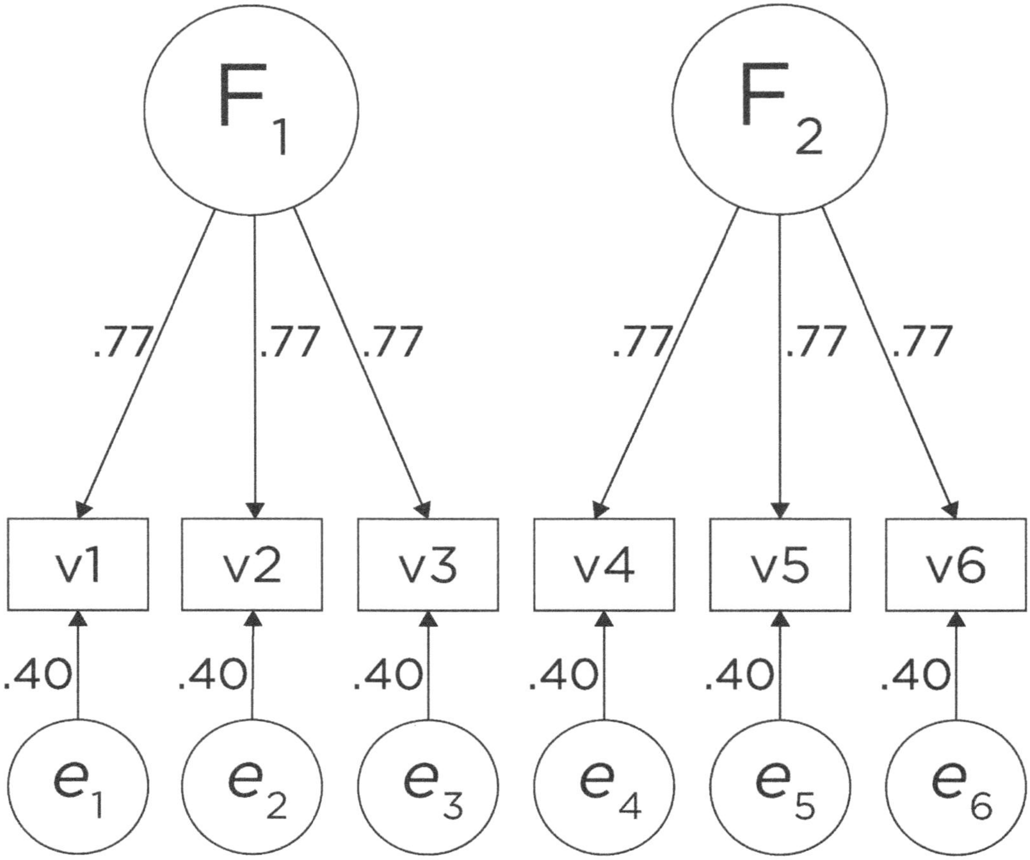

FIGURE 6.6 Example Confirmatory Factor Analysis Model: Two-Factor Model with Uncorrelated Factors.

	v1	v2	v3	v4	v5	v6
v1	1					
v2	.6	1				
v3	.6	.6	1			
v4	.3	.3	.3	1		
v5	.3	.3	.3	.6	1	
v6	.3	.3	.3	.6	.6	1

FIGURE 6.7 Example Correlation Matrix 4.

using path tracing rules (described in Section 3.1), the correlation of measures within a factor in this model is calculated as: $0.60 = .77 \times .77$. Using path tracing rules, the correlation of measures across factors in this model is calculated as: $.30 = .77 \times .50 \times .77$. In this model, each latent factor accounts for 60% of the variance in the indicators that load onto it: $\frac{.77^2+.77^2+.77^2}{3} = \frac{.60+.60+.60}{3} = .60$. Each latent factor accounts for 37% of the variance in all of the indicators: $\frac{.77^2+.77^2+.77^2+(.50^2\times.77^2)+(.50^2\times.77^2)+(.50^2\times.77^2)}{6} = \frac{.60+.60+.60+.15+.15+.15}{6} = .37$.

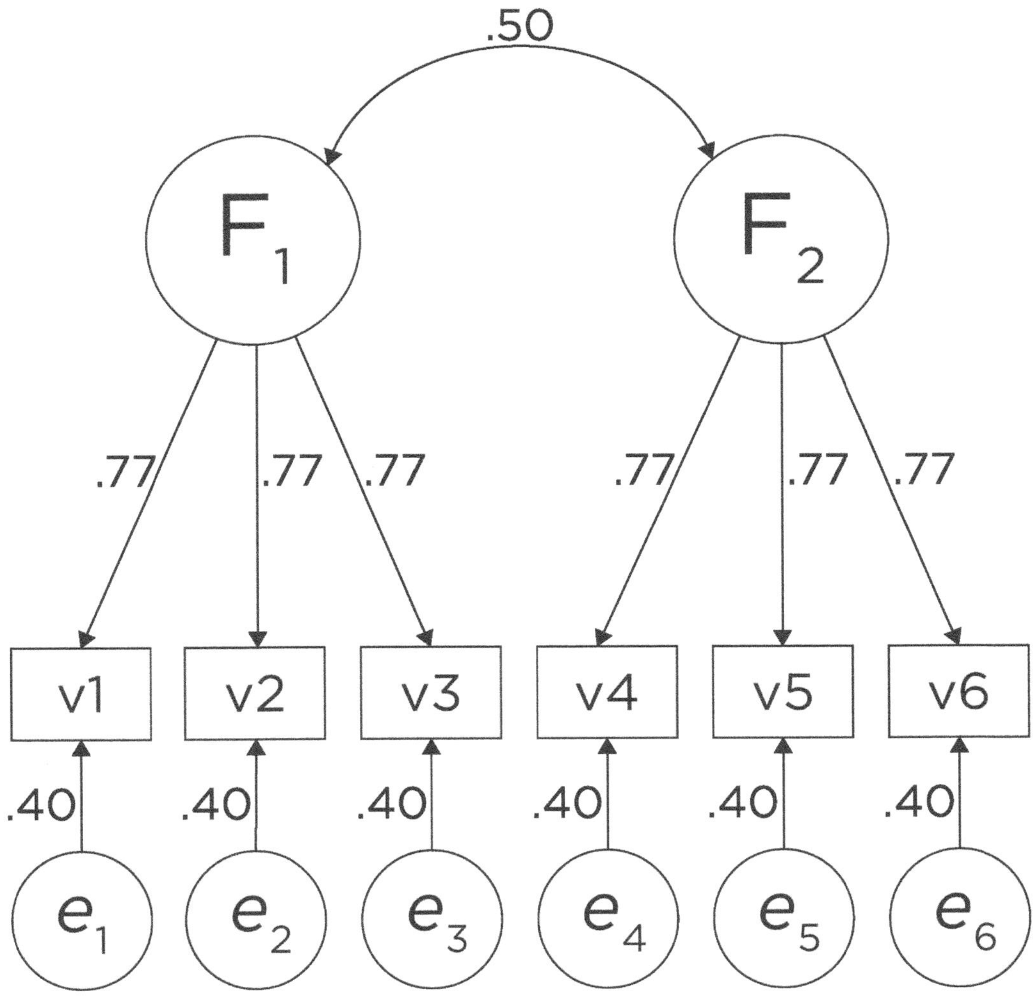

FIGURE 6.8 Example Confirmatory Factor Analysis Model: Two-Factor Model with Correlated Factors.

Although going from the model to the correlation matrix is deterministic, going from the correlation matrix to the model is not deterministic. If you know the correlation matrix, there may be many possible models. For instance, the model could also be the one depicted in Figure 6.9, with factor loadings of .77, residual error terms of .40, a regression path of .50, and a disturbance term of .75. The proportion of variance in Factor 2 that is explained by Factor 1 is calculated as: $.25 = .50 \times .50$. The disturbance term is calculated as $.75 = 1 - (.50 \times .50) = 1 - .25$. In this model, each latent factor accounts for 60% of the variance in the indicators that load onto it: $\frac{.77^2+.77^2+.77^2}{3} = \frac{.60+.60+.60}{3} = .60$. Factor 1 accounts for 15% of the variance in the indicators that load onto Factor 2: $\frac{(.50^2\times.77^2)+(.50^2\times.77^2)+(.50^2\times.77^2)}{3} = \frac{.15+.15+.15}{3} = .15$. This model has the exact same fit as the previous model, but it has different implications. Unlike the previous model, in this model, there is a "causal" pathway from Factor 1 to Factor 2. However, the causal effect of Factor 1 does not account for all of the variance in Factor 2 because the correlation is only .50.

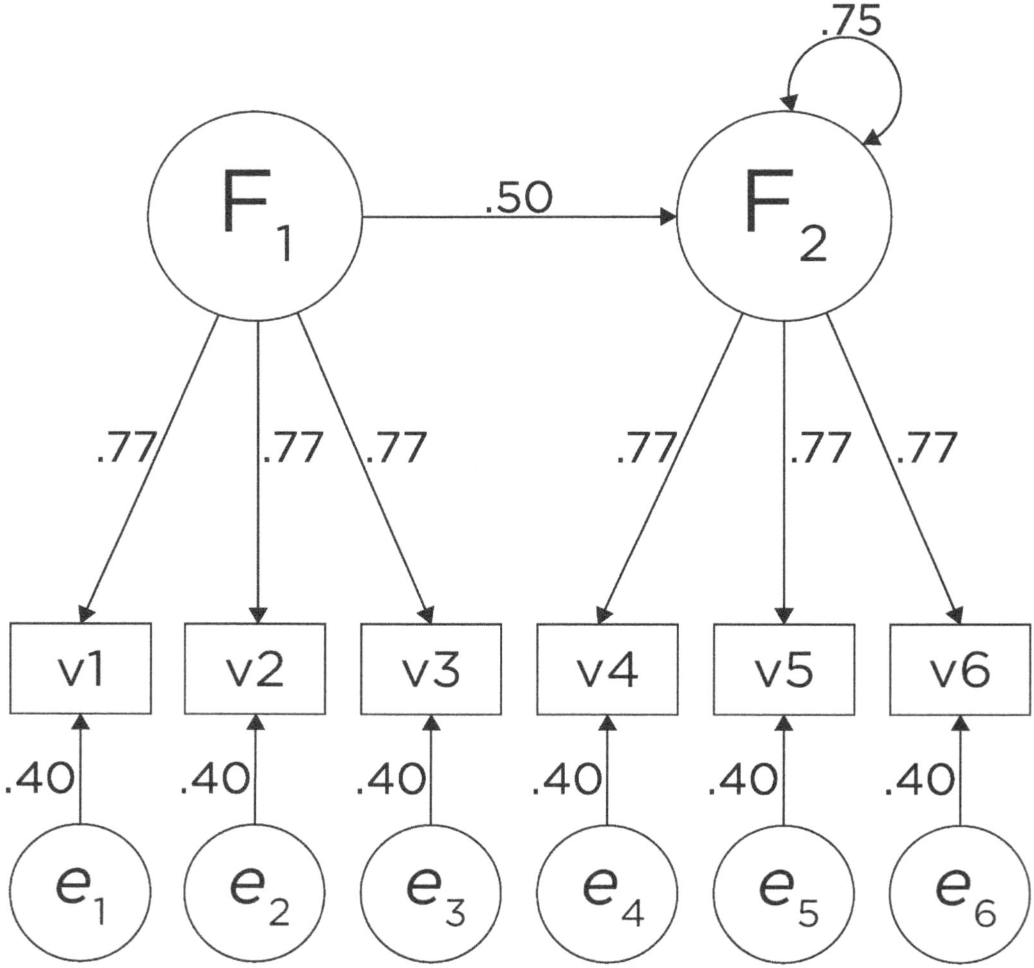

FIGURE 6.9 Example Confirmatory Factor Analysis Model: Two-Factor Model with Regression Path.

Alternatively, something else (e.g., another factor) could be explaining the data that we have not considered, as depicted in Figure 6.10. This is a higher-order factor model, in which there is a higher-order factor (A_1) that influences both lower-order factors, Factor 1 (F_1) and Factor 2 (F_2). The factor loadings from the lower order factors to the manifest variables are .77, the factor loading from the higher-order factor to the lower-order factors is .71, and the residual error terms are .40. This model has the exact same fit as the previous models. The proportion of variance in a lower-order factor (F_1 or F_2) that is explained by the higher-order factor (A_1) is calculated as: $.50 = .71 \times .71$. The disturbance term is calculated as $.50 = 1 - (.71 \times .71) = 1 - .50$. Using path tracing rules, the correlation of measures across factors in this model is calculated as: $.30 = .77 \times .71 \times .71 \times .77$. In this model, the higher-order factor (A_1) accounts for 30% of the variance in the indicators: $\frac{(.77^2 \times .71^2)+(.77^2 \times .71^2)+(.77^2 \times .71^2)+(.77^2 \times .71^2)+(.77^2 \times .71^2)+(.77^2 \times .71^2)}{6} = \frac{.30+.30+.30+.30+.30+.30}{6} = .30$.

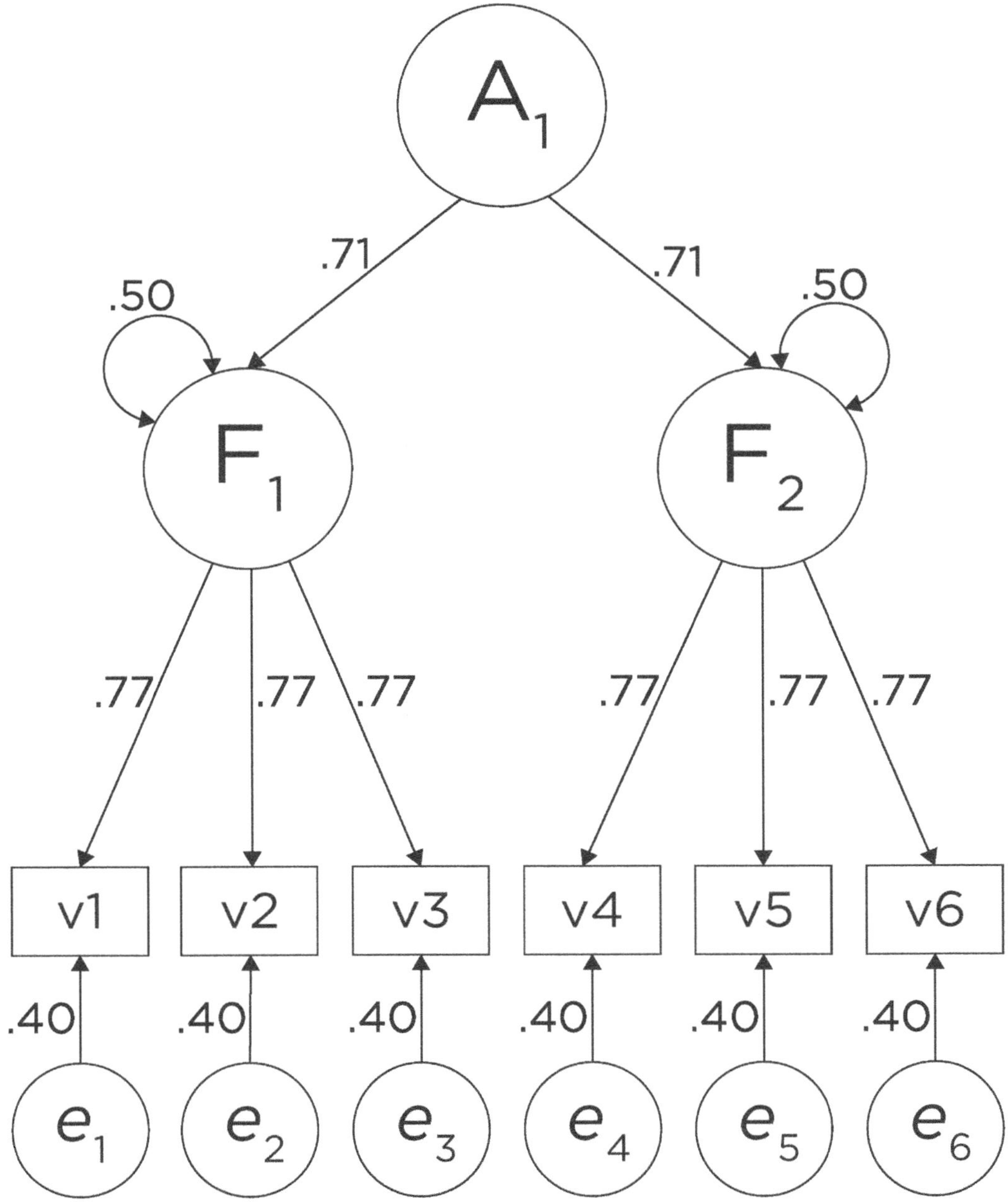

FIGURE 6.10 Example Confirmatory Factor Analysis Model: Higher-Order Factor Model.

Alternatively, there could be a single factor that ties measures 1, 2, and 3 together and measures 4, 5, and 6 together, as depicted in Figure 6.11. In this model, the measures no longer have random error: measures 1, 2, and 3 have correlated residuals—that is, they share error variance; likewise, measures 4, 5, and 6 have correlated residuals. This model has the exact same fit as the previous models. Using path tracing rules, the correlation of measures within a factor in this model is calculated as: $.60 = (.55 \times .55) + (.70 \times .43 \times .70) + (.70 \times .43 \times .43 \times .70)$. The correlation of measures across factors in this model is calculated as: $.30 = .55 \times .55$. In this model, the latent factor accounts for 30% of the variance in the indicators: $\frac{.55^2+.55^2+.55^2+.55^2+.55^2+.55^2}{6} = \frac{.30+.30+.30+.30+.30+.30}{6} = .30$.

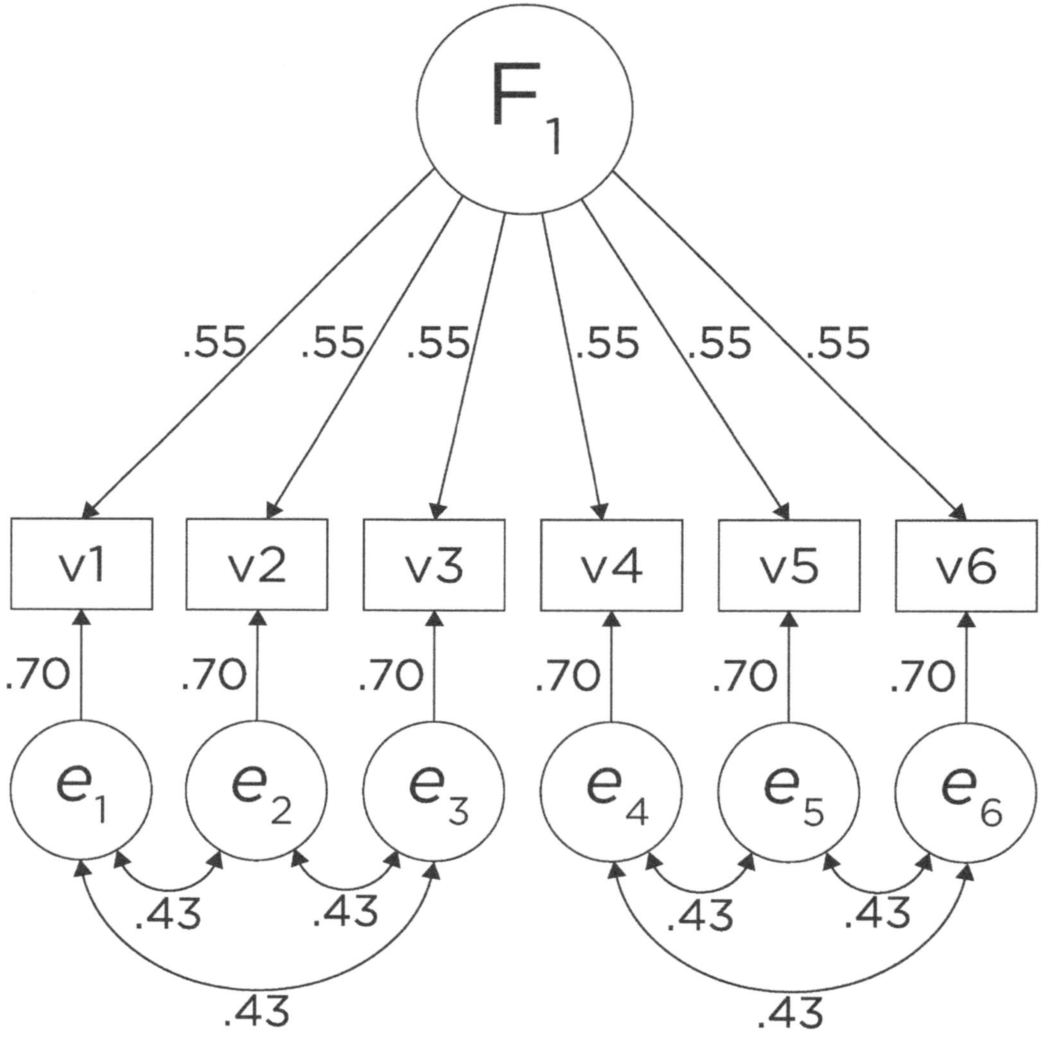

FIGURE 6.11 Example Confirmatory Factor Analysis Model: Unidimensional Model with Correlated Residuals.

6.1.2 Indeterminacy

There could be many more models that have the same fit to the data. Thus, factor analysis has *indeterminacy* because all of these models can explain these same data equally well, with all having different theoretical meaning. The goal of factor analysis is for the model to look at the data and induce the model. However, most data matrices in real life are very complicated—much more complicated than in these examples.

This is why we do not calculate our own factor analysis by hand; use a stats program! It is important to think about the possibility of other models to determine how confident you can be in your data model. For every fully specified factor model—i.e., where the relevant paths are all defined, there is one and only one predictive data matrix (correlation matrix). However, each data matrix can produce many different factor models. There is no way to distinguish which of these factor models is correct from the data matrix alone. Any given data matrix can predict an infinite number of factor models that accurately represent the data structure—so we make decisions that determine what type of factor solution our data will yield.

Many models could explain your data, and there are many more models that do not explain the data. For equally good-fitting models, decide based on interpretability. If you have strong theory, decide based on theory and things outside of factor analysis!

6.1.3 Practical Considerations

There are important considerations for doing factor analysis in real life with complex data. Traditionally, researchers had to consider what kind of data they have, and they often assumed interval-level data even though data in psychology are often not interval data. In the past, factor analysis was not good with categorical and dichotomous (e.g., True/False) data because the variance then is largely determined by the mean. So, we need something more complicated for dichotomous data. More solutions are available now for factor analysis with ordinal and dichotomous data, but it is generally best to have at least four ordered categories to perform factor analysis.

The necessary sample size depends on the complexity of the true factor structure. If there is a strong single factor for 30 items, then $N = 50$ is plenty. But if there are five factors and some correlated errors, then the sample size will need to be closer to ~5,000. Factor analysis can recover the truth when the world is simple. However, nature is often not simple, and it may end in the distortion of nature instead of nature itself.

Recommendations for factor analysis are described by Sellbom & Tellegen (2019).

6.1.4 Decisions To Make in Factor Analysis

There are many decisions to make in factor analysis. These decisions can have important impacts on the resulting solution. Decisions include things such as:

1. What variables to include in the model and how to scale them
2. Method of factor extraction: factor analysis or PCA
3. If factor analysis, the kind of factor analysis: EFA or CFA
4. How many factors to retain
5. If EFA or PCA, whether and how to rotate factors (factor rotation)
6. Model selection and interpretation

6.1.4.1 Variables To Include and their Scaling

The first decision when conducting a factor analysis is which variables to include and the scaling of those variables. What factors (or components) you extract can differ widely depending on what variables you include in the analysis. For example, if you include many variables from the same source (e.g., self-report), it is possible that you will extract a factor that represents the common variance among the variables from that source (i.e., the self-reported variables). This would be considered a method factor, which works against the goal of estimating latent factors that represent the constructs of interest (as opposed to the measurement methods used to estimate those constructs). An additional consideration is the scaling of the variables—whether to use the raw scaling or whether to standardize them to be on a more common metric (e.g., z-score metric with a mean of zero and standard deviation of one).

6.1.4.2 Method of Factor Extraction

The second decision is to select the method of factor extraction. This is the algorithm that is going to try to identify factors. There are two main families of factor or component extraction: analytic or principal components. The principal components approach is called principal component analysis (PCA). PCA is not really a form factor analysis; rather, it is useful for data reduction (Lilienfeld et al., 2015). The analytic family includes factor analysis approaches such as principal axis factoring and maximum likelihood factor analysis. The distinction between factor analysis and PCA is depicted in Figure 6.12.

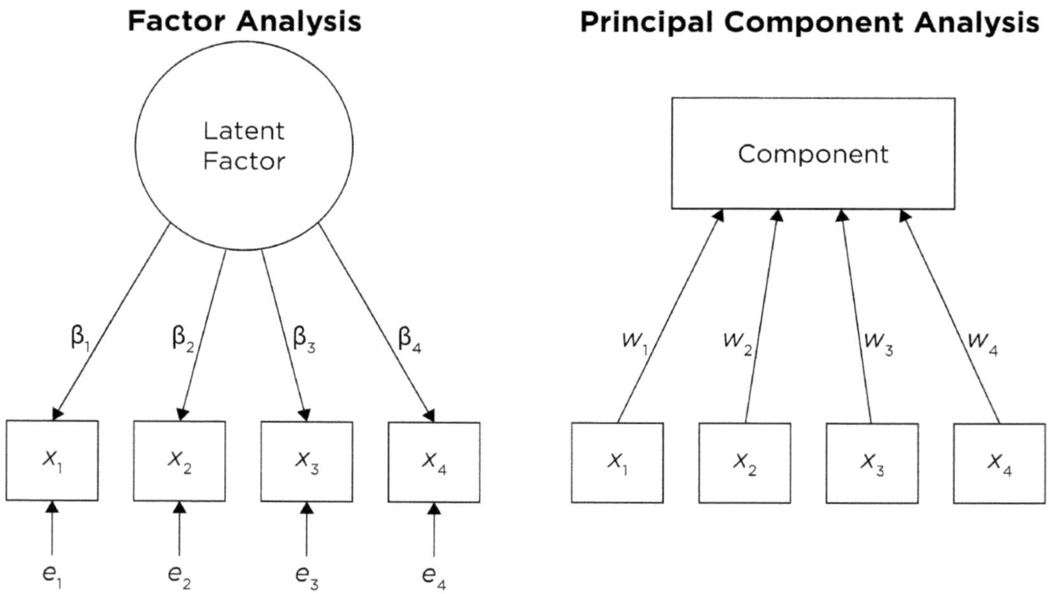

FIGURE 6.12 Distinction Between Factor Analysis and Principal Component Analysis.

6.1.4.2.1 Principal component analysis

Principal component analysis (PCA) is used if you want to reduce your data matrix. PCA composites represent the variances of an observed measure in as economical a fashion as possible, with no latent underlying variables. The goal of PCA is to identify a smaller number of components that explain as much variance in a set of variables as possible. It is an atheoretical way to decompose a matrix. PCA involves decomposition of a data matrix into a set of eigenvectors, which are transformations of the old variables.

The eigenvectors attempt to simplify the data in the matrix. PCA takes the data matrix and identifies the weighted sum of all variables that does the best job at explaining variance: these are the principal components, also called eigenvectors. Principal components reflect optimally weighted sums. In this way, PCA is a formative model (by contrast, factor analysis applies a reflective model).

PCA decomposes the data matrix into any number of components—as many as the number of variables, which will always account for all variance. After the model is fit, you can look at the results and discard the components which likely reflect error variance. Judgments about which factors to retain are based on empirical criteria in conjunction with theory to select a parsimonious number of components that account for the majority of variance.

The eigenvalue reflects the amount of variance explained by the component (eigenvector). When using a varimax (orthogonal) rotation, an eigenvalue for a component is calculated as the sum of squared standardized component loadings on that component. When using oblique rotation, however, the items explain more variance than is attributable to their factor loadings because the factors are correlated.

PCA pulls the first principal component out (i.e., the eigenvector that explains the most variance) and makes a new data matrix: i.e., new correlation matrix. Then the PCA pulls out the component that explains the next most variance—i.e., the eigenvector with the next largest eigenvalue, and it does this for all components, equal to the same number of variables. For instance, if there are six variables, it will iteratively extract an additional component up to six components. You can extract as many eigenvectors as there are variables. If you extract all six components, the data matrix left over will be the same as the correlation matrix in Figure 6.3. That is, the remaining variables will be entirely uncorrelated with the remaining variables, because six components explain 100% of the variance from six variables. In other words, you can explain (6) variables with (6) new things!

However, it does no good if you have to use all (6) components because there is no data reduction from the original number of variables, but hopefully the first few components will explain most of the variance.

The sum of all eigenvalues is equal to the number of variables in the analysis. PCA does not have the same assumptions as factor analysis, which assumes that measures are partly from common variance and error. But if you estimate (6) eigenvectors and only keep (2), the model is a two-component model and whatever left becomes error. Therefore, PCA does not have the same assumptions as factor analysis, but it often ends up in the same place.

Most people who want to conduct a factor analysis use PCA, but PCA is not really factor analysis (Lilienfeld et al., 2015). PCA is what SPSS can do quickly. But computers are so fast now—just do a real factor analysis! Factor analysis better handles error than PCA—factor analysis assumes that what is in the variable is the combination of common construct variance and error. By contrast, PCA assumes that the measures have no measurement error.

6.1.4.2.2 Factor analysis

Factor analysis is an analytic approach to factor extraction. Factor analysis is a special case of structural equation modeling (SEM). Factor analysis is an analytic technique that is interested in the factor structure of a measure or set of measures. Factor analysis is a theoretical approach that considers that there are latent theoretical constructs that influence the scores on particular variables. It assumes that part of the explanation for each variable is shared between variables, and that part of it is unique variance. The unique variance is considered error. The common variance is called the communality, which is the factor variance. Communality of a factor is estimated using the average variance extracted (AVE). The amount of variance due to error is: 1 – communality. There are several types of factor analysis, including principal axis factoring and maximum likelihood factor analysis.

Factor analysis can be used to test measurement/factorial invariance and for multitrait-multimethod designs. One example of a MTMM model in factor analysis is the correlated traits correlated methods model (Tackett, Lang, et al., 2019).

There are several differences between (real) factor analysis versus PCA. Factor analysis has greater sophistication than PCA, but greater sophistication often results in greater assumptions. Factor analysis does not always work; the data may not always fit to a factor analysis model; therefore, use PCA as a second/last option. PCA can decompose any data matrix; it always works. PCA is okay if you are not interested in the factor structure. PCA uses all variance of variables and assumes variables have no error, so it does not account for measurement error. PCA is good if you just want to form a linear composite and if the causal structure is formative (rather than reflective). However, if you are interested in the factor structure, use factor analysis, which estimates a latent variable that accounts for the common variance and discards error variance. Factor analysis is useful for the identification of latent constructs—i.e., underlying dimensions or factors that explain (cause) scores on items.

6.1.4.3 EFA or CFA

A third decision is the kind of factor analysis to use: exploratory factor analysis (EFA) or confirmatory factor analysis (CFA).

6.1.4.3.1 Exploratory factor analysis

Exploratory factor analysis (EFA) is used if you have no a priori hypotheses about the factor structure of the model, but you would like to understand the latent variables represented by your items.

EFA is partly induced from the data. You feed in the data and let the program build the factor model. You can set some parameters going in, including how to extract or rotate the factors. The factors are extracted from the data without specifying the number and pattern of loadings between the items and the latent factors (Bollen, 2002). All cross-loadings are freely estimated.

6.1.4.3.2 Confirmatory factor analysis

Confirmatory Factor Analysis (CFA) is used to confirm a priori hypotheses about the factor structure of the model. CFA is a test of the hypothesis. In CFA, you specify the model and ask how well this model represents the data. The researcher specifies the number, meaning, associations, and pattern of free parameters in the factor loading matrix (Bollen, 2002). A key advantage of CFA is the ability to directly compare alternative models (i.e., factor structures), which is valuable for theory testing (Strauss & Smith, 2009). For instance, you could use CFA to test whether the variance in several measures' scores is best explained with one factor or two factors. In CFA, cross-loadings are not estimated unless the researcher specifies them.

6.1.4.3.3 Exploratory structural equation modeling

In real life, there is not a clear distinction between EFA and CFA. In CFA, researchers often set only half of the constraints, and let the data fill in the rest. In EFA, researchers often set constraints and assumptions. Thus, the line between EFA and CFA is often blurred.

EFA and CFA can be considered special cases of exploratory structural equation modeling (ESEM), which combines features of EFA, CFA, and SEM (Marsh et al., 2014). ESEM can include any combination of exploratory (i.e., EFA) and confirmatory (CFA) factors. ESEM, unlike traditional CFA models, typically estimates all cross-loadings—at least for the exploratory factors. If a CFA model without cross-loadings and correlated residuals fits as well as an ESEM model with all cross-loadings, the CFA model should be retained for its simplicity. However, ESEM models often fit better than CFA models because requiring no cross-loadings is an unrealistic expectation of items from many psychological instruments (Marsh et al., 2014). The correlations between factors tend to be positively biased when fitting CFA models without cross-loadings, which leads to challenges in using CFA to establish discriminant validity (Marsh et al., 2014). Thus, compared to CFA, ESEM has the potential to more accurately estimate factor correlations and establish discriminant validity (Marsh et al., 2014). Moreover, ESEM can be useful in a multitrait-multimethod framework. We provide examples of ESEM in Section 6.4.3.

6.1.4.4 How Many Factors To Retain

A goal of factor analysis and PCA is simplification or parsimony, while still explaining as much variance as possible. The hope is that you can have fewer factors that explain the associations between the variables than the number of observed variables. But how do you decide on the number of factors (in factor analysis) or components (in PCA)?

There are a number of criteria that one can use to help determine how many factors/components to keep:

- Kaiser-Guttman criterion: in PCA, components with eigenvalues greater than 1 or, for factor analysis, factors with eigenvalues greater than zero
- Cattell's scree test: the "elbow" in a scree plot minus one; sometimes operationalized with optimal coordinates (OC) or the acceleration factor (AF)
- Parallel analysis: factors that explain more variance than randomly simulated data
- Very simple structure (VSS) criterion: larger is better
- Velicer's minimum average partial (MAP) test: smaller is better
- Akaike information criterion (AIC): smaller is better
- Bayesian information criterion (BIC): smaller is better
- Sample size-adjusted BIC (SABIC): smaller is better
- Root mean square error of approximation (RMSEA): smaller is better
- Chi-square difference test: smaller is better; a significant test indicates that the more complex model is significantly better fitting than the less complex model
- Standardized root mean square residual (SRMR): smaller is better
- Comparative Fit Index (CFI): larger is better
- Tucker Lewis Index (TLI): larger is better

There is not necessarily a "correct" criterion to use in determining how many factors to keep, so it is generally recommended that researchers use multiple criteria in combination with theory and interpretability.

A scree plot from a factor analysis or PCA provides lots of information. A scree plot has the factor number on the x-axis and the eigenvalue on the y-axis. The eigenvalue is the variance accounted for by a factor; when using a varimax (orthogonal) rotation, an eigenvalue (or factor variance) is calculated as the sum of squared standardized factor (or component) loadings on that factor. An example of a scree plot is in Figure 6.13.

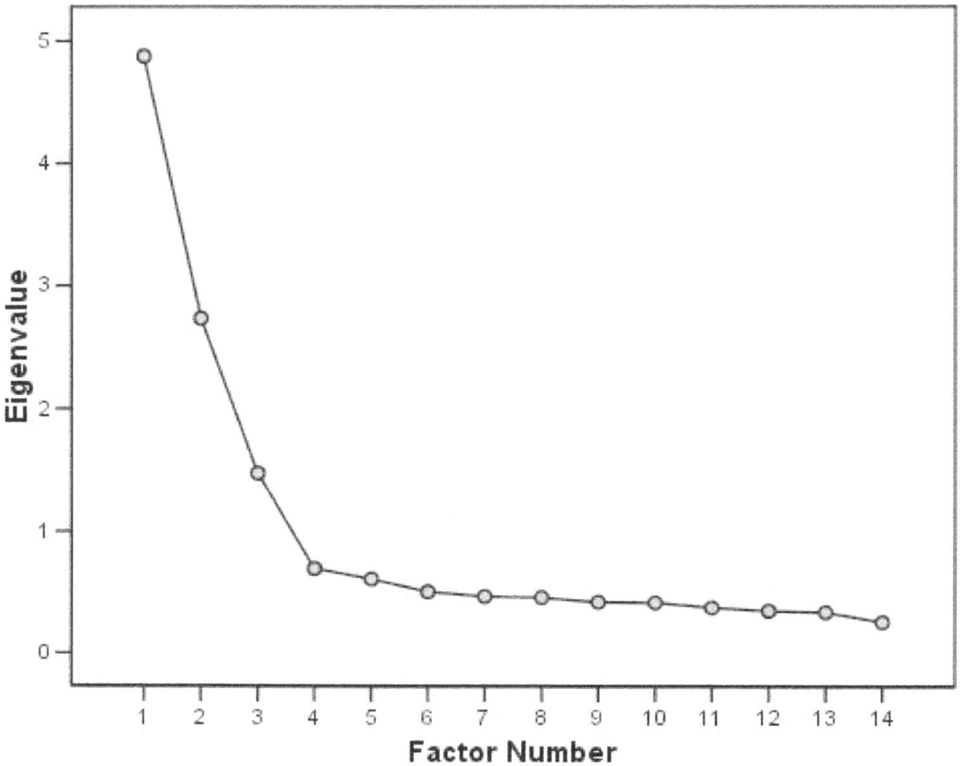

FIGURE 6.13 Example of a Scree Plot.

The total variance is equal to the number of variables you have, so one eigenvalue is approximately one variable's worth of variance. In a factor analysis and PCA, the first factor (or component) accounts for the most variance, the second factor accounts for the second-most variance, and so on. The more factors you add, the less variance is explained by the additional factor.

One criterion for how many factors to keep is the Kaiser-Guttman criterion. According to the Kaiser-Guttman criterion, you should keep any factors whose eigenvalue is greater than 1. That is, for the sake of simplicity, parsimony, and data reduction, you should take any factors that explain more than a single variable would explain. According to the Kaiser-Guttman criterion, we would keep three factors from Figure 6.13 that have eigenvalues greater than 1. The default in SPSS is to retain factors with eigenvalues greater than 1. However, keeping factors whose eigenvalue is greater than 1 is not the most correct rule. If you let SPSS do this, you may get many factors with eigenvalues around 1 (e.g., factors with an eigenvalue ~ 1.0001) that are not adding so much that it is worth the added complexity. The Kaiser-Guttman criterion usually results in keeping too many factors. Factors with small eigenvalues around 1 could reflect error shared across variables. For instance, factors with small eigenvalues could reflect method variance (i.e., method factor), such as a self-report factor that turns up as a factor in factor analysis, but that may be useless to you as a conceptual factor of a construct of interest.

Another criterion is Cattell's scree test, which involves selecting the number of factors from looking at the scree plot. "Scree" refers to the rubble of stones at the bottom of a mountain. According to Cattell's scree test, you should keep the factors before the last steep drop in eigenvalues—i.e., the factors before the rubble, where the slope approaches zero. The beginning of the scree (or rubble), where the slope approaches zero, is called the "elbow" of a scree plot. Using Cattell's scree test, you retain the number of factors that explain the most variance prior to the explained variance drop-off, because, ultimately, you want to include only as many factors in which you gain substantially more by the inclusion of these factors. That is, you would keep the number of factors at the elbow of the scree plot minus one. If the last steep drop occurs from Factor 4 to Factor 5 and the elbow is at Factor 5, we would keep four factors. In Figure 6.13, the last steep drop in eigenvalues occurs from Factor 3 to Factor 4; the elbow of the scree plot occurs at Factor 4. We would keep the number of factors at the elbow minus one. Thus, using Cattell's scree test, we would keep three factors based on Figure 6.13.

There are more sophisticated ways of using a scree plot, but they usually end up at a similar decision. Examples of more sophisticated tests include parallel analysis and very simple structure (VSS) plots. In a parallel analysis, you examine where the eigenvalues from observed data and random data converge, so you do not retain a factor that explains less variance than would be expected by random chance. A parallel analysis can be helpful when you have many variables and one factor accounts for the majority of the variance such that the elbow is at Factor 2 (which would result in keeping one factor), but you have theoretical reasons to select more than one factor. An example in which parallel analysis may be helpful is with neurophysiological data. For instance, parallel analysis can be helpful when conducting temporo-spatial PCA of event-related potential (ERP) data in which you want to separate multiple time windows and multiple spatial locations despite a predominant signal during a given time window and spatial location (Dien, 2012).

In general, my recommendation is to use Cattell's scree test, and then test the factor solutions with plus or minus one factor. You should never accept PCA components with eigenvalues less than one (or factors with eigenvalues less than zero), because they are likely to be largely composed of error. If you are using maximum likelihood factor analysis, you can compare the fit of various models with model fit criteria to see which model fits best for its parsimony. A model will always fit better when you add additional parameters or factors, so you examine if there is *significant* improvement in model fit when adding the additional factor—that is, we keep adding complexity until additional complexity does not buy us much. Always try a factor solution that is one less and one more than suggested by Cattell's scree test to buffer your final solution because the purpose of factor analysis is to explain things and to have interpretability. Even if all rules or indicators suggest to keep X number of factors, maybe $\pm$ one factor helps clarify things. Even though factor analysis is empirical, theory and interpretatability should also inform decisions.

6.1.4.5 Factor Rotation

The next step if using EFA or PCA is, possibly, to rotate the factors to make them more interpretable and simple, which is the whole goal. To interpret the results of a factor analysis, we examine the factor matrix. The columns refer to the different factors; the rows refer to the different observed variables. The cells in the table are the factor loadings—they are basically the correlation between the variable and the factor. Our goal is to achieve a model with simple structure because it is easily interpretable. *Simple structure* means that every variable loads perfectly on one and only one factor, as operationalized by a matrix of factor loadings with values of one and zero and nothing else. An example of a factor matrix that follows simple structure is depicted in Figure 6.14.

	Factor		
Variable	1	2	3
1	1	0	0
2	1	0	0
3	1	0	0
4	1	0	0
5	0	1	0
6	0	1	0
7	0	0	1
8	0	0	1

FIGURE 6.14 Example of a Factor Matrix That Follows Simple Structure.

An example of a measurement model that follows simple structure is depicted in Figure 6.15. Each variable loads onto one and only one factor, which makes it easy to interpret the meaning of each factor, because a given factor represents the common variance among the items that load onto it.

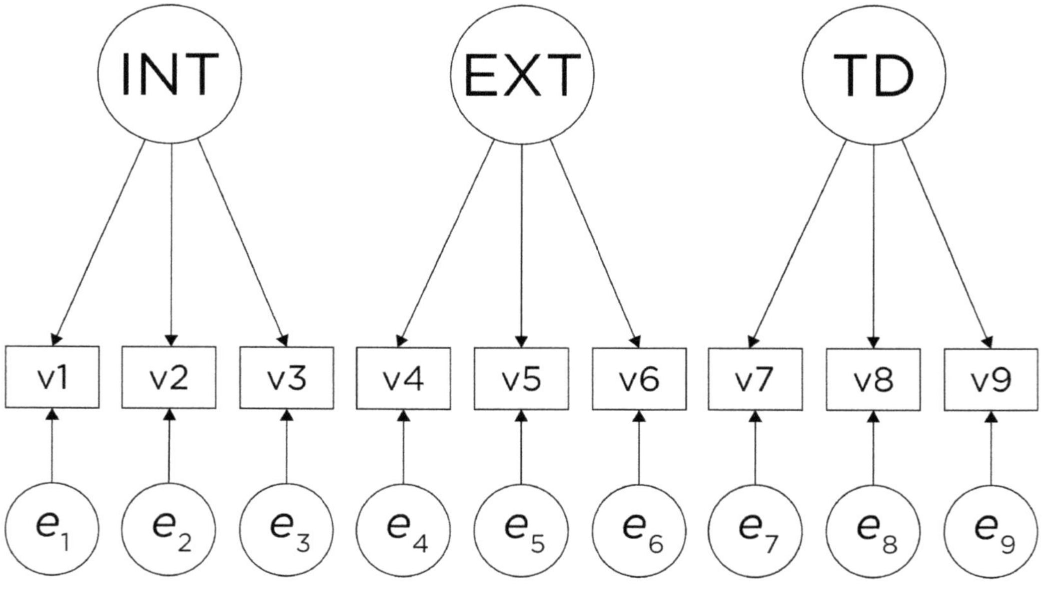

FIGURE 6.15 Example of a Measurement Model That Follows Simple Structure. INT = internalizing problems; EXT = externalizing problems; TD = thought-disordered problems.

However, pure simple structure only occurs in simulations, not in real-life data. In reality, our measurement model in an unrotated factor analysis model might look like the model in Figure 6.16. In this example, the measurement model does not show simple structure because the items have cross-loadings—that is, the items load onto more than one factor. The cross-loadings make it difficult to interpret the factors, because all of the items load onto all of the factors, so the factors are not very distinct from each other, which makes it difficult to interpret what the factors mean.

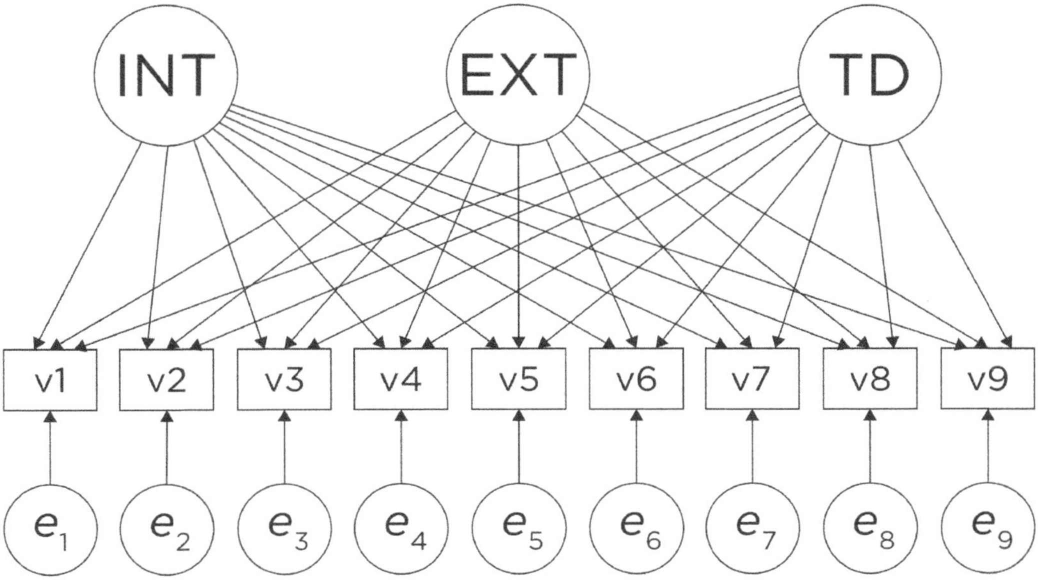

FIGURE 6.16 Example of a Measurement Model That Does Not Follow Simple Structure. INT = internalizing problems; EXT = externalizing problems; TD = thought-disordered problems.

As a result of the challenges of intepretability caused by cross-loadings, factor rotations are often performed. An example of an unrotated factor matrix is in Figure 6.17.

	Factor	
Variable	1	2
1	.50	.50
2	.45	.40
3	.40	.45
4	-.40	.50
5	-.50	.50
6	-.55	.40

FIGURE 6.17 Example of a Factor Matrix.

In the example factor matrix in Figure 6.17, the factor analysis is not very helpful—it tells us very little because it did not distinguish between the two factors. The variables have similar loadings on Factor 1 and Factor 2. An example of a unrotated factor solution is in Figure 6.18. In the figure, all of the variables are in the midst of the quadrants—they are not on the factors' axes. Thus, the factors are not very informative.

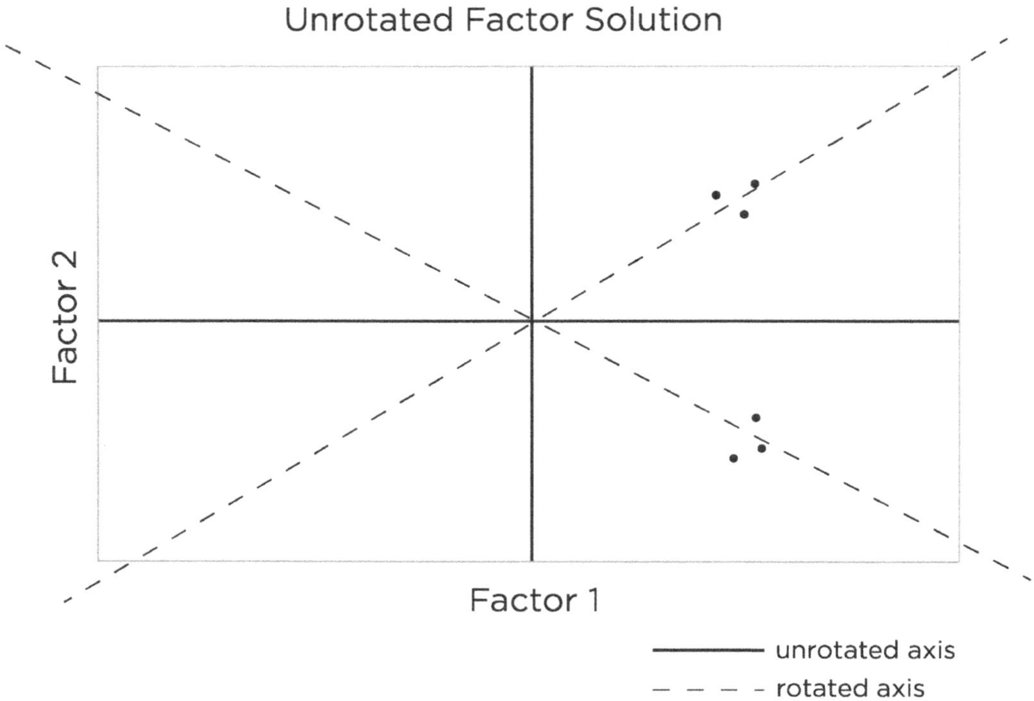

FIGURE 6.18 Example of an Unrotated Factor Solution.

As a result, to improve the interpretability of the factor analysis, we can do what is called rotation. *Rotation* involves changing the orientation of the factors by changing the axes so that variables end up with very high (close to one or negative one) or very low (close to zero) loadings, so that it is clear which factors include which variables. That is, it tries to identify the ideal solution (factor) for each variable. It searches for simple structure and keeps searching until it finds a minimum. After rotation, if the rotation was successful for imposing simple structure, each factor will have loadings close to one (or negative one) for some variables and close to zero for other variables. The goal of factor rotation is to achieve simple structure, to help make it easier to interpret the meaning of the factors. To perform factor rotation, orthogonal rotations are often used. Orthogonal rotations make the rotated factors uncorrelated. An example of a commonly used orthogonal rotation is varimax rotation.

An example of a factor matrix following an orthogonal rotation is depicted in Figure 6.19. An example of a factor solution following an orthogonal rotation is depicted in Figure 6.20.

An example of a factor matrix from SPSS following an orthogonal rotation is depicted in Figure 6.21.

An example of a factor structure from an orthogonal rotation is shown in Figure 6.22.

Sometimes, however, the two factors and their constituent variables may be correlated. Examples of two correlated factors may be depression and anxiety. When the two factors are correlated in reality, if we make them uncorrelated, this would result in an inaccurate model. Oblique rotation allows for factors to be correlated, but if the factors have low correlation (e.g., .2 or less), you can likely continue with orthogonal rotation. An example

	Factor	
Variable	1	2
1	.90	-.03
2	.85	.01
3	.95	.05
4	.05	.90
5	-.03	.92
6	-.05	.80

FIGURE 6.19 Example of a Rotated Factor Matrix.

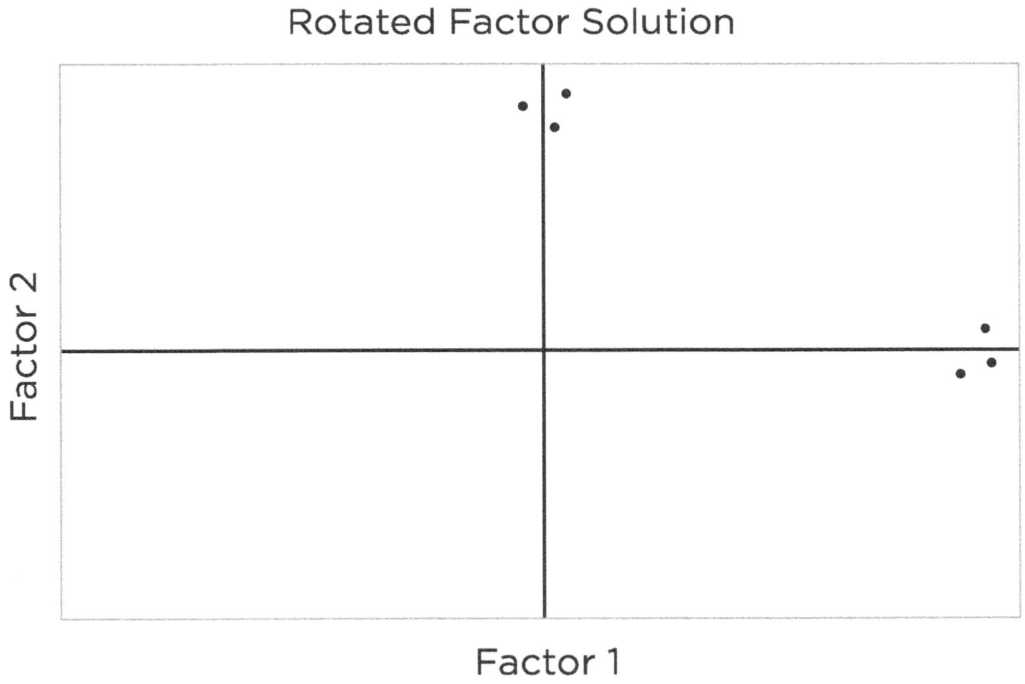

FIGURE 6.20 Example of a Rotated Factor Solution.

	Factor		
	1	2	3
Long distance last month	.062	-.121	.854
Toll free last month	.726	.018	.191
Equipment last month	.067	.831	.049
Calling card last month	.348	-.012	.431
Wireless last month	.530	.637	.146
Multiple lines	-.025	.384	.438
Voice mail	.455	.539	.054
Paging service	.468	.566	.044
Internet	-.049	.722	-.045
Caller ID	.787	.056	.008
Call waiting	.779	.033	.054
Call forwarding	.768	.062	.048
3-way calling	.743	.050	.078
Electronic billing	-.107	.686	-.080

FIGURE 6.21 Example of a Rotated Factor Matrix from SPSS.

of a factor structure from an oblique rotation is in Figure 6.23. Results from an oblique rotation are more complicated than orthogonal rotation—they provide lots of output and are more complicated to interpret. In addition, oblique rotation might not yield a smooth answer if you have a relatively small sample size.

As an example of rotation based on interpretability, consider the Five-Factor Model of Personality (the Big Five), which goes by the acronym, OCEAN: **O**penness, **C**onscientiousness, **E**xtraversion, **A**greeableness, and **N**euroticism. Although the five factors of personality are somewhat correlated, we can use rotation to ensure they are maximally independent. Upon rotation, extraversion and neuroticism are essentially uncorrelated, as depicted in Figure 6.24. The other pole of extraversion is intraversion and the other pole of neuroticism might be emotional stability or calmness.

Simple structure is achieved when each variable loads highly onto as few factors as possible (i.e., each item has only one significant or primary loading). Often this is not the case, so we choose our rotation method in order to decide if the factors can be correlated (an oblique rotation) or if the factors will be uncorrelated (an orthogonal rotation). If the factors are not correlated with each other, use an orthogonal rotation. The correlation between an item and a factor is a factor loading, which is simply a way to ask how much a variable is correlated with the underlying factor. However, its interpretation is more complicated if there are correlated factors!

An orthogonal rotation (e.g., varimax) can help with simplicity of interpretation because it seeks to yield simple structure without cross-loadings. Cross-loadings are instances where a variable loads onto multiple factors. My recommendation would always be to use an orthogonal rotation if you have reason to believe that finding simple structure in your data is possible; otherwise, the factors are extremely difficult to interpret—what exactly does a cross-loading even mean? However, you should always try an oblique rotation, too, to see how strongly the factors are correlated. Examples of oblique rotations include oblimin and promax.

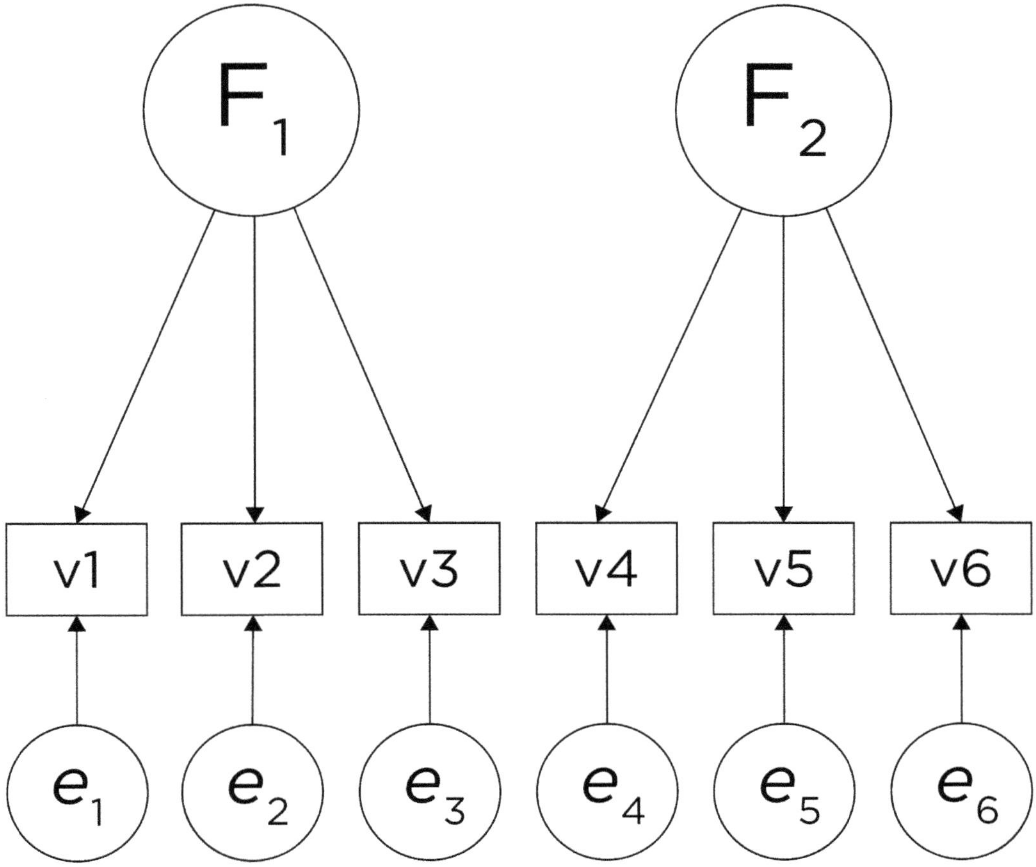

FIGURE 6.22 Example of a Factor Structure from an Orthogonal Rotation.

6.1.4.6 Model Selection and Interpretation

The next step of factor analysis is selecting and interpreting the model. One data matrix can lead to many different (correct) models—you must choose one based on the factor structure and theory. Use theory to interpret the model and label the factors. When interpreting others' findings, do not rely just on the factor labels—look at the actual items to determine what they assess. What they are called matters much less than what the actual items are!

6.1.5 The Downfall of Factor Analysis

The downfall of factor analysis is cross-validation. Cross-validating a factor structure would mean getting the same factor structure with a new sample. We want factor structures to show good replicability across samples. However, cross-validation often falls apart. The way to attempt to replicate a factor structure in an independent sample is to use CFA to set everything up and test the hypothesized factor structure in the independent sample.

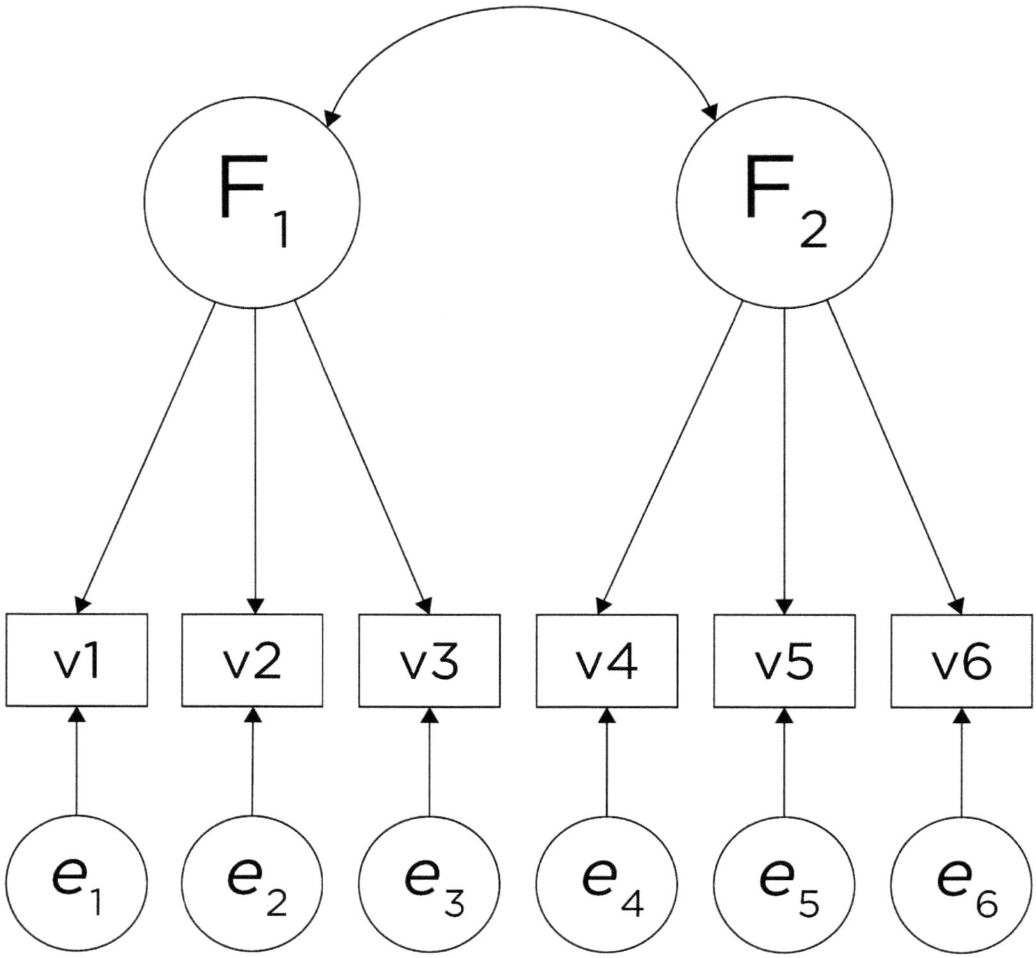

FIGURE 6.23 Example of a Factor Structure from an Oblique Rotation.

6.1.6 What to Do with Factors

What can you do with factors once you have them? In SEM, factors have meaning. You can use them as predictors, mediators, moderators, or outcomes. And, using latent factors in SEM helps disattenuate associations for measurement error, as described in Section 4.6.2. People often want to use factors outside of SEM, but there is confusion here: When researchers find that three variables load onto Factor A, the researchers often combine those three using a sum or average—but this is not accurate. If you just add or average them, this ignores the factor loadings and the error. Another solution is to form a linear composite by adding and weighting the variables by the factor loadings, which retains the differences in correlations (i.e., a weighted sum), but this still ignores the estimated error, so it still may not be generalizable and meaningful. At the same time, weighted sums may be less generalizable than unit-weighted composites where each variable is given equal weight because some variability in factor loadings likely reflects sampling error.

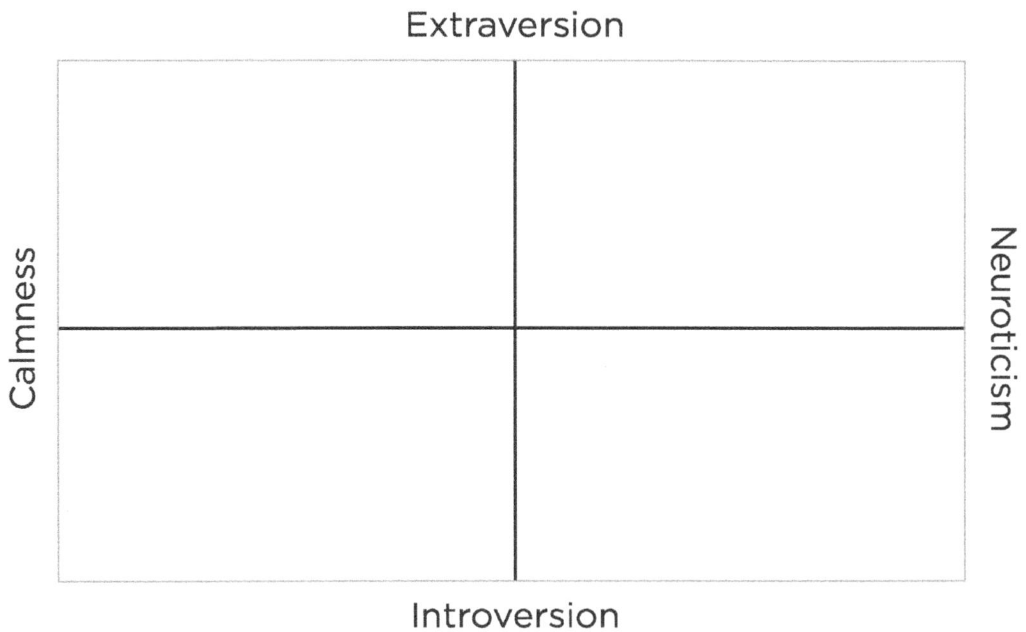

FIGURE 6.24 Example of a Factor Rotation of Neuroticism and Extraversion.

6.1.7 Missing Data Handling

The PCA default in SPSS is listwise deletion of missing data: if a participant is missing data on any variable, the subject gets excluded from the analysis, so you might end up with too few participants. Instead, use a correlation matrix with pairwise deletion for PCA with missing data. Maximum likelihood factor analysis can make use of all available data points for a participant, even if they are missing some data points. Mplus, which is often used for SEM and factor analysis, will notify you if you are removing many participants in CFA/EFA. The `lavaan` package (Rosseel et al., 2022) in `R` also notifies you if you are removing participants in CFA/SEM models.

6.2 Getting Started

6.2.1 Load Libraries

```
library("petersenlab")
library("lavaan")
library("psych")
library("corrplot")
library("nFactors")
library("semPlot")
library("lavaan")
```

```
library("semTools")
library("dagitty")
library("MOTE")
library("here")
library("tidyverse")
library("tinytex")
library("knitr")
library("kableExtra")
library("rmarkdown")
library("bookdown")
```

6.2.2 Prepare Data and Add Missing Data

Adding missing data to dataframes helps make examples more realistic to real-life data and helps you get in the habit of programming to account for missing data.

`HolzingerSwineford1939` is a data set from the `lavaan` package (Rosseel et al., 2022) that contains mental ability test scores (`x1`–`x9`) for seventh- and eighth-grade children.

```
set.seed(52242)

varNames <- names(HolzingerSwineford1939)
dimensionsDf <- dim(HolzingerSwineford1939)
unlistedDf <- unlist(HolzingerSwineford1939)
unlistedDf[sample(
  1:length(unlistedDf),
  size = .15 * length(unlistedDf))] <- NA
HolzingerSwineford1939 <- as.data.frame(matrix(
  unlistedDf,
  ncol = dimensionsDf[2]))
names(HolzingerSwineford1939) <- varNames
vars <- c("x1","x2","x3","x4","x5","x6","x7","x8","x9")
```

6.3 Descriptive Statistics and Correlations

Before conducting a factor analysis, it is important to examine descriptive statistics and correlations among variables.

6.3.1 Descriptive Statistics

Descriptive statistics are presented in Table 6.1.

TABLE 6.1 Descriptive Statistics.

	x1	x2	x3	x4	x5	x6	x7	x8	x9
n	251.00	265.00	255.00	252.00	259.00	248.00	266.00	259.00	257.00
missingness	16.61	11.96	15.28	16.28	13.95	17.61	11.63	13.95	14.62
M	4.97	6.05	2.22	3.12	4.34	2.16	4.17	5.51	5.39
SD	1.16	1.16	1.13	1.18	1.28	1.03	1.07	1.02	1.02
min	1.67	2.25	0.38	0.00	1.00	0.14	1.30	3.05	2.78
max	8.50	9.25	4.50	6.33	6.75	6.14	7.26	10.00	9.25
skewness	−0.11	0.51	0.41	0.23	−0.39	0.84	0.23	0.52	0.24
kurtosis	0.06	0.45	−0.91	0.09	−0.59	1.12	−0.39	1.38	0.28

6.3.2 Correlations

Correlation matrices of various types using the `cor.table()` from the `petersenlab` package (Petersen, 2024) are in Tables 6.2, 6.3, and 6.4.

```
cor.table(
  HolzingerSwineford1939[,vars],
  dig = 2)

cor.table(
  HolzingerSwineford1939[,vars],
  type = "manuscript",
  dig = 2)

cor.table(
  HolzingerSwineford1939[,vars],
  type = "manuscriptBig",
  dig = 2)
```

Pairs panel plots were generated using the `psych` package (Revelle, 2022). Correlation plots were generated using the `corrplot` package (Wei & Simko, 2021).

A pairs panel plot is shown in Figure 6.25.

```
pairs.panels(HolzingerSwineford1939[,vars])
```

A correlation plot is depicted in Figure 6.26.

```
corrplot(cor(
  HolzingerSwineford1939[,vars],
  use = "pairwise.complete.obs"),
  col = c("gray","black"))
```

TABLE 6.2 Correlation Matrix with r, n, and p-values.

	x1	x2	x3	x4	x5	x6	x7	x8	x9
1. x1.r	1.00	.32***	.46***	.40***	.31***	.32***	.04	.26***	.34***
2. sig	NA	.00	.00	.00	.00	.00	.52	.00	.00
3. n	251	221	211	208	215	205	221	219	215
4. x2.r	.32***	1.00	.34***	.15*	.19***	.17*	−.09	.09	.20***
5. sig	.00	NA	.00	.03	.00	.01	.18	.16	.00
6. n	221	265	225	227	228	216	234	227	229
7. x3.r	.46***	.34***	1.00	.18*	.15*	.19*	.09	.20***	.40***
8. sig	.00	.00	NA	.01	.03	.01	.19	.00	.00
9. n	211	225	255	211	215	206	227	219	220
10. x4.r	.40***	.15*	.18*	1.00	.73***	.68***	.15*	.13^{Ď}	.19***
11. sig	.00	.03	.01	NA	.00	.00	.03	.06	.00
12. n	208	227	211	252	216	209	224	217	215
13. x5.r	.31***	.19***	.15*	.73***	1.00	.69***	.11	.21***	.26***
14. sig	.00	.00	.03	.00	NA	.00	.11	.00	.00
15. n	215	228	215	216	259	217	226	222	219
16. x6.r	.32***	.17*	.19*	.68***	.69***	1.00	.10	.19*	.18*
17. sig	.00	.01	.01	.00	.00	NA	.15	.01	.01
18. n	205	216	206	209	217	248	218	214	209
19. x7.r	.04	−.09	.09	.15*	.11	.10	1.00	.49***	.35***
20. sig	.52	.18	.19	.03	.11	.15	NA	.00	.00
21. n	221	234	227	224	226	218	266	231	226
22. x8.r	.26***	.09	.20***	.13^{Ď}	.21***	.19*	.49***	1.00	.46***
23. sig	.00	.16	.00	.06	.00	.01	.00	NA	.00
24. n	219	227	219	217	222	214	231	259	222
25. x9.r	.34***	.20***	.40***	.19***	.26***	.18*	.35***	.46***	1.00
26. sig	.00	.00	.00	.00	.00	.01	.00	.00	NA
27. n	215	229	220	215	219	209	226	222	257

TABLE 6.3 Correlation Matrix with Asterisks for Significant Associations.

	x1	x2	x3	x4	x5	x6	x7	x8	x9
1. x1	1.00								
2. x2	.32***	1.00							
3. x3	.46***	.34***	1.00						
4. x4	.40***	.15*	.18*	1.00					
5. x5	.31***	.19***	.15*	.73***	1.00				
6. x6	.32***	.17*	.19*	.68***	.69***	1.00			
7. x7	.04	−.09	.09	.15*	.11	.10	1.00		
8. x8	.26***	.09	.20***	.13^{Ď}	.21***	.19*	.49***	1.00	
9. x9	.34***	.20***	.40***	.19***	.26***	.18*	.35***	.46***	1.00

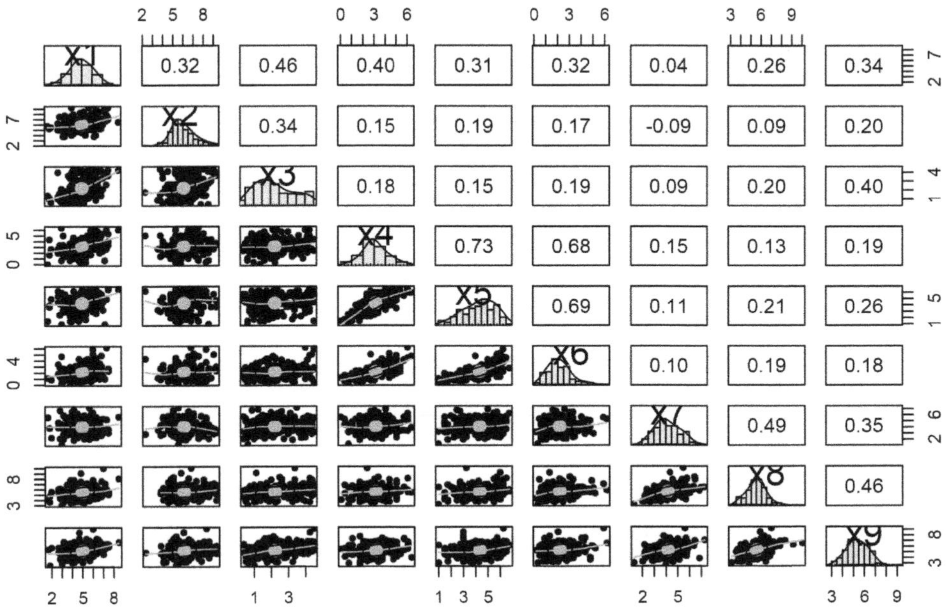

FIGURE 6.25 Pairs Panel Plot.

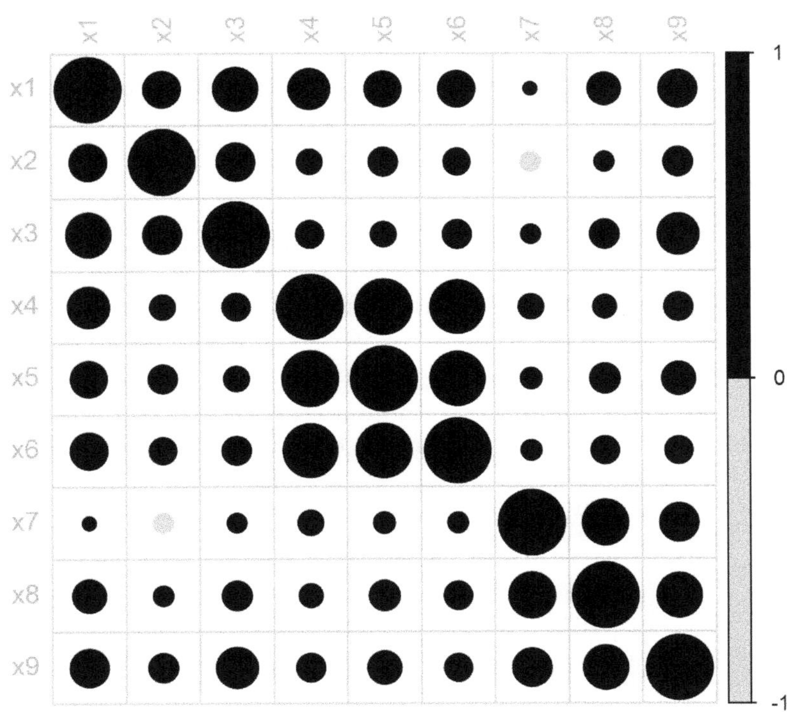

FIGURE 6.26 Correlation Plot.

TABLE 6.4 Correlation Matrix.

	x1	x2	x3	x4	x5	x6	x7	x8	x9
1. x1	1.00								
2. x2	.32	1.00							
3. x3	.46	.34	1.00						
4. x4	.40	.15	.18	1.00					
5. x5	.31	.19	.15	.73	1.00				
6. x6	.32	.17	.19	.68	.69	1.00			
7. x7	.04	−.09	.09	.15	.11	.10	1.00		
8. x8	.26	.09	.20	.13	.21	.19	.49	1.00	
9. x9	.34	.20	.40	.19	.26	.18	.35	.46	1.00

6.4 Factor Analysis

6.4.1 Exploratory Factor Analysis

We introduced exploratory factor analysis (EFA) models in Section 6.1.4.3.1.

6.4.1.1 Determine Number of Factors

Determine the number of factors to retain using the Scree plot and Very Simple Structure plot.

6.4.1.1.1 Scree plot

Scree plots were generated using the `psych` (Revelle, 2022) and `nFactors` (Raiche & Magis, 2020) packages. The optimal coordinates and the acceleration factor attempt to operationalize the Cattell scree test: i.e., the "elbow" of the scree plot (Ruscio & Roche, 2012). The optimal coordinators factor is quantified using a series of linear equations to determine whether observed eigenvalues exceed the predicted values. The acceleration factor is quantified using the acceleration of the curve, that is, the second derivative. The Kaiser-Guttman rule states to keep principal components whose eigenvalues are greater than 1. However, for exploratory factor analysis (as opposed to PCA), the criterion is to keep the factors whose eigenvalues are greater than zero (i.e., not the factors whose eigenvalues are greater than 1) (Dinno, 2014).

The number of factors to keep would depend on which criteria one uses. Based on the rule to keep factors whose eigenvalues are greater than zero and based on the parallel test, we would keep three factors. However, based on the Cattell scree test (as operationalized by the optimal coordinates and acceleration factor), we would keep one factor. Therefore, interpretability of the factors would be important for deciding between whether to keep one, two, or three factors.

A scree plot from a parallel analysis is depicted in Figure 6.27.

```
fa.parallel(
  x = HolzingerSwineford1939[,vars],
```

```
  fm = "ml",
  fa = "fa")
```

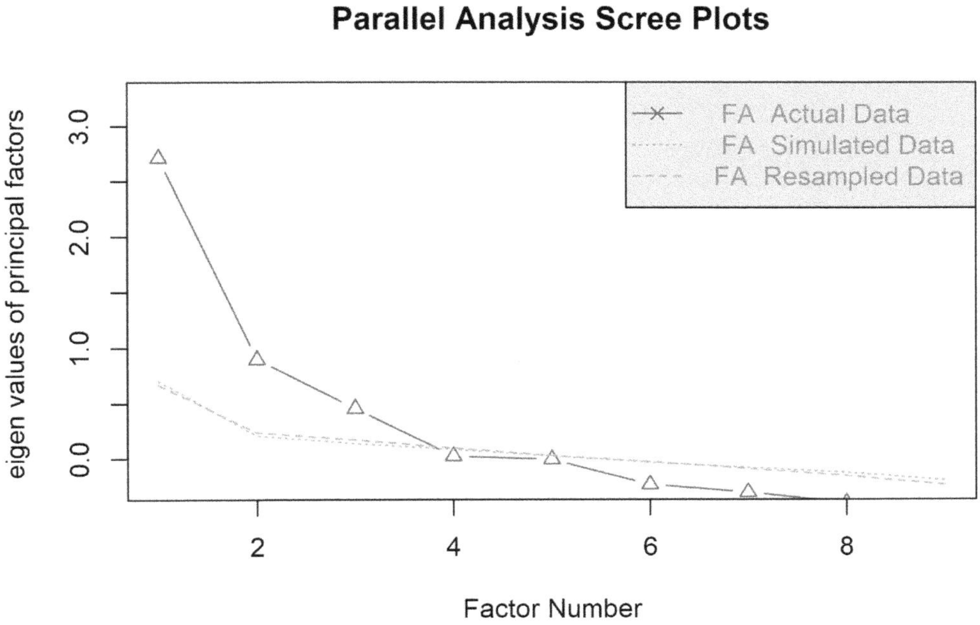

FIGURE 6.27 Scree Plot from Parallel Analysis in Exploratory Factor Analysis.

```
Parallel analysis suggests that the number of factors = 3  and the number of components = NA
```

6.4.1.1.2 Very simple structure plot

The very simple structure (VSS) is another criterion that can be used to determine the optimal number of factors or components to retain. Using the VSS criterion, the optimal number of factors to retain is the number of factors that maximizes the VSS criterion (Revelle & Rocklin, 1979). The VSS criterion is evaluated with models in which factor loadings for a given item that are less than the maximum factor loading for that item are suppressed to zero, thus forcing simple structure (i.e., no cross-loadings). The goal is finding a factor structure with interpretability so that factors are clearly distinguishable. Thus, we want to identify the number of factors with the highest VSS criterion (i.e., the highest line). VSS plots were generated using the `psych` package (Revelle, 2022).

The output also provides additional criteria by which to determine the optimal number of factors, each for which lower values are better, including the Velicer minimum average partial (MAP) test, the Bayesian information criterion (BIC), the sample size-adjusted BIC (SABIC), and the root mean square error of approximation (RMSEA).

In the example with orthogonal rotation below, the VSS criterion is highest with 3 or 4 factors. A three-factor solution is supported by the lowest BIC, whereas a four-factor solution is supported by the lowest SABIC.

A VSS plot is shown in Figure 6.28.

```
vss(
  HolzingerSwineford1939[,vars],
  rotate = "varimax",
  fm = "ml")
```

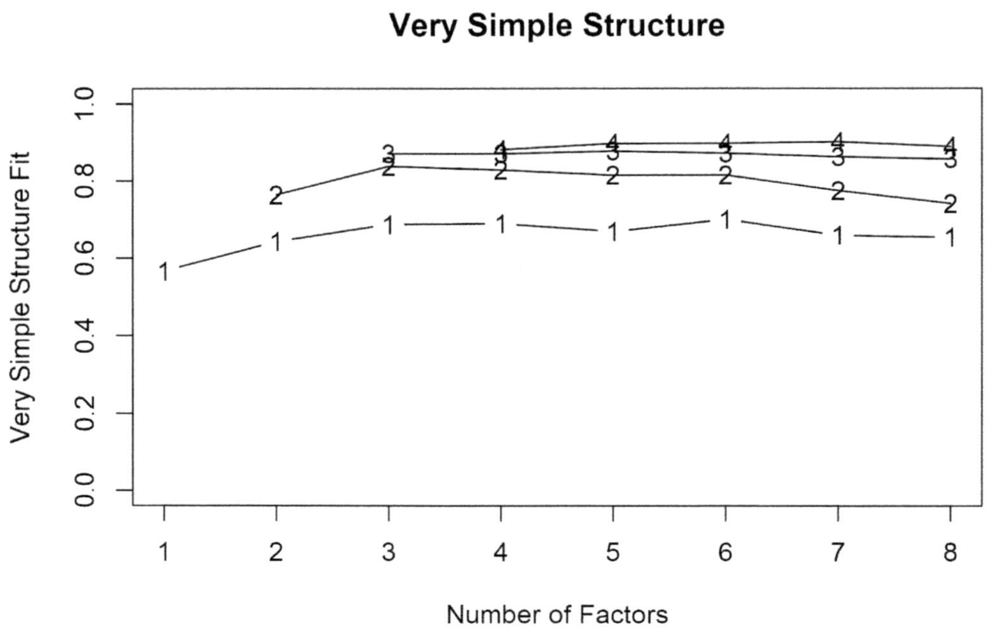

FIGURE 6.28 Very Simple Structure Plot with Orthogonal Rotation in Exploratory Factor Analysis.

```
Very Simple Structure
Call: vss(x = HolzingerSwineford1939[, vars], rotate = "varimax", fm = "ml")
Although the VSS complexity 1 shows  6  factors, it is probably more reasonable to
think about  4  factors
VSS complexity 2 achieves a maximimum of 0.84  with  3  factors

The Velicer MAP achieves a minimum of 0.07  with  2  factors
BIC achieves a minimum of  -32.61  with  3  factors
Sample Size adjusted BIC achieves a minimum of  -5.65  with  4  factors

Statistics by number of factors
  vss1 vss2   map dof   chisq     prob sqresid  fit RMSEA   BIC  SABIC
1 0.57 0.00 0.078  27 3.2e+02 2.3e-52     7.1 0.57 0.191 168.4 254.05
2 0.64 0.76 0.067  19 1.4e+02 1.2e-20     3.9 0.76 0.146  32.5  92.75
3 0.69 0.84 0.071  12 3.6e+01 3.4e-04     2.1 0.87 0.081 -32.6   5.45
4 0.69 0.83 0.125   6 9.6e+00 1.4e-01     2.0 0.88 0.044 -24.7  -5.65
5 0.67 0.81 0.199   1 1.8e+00 1.8e-01     1.6 0.90 0.050  -3.9  -0.77
```

```
6 0.70 0.82 0.403  -3 2.6e-08        NA      1.6 0.91     NA     NA      NA
7 0.66 0.78 0.447  -6 5.2e-13        NA      1.4 0.91     NA     NA      NA
8 0.65 0.74 1.000  -8 0.0e+00        NA      1.3 0.92     NA     NA      NA
  complex  eChisq     SRMR eCRMS  eBIC
1     1.0 5.5e+02 1.6e-01 0.184 396.3
2     1.2 1.6e+02 8.7e-02 0.119  53.8
3     1.3 1.2e+01 2.3e-02 0.040 -56.7
4     1.4 4.5e+00 1.4e-02 0.035 -29.7
5     1.5 8.0e-01 6.1e-03 0.036  -4.9
6     1.5 1.3e-08 7.7e-07    NA    NA
7     1.6 2.1e-13 3.1e-09    NA    NA
8     1.7 2.1e-16 1.0e-10    NA    NA
```

6.4.1.2 Run Factor Analysis

Exploratory factor analysis (EFA) models were fit using the `fa()` function of the `psych` package (Revelle, 2022) and the `sem()` and `efa()` functions of the `lavaan` package (Rosseel et al., 2022).

6.4.1.2.1 Orthogonal (Varimax) rotation

The `efa()` wrapper can fit multiple orthogonal EFA models in one function call:

```
efaOrthogonalLavaan_fit <- efa(
  data = HolzingerSwineford1939,
  ov.names = vars,
  nfactors = 1:5,
  rotation = "varimax",
  missing = "ML",
  estimator = "MLR",
  meanstructure = TRUE,
  rotation.args = list(orthogonal = TRUE)
)
```

The `efa()` wrapper can also fit individual orthogonal EFA models (with `output = "lavaan"`):

```
efaFactor3OrthogonalLavaan_fit <- efa(
  data = HolzingerSwineford1939,
  ov.names = vars,
  nfactors = 3,
  rotation = "varimax",
  missing = "ML",
  estimator = "MLR",
  meanstructure = TRUE,
  rotation.args = list(orthogonal = TRUE),
  output = "lavaan"
)
```

6.4.1.2.2 Oblique (Oblimin) rotation

The `efa()` wrapper can fit multiple oblique EFA models in one function call:

```
# settings to mimic Mplus
mplusRotationArgs <-
  list(
    rstarts = 30,
    row.weights = "none",
    algorithm = "gpa",
    orthogonal = FALSE,
    jac.init.rot = TRUE,
    std.ov = TRUE, # row standard = correlation
    geomin.epsilon = 0.0001)

efaObliqueLavaan_fit <- efa(
  data = HolzingerSwineford1939,
  ov.names = vars,
  nfactors = 1:5,
  rotation = "geomin",
  missing = "ML",
  estimator = "MLR",
  meanstructure = TRUE,
  rotation.args = mplusRotationArgs
)
```

The `efa()` wrapper can also fit individual oblique EFA models (with `output = "lavaan"`):

```
efaFactor3ObliqueLavaan_fit <- efa(
  data = HolzingerSwineford1939,
  ov.names = vars,
  nfactors = 3,
  rotation = "geomin",
  missing = "ML",
  estimator = "MLR",
  meanstructure = TRUE,
  rotation.args = mplusRotationArgs,
  output = "lavaan"
)
```

6.4.1.3 Factor Loadings

The factor loadings and summaries of the orthogonal models are below:

```
summary(
  efaOrthogonalLavaan_fit)
```

```
This is lavaan 0.6.17 -- running exploratory factor analysis

  Estimator                                         ML
  Rotation method                   VARIMAX ORTHOGONAL
  Rotation algorithm (rstarts)                GPA (30)
  Standardized metric                             TRUE
```

```
  Row weights                                  Kaiser

  Number of observations                          301
  Number of missing patterns                       75

Overview models:
                aic  bic sabic  chisq df pvalue   cfi rmsea
  nfactors = 1 6656 6756  6670 235.32 27  0.000 0.664 0.190
  nfactors = 2 6536 6666  6555 113.00 19  0.000 0.863 0.144
  nfactors = 3 6469 6624  6491  23.72 12  0.022 0.980 0.070
  nfactors = 4 6465 6643  6490     NA  6     NA 0.999 0.022
  nfactors = 5 6469 6666  6498     NA  1     NA 0.999 0.066

Eigenvalues correlation matrix:

    ev1     ev2     ev3     ev4     ev5     ev6     ev7     ev8     ev9
  3.220   1.621   1.380   0.689   0.569   0.542   0.461   0.289   0.229

Number of factors:  1

Standardized loadings: (* = significant at 1% level)

       f1       unique.var   communalities
x1  0.447*           0.800           0.200
x2      .*           0.944           0.056
x3      .*           0.928           0.072
x4  0.829*           0.313           0.687
x5  0.851*           0.276           0.724
x6  0.817*           0.332           0.668
x7      .*           0.964           0.036
x8      .*           0.926           0.074
x9  0.335*           0.888           0.112

                             f1
Sum of squared loadings 2.629
Proportion of total     1.000
Proportion var          0.292
Cumulative var          0.292

Number of factors:  2

Standardized loadings: (* = significant at 1% level)

       f1      f2       unique.var   communalities
x1  0.323*  0.427*           0.714           0.286
x2       .       .           0.907           0.093
x3       .  0.495*           0.742           0.258
x4  0.840*       .           0.279           0.721
x5  0.842*      .*           0.259           0.741
x6  0.796*       .           0.333           0.667
x7          0.438*           0.804           0.196
```

```
x8          0.612*           0.619            0.381
x9       .  0.737*           0.441            0.559

                              f1    f2 total
Sum of sq (ortho) loadings 2.215 1.686 3.900
Proportion of total        0.568 0.432 1.000
Proportion var             0.246 0.187 0.433
Cumulative var             0.246 0.433 0.433

Number of factors:  3

Standardized loadings: (* = significant at 1% level)

       f1      f2      f3       unique.var   communalities
x1  0.620*      .*      .            0.531           0.469
x2  0.497*      .                    0.741           0.259
x3  0.689*              .            0.493           0.507
x4      .   0.830*                   0.284           0.716
x5      .   0.854*      .            0.241           0.759
x6      .*  0.782*                   0.336           0.664
x7                  0.706*           0.487           0.513
x8      .           0.689*           0.488           0.512
x9  0.402*      .   0.536*           0.533           0.467

                              f2    f1    f3 total
Sum of sq (ortho) loadings 2.143 1.385 1.338 4.865
Proportion of total        0.440 0.285 0.275 1.000
Proportion var             0.238 0.154 0.149 0.541
Cumulative var             0.238 0.392 0.541 0.541

Number of factors:  4

Standardized loadings: (* = significant at 1% level)

       f1      f2      f3      f4       unique.var   communalities
x1  0.634*              .       .            0.516           0.484
x2  0.502                                    0.733           0.267
x3  0.677*                      .            0.506           0.494
x4      .   0.435   0.886                    0.000           1.000
x5      .       .   0.943       .            0.000           1.000
x6      .           0.718       .            0.422           0.578
x7      .       .           0.756            0.396           0.604
x8      .                   0.657            0.521           0.479
x9  0.414               .   0.527*           0.522           0.478

                              f3    f1    f4    f2 total
Sum of sq (ortho) loadings 2.293 1.417 1.357 0.317 5.384
Proportion of total        0.426 0.263 0.252 0.059 1.000
Proportion var             0.255 0.157 0.151 0.035 0.598
Cumulative var             0.255 0.412 0.563 0.598 0.598
```

```
Number of factors:  5

Standardized loadings: (* = significant at 1% level)

       f1      f2      f3      f4      f5        unique.var
x1  0.603       .               .       .             0.517
x2  0.473       .                                     0.748
x3  0.462   0.871                       .             0.000
x4      .           0.444   0.882                     0.000
x5      .               .   0.942       .             0.000
x6      .                   0.719       .             0.423
x7      .               .           0.761             0.333
x8      .                           0.688             0.475
x9  0.338*      .               .   0.534*            0.547
     communalities
x1           0.483
x2           0.252
x3           1.000
x4           1.000
x5           1.000
x6           0.577
x7           0.667
x8           0.525
x9           0.453

                                f4    f5    f1    f2    f3 total
Sum of sq (ortho) loadings 2.282 1.418 1.092 0.847 0.316 5.955
Proportion of total        0.383 0.238 0.183 0.142 0.053 1.000
Proportion var             0.254 0.158 0.121 0.094 0.035 0.662
Cumulative var             0.254 0.411 0.533 0.627 0.662 0.662
```

6.4.1.4 Estimates of Model Fit

Fit indices for the orthogonal models are extracted using the syntax below and are shown in Table 6.5.

```
efaOrthogonalLavaan_fitIndices <- fitMeasures(
  efaOrthogonalLavaan_fit,
  fit.measures = c(
    "chisq", "df", "pvalue",
    "chisq.scaled", "df.scaled", "pvalue.scaled",
    "chisq.scaling.factor",
    "baseline.chisq","baseline.df","baseline.pvalue",
    "rmsea", "cfi", "tli", "srmr",
    "rmsea.robust", "cfi.robust", "tli.robust"))
```

6.4.1.5 Factor Scores

Factor scores are extracted using the following syntax:

TABLE 6.5 Fit Indices from EFA with Orthogonal Rotation.

	nfactors = 1	nfactors = 2	nfactors = 3	nfactors = 4	nfactors = 5
chisq	239.990	104.454	23.051	7.171	1.736
df	27.000	19.000	12.000	6.000	1.000
pvalue	0.000	0.000	0.027	0.305	0.188
chisq.scaled	235.316	112.999	23.723	NA	NA
df.scaled	27.000	19.000	12.000	6.000	1.000
pvalue.scaled	0.000	0.000	0.022	NA	NA
chisq.scaling.factor	1.020	0.924	0.972	NA	NA
baseline.chisq	693.305	693.305	693.305	693.305	693.305
baseline.df	36.000	36.000	36.000	36.000	36.000
baseline.pvalue	0.000	0.000	0.000	0.000	0.000
rmsea	0.162	0.122	0.055	0.025	0.049
cfi	0.676	0.870	0.983	0.998	0.999
tli	0.568	0.754	0.950	0.989	0.960
srmr	0.129	0.073	0.020	0.012	0.006
rmsea.robust	0.190	0.144	0.070	0.022	0.066
cfi.robust	0.664	0.863	0.980	0.999	0.999
tli.robust	0.552	0.741	0.939	0.994	0.946

```
fa3Orthogonal_lavaan <- lavPredict(efaFactor3OrthogonalLavaan_fit)
```

6.4.1.6 Plots

Pairs panel plots were generated using the `psych` package (Revelle, 2022).

A scree plot based on factor loadings from the orthogonal model is in Figure 6.29. When the factors are uncorrelated (orthogonal rotation), the eigenvalue for a factor is calculated as the sum of squared standardized factor loadings across all items, as described in Section 6.1.4.2.1.

A pairs panel plot is illustrated in Figure 6.30.

```
pairs.panels(fa3Orthogonal_lavaan)
```

6.4.2 Confirmatory Factor Analysis

The confirmatory factor analysis (CFA) models were fit in the `lavaan` package (Rosseel et al., 2022). The examples were adapted from the `lavaan` documentation: https://lavaan.ugent.be/tutorial/cfa.html (archived at https://perma.cc/GKY3-9YE4)

6.4.2.1 Specify the Model

```
cfaModel_syntax <- '
 visual  =~ x1 + x2 + x3
 textual =~ x4 + x5 + x6
```

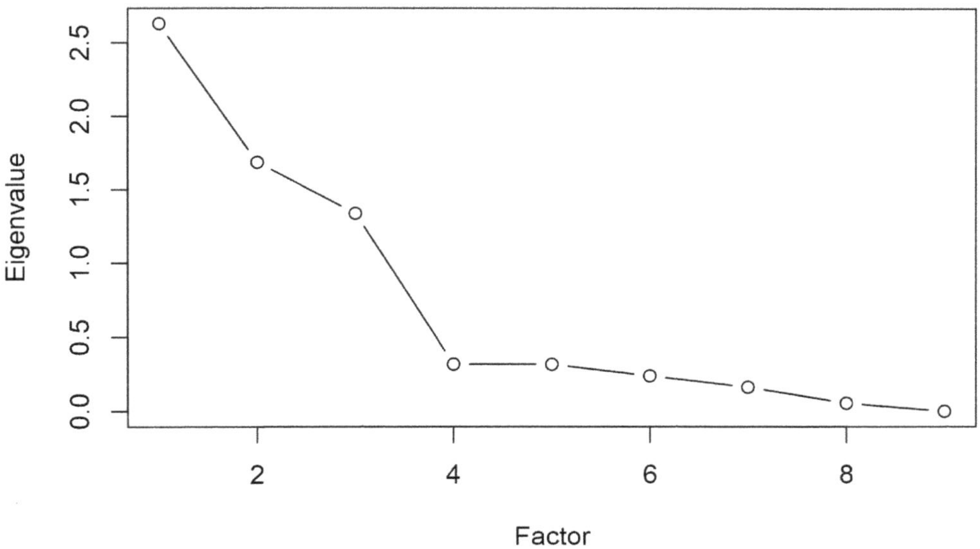

FIGURE 6.29 Scree Plot with Orthogonal Rotation in Exploratory Factor Analysis.

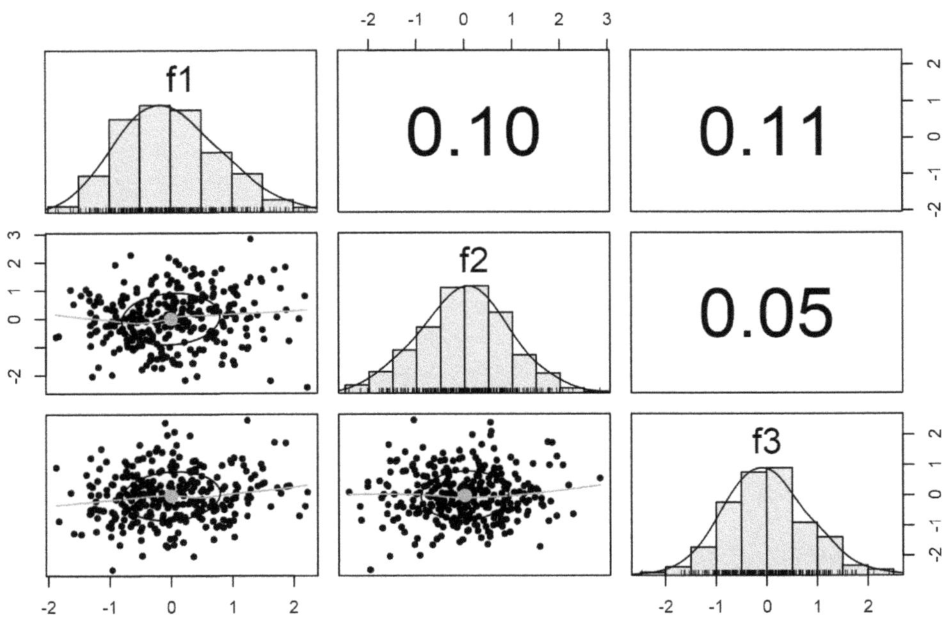

FIGURE 6.30 Pairs Panel Plot with Orthogonal Rotation in Exploratory Factor Analysis.

```
 speed   =~ x7 + x8 + x9
'
```

6.4.2.2 Fit the Model

```
cfaModelFit <- cfa(
  cfaModel_syntax,
  data = HolzingerSwineford1939,
  missing = "ML",
  estimator = "MLR",
  std.lv = TRUE)
```

6.4.2.3 Display Summary Output

```
summary(
  cfaModelFit,
  standardized = TRUE)
```

```
lavaan 0.6.17 ended normally after 40 iterations

  Estimator                                         ML
  Optimization method                           NLMINB
  Number of model parameters                        30

  Number of observations                           301
  Number of missing patterns                        75

Model Test User Model:
                                              Standard      Scaled
  Test Statistic                                65.643      63.641
  Degrees of freedom                                24          24
  P-value (Chi-square)                           0.000       0.000
  Scaling correction factor                                  1.031
    Yuan-Bentler correction (Mplus variant)

Parameter Estimates:

  Standard errors                             Sandwich
  Information bread                           Observed
  Observed information based on                Hessian

Latent Variables:
                   Estimate  Std.Err  z-value  P(>|z|)   Std.lv
  visual =~
    x1                0.885    0.108    8.183    0.000    0.885
    x2                0.521    0.086    6.037    0.000    0.521
    x3                0.712    0.088    8.065    0.000    0.712
```

```
  textual =~
    x4                0.989    0.067   14.690    0.000    0.989
    x5                1.121    0.066   16.890    0.000    1.121
    x6                0.849    0.065   12.991    0.000    0.849
  speed =~
    x7                0.596    0.084    7.092    0.000    0.596
    x8                0.742    0.096    7.703    0.000    0.742
    x9                0.686    0.099    6.939    0.000    0.686
  Std.all

    0.762
    0.451
    0.632

    0.842
    0.866
    0.818

    0.557
    0.733
    0.673

Covariances:
                   Estimate  Std.Err  z-value  P(>|z|)   Std.lv
  visual ~~
    textual           0.430    0.080    5.386    0.000    0.430
    speed             0.465    0.110    4.213    0.000    0.465
  textual ~~
    speed             0.314    0.084    3.746    0.000    0.314
  Std.all

    0.430
    0.465

    0.314

Intercepts:
                   Estimate  Std.Err  z-value  P(>|z|)   Std.lv
   .x1                4.977    0.071   69.850    0.000    4.977
   .x2                6.050    0.070   85.953    0.000    6.050
   .x3                2.227    0.069   32.218    0.000    2.227
   .x4                3.097    0.071   43.828    0.000    3.097
   .x5                4.344    0.077   56.058    0.000    4.344
   .x6                2.187    0.064   34.391    0.000    2.187
   .x7                4.180    0.065   64.446    0.000    4.180
   .x8                5.517    0.062   89.668    0.000    5.517
   .x9                5.405    0.063   86.063    0.000    5.405
  Std.all
    4.289
    5.235
    1.976
```

```
    2.634
    3.355
    2.108
    3.904
    5.451
    5.298

Variances:
                   Estimate  Std.Err  z-value  P(>|z|)   Std.lv
   .x1                0.564    0.169    3.345    0.001    0.564
   .x2                1.064    0.119    8.935    0.000    1.064
   .x3                0.763    0.118    6.454    0.000    0.763
   .x4                0.403    0.063    6.363    0.000    0.403
   .x5                0.420    0.074    5.664    0.000    0.420
   .x6                0.356    0.056    6.415    0.000    0.356
   .x7                0.790    0.093    8.512    0.000    0.790
   .x8                0.474    0.128    3.693    0.000    0.474
   .x9                0.570    0.122    4.660    0.000    0.570
    visual            1.000                               1.000
    textual           1.000                               1.000
    speed             1.000                               1.000
  Std.all
    0.419
    0.797
    0.601
    0.292
    0.251
    0.331
    0.690
    0.463
    0.548
    1.000
    1.000
    1.000
```

6.4.2.4 Estimates of Model Fit

```
fitMeasures(
  cfaModelFit,
  fit.measures = c(
    "chisq", "df", "pvalue",
    "chisq.scaled", "df.scaled", "pvalue.scaled",
    "chisq.scaling.factor",
    "baseline.chisq","baseline.df","baseline.pvalue",
    "rmsea", "cfi", "tli", "srmr",
    "rmsea.robust", "cfi.robust", "tli.robust"))
```

```
          chisq                 df             pvalue
         65.643             24.000              0.000
   chisq.scaled          df.scaled      pvalue.scaled
```

```
           63.641              24.000               0.000
chisq.scaling.factor       baseline.chisq         baseline.df
            1.031             693.305              36.000
     baseline.pvalue            rmsea                 cfi
            0.000               0.076               0.937
              tli                srmr         rmsea.robust
            0.905               0.061               0.092
       cfi.robust          tli.robust
            0.930               0.894
```

6.4.2.5 Residuals

```
residuals(cfaModelFit, type = "cor")
```

```
$type
[1] "cor.bollen"

$cov
       x1     x2     x3     x4     x5     x6     x7     x8     x9
x1  0.000
x2 -0.020  0.000
x3 -0.019  0.053  0.000
x4  0.077 -0.035 -0.083  0.000
x5  0.015 -0.006 -0.119  0.004  0.000
x6  0.044  0.038 -0.002 -0.005  0.002  0.000
x7 -0.178 -0.215 -0.073  0.005 -0.061 -0.032  0.000
x8 -0.017 -0.053 -0.013 -0.088 -0.018 -0.008  0.062  0.000
x9  0.103  0.067  0.192  0.003  0.084  0.043 -0.031 -0.044  0.000

$mean
    x1     x2     x3     x4     x5     x6     x7     x8     x9
 0.001 -0.003 -0.002 -0.004 -0.003  0.006  0.000  0.002  0.000
```

6.4.2.6 Factor Scores

```
cfaFactorScores <- lavPredict(cfaModelFit)
```

6.4.2.6.1 Compare CFA factor scores to EFA factor scores

As would be expected, the factor scores from the CFA model are highly correlated with the factor scores from the EFA model.

```
cor(
  x = cfaFactorScores[,"visual"],
  y = fa3Orthogonal_lavaan[,"f1"],
  use = "pairwise.complete.obs")
```

```
[1] 0.9051
```

```
cor(
  x = cfaFactorScores[,"textual"],
  y = fa3Orthogonal_lavaan[,"f2"],
  use = "pairwise.complete.obs")
```

```
[1] 0.9792
```

```
cor(
  x = cfaFactorScores[,"speed"],
  y = fa3Orthogonal_lavaan[,"f3"],
  use = "pairwise.complete.obs")
```

```
[1] 0.9187
```

6.4.2.7 Internal Consistency Reliability

Internal consistency reliability of items composing the latent factors, as quantified by omega (ω) and average variance extracted (AVE), was estimated using the `semTools` package (Jorgensen et al., 2021).

```
compRelSEM(cfaModelFit)
```

```
 visual textual   speed
  0.652   0.878   0.695
```

```
AVE(cfaModelFit)
```

```
 visual textual   speed
  0.397   0.713   0.430
```

6.4.2.8 Path Diagram

A path diagram of the model is in Figure 6.31.

```
semPaths(
  cfaModelFit,
  what = "std",
  layout = "tree2",
  edge.label.cex = 1.3)
```

6.4.2.9 Examples

```
standardDeviations <- rep(1, 6)
sampleSize <- 300
```

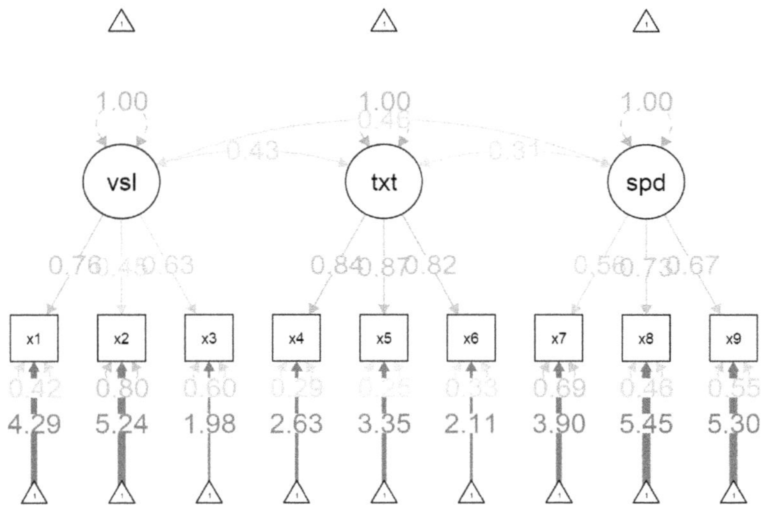

FIGURE 6.31 Confirmatory Factor Analysis Model Diagram.

6.4.2.9.1 Create the covariance matrix

```
correlationMatrixModel3 <- matrix(c(
  1,.6,.6,0,0,0,
  .6,1,.6,0,0,0,
  0,0,1,0,0,0,
  0,0,0,1,.6,.6,
  0,0,0,.6,1,.6,
  0,0,0,.6,.6,1),
  nrow = 6,
  ncol = 6)
rownames(correlationMatrixModel3) <-
  colnames(correlationMatrixModel3) <-
  paste("V", 1:6, sep = "")

covarianceMatrixModel3 <- psych::cor2cov(
  correlationMatrixModel3,
  sigma = standardDeviations)
covarianceMatrixModel3
```

```
    V1  V2 V3  V4  V5  V6
V1 1.0 0.6  0 0.0 0.0 0.0
V2 0.6 1.0  0 0.0 0.0 0.0
V3 0.6 0.6  1 0.0 0.0 0.0
```

```
V4 0.0 0.0  0 1.0 0.6 0.6
V5 0.0 0.0  0 0.6 1.0 0.6
V6 0.0 0.0  0 0.6 0.6 1.0
```

6.4.2.9.2 Specify the model

```
cfaModel3A <- '
 f1 =~ V1 + V2 + V3 + V4 + V5 + V6
'

cfaModel3B <- '
 f1 =~ V1 + V2 + V3
 f2 =~ V4 + V5 + V6
'
```

6.4.2.9.3 Fit the model

```
cfaModel3AFit <- cfa(
  cfaModel3A,
  sample.cov = covarianceMatrixModel3,
  sample.nobs = sampleSize,
  estimator = "ML",
  std.lv = TRUE)

cfaModel3BFit <- cfa(
  cfaModel3B,
  sample.cov = covarianceMatrixModel3,
  sample.nobs = sampleSize,
  estimator = "ML",
  std.lv = TRUE)
```

6.4.2.9.4 Estimates of model fit

```
fitMeasures(
  cfaModel3AFit,
  fit.measures = c(
    "chisq", "df", "pvalue",
    "rmsea", "cfi", "tli", "srmr"))
```

```
  chisq      df  pvalue   rmsea     cfi     tli    srmr
313.237   9.000   0.000   0.336   0.502   0.171   0.227
```

```
fitMeasures(
  cfaModel3BFit,
  fit.measures = c(
    "chisq", "df", "pvalue",
    "rmsea", "cfi", "tli", "srmr"))
```

```
  chisq      df pvalue  rmsea    cfi    tli   srmr
  0.000   8.000  1.000  0.000  1.000  1.025  0.000
```

6.4.2.9.5 Compare model fit

Below is a test of whether the two-factor model fits better than the one-factor model. A significant chi-square difference test indicates that the two-factor model fits significantly better than the one-factor model.

```
anova(cfaModel3BFit, cfaModel3AFit)
```

```

Chi-Squared Difference Test

              Df  AIC  BIC Chisq Chisq diff RMSEA Df diff Pr(>Chisq)
cfaModel3BFit  8 4502 4550     0
cfaModel3AFit  9 4813 4857   313        313  1.02       1     <2e-16

cfaModel3BFit
cfaModel3AFit ***
---
Signif. codes:  0 '***' 0.001 '**' 0.01 '*' 0.05 '.' 0.1 ' ' 1
```

6.4.2.9.6 Equivalently fitting models

Markov equivalent directed acyclic graphs (DAGs) of equivalent models can be generated using the `dagitty` package (Textor et al., 2021).

```
dagModel <- lavaanToGraph(cfaModel3BFit)
lapply(equivalentDAGs(dagModel, n = 16), plot)
```

6.4.2.10 Higher-Order Factor Model

A higher-order (or hierarchical) factor model is a model in which a higher-order latent factor is thought to influence lower-order latent factors. Higher-order factor models are depicted in Figure 6.10. An analysis example of a higher-order factor model is below.

6.4.2.10.1 Create the covariance matrix

```
correlationMatrixModel4 <- matrix(c(
  1,.6,.6,.3,.3,.3,
  .6,1,.6,.3,.3,.3,
  .3,.3,1,.3,.3,.3,
  .3,.3,.3,1,.6,.6,
  .3,.3,.3,.6,1,.6,
  .3,.3,.3,.6,.6,1),
  nrow = 6,
  ncol = 6)
rownames(correlationMatrixModel4) <- colnames(correlationMatrixModel4) <-
  paste("V", 1:6, sep = "")
```

```
covarianceMatrixModel4 <- psych::cor2cov(
  correlationMatrixModel4,
  sigma = standardDeviations)
covarianceMatrixModel4
```

```
    V1  V2  V3  V4  V5  V6
V1 1.0 0.6 0.3 0.3 0.3 0.3
V2 0.6 1.0 0.3 0.3 0.3 0.3
V3 0.6 0.6 1.0 0.3 0.3 0.3
V4 0.3 0.3 0.3 1.0 0.6 0.6
V5 0.3 0.3 0.3 0.6 1.0 0.6
V6 0.3 0.3 0.3 0.6 0.6 1.0
```

6.4.2.10.2 Specify the model

```
cfaModel4C <- '
 f1 =~ V1 + V2 + V3
 f2 =~ V4 + V5 + V6

 #Higher-order factor
 A1 =~ fixloading*f1 + fixloading*f2
'
```

6.4.2.10.2.1 Fit the model

```
cfaModel4CFit <- cfa(
  cfaModel4C,
  sample.cov = covarianceMatrixModel4,
  sample.nobs = sampleSize,
  missing = "ML",
  std.lv = TRUE)
```

6.4.2.11 Bifactor Model

A bifactor model is a model in which both a general latent factor and specific latent factors are extracted from items (Markon, 2019). The general factor represents the common variance among all items, whereas the specific factor represents the common variance among the specific items that load on the specific factor, after extracting the general factor variance. As estimated below, the general factor is orthogonal to the specific factors. Some modified versions of the bifactor allow the specific factors to inter-correlate (in addition to estimating the general factor).

6.4.2.11.1 Specify the model

```
cfaModelBifactor_syntax <- '
 Verbal =~
```

```
    VO1 + VO2 + VO3 +
    VW1 + VW2 + VW3 +
    VM1 + VM2 + VM3
  Spatial =~
    SO1 + SO2 + SO3 +
    SW1 + SW2 + SW3 +
    SM1 + SM2 + SM3
  Quant =~
    QO1 + QO2 + QO3 +
    QW1 + QW2 + QW3 +
    QM1 + QM2 + QM3
  g =~
    VO1 + VO2 + VO3 +
    VW1 + VW2 + VW3 +
    VM1 + VM2 + VM3 +
    SO1 + SO2 + SO3 +
    SW1 + SW2 + SW3 +
    SM1 + SM2 + SM3 +
    QO1 + QO2 + QO3 +
    QW1 + QW2 + QW3 +
    QM1 + QM2 + QM3
'
```

6.4.2.11.2 Fit the model

```
cfaModelBifactorFit <- cfa(
  cfaModelBifactor_syntax,
  data = MTMM_data,
  orthogonal = TRUE,
  std.lv = TRUE,
  missing = "ML",
  estimator = "MLR")
```

6.4.2.11.3 Path diagram

A path diagram of the model is shown in Figure 6.32.

```
semPaths(
  cfaModelBifactorFit,
  what = "std",
  layout = "tree3",
  bifactor = c("g"),
  edge.label.cex = 1.3)
```

6.4.2.12 Multitrait-Multimethod Model

6.4.2.12.1 Simulate the data

We simulated the data for the multitrait-multimethod model (MTMM) in Section 4.3.1.4.2.3.

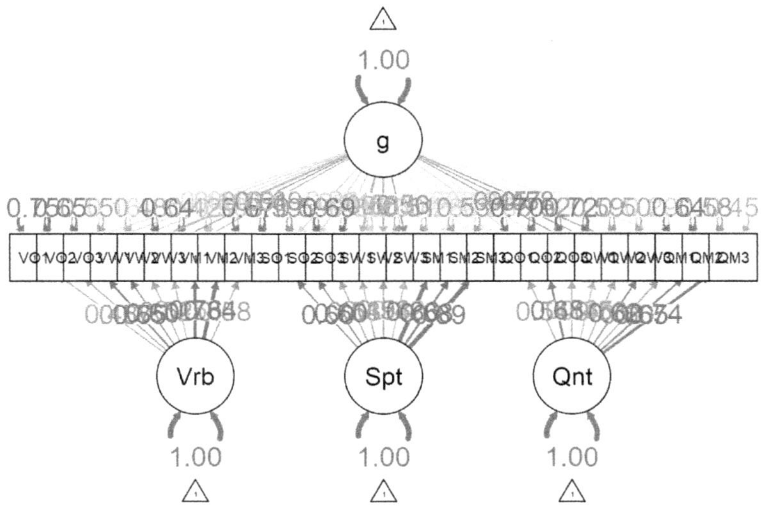

FIGURE 6.32 Bifactor Model.

6.4.2.12.2 Specify the model

This example is courtesy of W. Joel Schneider.

```
cfaModelMTMM_syntax <- '
 g =~ Verbal + Spatial + Quant
 Verbal =~
   VO1 + VO2 + VO3 +
   VW1 + VW2 + VW3 +
   VM1 + VM2 + VM3
 Spatial =~
   SO1 + SO2 + SO3 +
   SW1 + SW2 + SW3 +
   SM1 + SM2 + SM3
 Quant =~
   QO1 + QO2 + QO3 +
   QW1 + QW2 + QW3 +
   QM1 + QM2 + QM3
 Oral =~
   VO1 + VO2 + VO3 +
   SO1 + SO2 + SO3 +
   QO1 + QO2 + QO3
 Written =~
   VW1 + VW2 + VW3 +
```

```
    SW1 + SW2 + SW3 +
    QW1 + QW2 + QW3
  Manipulative =~
    VM1 + VM2 + VM3 +
    SM1 + SM2 + SM3 +
    QM1 + QM2 + QM3
'
```

6.4.2.12.3 Fit the model

```
cfaModelMTMMFit <- cfa(
  cfaModelMTMM_syntax,
  data = MTMM_data,
  orthogonal = TRUE,
  std.lv = TRUE,
  missing = "ML",
  estimator = "MLR")
```

6.4.3 Exploratory Structural Equation Model

6.4.3.1 Example 1

6.4.3.1.1 Specify the model

To specify an exploratory structural equation model (ESEM), you use the factor loadings from an EFA model as the starting values in a structural equation model. In this example, we use the factor loadings from the three-factor EFA model, as specified in Section 6.4.1.2.2. The factor loadings are in Table 6.6.

```
esem_loadings <- parameterEstimates(
  efaFactor3ObliqueLavaan_fit,
  standardized = TRUE
) %>%
  dplyr::filter(efa == "efa") %>%
  dplyr::select(lhs, rhs, est) %>%
  dplyr::rename(item = rhs, latent = lhs, loading = est)
```

In ESEM, you specify one anchor item for each latent factor. You want the anchor item to be an item that has a strong loading on one latent factor and to have weak loadings on every other latent factor. The cross-loadings for the anchor item are fixed to the respective loadings from the original EFA model. We specify an anchor item for each latent factor below:

```
anchors <- c(f1 = "x3", f2 = "x5", f3 = "x7")
```

The `petersenlab` package (Petersen, 2024) includes the `make_esem_model()` function that creates `lavaan` syntax for an ESEM model from the factor loadings of an EFA model, as

TABLE 6.6 Factor Loadings from Exploratory Factor Analysis for Use in Exploratory Structural Equation Modeling.

Item	Latent	Loading
f1	x1	0.732
f1	x2	0.584
f1	x3	0.848
f1	x4	0.006
f1	x5	−0.005
f1	x6	0.097
f1	x7	−0.001
f1	x8	0.284
f1	x9	0.496
f2	x1	0.139
f2	x2	−0.008
f2	x3	−0.145
f2	x4	0.991
f2	x5	1.127
f2	x6	0.804
f2	x7	0.060
f2	x8	−0.008
f2	x9	0.008
f3	x1	−0.043
f3	x2	−0.180
f3	x3	0.006
f3	x4	0.007
f3	x5	0.034
f3	x6	−0.001
f3	x7	0.756
f3	x8	0.638
f3	x9	0.432

adapted from Mateus Silvestrin: https://msilvestrin.me/post/esem (archived at https://perma.cc/FA8D-4NB9)

```
esemModel_syntax <- make_esem_model(
  esem_loadings,
  anchors)
```

6.4.3.1.2 Fit the model

```
esemModelFit <- sem(
  esemModel_syntax,
  data = HolzingerSwineford1939,
  missing = "ML",
  estimator = "MLR")
```

6.4.3.1.3 Nested model comparison

A nested model comparison indicates that the ESEM model fits significantly better than the CFA model.

```
anova(cfaModelFit, esemModelFit)
```

```

Scaled Chi-Squared Difference Test (method = "satorra.bentler.2001")

lavaan NOTE:
    The "Chisq" column contains standard test statistics, not the
    robust test that should be reported per model. A robust difference
    test is a function of two standard (not robust) statistics.

             Df  AIC  BIC Chisq Chisq diff Df diff Pr(>Chisq)
esemModelFit 12 6469 6624  23.1
cfaModelFit  24 6487 6598  65.6         39      12      1e-04 ***
---
Signif. codes:  0 '***' 0.001 '**' 0.01 '*' 0.05 '.' 0.1 ' ' 1
```

6.4.3.2 Example 2

6.4.3.2.1 Specify the model

Another way to fit a ESEM model in `lavaan` is to fit exploratory factors, confirmatory factors, and structural components in the same model. For instance, below is the syntax for a model with exploratory factors, confirmatory factors, and structural components:

```
esem_syntax <- '
 # exploratory factors: EFA Block 1
 efa("efa1")*f1 +
 efa("efa1")*f2 =~ x1 + x2 + x3 + x4 + x5 + x6

 # confirmatory factors
 speed =~ x7 + x8 + x9

 # regression paths
 speed ~ f1 + f2
'
```

6.4.3.2.2 Fit the model

```
esem_fit <- sem(
  esem_syntax,
  data = HolzingerSwineford1939,
  rotation = "geomin",
  missing = "ML",
  estimator = "MLR")
```

6.5 Principal Component Analysis

Principal component analysis (PCA) is a technique for data reduction. PCA seeks to identify the principal components of the data, so that data can be reduced to that smaller set of components. That is, PCA seeks to identify the smallest set of components that explain the most variance in the variables. Although PCA is sometimes referred to as factor analysis, PCA is not factor analysis (Lilienfeld et al., 2015). PCA uses the *total* variance of all variables, whereas factor analysis uses the *common* variance among the variables.

6.5.1 Determine Number of Components

Determine the number of components to retain using the Scree plot and Very Simple Structure (VSS) plot.

6.5.1.1 Scree Plot

Scree plots were generated using the **psych** (Revelle, 2022) and **nFactors** (Raiche & Magis, 2020) packages. Note that eigenvalues of factors in PCA models are higher than factors from EFA models, because PCA components include *common* variance among the indicators in addition to *error* variance, whereas EFA factors include only the common variance among the indicators. A scree plot based on parallel analysis is shown in Figure 6.33.

The number of components to keep would depend on which criteria one uses. Based on the rule to keep components whose eigenvalues are greater than 1 and based on the parallel test, we would keep three factors. However, based on the Cattell scree test (as operationalized by the optimal coordinates and acceleration factor), we would keep one or three factors. Therefore, interpretability of the factors would be important for deciding between whether to keep one, two, or three factors.

```
fa.parallel(
  x = HolzingerSwineford1939[,vars],
  fm = "ml",
  fa = "pc")
```

```
Parallel analysis suggests that the number of factors =  NA  and the number of
components =  3
```

A scree plot is shown in Figure 6.34.

```
plot(nScree(
  x = cor(
    HolzingerSwineford1939[,vars],
    use = "pairwise.complete.obs"),
  model = "components"))
```

6.5.1.2 Very Simple Structure Plot

In the example with orthogonal rotation below, the very simple structure (VSS) criterion is highest with three or four components.

A VSS plot of PCA with orthogonal rotation is shown in Figure 6.35.

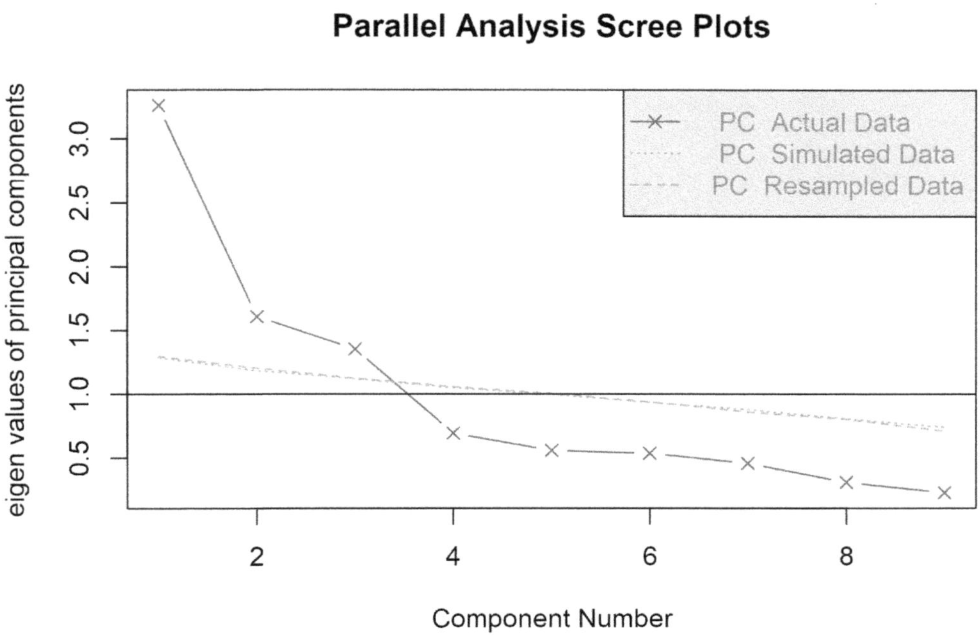

FIGURE 6.33 Scree Plot Based on Parallel Analysis in Principal Component Analysis.

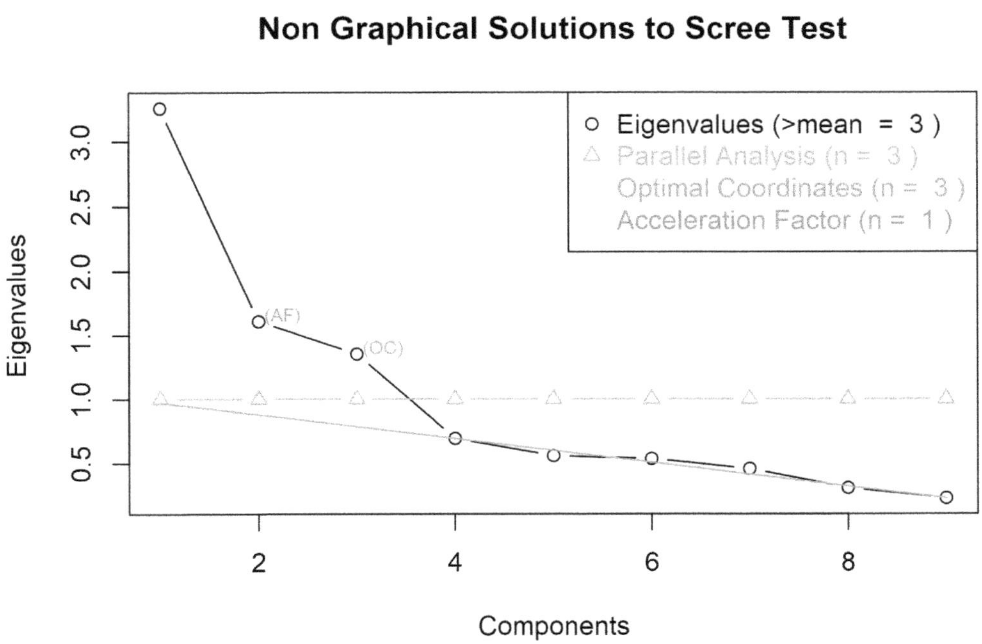

FIGURE 6.34 Scree Plot in Principal Component Analysis.

```
vss(
  HolzingerSwineford1939[,vars],
  rotate = "varimax",
  fm = "pc")
```

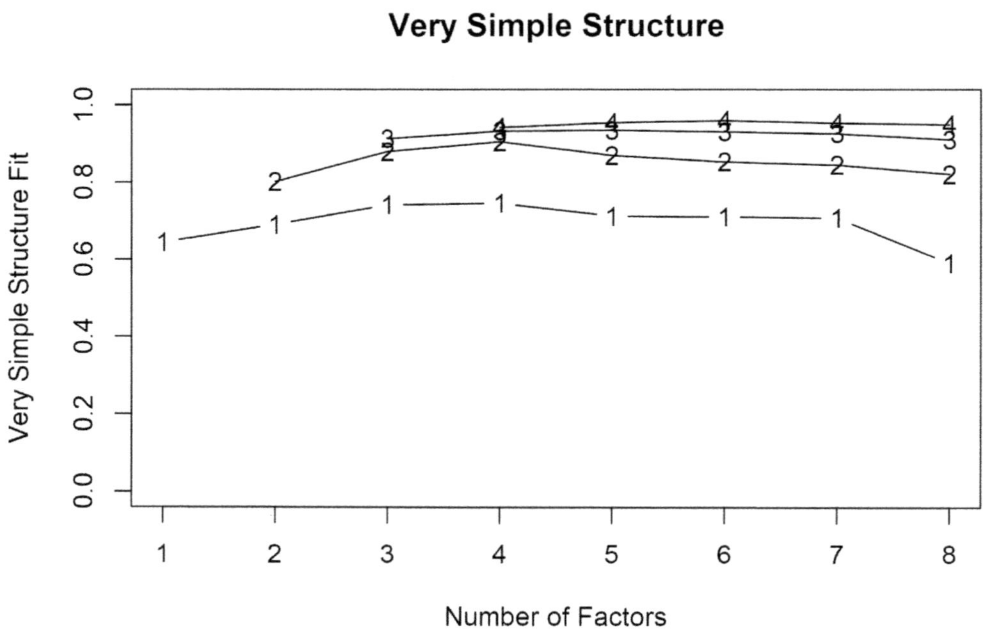

FIGURE 6.35 Very Simple Structure Plot with Orthogonal Rotation in Principal Component Analysis.

```
Very Simple Structure
Call: vss(x = HolzingerSwineford1939[, vars], rotate = "varimax", fm = "pc")
VSS complexity 1 achieves a maximimum of 0.75  with  4  factors
VSS complexity 2 achieves a maximimum of 0.91  with  4  factors

The Velicer MAP achieves a minimum of 0.07  with  2  factors
BIC achieves a minimum of  Inf  with    factors
Sample Size adjusted BIC achieves a minimum of  Inf  with    factors

Statistics by number of factors
  vss1 vss2   map dof chisq prob sqresid  fit RMSEA BIC SABIC complex
1 0.64 0.00 0.078   0    NA   NA   5.853 0.64    NA  NA    NA      NA
2 0.69 0.80 0.067   0    NA   NA   3.266 0.80    NA  NA    NA      NA
3 0.74 0.88 0.071   0    NA   NA   1.434 0.91    NA  NA    NA      NA
4 0.75 0.91 0.125   0    NA   NA   0.954 0.94    NA  NA    NA      NA
5 0.71 0.87 0.199   0    NA   NA   0.643 0.96    NA  NA    NA      NA
6 0.71 0.85 0.403   0    NA   NA   0.356 0.98    NA  NA    NA      NA
```

```
7 0.71 0.84 0.447    0     NA    NA    0.147 0.99     NA  NA     NA        NA
8 0.59 0.82 1.000    0     NA    NA    0.052 1.00     NA  NA     NA        NA
  eChisq SRMR eCRMS eBIC
1     NA   NA    NA   NA
2     NA   NA    NA   NA
3     NA   NA    NA   NA
4     NA   NA    NA   NA
5     NA   NA    NA   NA
6     NA   NA    NA   NA
7     NA   NA    NA   NA
8     NA   NA    NA   NA
```

6.5.2 Run the Principal Component Analysis

Principal component analysis (PCA) models were fit using the `psych` package (Revelle, 2022).

6.5.2.1 Orthogonal (Varimax) Rotation

```
pca1factorOrthogonal <- principal(
  HolzingerSwineford1939[,vars],
  nfactors = 1,
  rotate = "varimax")

pca2factorOrthogonal <- principal(
  HolzingerSwineford1939[,vars],
  nfactors = 2,
  rotate = "varimax")

pca3factorOrthogonal <- principal(
  HolzingerSwineford1939[,vars],
  nfactors = 3,
  rotate = "varimax")
```

6.5.2.2 Oblique (Oblimin) Rotation

An oblique (oblimin) rotation can be obtained by specifying `rotate = "oblimin"`.

```
pca3factorOblique <- principal(
  HolzingerSwineford1939[,vars],
  nfactors = 3,
  rotate = "oblimin")
```

6.5.3 Component Loadings

The component loadings can be extracted using the following syntax:

```
pca1factorOrthogonal
pca2factorOrthogonal
pca3factorOrthogonal
```

The component loadings for the three-component orthogonal model are below:

```
pca3factorOrthogonal
```

6.5.4 Component Scores

```
pca3Orthogonal <- pca3factorOrthogonal$scores
```

6.5.5 Plots

A biplot of the two-component orthogonal model is shown in Figure 6.36.

```
biplot(pca2factorOrthogonal)
abline(h = 0, v = 0, lty = 2)
```

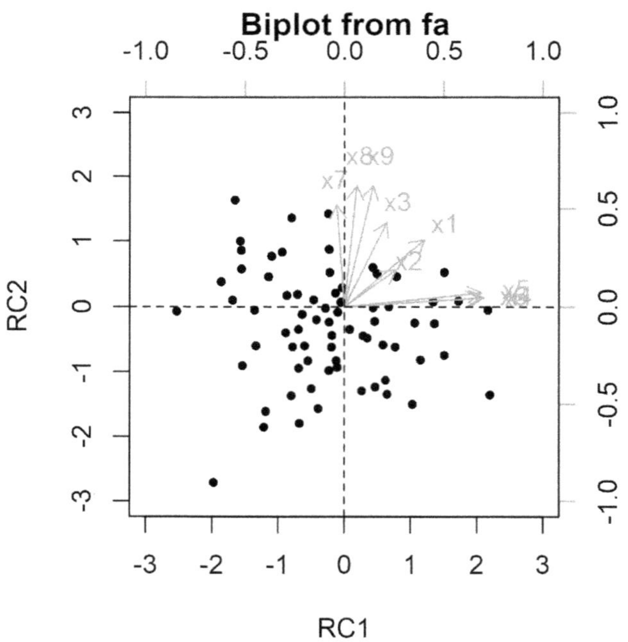

FIGURE 6.36 Biplot Using Orthogonal Rotation in Principal Component Analysis.

A pairs panel plot of the three-component orthogonal model is depicted in Figure 6.37.

```
pairs.panels(pca3Orthogonal)
```

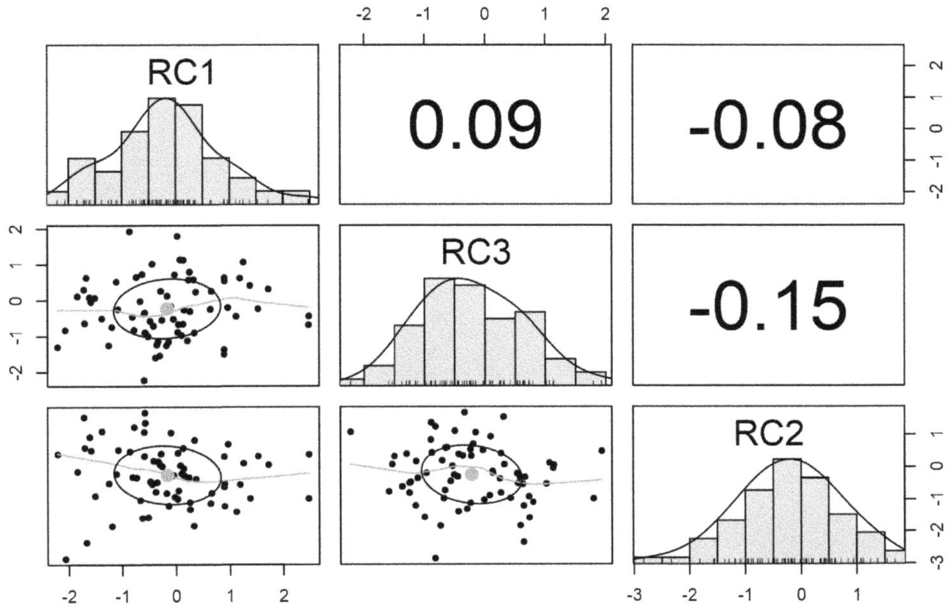

FIGURE 6.37 Pairs Panel Plot Using Orthogonal Rotation in Principal Component Analysis.

6.6 Conclusion

PCA is not factor analysis. PCA is a technique for data reduction, whereas factor analysis uses latent variables and can be used to identify the structure of measures/constructs or for data reduction. Many people use PCA when they should use factor analysis instead, such as when they are assessing latent constructs. Nevertheless, factor analysis has weaknesses including indeterminacy—i.e., a given data matrix can produce many different factor models, and you cannot determine which one is correct based on the data matrix alone. There are many decisions to make in factor analysis. These decisions can have important impacts on the resulting solution. Thus, it can be helpful for theory and interpretability to help guide decision-making when conducting factor analysis.

6.7 Suggested Readings

Floyd & Widaman (1995)

7

Structural Equation Modeling

> All models are wrong, but some are useful.
>
> — George Box (1979, p. 202)

7.1 Overview

Structural equation modeling is an advanced modeling approach that allows estimating latent variables to account for measurement error and to get purer estimates of constructs.

7.2 Getting Started

7.2.1 Load Libraries

```
library("petersenlab")
library("lavaan")
library("semTools")
library("semPlot")
library("simsem")
library("snow")
library("mice")
library("quantreg")
library("nonnest2")
library("MOTE")
library("here")
library("tidyverse")
library("tinytex")
library("knitr")
library("kableExtra")
```

```
library("rmarkdown")
library("bookdown")
```

7.2.2 Prepare Data

7.2.2.1 Simulate Data

`PoliticalDemocracy` refers to the Industrialization and Political Democracy data set from the `lavaan` package (Rosseel et al., 2022), and it contains measures of political democracy and industrialization in developing countries.

```
sampleSize <- 300

set.seed(52242)

v1 <- complement(PoliticalDemocracy$y1, .4)
v2 <- complement(PoliticalDemocracy$y1, .4)
v3 <- complement(PoliticalDemocracy$y1, .4)
v4 <- complement(PoliticalDemocracy$y1, .4)

PoliticalDemocracy$v1 <- v1
PoliticalDemocracy$v2 <- v2
PoliticalDemocracy$v3 <- v3
PoliticalDemocracy$v4 <- v4

measure1 <- rnorm(n = sampleSize, mean = 50, sd = 10)
measure2 <- measure1 + rnorm(n = sampleSize, mean = 0, sd = 15)
measure3 <- measure1 + measure2 + rnorm(n = sampleSize, mean = 0, sd = 15)
```

7.2.2.2 Add Missing Data

Adding missing data to dataframes helps make examples more realistic to real-life data and helps you get in the habit of programming to account for missing data.

```
measure1[c(5,10)] <- NA
measure2[c(10,15)] <- NA
measure3[c(10)] <- NA
PoliticalDemocracy <-
  as.data.frame(lapply(
    PoliticalDemocracy,
    function(cc) cc[ sample(
      c(TRUE, NA),
      prob = c(0.9, 0.1),
      size = length(cc),
      replace = TRUE)]))
```

7.2.2.3 Combine Data into Dataframe

```
mydataSEM <- data.frame(measure1, measure2, measure3)
```

7.3 Types of Models

7.3.1 Path Analysis Model

To understand structural equation modeling (SEM), it is helpful to first understand *path analysis*. Path analysis is similar to multiple regression. Path analysis allows examining the association between multiple predictor variables (or independent variables) in relation to an outcome variable (or dependent variable). Unlike multiple regression, however, path analysis also allows inclusion of multiple *dependent* variables in the same model. Unlike SEM, path analysis uses only manifest (observed) variables, not latent variables (described next). SEM is path analysis, but with latent (unobserved) variables. That is, a SEM model is a model that includes latent variables in addition to observed variables, where one attempts to model (i.e., explain) the *structure* of associations between variance using a series of equations (hence structural equation modeling).

7.3.2 Components of a Structural Equation Model

7.3.2.1 Measurement Model

The measurement model is a crucial sub-component of any SEM model. A SEM model consists of two components: a measurement model and a structural model. The *measurement model* is a confirmatory factor analysis (CFA) model that identifies how many latent factors are estimated, and which items load onto which latent factor. The measurement model can also specify correlated residuals. Basically, the measurement model specifies your best understanding of the structure of the latent construct(s) given how they were assessed. Before fitting the structural component of a SEM, it is important to have a well-fitting measurement model for each construct in the model. In Section 7.3.2.1, we present an example of a measurement model.

7.3.2.2 Structural Model

The *structural component* of a SEM model includes the regression paths that specify the hypothesized causal relations among the latent variables.

7.3.3 Confirmatory Factor Analysis Model

Confirmatory factor analysis (CFA) is a subset of SEM. CFA includes the measurement model but not the structural component of the model. In Section 7.8, we present an example of a CFA model. We discuss CFA models in greater depth in Chapter 6.

7.3.4 Structural Equation Model

SEM is CFA, but it adds regression paths that specify hypothesized causal relations between the latent variables, which is called the structural component of the model. The structural model includes the hypothesized causal relations between latent variables. A SEM model includes both the measurement model and the structural model (see Figure 7.1, Civelek, 2018). SEM fits a model to observed data, or the variance-covariance matrix, and evaluates the degree of model misfit. That is, fit indices evaluate how likely it is that a given model gave rise to the observed data. In Section 7.9, we present an example of a SEM model.

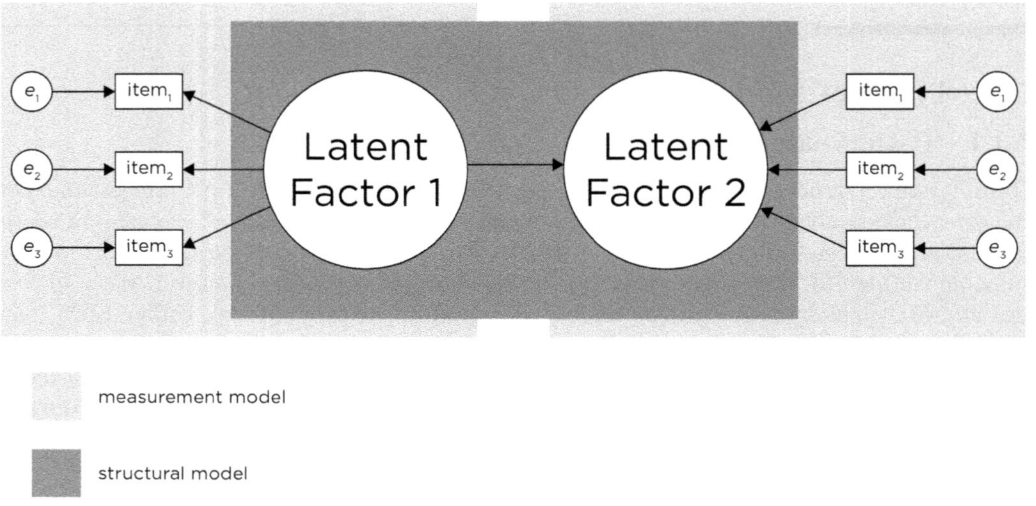

FIGURE 7.1 Demarcation Between Measurement Model and Structural Model. (Figure adapted from Civelek (2018), figure 1, p. 7. Civelek, M. E. (2018). *Essentials of structural equation modeling*. Zea E-Books. https://doi.org/10.13014/K2SJ1HR5)

SEM is flexible in allowing you to specify measurement error and correlated errors. Thus, you do not need the same assumptions as in classical test theory, which assumes that errors are random and uncorrelated. But the flexibility of SEM also poses challenges because you must explicitly decide what to include—and not include—in your model. This flexibility can be both a blessing and a curse. If the model fit is unacceptable, you can try fitting a different model to see which fits better. Nevertheless, it is important to use theory as a guide when specifying and comparing competing models, and not just rely solely on model fit comparison. For example, the model you fit should depend on how you conceptualize each construct: as reflective or formative.

7.4 Estimating Latent Factors

7.4.1 Model Identification

7.4.1.1 Types of Model Identification

There are important practical issues to consider with both reflective and formative models. An important practical issue is model identification—adding enough constraints so that there is only one, best answer. The model is identified when each of the estimated parameters has a unique solution.

Degrees of freedom in a SEM model is the number of known values minus the number of estimated parameters. The number of known values in a SEM model is the number of variances and covariances in the variance-covariance matrix of the manifest (observed) variables in addition to the number of means (i.e., the number of manifest variables), which can be calculated as: $\frac{m(m+1)}{2} + m$, where $m =$ the number of manifest variables. You can never estimate more parameters than the number of known values. A model with zero degrees of freedom is considered "saturated"—it will have perfect fit because the model estimates as many parameters as there are known values. All things equal (i.e., in terms of model fit with the same number of manifest variables), a model with more degrees of freedom is preferred for its parsimony, because fewer parameters are estimated.

Based on the number of known values compared to the number of estimated parameters, a model can be considered either just identified, under-identified, or over-identified. A *just identified model* is a model in which the number of known values is equal to the number of parameters to be estimated (degrees of freedom $= 0$). An *under-identified model* is a model in which the number of known values is less than the number of parameters to be estimated (degrees of freedom < 0). An *over-identified model* is a model in which the number of known values is greater than the number of parameters to be estimated (degrees of freedom > 0).

As an example, there are 14 known values for a model with 4 manifest variables ($\frac{4(4+1)}{2} + 4 = 14$): 4 variances, 6 covariances, and 4 means.

Here is the variance-covariance matrix:

```
vcovMatrix4measures <- cov(
  PoliticalDemocracy[,c("y1","y2","y3","y4")],
  use = "pairwise.complete.obs")

vcovMatrix4measures[upper.tri(vcovMatrix4measures)] <- NA

vcovMatrix4measures
```

```
      y1     y2     y3    y4
y1 6.387     NA     NA    NA
y2 6.060 16.425     NA    NA
y3 5.613  6.329 11.066    NA
y4 5.394  9.911  7.152 11.22
```

Here are the variances:

```
variances4measures <- diag(vcovMatrix4measures)

variances4measures
```

```
    y1     y2     y3     y4
 6.387 16.425 11.066 11.221
```

Here are the covariances:

```
covariances4measures <- vcovMatrix4measures[lower.tri(vcovMatrix4measures)]

covariances4measures
```

```
[1] 6.060 5.613 5.394 6.329 9.911 7.152
```

Here are the means:

```
means4Measures <- apply(
  PoliticalDemocracy[,c("y1","y2","y3","y4")],
  2, mean, na.rm = TRUE)

means4Measures
```

```
   y1    y2    y3    y4
5.347 4.285 6.367 4.357
```

7.4.1.2 Approaches to Model Identification

The three most widely used approaches to identifying latent factors are:

1. Marker variable
2. Effects coding
3. Standardized latent factor

7.4.1.2.1 Marker variable method

In the marker variable method, one of the indicators (i.e., manifest variables) is set to have a loading of 1. Here are examples of using the marker variable method for identification of a latent variable:

```
markerVariable_syntax <- '
 latentFactor =~ y1 + y2 + y3 + y4
'

markerVariableModelFit <- sem(
  markerVariable_syntax,
  data = PoliticalDemocracy,
  missing = "ML",
  estimator = "MLR")
```

7.4.1.2.2 Effects coding method

In the effects coding method, the average of the factor loadings is set to be 1. The effects coding method is useful if you are interested in the means or variances of the latent factor, because the metric of the latent factor is on the metric of the indicators. Here are examples of using the effects coding method for identification of a latent variable:

```
effectsCoding_abbreviatedSyntax <- '
 latentFactor =~ y1 + y2 + y3 + y4
'

effectsCodingModelFit_abbreviated <- sem(
  effectsCoding_abbreviatedSyntax,
  data = PoliticalDemocracy,
```

```
  effect.coding = "loadings",
  missing = "ML",
  estimator = "MLR")
```

7.4.1.2.3 Standardized latent factor method

In the standardized latent factor method, the latent factor is set to have a mean of 0 and a standard deviation of 1. The standardized latent factor method is a useful approach if you are not interested in the means or variances of the latent factors and want to freely estimate the factor loadings. Here are examples of using the standardized latent factor method for identification of a latent variable:

```
standardizedLatent_abbreviatedsyntax <- '
 latentFactor =~ y1 + y2 + y3 + y4
'

standardizedLatentFit_abbreviated <- sem(
  standardizedLatent_abbreviatedsyntax,
  data = PoliticalDemocracy,
  std.lv = TRUE,
  missing = "ML",
  estimator = "MLR")
```

7.4.2 Types of Latent Factors

7.4.2.1 Reflective Latent Factors

For a reflective model with 4 indicators, we would need to estimate 12 parameters: a factor loading, error term, and intercept for each of the 4 indicators. Here are the parameters estimated:

```
reflectiveModel_syntax <- '
 #Reflective model factor loadings
 reflective =~ y1 + y2 + y3 + y4
'

reflectiveModelFit <- sem(
  reflectiveModel_syntax,
  data = PoliticalDemocracy,
  missing = "ML",
  estimator = "MLR",
  std.lv = TRUE)

reflectiveModelParameters <- parameterEstimates(
  reflectiveModelFit)[!is.na(parameterEstimates(reflectiveModelFit)$z),]

row.names(reflectiveModelParameters) <- NULL
```

Here are the degrees of freedom:

```
fitMeasures(reflectiveModelFit, "df")
```

```
df
 2
```

Thus, for a reflective model, we only have to estimate a small number of parameters to specify what is happening in our model, so the model is parsimonious. With 4 indicators, the number of known values (14) is greater than the number of parameters (12). We have 2 degrees of freedom ($14 - 12 = 2$). Because the degrees of freedom is greater than 0, it is easy to identify the model—the model is over-identified. A reflective model with 3 indicators would have 9 known values ($\frac{3(3+1)}{2} + 3 = 9$), 9 parameters (3 factor loadings, 3 error terms, 3 intercepts), and 0 degrees of freedom, and it would be identifiable because it would be just-identified.

7.4.2.2 Formative Latent Factors

However, for a formative model, we must specify more parameters: a factor loading, intercept, and variance for each of the 4 indicators, all 6 permissive correlations, and 1 error term for the latent variable, for a total of 19 parameters. Here are the parameters estimated:

```
formativeModel_syntax <- '
 #Formative model factor loadings
 formative <~ v1 + v2 + v3 + v4

 formative ~~ formative
'

formativeModelFit <- sem(
  formativeModel_syntax,
  data = PoliticalDemocracy,
  missing = "ML",
  estimator = "MLR")

formativeModelParameters <- parameterEstimates(formativeModelFit)
```

For a formative model with 4 measures, the number of known values (14) is less than the number of parameters (19). The number of degrees of freedom is negative ($14 - 19 = -5$), thus the model is not able to be identified—the model is under-identified.

Thus, for a formative model, we need more parameters than we have data—the model is under-identified. Therefore, to estimate a formative model with 4 indicators, we must add assumptions and other variables that are consequences of the formative construct. Options for identifying a formative construct are described by Treiblmaier et al. (2011). See below for an example formative model that is identified because of additional assumptions.

```
formativeModel2_syntax <- '
 #Formative model factor loadings
 formative <~ 1*v1 + v2 + v3 + v4
 reflective =~ y1 + y2 + y3 + y4
```

```
 formative ~~ 1*formative
 reflective ~ formative
'

formativeModel2Fit <- sem(
  formativeModel2_syntax,
  data = PoliticalDemocracy,
  missing = "ML",
  estimator = "MLR")

formativeModel2Parameters <- parameterEstimates(formativeModel2Fit)

fitMeasures(formativeModel2Fit, "df")
```

```
df
14
```

Thus, formative constructs are challenging to use in a SEM framework. To estimate a formative construct in a SEM framework, the formative construct must be used in the context of a model that allows some constraints. A formative latent factor includes a disturbance term, and is thus not entirely determined by the causal indicators (Bollen & Bauldry, 2011). A composite (such as in principal component analysis), by contrast, has no disturbance term and is therefore completely determined by the composite indicators (Bollen & Bauldry, 2011). Emerging techniques such as confirmatory composite analysis allow estimation of formative composites (Schuberth, 2023; Yu et al., 2023).

7.5 Additional Types of SEM

Up to this point, we have discussed SEM with dimensional constructs. It also worth knowing about additional types of SEM models, including latent class models and mixture models, that handle categorical constructs. However, most disorders are more accurately conceptualized as dimensional than as categorical (Markon et al., 2011), so just because you can estimate categorical latent factors does not necessarily mean that one should.

7.5.1 Latent Class Models

In *latent class models*, the construct is not dimensional, but rather categorical. The categorical constructs are latent classifications and are called latent classes. For instance, the construct could be a diagnosis that influences scores on the measures. Latent class models examine qualitative differences in kind, rather than quantitative differences in degree.

7.5.2 Mixture Models

Mixture models allow for a combination of latent categorical constructs (classes) and latent dimensional constructs. That is, it allows for both qualitative and quantitative differences. However, this additional model complexity also necessitates a larger sample size for estimation. SEM generally requires a 3-digit sample size ($N = 100+$), whereas mixture models typically require a 4- or 5-digit sample size ($N = 1,000+$).

7.5.3 Exploratory Structural Equation Models

We describe exploratory structural equation models in Section 6.1.4.3.3.

7.6 Model Fit Indices

Various model fit indices can be used for evaluating how well a model fits the data and for comparing the fit of two competing models. Fit indices known as absolute fit indices compare whether the model fits better than the best-possible fitting model (i.e., a saturated model). Examples of absolute fit indices include the chi-square test, root mean square error of approximation (RMSEA), and the standardized root mean square residual (SRMR).

The chi-square test evaluates whether the model has a significant degree of misfit relative to the best-possible fitting model (a saturated model that fits as many parameters as possible; i.e., as many parameters as there are degrees of freedom); the null hypothesis of a chi-square test is that there is no difference between the predicted data (i.e., the data that would be observed if the model were true) and the observed data. Thus, a non-significant chi-square test indicates good model fit. However, because the null hypothesis of the chi-square test is that the model-implied covariance matrix is exactly equal to the observed covariance matrix (i.e., a model of perfect fit), this may be an unrealistic comparison. Models are simplifications of reality, and our models are virtually never expected to be a perfect description of reality. Thus, we would say a model is "useful" and partially validated if "it helps us to understand the relation between variables and does a 'reasonable' job of matching the data...A perfect fit may be an inappropriate standard, and a high chi-square estimate may indicate what we already know—that the hypothesized model holds approximately, not perfectly." (Bollen, 1989, p. 268). The power of the chi-square test depends on sample size, and a large sample will likely detect small differences as significantly worse than the best-possible fitting model (Bollen, 1989).

RMSEA is an index of absolute fit. Lower values indicate better fit.

SRMR is an index of absolute fit with no penalty for model complexity. Lower values indicate better fit.

There are also various fit indices known as incremental, comparative, or relative fit indices that compare whether the model fits better than the worst-possible fitting model (i.e., a "baseline" or "null" model). Incremental fit indices include a chi-square difference test, the comparative fit index (CFI), and the Tucker-Lewis index (TLI). Unlike the chi-square test comparing the model to the best-possible fitting model, a significant chi-square test of the relative fit index indicates better fit—i.e., that the model fits better than the worst-possible fitting model.

CFI is another relative fit index that compares the model to the worst-possible fitting model. Higher values indicate better fit.

TLI is another relative fit index. Higher values indicate better fit.

Parsimony fit include fit indices that use information criteria fit indices, including the Akaike Information Criterion (AIC) and the Bayesian Information Criterion (BIC). BIC penalizes model complexity more so than AIC. Lower AIC and BIC values indicate better fit.

Chi-square difference tests and CFI can be used to compare two nested models. AIC and BIC can be used to compare two non-nested models.

Criteria for acceptable fit and good fit of SEM models are shown in Table 7.1. In addition, dynamic fit indexes have been proposed based on simulation to identify fit index cutoffs that are tailored to the characteristics of the specific model and data (McNeish & Wolf, 2023).

TABLE 7.1 Criteria for Acceptable and Good Fit of Structural Equation Models Based on Fit Indices.

SEM Fit Index	Acceptable Fit	Good Fit
RMSEA	$\leq .08$	$\leq .05$
CFI	$\geq .90$	$\geq .95$
TLI	$\geq .90$	$\geq .95$
SRMR	$\leq .10$	$\leq .08$

However, good model fit does not necessarily indicate a true model.

In addition to fit indices, it can be helpful to examine model correlation residuals. Correlation residuals greater than $|.10|$ are possible evidence for poor local fit (Kline, 2023). If a correlation residual is positive, it suggests that the model underpredicts the observed association between the two variables. If a correlation residual is negative, it suggests that the model overpredicts their observed association between the two variables. If the two variables are connected by only indirect pathways, it may be helpful to respecify the model with direct pathways between the two variables, such as a direct effect (i.e., regression path) or a covariance path.

7.7 Measurement Model (of a Given Construct)

In the measurement model below, we present a simple one-factor model with three measures. The measurement model is what we settle on as the estimation of each construct before we add the structural component to estimate the relations among latent variables. Basically, we add the structural component onto the measurement model. In Section 7.8, we present a CFA model with multiple latent factors.

The measurement models were fit in the `lavaan` package (Rosseel et al., 2022).

7.7.1 Specify the Model

```
measurementModel_syntax <- '
 latentFactor =~ measure1 + measure2 + measure3
'
```

7.7.2 Fit the Model

```
measurementModelFit <- cfa(
  measurementModel_syntax,
  data = mydataSEM,
  missing = "ML",
  estimator = "MLR",
  std.lv = TRUE)
```

7.7.3 Display Summary Output

This measurement model with three indicators is just-identified—the number of parameters estimated is equal to the number of known values, thus leaving 0 degrees of freedom. In the model, all three indicators load strongly on the latent factor (measure 1: $\beta = 0.69$; measure 2: $\beta = 0.79$; measure 3: $\beta = 0.98$). Thus, the loadings of this measurement model would be consistent with a reflective latent construct. In terms of interpretation, all three indicators loaded positively on the latent factor, so higher levels of the latent factor are indicated by higher levels on the indicators. However, one of the estimated observed variances is negative, so the model is not able to be estimated accurately. Thus, we would need to make additional adjustments in order to estimate the model. Because the model is just-identified, many fit statistics are not able to be estimated.

7.7.4 Internal Consistency Reliability

Internal consistency reliability of items composing the latent factors, as quantified by omega (ω) and average variance extracted (AVE), was estimated using the `semTools` package (Jorgensen et al., 2021).

```
compRelSEM(measurementModelFit)
```

```
latentFactor
       0.925
```

```
AVE(measurementModelFit)
```

```
latentFactor
       0.841
```

7.8 Confirmatory Factor Analysis

The confirmatory factor analysis (CFA) models were fit in the `lavaan` package (Rosseel et al., 2022). The examples were adapted from the `lavaan` documentation: http://lavaan.ugent.be/tutorial/cfa.html (archived at https://perma.cc/GKY3-9YE4).

In this CFA model, we estimate three latent factors with three indicators loading on each latent factor.

7.8.1 Specify the Model

```
cfaModel_syntax <- '
 visual  =~ x1 + x2 + x3
 textual =~ x4 + x5 + x6
 speed   =~ x7 + x8 + x9
'
```

7.8.2 Fit the Model

```
cfaModelFit <- cfa(
  cfaModel_syntax,
  data = HolzingerSwineford1939,
  missing = "ML",
  estimator = "MLR",
  std.lv = TRUE)
```

7.8.3 Display Summary Output

In this model, all nine indicators load strongly on their respective latent factor. Thus, this measurement model would be defensible. In terms of interpretation, all indicators load positively on their respective latent factor, so higher levels of the latent factor are indicated by higher levels on the indicators.

```
summary(
  cfaModelFit,
  fit.measures = TRUE,
  standardized = TRUE,
  rsquare = TRUE)
```

```
lavaan 0.6.17 ended normally after 40 iterations

  Estimator                                         ML
  Optimization method                           NLMINB
  Number of model parameters                        30

  Number of observations                           301
  Number of missing patterns                        75

Model Test User Model:
                                              Standard      Scaled
  Test Statistic                                65.643      63.641
  Degrees of freedom                                24          24
  P-value (Chi-square)                           0.000       0.000
  Scaling correction factor                                  1.031
    Yuan-Bentler correction (Mplus variant)

Model Test Baseline Model:

  Test statistic                               693.305     646.574
  Degrees of freedom                                36          36
  P-value                                        0.000       0.000
  Scaling correction factor                                  1.072

User Model versus Baseline Model:

  Comparative Fit Index (CFI)                    0.937       0.935
```

```
  Tucker-Lewis Index (TLI)                        0.905       0.903

  Robust Comparative Fit Index (CFI)                          0.930
  Robust Tucker-Lewis Index (TLI)                             0.894

Loglikelihood and Information Criteria:

  Loglikelihood user model (H0)               -3213.600   -3213.600
  Scaling correction factor                                   1.090
      for the MLR correction
  Loglikelihood unrestricted model (H1)       -3180.778   -3180.778
  Scaling correction factor                                   1.064
      for the MLR correction

  Akaike (AIC)                                 6487.199    6487.199
  Bayesian (BIC)                               6598.413    6598.413
  Sample-size adjusted Bayesian (SABIC)        6503.270    6503.270

Root Mean Square Error of Approximation:

  RMSEA                                           0.076       0.074
  90 Percent confidence interval - lower          0.054       0.053
  90 Percent confidence interval - upper          0.098       0.096
  P-value H_0: RMSEA <= 0.050                     0.026       0.034
  P-value H_0: RMSEA >= 0.080                     0.403       0.349

  Robust RMSEA                                                0.092
  90 Percent confidence interval - lower                      0.064
  90 Percent confidence interval - upper                      0.120
  P-value H_0: Robust RMSEA <= 0.050                          0.008
  P-value H_0: Robust RMSEA >= 0.080                          0.780

Standardized Root Mean Square Residual:

  SRMR                                            0.061       0.061

Parameter Estimates:

  Standard errors                              Sandwich
  Information bread                            Observed
  Observed information based on                 Hessian

Latent Variables:
                   Estimate  Std.Err  z-value  P(>|z|)   Std.lv
  visual =~
    x1                0.885    0.108    8.183    0.000    0.885
    x2                0.521    0.086    6.037    0.000    0.521
    x3                0.712    0.088    8.065    0.000    0.712
  textual =~
    x4                0.989    0.067   14.690    0.000    0.989
    x5                1.121    0.066   16.890    0.000    1.121
```

```
    x6                 0.849    0.065   12.991    0.000    0.849
  speed =~
    x7                 0.596    0.084    7.092    0.000    0.596
    x8                 0.742    0.096    7.703    0.000    0.742
    x9                 0.686    0.099    6.939    0.000    0.686
  Std.all

    0.762
    0.451
    0.632

    0.842
    0.866
    0.818

    0.557
    0.733
    0.673

Covariances:
                   Estimate  Std.Err  z-value  P(>|z|)   Std.lv
  visual ~~
    textual            0.430    0.080    5.386    0.000    0.430
    speed              0.465    0.110    4.213    0.000    0.465
  textual ~~
    speed              0.314    0.084    3.746    0.000    0.314
  Std.all

    0.430
    0.465

    0.314

Intercepts:
                   Estimate  Std.Err  z-value  P(>|z|)   Std.lv
   .x1                 4.977    0.071   69.850    0.000    4.977
   .x2                 6.050    0.070   85.953    0.000    6.050
   .x3                 2.227    0.069   32.218    0.000    2.227
   .x4                 3.097    0.071   43.828    0.000    3.097
   .x5                 4.344    0.077   56.058    0.000    4.344
   .x6                 2.187    0.064   34.391    0.000    2.187
   .x7                 4.180    0.065   64.446    0.000    4.180
   .x8                 5.517    0.062   89.668    0.000    5.517
   .x9                 5.405    0.063   86.063    0.000    5.405
  Std.all
    4.289
    5.235
    1.976
    2.634
    3.355
    2.108
```

```
    3.904
    5.451
    5.298

Variances:
                   Estimate  Std.Err  z-value  P(>|z|)   Std.lv
   .x1                0.564    0.169    3.345    0.001    0.564
   .x2                1.064    0.119    8.935    0.000    1.064
   .x3                0.763    0.118    6.454    0.000    0.763
   .x4                0.403    0.063    6.363    0.000    0.403
   .x5                0.420    0.074    5.664    0.000    0.420
   .x6                0.356    0.056    6.415    0.000    0.356
   .x7                0.790    0.093    8.512    0.000    0.790
   .x8                0.474    0.128    3.693    0.000    0.474
   .x9                0.570    0.122    4.660    0.000    0.570
    visual            1.000                               1.000
    textual           1.000                               1.000
    speed             1.000                               1.000
  Std.all
    0.419
    0.797
    0.601
    0.292
    0.251
    0.331
    0.690
    0.463
    0.548
    1.000
    1.000
    1.000

R-Square:
                   Estimate
    x1                0.581
    x2                0.203
    x3                0.399
    x4                0.708
    x5                0.749
    x6                0.669
    x7                0.310
    x8                0.537
    x9                0.452
```

7.8.4 Estimates of Model Fit

According to model fit estimates, the model fit is good according to SRMR and acceptable according to CFI, but the model fit is weaker according to RMSEA and TLI. Thus, we may want to consider adjustments to improve the model fit. In general, we want to make decisions regarding what parameters to estimate based on theory in conjunction with empiricism.

```r
fitMeasures(
  cfaModelFit,
  fit.measures = c(
    "chisq", "df", "pvalue",
    "chisq.scaled", "df.scaled", "pvalue.scaled",
    "chisq.scaling.factor",
    "baseline.chisq","baseline.df","baseline.pvalue",
    "rmsea", "cfi", "tli", "srmr",
    "rmsea.robust", "cfi.robust", "tli.robust"))
```

```
                 chisq                     df                 pvalue 
                65.643                 24.000                  0.000 
          chisq.scaled              df.scaled          pvalue.scaled 
                63.641                 24.000                  0.000 
  chisq.scaling.factor         baseline.chisq            baseline.df 
                 1.031                693.305                 36.000 
       baseline.pvalue                  rmsea                    cfi 
                 0.000                  0.076                  0.937 
                   tli                   srmr           rmsea.robust 
                 0.905                  0.061                  0.092 
            cfi.robust             tli.robust 
                 0.930                  0.894 
```

7.8.5 Residuals

```r
residuals(cfaModelFit, type = "cor")
```

```
$type
[1] "cor.bollen"

$cov
       x1     x2     x3     x4     x5     x6     x7     x8     x9
x1  0.000                                                        
x2 -0.020  0.000                                                 
x3 -0.019  0.053  0.000                                          
x4  0.077 -0.035 -0.083  0.000                                   
x5  0.015 -0.006 -0.119  0.004  0.000                            
x6  0.044  0.038 -0.002 -0.005  0.002  0.000                     
x7 -0.178 -0.215 -0.073  0.005 -0.061 -0.032  0.000              
x8 -0.017 -0.053 -0.013 -0.088 -0.018 -0.008  0.062  0.000       
x9  0.103  0.067  0.192  0.003  0.084  0.043 -0.031 -0.044  0.000

$mean
    x1     x2     x3     x4     x5     x6     x7     x8     x9 
 0.001 -0.003 -0.002 -0.004 -0.003  0.006  0.000  0.002  0.000 
```

TABLE 7.2 Modification Indices from Confirmatory Factor Analysis Model.

	lhs	op	rhs	mi	epc	sepc.lv	sepc.all	sepc.nox
42	visual	=~	x9	22.57	0.48	0.48	0.47	0.47
88	x7	~~	x8	21.07	0.46	0.46	0.75	0.75
40	visual	=~	x7	17.00	−0.40	−0.40	−0.37	−0.37
90	x8	~~	x9	12.70	−0.45	−0.45	−0.87	−0.87
75	x3	~~	x9	10.57	0.19	0.19	0.29	0.29
67	x2	~~	x7	7.75	−0.19	−0.19	−0.21	−0.21

7.8.6 Modification Indices

Modification indices indicate potential additional parameters that could be estimated and that would improve model fit. For instance, the modification indices in Table 7.2 (generated from the syntax below) indicate a few additional factor loadings (i.e., cross-loadings) or correlated residuals that could substantially improve model fit. However, it is generally not recommended to blindly estimate additional parameters solely based on modification indices. Rather, it is generally advised to consider modification indices in light of theory.

```
cfaModelFitIndices <- modificationindices(cfaModelFit, sort. = TRUE)
```

7.8.7 Internal Consistency Reliability

Internal consistency reliability of items composing the latent factors, as quantified by omega (ω) and average variance extracted (AVE), was estimated using the `semTools` package (Jorgensen et al., 2021).

```
compRelSEM(cfaModelFit)
```

```
 visual textual   speed 
  0.652   0.878   0.695 
```

```
AVE(cfaModelFit)
```

```
 visual textual   speed 
  0.397   0.713   0.430 
```

7.8.8 Modify Model Based on Modification Indices

In the model below, we modified the model based on estimating an additional factor loading (assuming the additional factor loading is theoretically supported). This could be supported, for instance, if a given test involves considerable skills in both the visual domain and in speed of processing. When the same indicator loads simultaneously on two factors, this is called a *cross-loading*. Cross-loadings can complicate the interpretation of latent factors, as discussed in Section 6.1.4.5 of the chapter on factor analysis.

7.8.8.1 Specify the Model

```
cfaModel2_syntax <- '
 textual =~ x4 + x5 + x6
 visual  =~ x1 + x2 + x3 + x9
 speed   =~ x7 + x8 + x9
'
```

7.8.8.2 Fit the Model

```
cfaModel2Fit <- cfa(
  cfaModel2_syntax,
  data = HolzingerSwineford1939,
  missing = "ML",
  estimator = "MLR",
  std.lv = TRUE)
```

7.8.8.3 Estimates of Model Fit

After fitting the additional factor loading, the model fits well according to RMSEA, CFI, and SRMR, and the model fit is acceptable according to TLI. Thus, this model could be defensible.

```
fitMeasures(
  cfaModel2Fit,
  fit.measures = c(
    "chisq", "df", "pvalue",
    "chisq.scaled", "df.scaled", "pvalue.scaled",
    "chisq.scaling.factor",
    "baseline.chisq","baseline.df","baseline.pvalue",
    "rmsea", "cfi", "tli", "srmr",
    "rmsea.robust", "cfi.robust", "tli.robust"))
```

```
               chisq                   df               pvalue
              44.101               23.000                0.005
        chisq.scaled            df.scaled        pvalue.scaled
              41.745               23.000                0.010
chisq.scaling.factor       baseline.chisq          baseline.df
               1.056              693.305               36.000
     baseline.pvalue                rmsea                  cfi
               0.000                0.055                0.968
                 tli                 srmr         rmsea.robust
               0.950                0.045                0.069
          cfi.robust           tli.robust
               0.962                0.941
```

7.8.8.4 Compare Model Fit

The modified model with the cross-loading and the original model are considered "nested" models. The original model is nested within the modified model because the modified model includes all of the terms of the original model along with additional terms. Model fit of nested models can be compared with a chi-square difference test.

```
anova(cfaModelFit, cfaModel2Fit)
```

```

Scaled Chi-Squared Difference Test (method = "satorra.bentler.2001")

lavaan NOTE:
    The "Chisq" column contains standard test statistics, not the
    robust test that should be reported per model. A robust difference
    test is a function of two standard (not robust) statistics.

             Df  AIC  BIC Chisq Chisq diff Df diff Pr(>Chisq)
cfaModel2Fit 23 6468 6583  44.1
cfaModelFit  24 6487 6598  65.6       47.2       1    6.4e-12 ***
---
Signif. codes:  0 '***' 0.001 '**' 0.01 '*' 0.05 '.' 0.1 ' ' 1
```

In this case, the model with the cross-loading fits significantly better (i.e., has a significantly smaller chi-square value) than the model without the cross-loading.

One can also compare nested models using a robust likelihood ratio test:

```
cfaModelFitML <- cfa(
  cfaModel_syntax,
  data = HolzingerSwineford1939,
  missing = "ML",
  estimator = "ML",
  std.lv = TRUE)

cfaModel2FitML <- cfa(
  cfaModel2_syntax,
  data = HolzingerSwineford1939,
  missing = "ML",
  estimator = "ML",
  std.lv = TRUE)

vuongtest(
  cfaModelFitML,
  cfaModel2FitML,
  nested = TRUE)
```

```

Model 1
 Class: lavaan
 Call: lavaan::lavaan(model = cfaModel2_syntax, data = HolzingerSwineford1939, ...
```

```
Model 2
 Class: lavaan
 Call: lavaan::lavaan(model = cfaModel_syntax, data = HolzingerSwineford1939, ...

Variance test
  H0: Model 1 and Model 2 are indistinguishable
  H1: Model 1 and Model 2 are distinguishable
    w2 = 0.075,   p = 0.00123

Robust likelihood ratio test of distinguishable models
  H0: Model 2 fits as well as Model 1
  H1: Model 1 fits better than Model 2
    LR = 21.541,   p = 1.18e-05
```

For non-nested models, one can compare model fit with AIC, BIC, or the Vuong test.

```
fitMeasures(
  cfaModelFitML,
  fit.measures = c(
    "aic","bic","bic2"))
```

```
 aic  bic bic2
6487 6598 6503
```

```
fitMeasures(
  cfaModel2FitML,
  fit.measures = c(
    "aic","bic","bic2"))
```

```
 aic  bic bic2
6468 6583 6484
```

```
vuongtest(
  cfaModelFitML,
  cfaModel2FitML,
  nested = FALSE)
```

```
Model 1
 Class: lavaan
 Call: lavaan::lavaan(model = cfaModel_syntax, data = HolzingerSwineford1939, ...

Model 2
 Class: lavaan
 Call: lavaan::lavaan(model = cfaModel2_syntax, data = HolzingerSwineford1939, ...

Variance test
  H0: Model 1 and Model 2 are indistinguishable
  H1: Model 1 and Model 2 are distinguishable
    w2 = 0.075,   p = 0.00123
```

```
Non-nested likelihood ratio test
  H0: Model fits are equal for the focal population
  H1A: Model 1 fits better than Model 2
    z = -2.270,    p = 0.988
  H1B: Model 2 fits better than Model 1
    z = -2.270,    p = 0.01161
```

7.9 Structural Equation Model

The structural equation models were fit in the `lavaan` package (Rosseel et al., 2022). The examples were adapted from the `lavaan` documentation: http://lavaan.ugent.be/tutorial/sem.html (archived at https://perma.cc/8NG9-7JAG).

In this model, we fit a measurement model with three latent factors in addition to a structural model with regressions estimated among the latent factors.

7.9.1 Specify the Model

```
semModel_syntax <- '
 #Measurement model factor loadings
 ind60 =~ x1 + x2 + x3
 dem60 =~ y1 + y2 + y3 + y4
 dem65 =~ y5 + y6 + y7 + y8

 #Regression paths
 dem60 ~ ind60
 dem65 ~ ind60 + dem60

 #Covariances among residual variances (correlated errors)
 y1 ~~ y5
 y2 ~~ y4 + y6
 y3 ~~ y7
 y4 ~~ y8
 y6 ~~ y8
'
```

7.9.2 Fit the Model

```
semModelFit <- sem(
  semModel_syntax,
  data = PoliticalDemocracy,
  missing = "ML",
  estimator = "MLR",
  std.lv = TRUE)
```

7.9.3 Display Summary Output

7.9.3.1 Interpreting `lavaan` Output

Output from a SEM model includes information such as regression coefficients, intercepts, variances, and model fit indices. As noted above, there are two chi-square tests. In `lavaan` syntax, one is labeled "Model Test User Model" and the other is labeled "Model Test Baseline Model." The chi-square test labeled "Model Test User Model" refers to the chi-square test of whether the model fits worse than the best-possible fitting model. In this case, the p-value of the robust chi-square test is 0.17. Thus, the model does not show significant misfit—i.e., the model does not fit significantly worse than the best-possible fitting model. The chi-square test labeled "Model Test Baseline Model" refers to the chi-square test of whether the model fits better than the worst-possible fitting model. In this case, the p-value of the robust chi-square test in comparison to the worse-possible fitting model is $< .05$. Thus, the model fits significantly better than the worst-possible-fitting model.

In terms of the model findings, `ind60` was significantly positively associated with `dem60`, `dem60` was significantly positively associated with `dem65`, and `ind60` was marginally significantly positively associated with `dem65`.

```
summary(
  semModelFit,
  fit.measures = TRUE,
  standardized = TRUE,
  rsquare = TRUE)
```

```
lavaan 0.6.17 ended normally after 82 iterations

  Estimator                                         ML
  Optimization method                           NLMINB
  Number of model parameters                        42

  Number of observations                            75
  Number of missing patterns                        36

Model Test User Model:
                                              Standard      Scaled
  Test Statistic                                38.748      42.709
  Degrees of freedom                                35          35
  P-value (Chi-square)                           0.304       0.174
  Scaling correction factor                                  0.907
    Yuan-Bentler correction (Mplus variant)

Model Test Baseline Model:

  Test statistic                               601.314     594.441
  Degrees of freedom                                55          55
  P-value                                        0.000       0.000
  Scaling correction factor                                  1.012

User Model versus Baseline Model:
```

```
  Comparative Fit Index (CFI)                    0.993       0.986
  Tucker-Lewis Index (TLI)                       0.989       0.978

  Robust Comparative Fit Index (CFI)                         0.988
  Robust Tucker-Lewis Index (TLI)                            0.981

Loglikelihood and Information Criteria:

  Loglikelihood user model (H0)              -1418.424   -1418.424
  Scaling correction factor                                  0.989
      for the MLR correction
  Loglikelihood unrestricted model (H1)      -1399.050   -1399.050
  Scaling correction factor                                  0.952
      for the MLR correction

  Akaike (AIC)                                2920.848    2920.848
  Bayesian (BIC)                              3018.183    3018.183
  Sample-size adjusted Bayesian (SABIC)       2885.810    2885.810

Root Mean Square Error of Approximation:

  RMSEA                                          0.038       0.054
  90 Percent confidence interval - lower         0.000       0.000
  90 Percent confidence interval - upper         0.094       0.106
  P-value H_0: RMSEA <= 0.050                    0.585       0.424
  P-value H_0: RMSEA >= 0.080                    0.126       0.240

  Robust RMSEA                                               0.055
  90 Percent confidence interval - lower                     0.000
  90 Percent confidence interval - upper                     0.113
  P-value H_0: Robust RMSEA <= 0.050                         0.422
  P-value H_0: Robust RMSEA >= 0.080                         0.279

Standardized Root Mean Square Residual:

  SRMR                                           0.046       0.046

Parameter Estimates:

  Standard errors                             Sandwich
  Information bread                           Observed
  Observed information based on                Hessian

Latent Variables:
                   Estimate  Std.Err  z-value  P(>|z|)   Std.lv
  ind60 =~
    x1                0.645    0.056   11.566    0.000    0.645
    x2                1.495    0.124   12.084    0.000    1.495
    x3                1.189    0.112   10.581    0.000    1.189
  dem60 =~
    y1                1.879    0.239    7.858    0.000    2.143
```

```
    y2                2.477    0.308    8.043    0.000    2.825
    y3                2.134    0.330    6.469    0.000    2.434
    y4                2.523    0.254    9.918    0.000    2.879
  dem65 =~
    y5                0.547    0.228    2.398    0.016    2.090
    y6                0.656    0.275    2.390    0.017    2.509
    y7                0.715    0.315    2.265    0.024    2.732
    y8                0.696    0.311    2.240    0.025    2.660
  Std.all

    0.908
    0.991
    0.863

    0.834
    0.714
    0.733
    0.864

    0.791
    0.753
    0.830
    0.805

Regressions:
                   Estimate  Std.Err  z-value  P(>|z|)   Std.lv
  dem60 ~
    ind60             0.549    0.162    3.381    0.001    0.481
  dem65 ~
    ind60             0.690    0.391    1.766    0.077    0.180
    dem60             2.900    1.362    2.129    0.033    0.865
  Std.all

    0.481

    0.180
    0.865

Covariances:
                   Estimate  Std.Err  z-value  P(>|z|)   Std.lv
 .y1 ~~
   .y5                0.728    0.511    1.427    0.154    0.728
 .y2 ~~
   .y4                1.087    0.847    1.284    0.199    1.087
   .y6                1.672    0.957    1.747    0.081    1.672
 .y3 ~~
   .y7                0.343    0.750    0.457    0.647    0.343
 .y4 ~~
   .y8                0.501    0.457    1.097    0.273    0.501
 .y6 ~~
   .y8                1.720    0.843    2.040    0.041    1.720
```

```
  Std.all

    0.318

    0.234
    0.275

    0.083

    0.153

    0.400

Intercepts:
                   Estimate  Std.Err  z-value  P(>|z|)   Std.lv
   .x1                5.064    0.084   60.554    0.000    5.064
   .x2                4.829    0.176   27.401    0.000    4.829
   .x3                3.524    0.163   21.557    0.000    3.524
   .y1                5.512    0.300   18.389    0.000    5.512
   .y2                4.273    0.468    9.127    0.000    4.273
   .y3                6.558    0.385   17.026    0.000    6.558
   .y4                4.391    0.392   11.214    0.000    4.391
   .y5                5.132    0.312   16.434    0.000    5.132
   .y6                2.979    0.390    7.642    0.000    2.979
   .y7                6.310    0.387   16.315    0.000    6.310
   .y8                4.019    0.392   10.247    0.000    4.019
  Std.all
    7.131
    3.202
    2.557
    2.145
    1.080
    1.974
    1.319
    1.942
    0.894
    1.918
    1.217

Variances:
                   Estimate  Std.Err  z-value  P(>|z|)   Std.lv
   .x1                0.088    0.023    3.792    0.000    0.088
   .x2                0.040    0.097    0.410    0.682    0.040
   .x3                0.486    0.090    5.418    0.000    0.486
   .y1                2.009    0.506    3.973    0.000    2.009
   .y2                7.675    1.433    5.354    0.000    7.675
   .y3                5.116    1.157    4.420    0.000    5.116
   .y4                2.803    0.883    3.175    0.001    2.803
   .y5                2.618    0.686    3.815    0.000    2.618
   .y6                4.819    0.987    4.884    0.000    4.819
   .y7                3.362    0.714    4.709    0.000    3.362
```

```
   .y8              3.835    1.001    3.831    0.000    3.835
    ind60           1.000                               1.000
   .dem60           1.000                               0.768
   .dem65           1.000                               0.068
  Std.all
    0.175
    0.017
    0.256
    0.304
    0.490
    0.463
    0.253
    0.375
    0.434
    0.311
    0.352
    1.000
    0.768
    0.068

R-Square:
                 Estimate
    x1              0.825
    x2              0.983
    x3              0.744
    y1              0.696
    y2              0.510
    y3              0.537
    y4              0.747
    y5              0.625
    y6              0.566
    y7              0.689
    y8              0.648
    dem60           0.232
    dem65           0.932
```

7.9.4 Estimates of Model Fit

You can extract specific fit indices using the following syntax:

```
fitMeasures(
  semModelFit,
  fit.measures = c(
    "chisq", "df", "pvalue",
    "chisq.scaled", "df.scaled", "pvalue.scaled",
    "chisq.scaling.factor",
    "baseline.chisq","baseline.df","baseline.pvalue",
    "rmsea", "cfi", "tli", "srmr",
    "rmsea.robust", "cfi.robust", "tli.robust"))
```

```
               chisq                     df                 pvalue
              38.748                 35.000                  0.304
        chisq.scaled              df.scaled          pvalue.scaled
              42.709                 35.000                  0.174
chisq.scaling.factor         baseline.chisq            baseline.df
               0.907                601.314                 55.000
     baseline.pvalue                  rmsea                    cfi
               0.000                  0.038                  0.993
                 tli                   srmr           rmsea.robust
               0.989                  0.046                  0.055
          cfi.robust             tli.robust
               0.988                  0.981
```

7.9.5 Residuals

```
residuals(semModelFit, type = "cor")
```

```
$type
[1] "cor.bollen"

$cov
       x1     x2     x3     y1     y2     y3     y4     y5     y6
x1  0.000
x2 -0.005  0.000
x3  0.000  0.007  0.000
y1  0.031 -0.025 -0.099  0.000
y2 -0.091 -0.076 -0.082  0.000  0.000
y3  0.017 -0.012 -0.086  0.072 -0.076  0.000
y4  0.103  0.067  0.033 -0.050  0.019 -0.015  0.000
y5  0.150  0.101  0.013 -0.026 -0.001 -0.026 -0.012  0.000
y6 -0.027 -0.056 -0.071  0.062  0.011 -0.147  0.049 -0.010  0.000
y7 -0.038 -0.058 -0.059 -0.001  0.012 -0.017 -0.001  0.016 -0.003
y8  0.032 -0.029 -0.081 -0.013  0.027 -0.058  0.031 -0.047  0.013
       y7     y8
x1
x2
x3
y1
y2
y3
y4
y5
y6
y7  0.000
y8  0.035  0.000

$mean
    x1     x2     x3     y1     y2     y3     y4     y5     y6     y7
 0.009  0.005 -0.014 -0.001  0.004 -0.012 -0.010  0.005 -0.001 -0.004
```

TABLE 7.3 Modification Indices from Structural Equation Model.

	lhs	op	rhs	mi	epc	sepc.lv	sepc.all	sepc.nox
53	ind60	=	y5	4.91	0.67	0.67	0.25	0.25
99	y1		y3	4.46	1.08	1.08	0.34	0.34
52	ind60	=	y4	3.98	0.57	0.57	0.17	0.17
70	dem65	=	y4	3.82	0.78	3.00	0.90	0.90
110	y3		y6	3.51	−1.14	−1.14	−0.23	−0.23
101	y1		y6	2.50	0.62	0.62	0.20	0.20

```
   y8
0.000
```

7.9.6 Modification Indices

Modification indices are generated using the syntax below and are presented in Table 7.3.

```
semModelFitIndices <- modificationindices(semModelFit, sort. = TRUE)
```

7.9.7 Internal Consistency Reliability

Internal consistency reliability of items composing the latent factors, as quantified by omega (ω) and average variance extracted (AVE), was estimated using the `semTools` package (Jorgensen et al., 2021).

```
compRelSEM(semModelFit)
```

```
ind60 dem60 dem65
0.938 0.855 0.843
```

```
AVE(semModelFit)
```

```
ind60 dem60 dem65
0.861 0.605 0.632
```

7.9.8 Path Diagram

A path diagram of the model is shown in Figure 7.2.

```
semPaths(
  semModelFit,
  what = "Std.all",
  layout = "tree2",
  edge.label.cex = 0.7)
```

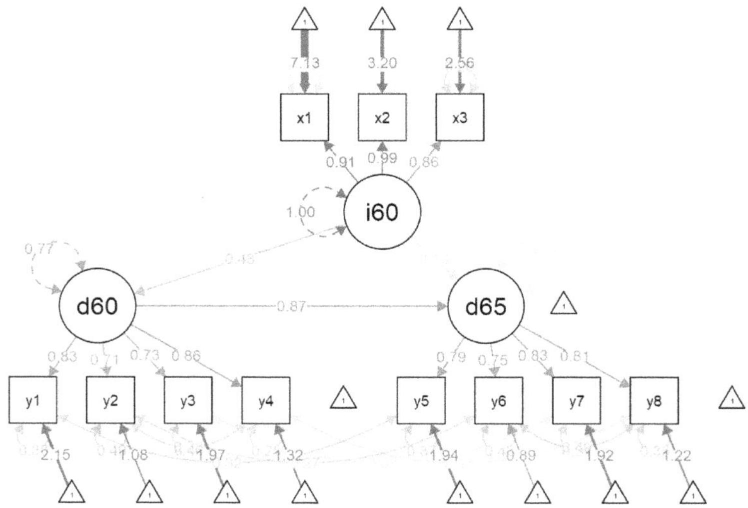

FIGURE 7.2 Example Structural Equation Model.

7.10 Benefits of SEM

There are many benefits of fitting a model in SEM (or in other latent variable approaches). First, unlike classical test theory, SEM can allow correlated errors. With SEM, you do not need to make as restrictive assumptions as in classical test theory. Second, unlike multiple regression, SEM can handle multiple dependent variables simultaneously. Third, SEM uses all available information (data) using a technique called full information maximum likelihood (FIML), even if participants have missing scores on some variables. By contrast, multiple regression and many other statistical analyses use listwise deletion, in which they discard participants if they have a missing score on any of the model variables. Fourth, as described in the next section (7.10.1), SEM can be used to account for different forms of measurement error (e.g., method bias). Accounting for measurement error allows disattenuating associations with other constructs. We provide an example showing that SEM disattenuates associations for measurement error in Section 4.6.2. All of these benefits allow SEM to generate purer estimation of constructs, more accurate estimates of people's levels on constructs, and more accurate estimates of associations between constructs.

7.10.1 Accounting for Method Bias

SEM/CFA can be used to account for method biases and other forms of measurement error. You can use indicators that reflect different method biases, so that the method biases are discarded as unique errors, and are not combined in the "common variance" of the latent construct. SEM/CFA can be used to fit a multitrait-multimethod matrix to account for method variance. We provide an example of fitting a multitrait-multimethod matrix in CFA in Sections 4.3.1.4.2.5 and 6.4.2.12. But estimation of a multitrait-multimethod matrix in CFA can be challenging without making additional constraints/assumptions.

A more practical utility of SEM is that it allows one to obtain "purer" estimates of latent constructs (and people's standing on them) by discarding measurement error, and you do not have to assume all errors are uncorrelated!

7.11 Generalizability Theory

There are also SEM approaches for performing generalizability theory analyses. The reader is referred to examples by Vispoel et al. (2018), Vispoel et al. (2019), Vispoel et al. (2022), and Vispoel et al. (2023).

7.12 Conclusion

Structural equation modeling (SEM) is an advanced modeling approach that allows estimating latent variables as the common variance from multiple measures. SEM holds promise to account for measurement error and method biases, which allows one to get more accurate estimates of constructs, people's standing on constructs (i.e., individual differences), and associations between constructs.

7.13 Suggested Readings

MacCallum & Austin (2000)

8

Item Response Theory

In the chapter on reliability, we introduced classical test theory (CTT). Classical test theory is a measurement theory of how test scores relate to a construct. Classical test theory provides a way to estimate the relation between the measure (or item) and the construct. For instance, with a CTT approach, to estimate the relation between an item and the construct, you would compute an item–total correlation. An item–total correlation is the correlation of an item with the total score on the measure (e.g., sum score). The item–total correlation approximates the relation between an item and the construct. However, the item–total correlation is a crude estimate of the relation between an item and the construct. And there are many other ways to characterize the relation between an item and a construct. One such way is with item response theory (IRT).

8.1 Overview

Unlike CTT, which is a measurement theory of how test scores relate to a construct, IRT is a measurement theory that describes how an *item* is related to a construct. For instance, given a particular person's level on the construct, what is their chance of answering "TRUE" on a particular item?

IRT is an approach to latent variable modeling. In IRT, we estimate a person's construct score (i.e., level on the construct) based on their item responses. The construct is estimated as a latent factor that represents the common variance among all items as in structural equation modeling or confirmatory factor analysis. The person's level on the construct is called theta (θ). When dealing with performance-based tests, theta is sometimes called "ability."

8.1.1 Item Characteristic Curve

In IRT, we can plot an *item characteristic curve* (ICC). The ICC is a plot of the model-derived probability of a symptom being present (or a correct response) as a function of a person's standing on a latent continuum. For instance, we can create empirical ICCs that can take any shape (see Figure 8.1).

In a model-implied ICC, we fit a logistic (sigmoid) curve to each item's probability of a symptom being present as a function of a person's level on the latent construct. The model-implied ICCs for the same 10 items from Figure 8.1 are depicted in Figure 8.2.

ICCs can be summed across items to get the test characteristic curve (TCC):

An ICC provides more information than an item–total correlation. Visually, we can see the utility of various items by looking at the items' ICC plots. For instance, consider what

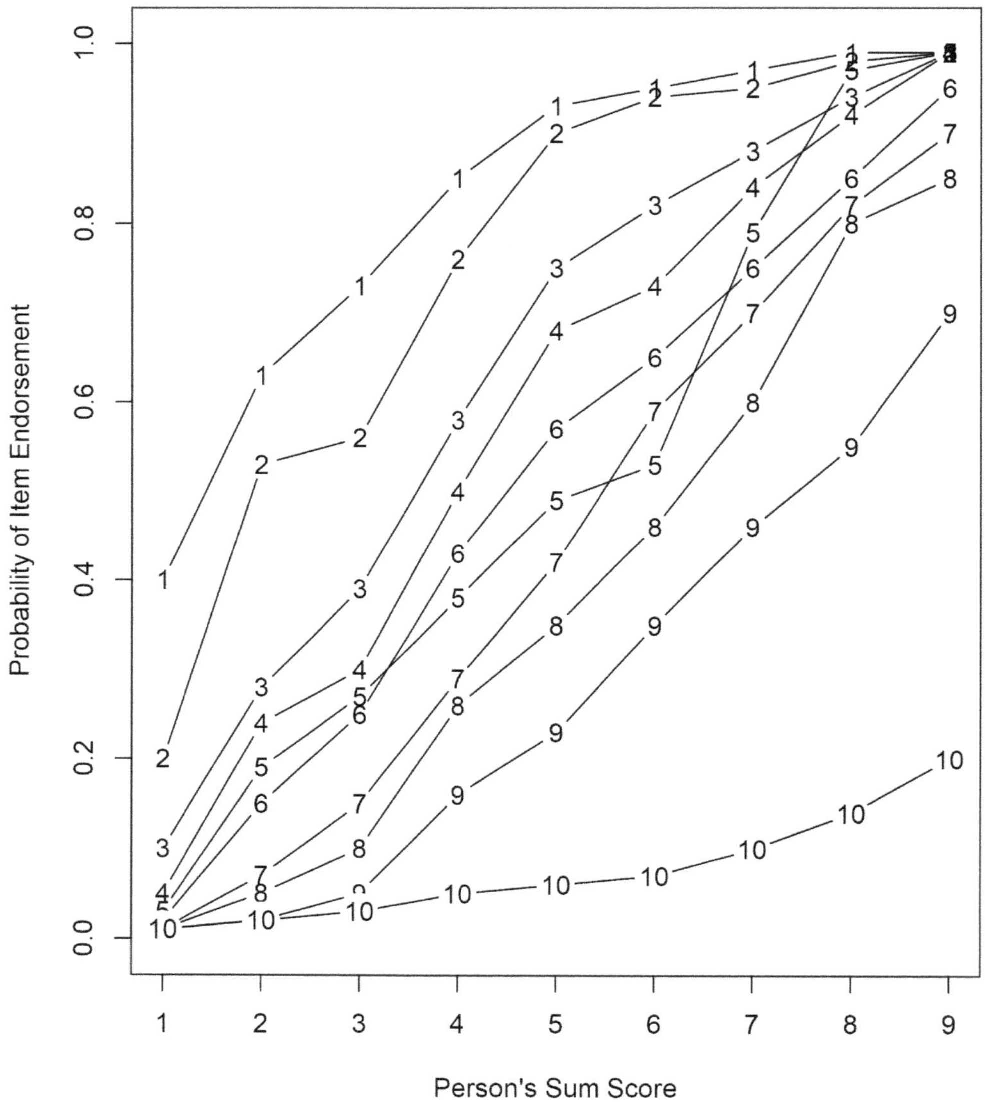

FIGURE 8.1 Empirical Item Characteristic Curves of the Probability of Endorsement of a Given Item as a Function of the Person's Sum Score.

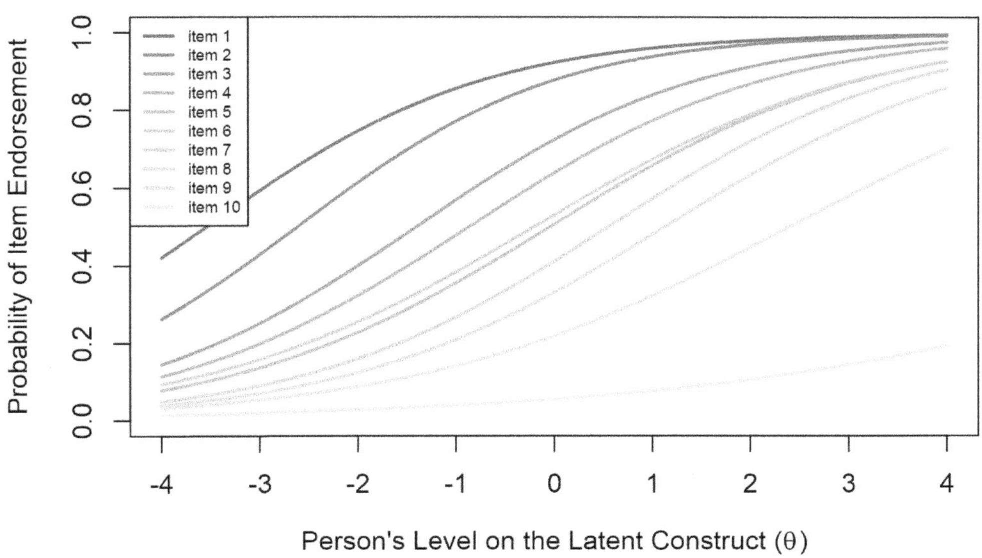

FIGURE 8.2 Item Characteristic Curves of the Probability of Endorsement of a Given Item as a Function of the Person's Level on the Latent Construct.

might be a useless item for diagnostic purposes. For a particular item, among those with a low total score (level on the construct), 90% respond with "TRUE" to the item, whereas among everyone else, 100% respond with "TRUE" (see Figure 8.4). This item has a ceiling effect and provides only a little information about who would be considered above clinical threshold for a disorder. So, the item is not very clinically useful.

Now, consider a different item. For those with a low level on the construct, 0% respond "TRUE", so it has a floor effect and tells us nothing about the lower end of the construct. But for those with a higher level on the construct, 70% respond true (see Figure 8.5). So, the item tells us something about the higher end of the distribution, and could be diagnostically useful. Thus, an ICC allows us to immediately tell the utility of items.

8.1.2 Parameters

We can estimate up to four parameters in an IRT model and can glean up to four key pieces of information from an item's ICC:

1. Difficulty (severity)
2. Discrimination
3. Guessing
4. Inattention/careless errors

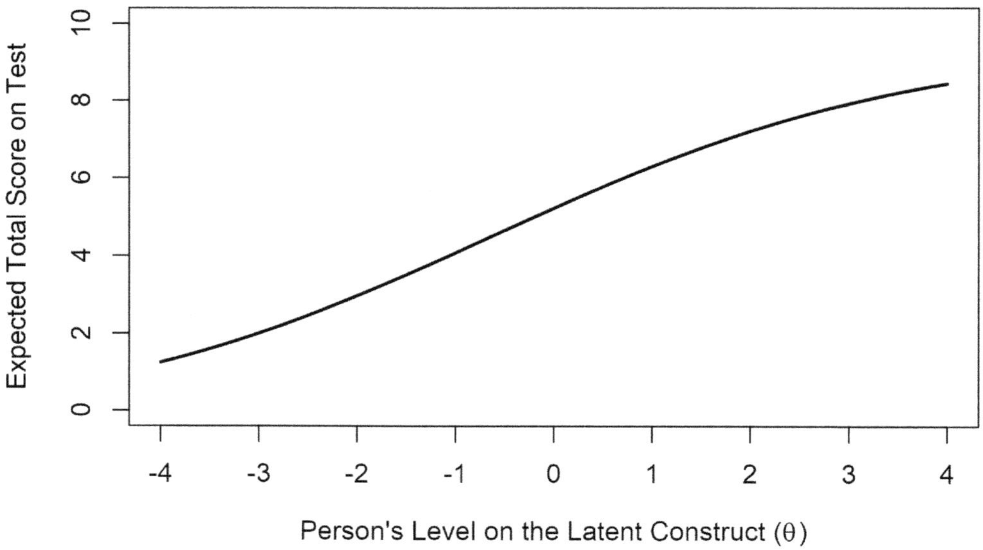

FIGURE 8.3 Test Characteristic Curve of the Expected Total Score on the Test as a Function of the Person's Level on the Latent Construct.

8.1.2.1 Difficulty (Severity)

The item's *difficulty* parameter is the item's location on the latent construct. It is quantified by the intercept, i.e., the location on the x-axis of the inflection point of the ICC. In a 1- or 2-parameter model, the inflection point is where 50% of the sample endorses the item (or gets the item correct), that is, the point on the x-axis where the ICC crosses .5 probability on the y-axis (i.e., the level on the construct at which the probability of endorsing the item is equal to the probability of not endorsing the item). Item difficulty is similar to item means or intercepts in structural equation modeling or factor analysis. Some items are more useful at the higher levels of the construct, whereas other items are more useful at the lower levels of the construct. See Figure 8.6 for an example of an item with a low difficulty and an item with a high difficulty.

When dealing with a measure of clinical symptoms (e.g., depression), the difficulty parameter is sometimes called severity, because symptoms that are endorsed less frequently tend to be more severe [e.g., suicidal behavior; Krueger et al. (2004)]. One way of thinking about the severity parameter of an item is: "How severe does your psychopathology have to be for half of people to endorse the symptom?"

When dealing with a measure of performance, aptitude, or intelligence, the parameter would be more likely to be called difficulty: "How high does your ability have to be for half of people to pass the item?" An item with a low difficulty would be considered easy, because even people with a low ability tend to pass the item. An item with a high difficulty would be considered difficult, because only people with a high ability tend to pass the item.

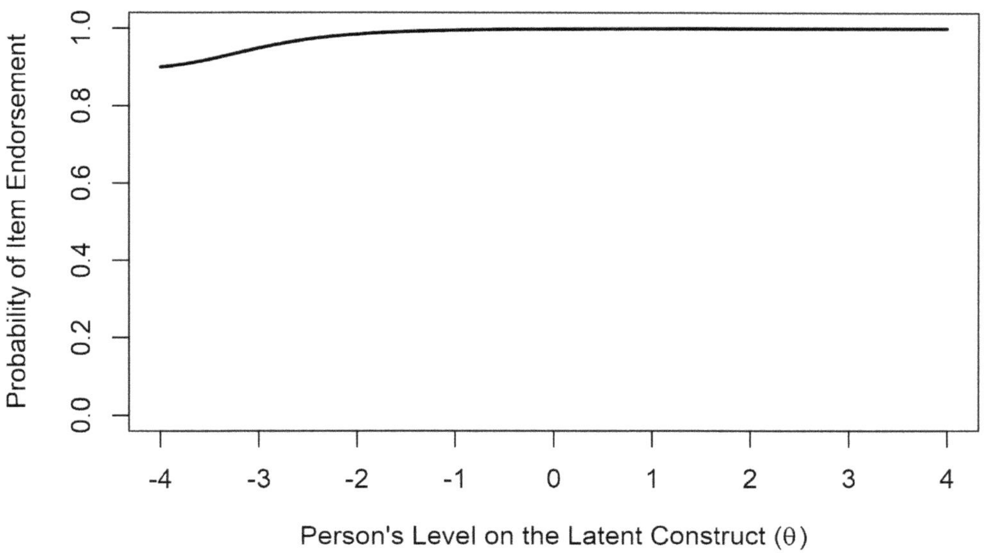

FIGURE 8.4 Item Characteristic Curve of an Item with a Ceiling Effect That Is Not Diagnostically Useful.

8.1.2.2 Discrimination

The item's *discrimination* parameter is how well the item can distinguish between those who were higher versus lower on the construct, that is, how strongly the item is correlated with the construct (i.e., the latent factor). It is similar to the factor loading in structural equation modeling or factor analysis. It is quantified by the slope of the ICC, i.e., the steepness of the line at its steepest point. The slope reflects the inverse of how much range of construct levels it would take to flip 50/50 whether a person is likely to pass or fail an item.

Some items have ICCs that go up fast (have a steep slope). These items provide a fine distinction between people with lower versus higher levels on the construct and therefore have high discrimination. Some items go up gradually (less steep slope), so it provides less precision and information, and has a low discrimination. See Figure 8.7 for an example of an item with a low discrimination and an item with a high discrimination.

8.1.2.3 Guessing

The item's *guessing* parameter is reflected by the lower asymptote of the ICC. If the item has a lower asymptote above zero, it suggests that the probability of getting the item correct (or endorsing the item) never reaches zero, for any level of the construct. On an educational test, this could correspond to the person's likelihood of being able to answer the item correctly by chance just by guessing. For example, for a 4-option multiple choice test, a respondent would be expected to get a given item correct 25% of the time just by guessing. See Figure 8.8 for an example of an item from a true/false exam and Figure 8.9 for an example of an item from a 4-option multiple choice exam.

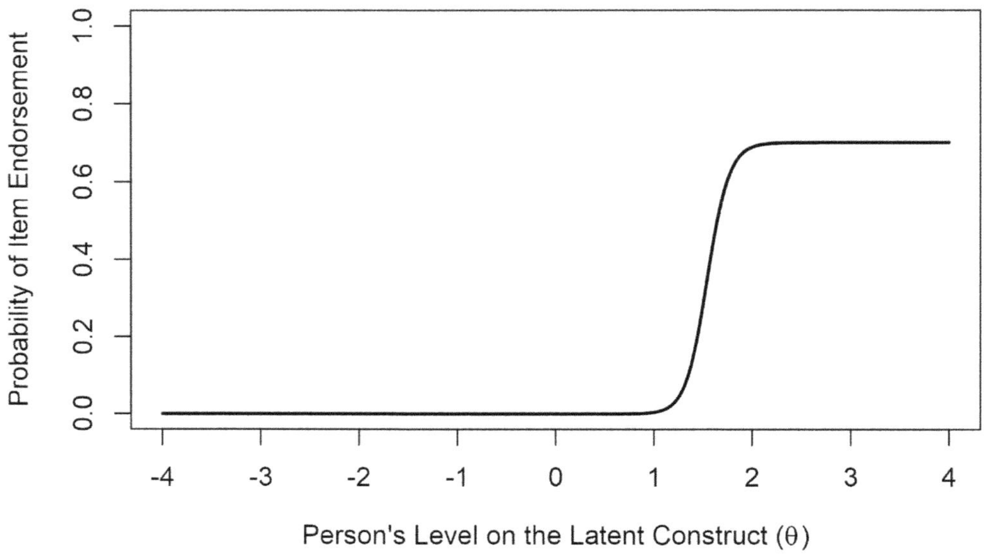

FIGURE 8.5 Item Characteristic Curve of an Item with a Floor Effect That Is Diagnostically Useful.

8.1.2.4 Inattention/Careless Errors

The item's *inattention* (or *careless error*) parameter is the reflected by the upper asymptote of the ICC. If the item has an upper asymptote below one, it suggests that the probability of getting the item correct (or endorsing the item) never reaches one, for any level on the construct. See Figure 8.10 for an example of an item whose probability of endorsement (or getting it correct) exceeds .85.

8.1.3 Models

IRT models can be fit that estimate one or more of these four item parameters.

8.1.3.1 One-Parameter and Rasch Models

A Rasch model estimates the item difficulty parameter and holds everything else fixed across items. It fixes the item discrimination to be one for each item. In the Rasch model, the probability that a person j with a level on the construct of θ gets a score of one (instead of zero) on item i, based on the difficulty (b) of the item, is estimated using Equation (8.1):

$$P(X = 1|\theta_j, b_i) = \frac{e^{\theta_j - b_i}}{1 + e^{\theta_j - b_i}} \tag{8.1}$$

The `petersenlab` package (Petersen, 2024) contains the `fourPL()` function that estimates the probability of item endorsement as function of the item characteristics from the Rasch model

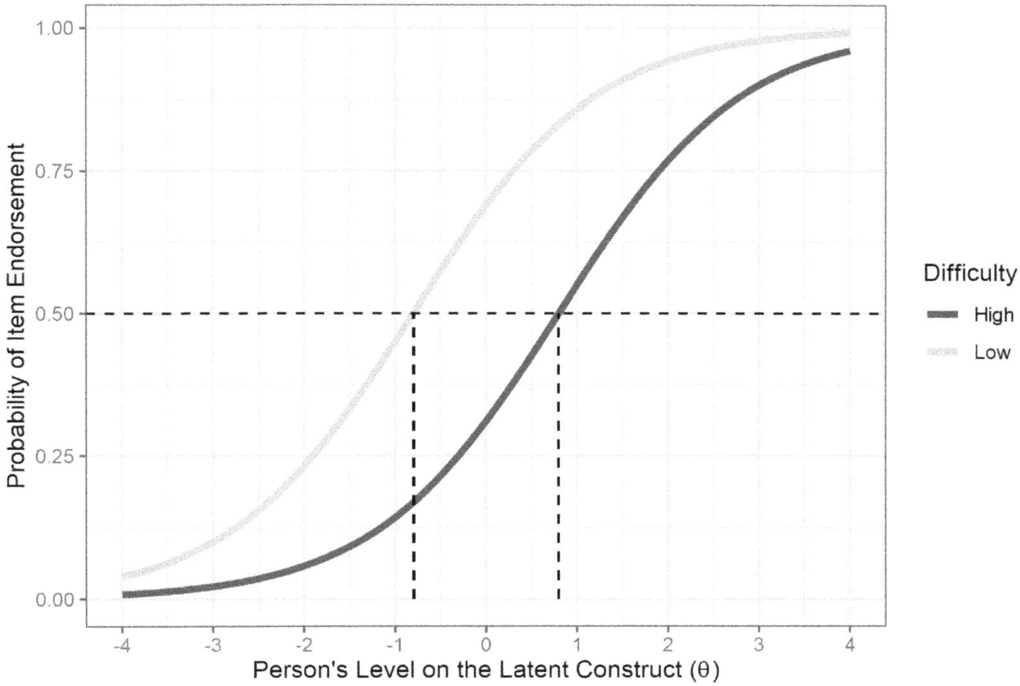

FIGURE 8.6 Item Characteristic Curves of an Item with Low Difficulty Versus High Difficulty. The dashed horizontal line indicates a probability of item endorsement of .50. The dashed vertical line is the item difficulty, i.e., the person's level on the construct (the location on the x-axis) at the inflection point of the item characteristic curve. In a two-parameter logistic model, the inflection point corresponds to the probability of item endorsement is 50%. Thus, in a two-parameter logistic model, the difficulty of an item is the person's level on the construct where the probability of endorsing the item is 50%.

and the person's level on the construct (theta). To estimate the probability of endorsement from the Rasch model, specify b and θ, while keeping the defaults for the other parameters.

```
library("petersenlab")
```

```
fourPL(b = 1, theta = 0)
```

```
[1] 0.2689
```

A one-parameter logistic (1-PL) IRT model, similar to a Rasch model, estimates the item difficulty parameter, and holds everything else fixed across items (see Figure 8.11). The 1-PL model holds the item discrimination fixed across items, but does not fix it to one, unlike the Rasch model.

In the 1-PL model, the probability that a person j with a level on the construct of θ gets a score of one (instead of zero) on item i, based on the difficulty (b) of the item and the items' (fixed) discrimination (a), is estimated using Equation (8.2):

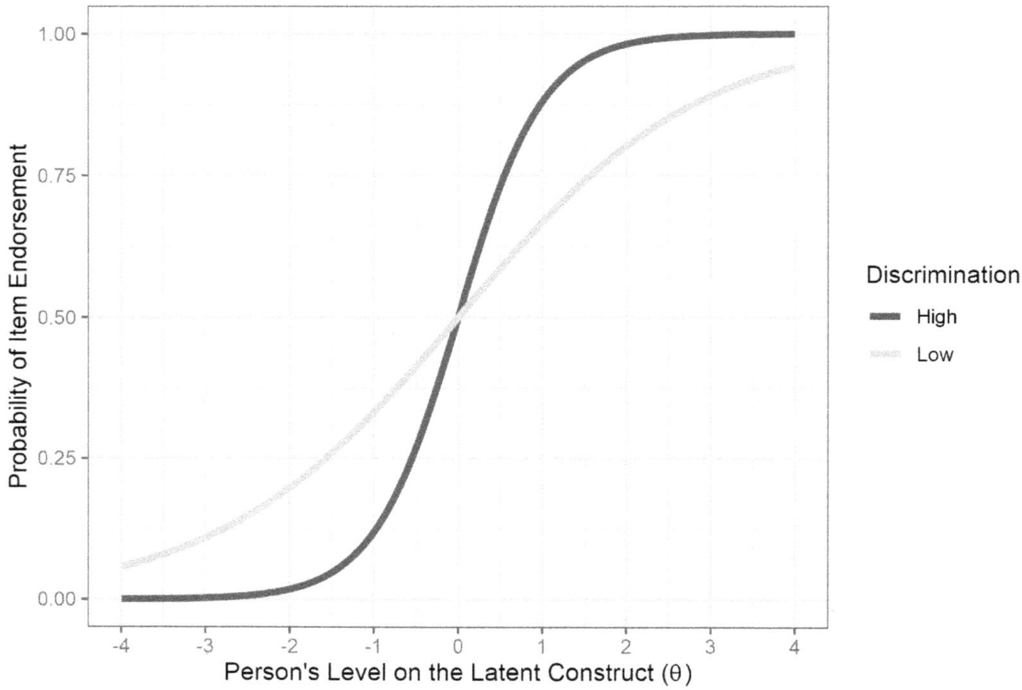

FIGURE 8.7 Item Characteristic Curves of an Item with Low Discrimination Versus High Discrimination. The discrimination of an item is the slope of the line at its inflection point.

$$P(X = 1|\theta_j, b_i, a) = \frac{e^{a(\theta_j - b_i)}}{1 + e^{a(\theta_j - b_i)}} \tag{8.2}$$

To estimate the probability of endorsement from the 1-PL model, specify a, b, and θ, while keeping the defaults for the other parameters.

```
fourPL(a, b, theta)
```

Rasch and 1-PL models are common and are the easiest to fit. However, they make fairly strict assumptions. They assume that items have the same discrimination.

A 1-PL model is only valid if there is no crossing of lines in empirical ICCs (see Figure 8.12).

8.1.3.2 Two-Parameter

A two-parameter logistic (2-PL) IRT model estimates item difficulty and discrimination, and it holds the asymptotes fixed across items (see Figure 8.13). Like 1-PL models, 2-PL models are also common.

In the 2-PL model, the probability that a person j with a level on the construct of θ gets a score of one (instead of zero) on item i, based on the difficulty (b) and discrimination (a) of the item, is estimated using Equation (8.3):

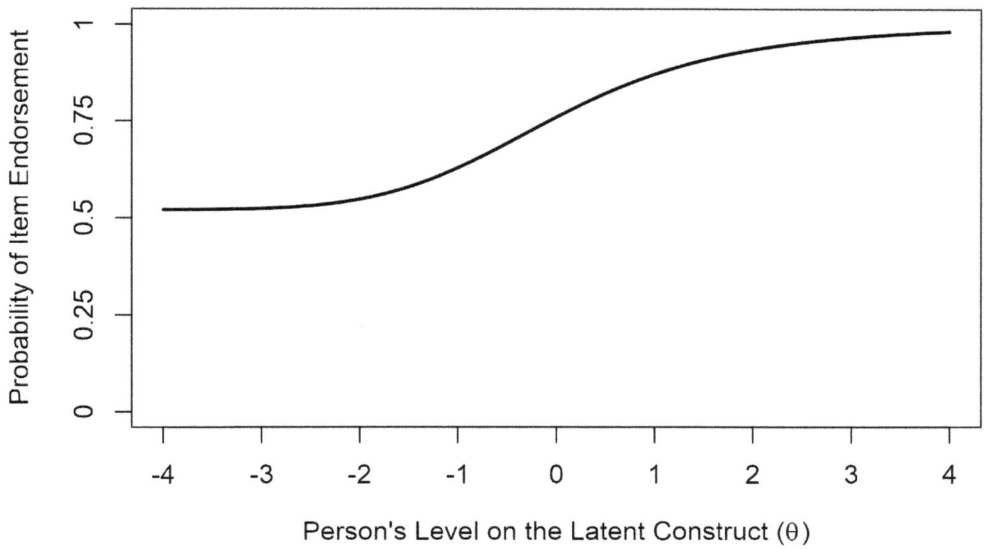

FIGURE 8.8 Item Characteristic Curve of an Item from a True/False Exam, Where Test Takers Get the Item Correct at Least 50% of the Time.

$$P(X = 1|\theta_j, b_i, a_i) = \frac{e^{a_i(\theta_j - b_i)}}{1 + e^{a_i(\theta_j - b_i)}} \tag{8.3}$$

To estimate the probability of endorsement from the 2-PL model, specify a, b, and θ, while keeping the defaults for the other parameters.

```
fourPL(a = 0.6, b = 0, theta = -1)
```

```
[1] 0.3543
```

8.1.3.3 Three-Parameter

A three-parameter logistic (3-PL) IRT model estimates item difficulty, discrimination, and guessing (lower asymptote), and it holds the upper asymptote fixed across items (see Figure 8.14). This model would provide information about where an item drops out. Three-parameter logistic models are less common to estimate because this adds considerable computational complexity and requires a large sample size, and the guessing parameter is often not as important as difficulty and discrimination. Nevertheless, 3-PL models are sometimes estimated in the education literature to account for getting items correct by random guessing.

In the 3-PL model, the probability that a person j with a level on the construct of θ gets a score of one (instead of zero) on item i, based on the difficulty (b), discrimination (a), and guessing parameter (c) of the item, is estimated using Equation (8.4):

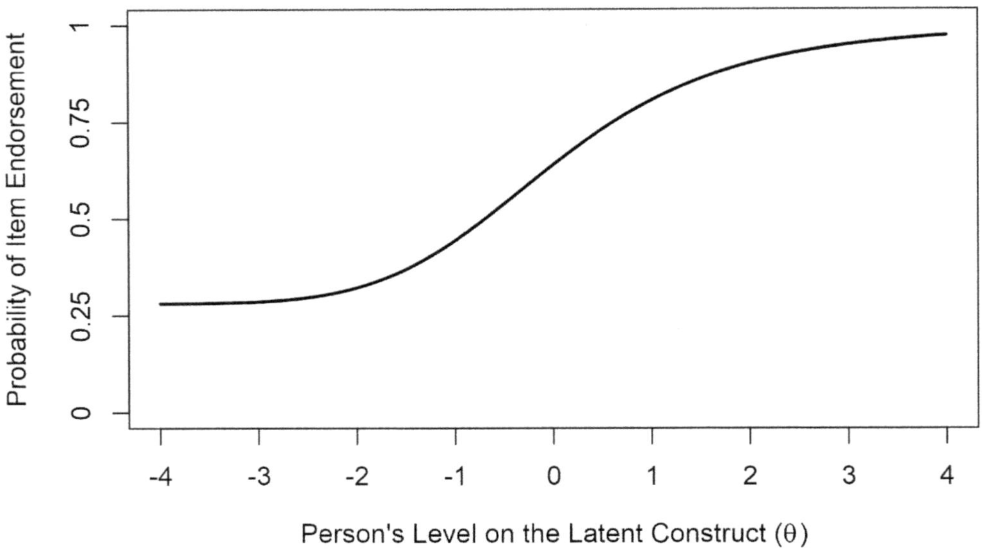

FIGURE 8.9 Item Characteristic Curve of an Item from a 4-Option Multiple Choice Exam, Where Test Takers Get the Item Correct at Least 25% of the Time.

$$P(X = 1|\theta_j, b_i, a_i, c_i) = c_i + (1 - c_i)\frac{e^{a_i(\theta_j - b_i)}}{1 + e^{a_i(\theta_j - b_i)}} \tag{8.4}$$

To estimate the probability of endorsement from the 3-PL model, specify a, b, c, and θ, while keeping the defaults for the other parameters.

```
fourPL(a = 0.8, b = -1, c = .25, theta = -1)
```

```
[1] 0.625
```

8.1.3.4 Four-Parameter

A four-parameter logistic (4-PL) IRT model estimates item difficulty, discrimination, guessing, and careless errors (see Figure 8.15). The fourth parameter adds considerable computational complexity and is rare to estimate.

In the 4-PL model, the probability that a person j with a level on the construct of θ gets a score of one (instead of zero) on item i, based on the difficulty (b), discrimination (a), guessing parameter (c), and careless error parameter (d) of the item, is estimated using Equation (8.5) (Magis, 2013):

$$P(X = 1|\theta_j, b_i, a_i, c_i, d_i) = c_i + (d_i - c_i)\frac{e^{a_i(\theta_j - b_i)}}{1 + e^{a_i(\theta_j - b_i)}} \tag{8.5}$$

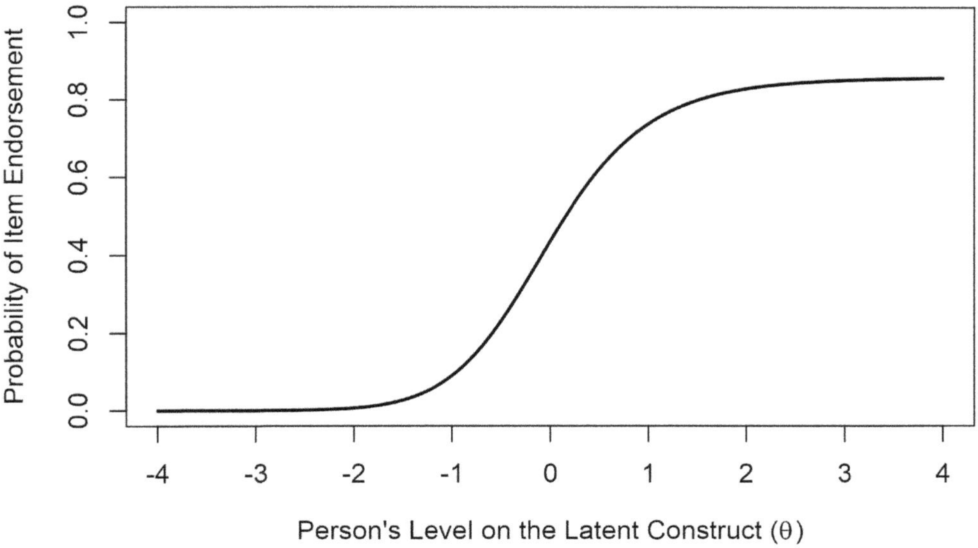

FIGURE 8.10 Item Characteristic Curve of an Item Where the Probability of Getting an Item Correct Never Exceeds .85.

To estimate the probability of endorsement from the 4-PL model, specify a, b, c, d, and θ.

```
fourPL(a = 1.5, b = 1, c = .15, d = 0.85, theta = 3)
```

```
[1] 0.8168
```

8.1.3.5 Graded Response Model

Graded response models and *generalized partial credit models* can be estimated with one, two, three, or four parameters. However, they use polytomous data (not dichotomous data), as described in the section below.

The two-parameter graded response model takes the general form of Equation (8.6):

$$P(X_{ji} = x_{ji}|\theta_j) = P^*_{x_{ji}}(\theta_j) - P^*_{x_{ji}+1}(\theta_j) \tag{8.6}$$

where:

$$P^*_{x_{ji}}(\theta_j) = P(X_{ji} \geq x_{ji}|\theta_j, b_{ic}, a_i) = \frac{1}{1 + e^{a_i(\theta_j - b_{ic})}} \tag{8.7}$$

In the model, a_i an item-specific discrimination parameter, b_{ic} is an item- and category-specific difficulty parameter, and θ_n is an estimate of a person's standing on the latent

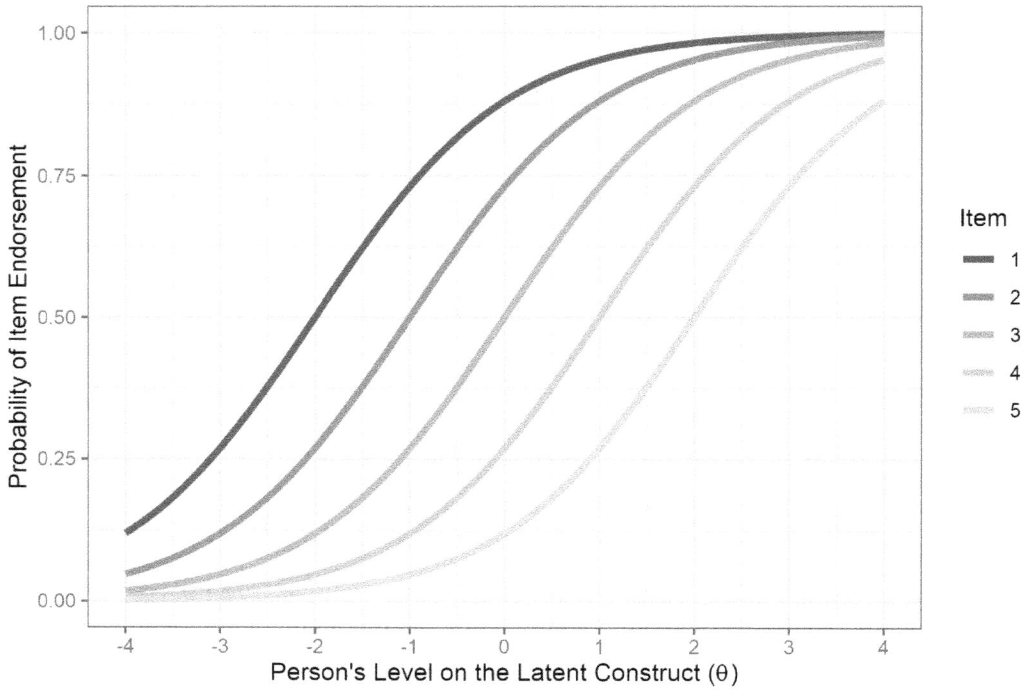

FIGURE 8.11 One-Parameter Logistic Model in Item Response Theory.

variable. In the model, i represents unique items, c represents different categories that are rated, and j represents participants.

8.1.4 Type of Data

IRT models are most commonly estimated with binary or dichotomous data. For example, the measures have questions or items that can be considered collapsed into two groups (e.g., true/false, correct/incorrect, endorsed/not endorsed). IRT models can also be estimated with polytomous data (e.g., likert scale), which adds computational complexity. IRT models with polytomous data can be fit with a graded response model or generalized partial credit model.

For example, see Figure 8.16 for an example of an item boundary characteristic curve for an item from a 5-level likert scale (based on a cumulative distribution). If an item has k response categories, it has $k - 1$ thresholds. For example, an item with 5-level likert scale (1 = strongly disagree; 2 = disagree; 3 = neither agree nor disagree; 4 = agree; 5 = strongly agree) has 4 thresholds: one from 1–2, one from 2–3, one from 3–4, and one from 4–5. The item boundary characteristic curve is the probability that a person selects a response category higher than k of a polytomous item. As depicted, one likert scale item does equivalent work as 4 binary items. See Figure 8.17 for the same 5-level likert scale item plotted with an item response category characteristic curve (based on a static, non-cumulative distribution).

IRT does not handle continuous data well, with some exceptions (Y. Chen et al., 2019) such as in a Bayesian framework (Bürkner, 2021). If you want to use continuous data, you might consider moving to a factor analysis framework.

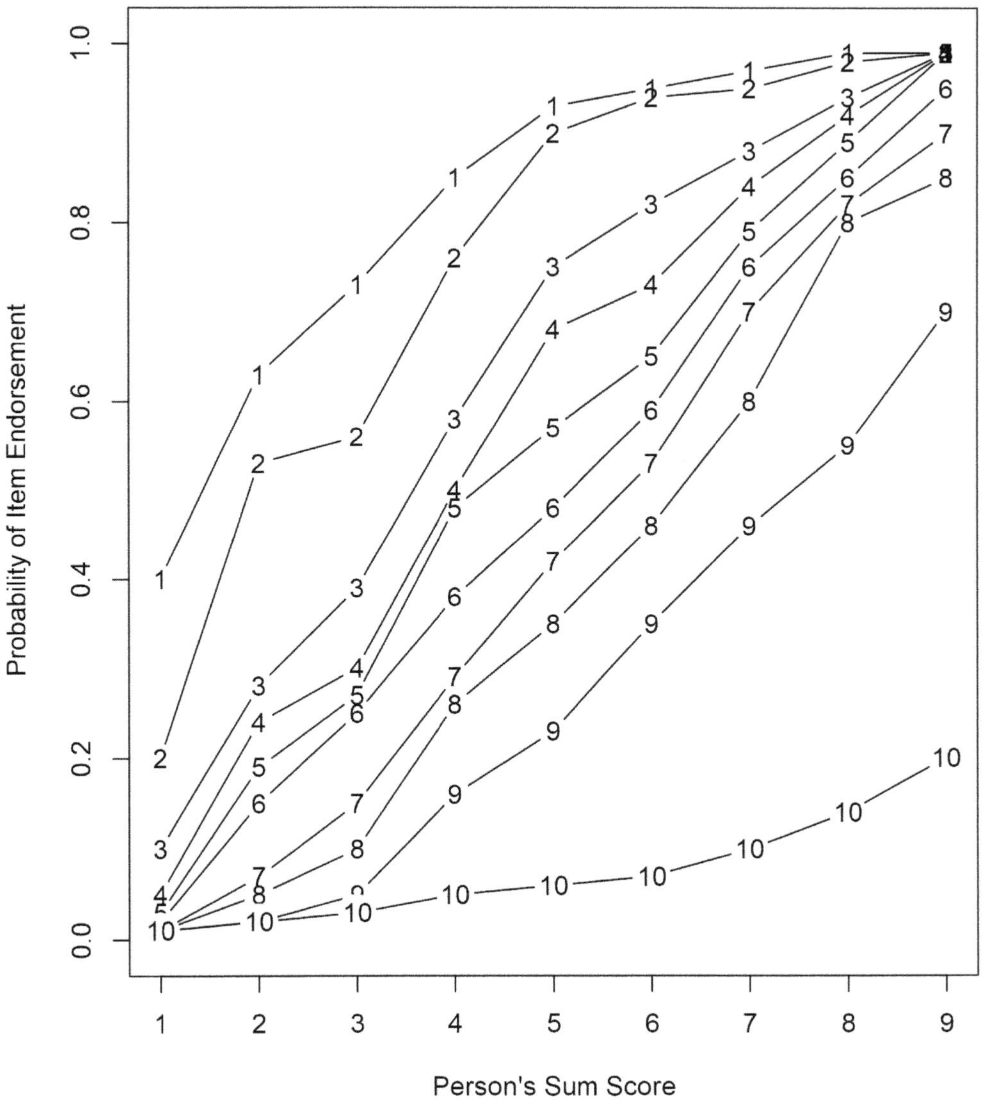

FIGURE 8.12 Empirical Item Characteristic Curves of the Probability of Endorsement of a Given Item as a Function of the Person's Sum Score. The empirical item characteristic curves of these items do not cross each other.

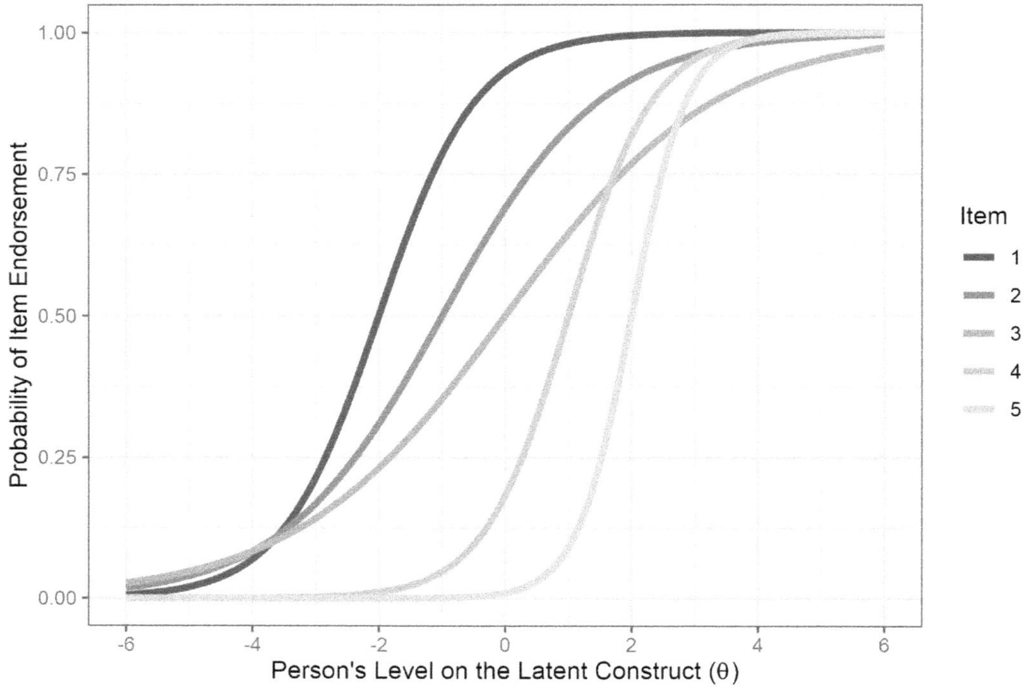

FIGURE 8.13 Two-Parameter Logistic Model in Item Response Theory.

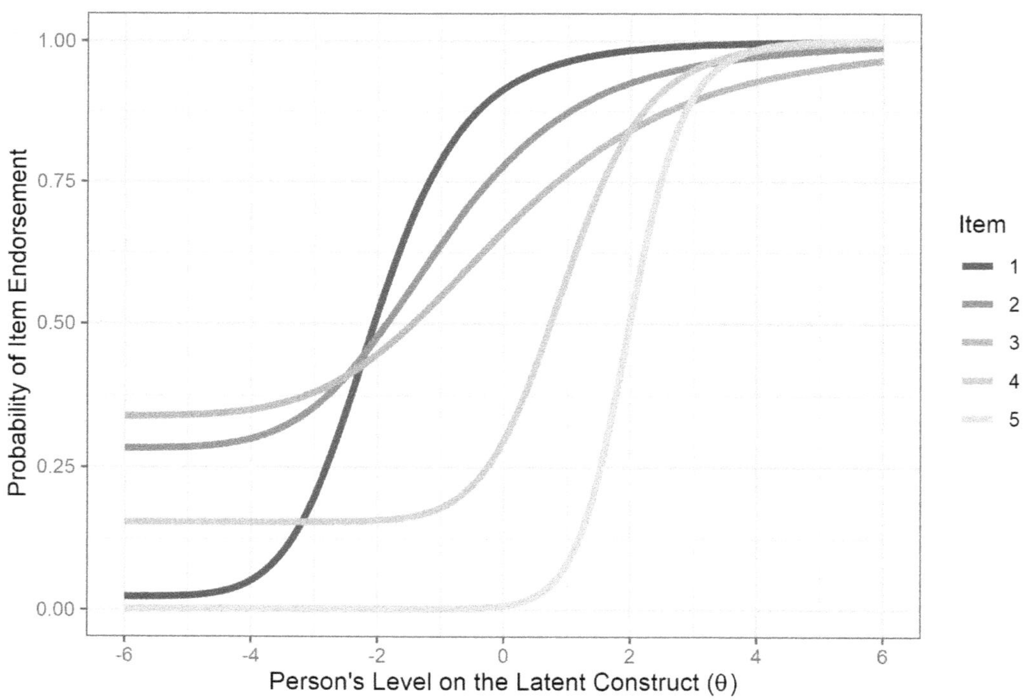

FIGURE 8.14 Three-Parameter Logistic Model in Item Response Theory.

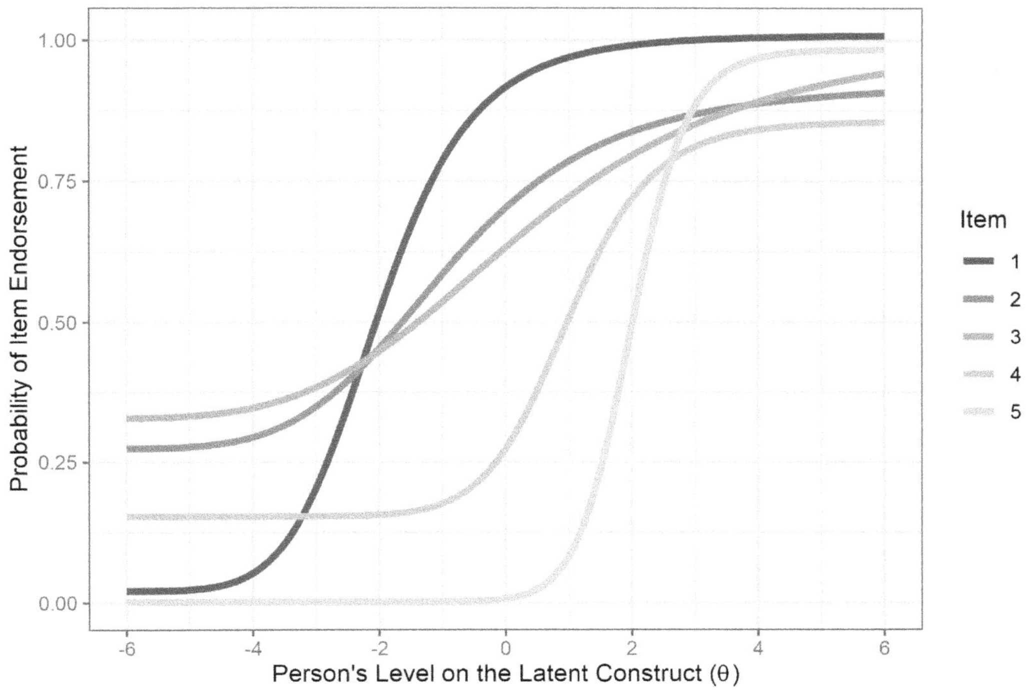

FIGURE 8.15 Four-Parameter Logistic Model in Item Response Theory.

8.1.5 Sample Size

Sample size requirements depend on the complexity of the model. A 1-parameter model often requires ~100 participants. A 2-parameter model often requires ~1,000 participants. A 3-parameter model often requires ~10,000 participants.

8.1.6 Reliability (Information)

IRT conceptualizes reliability in a different way than classical test theory does. Both IRT and classical test theory conceptualize reliability as involving the *precision* of a measure's scores. In classical test theory, (im)precision—as operationalized by the standard error of measurement—is estimated with a single index across the whole range of the construct. That is, in classical test theory, the same standard error of measurement applies to all scores in the population (Embretson, 1996). However, IRT estimates how much measurement precision (information) or imprecision (standard error of measurement) each item, and the test as a whole, has at different construct levels. This allows IRT to conceptualize reliability in such a way that precision/reliability can *differ* at different construct levels, unlike in classical test theory (Embretson, 1996). Thus, IRT does not have one index of reliability; rather, its estimate of reliability differs at different levels on the construct.

Based on an item's difficulty and discrimination, we can calculate how much information each item provides. In IRT, *information* is how much measurement precision or consistency an item (or the measure) provides. In other words, information is the degree to which an item (or measure) reduces the standard error of measurement, that is, how much it reduces

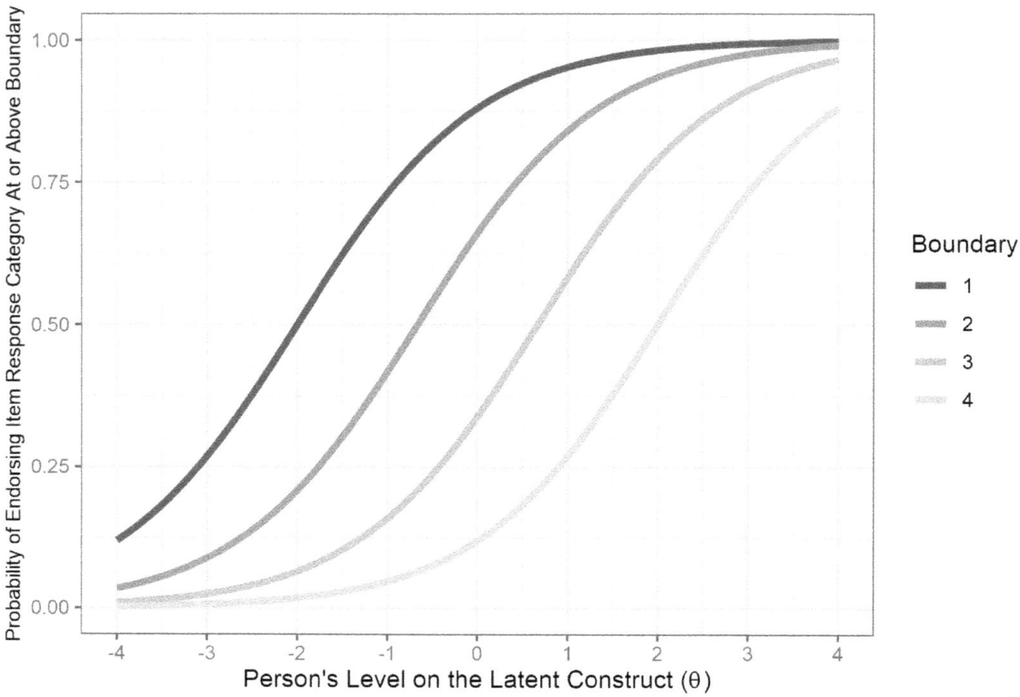

FIGURE 8.16 Item Boundary Characteristic Curves from Two-Parameter Graded Response Model in Item Response Theory.

uncertainty of a person's level on the construct. As a reminder (from Equation (3.11)), the standard error of measurement is calculated as:

$$\text{standard error of measurement (SEM)} = \sigma_x \sqrt{1 - r_{xx}}$$

where σ_x = standard deviation of observed scores on the item x, and r_{xx} = reliability of the item x. The standard error of measurement is used to generate confidence intervals for people's scores. In IRT, the standard error of measurement (at a given construct level) can be calculated as the inverse of the square root of the amount of test information at that construct level, as in Equation (8.8):

$$\text{SEM}(\theta) = \frac{1}{\sqrt{\text{information}(\theta)}} \tag{8.8}$$

The `petersenlab` package (Petersen, 2024) contains the `standardErrorIRT()` function that estimates the standard error of measurement at a person's level on the construct (theta) from the amount of information that the item (or test) provides.

```
standardErrorIRT(0.6)
```

```
[1] 1.291
```

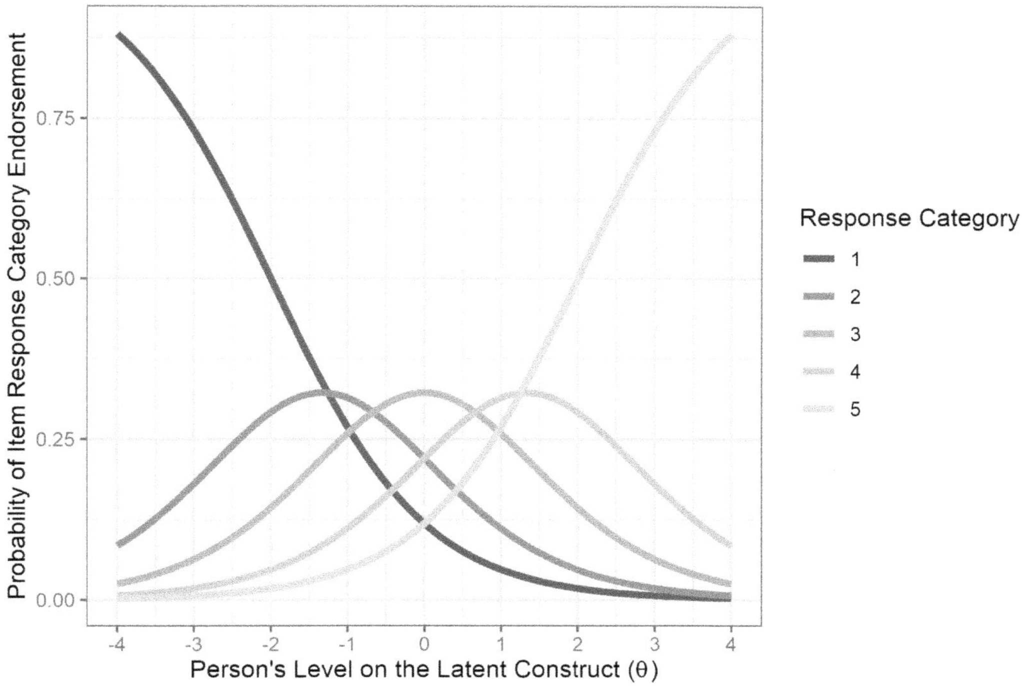

FIGURE 8.17 Item Response Category Characteristic Curves from Two-Parameter Graded Response Model in Item Response Theory.

The standard error of measurement tends to be higher (i.e., reliability/information tends to be lower) at the extreme levels of the construct where there are fewer items.

The formula for information for item i at construct level θ in a Rasch model is in Equation (8.9) (Baker & Kim, 2017):

$$\text{information}_i(\theta) = P_i(\theta)Q_i(\theta) \tag{8.9}$$

where $P_i(\theta)$ is the probability of getting a one instead of a zero on item i at a given level on the latent construct, and $Q_i(\theta) = 1 - P_i(\theta)$.

The `petersenlab` package (Petersen, 2024) contains the `itemInformation()` function that estimates the amount of information an item provides as function of the item characteristics from the Rasch model and the person's level on the construct (theta). To estimate the amount of information an item provides in a Rasch model, specify b and θ, while keeping the defaults for the other parameters.

```
itemInformation(b = 1, theta = 0)
```

```
[1] 0.1966
```

The formula for information for item i at construct level θ in a two-parameter logistic model is in Equation (8.10) (Baker & Kim, 2017):

$$\text{information}_i(\theta) = a_i^2 P_i(\theta) Q_i(\theta) \tag{8.10}$$

To estimate the amount of information an item provides in a two-parameter logistic model, specify a, b, and θ, while keeping the defaults for the other parameters.

```
itemInformation(a = 0.6, b = 0, theta = -1)
```

```
[1] 0.08236
```

The formula for information for item i at construct level θ in a three-parameter logistic model is in Equation (8.11) (Baker & Kim, 2017):

$$\text{information}_i(\theta) = a_i^2 \left[\frac{Q_i(\theta)}{P_i(\theta)}\right] \left[\frac{(P_i(\theta) - c_i)^2}{(1 - c_i)^2}\right] \tag{8.11}$$

To estimate the amount of information an item provides in a three-parameter logistic model, specify a, b, c, and θ, while keeping the defaults for the other parameters.

```
itemInformation(a = 0.8, b = -1, c = .25, theta = -1)
```

```
[1] 0.096
```

The formula for information for item i at construct level θ in a four-parameter logistic model is shown in Equation (8.12) (Magis, 2013):

$$\text{information}_i(\theta) = \frac{a_i^2 [P_i(\theta) - c_i]^2 [d_i - P_i(\theta)^2]}{(d_i - c_i)^2 P_i(\theta) [1 - P_i(\theta)]} \tag{8.12}$$

To estimate the amount of information an item provides in a four-parameter logistic model, specify a, b, c, d, and θ.

```
itemInformation(a = 1.5, b = 1, c = .15, d = 0.85, theta = 3)
```

```
[1] 0.01504
```

Reliability at a given level of the construct (θ) can be estimated as in Equation (8.13):

$$\begin{aligned} \text{reliability}(\theta) &= \frac{\text{information}(\theta)}{\text{information}(\theta) + \sigma^2(\theta)} \\ &= \frac{\text{information}(\theta)}{\text{information}(\theta) + 1} \end{aligned} \tag{8.13}$$

where $\sigma^2(\theta)$ is the variance of theta, which is fixed to one in most IRT models.

The `petersenlab` package (Petersen, 2024) contains the `reliabilityIRT()` function that estimates the amount of reliability an item or a measure provides as function of its information and the variance of people's construct levels (θ).

```
reliabilityIRT(10)
```

```
[1] 0.9091
```

Consider some hypothetical items depicted with ICCs in Figure 8.18.

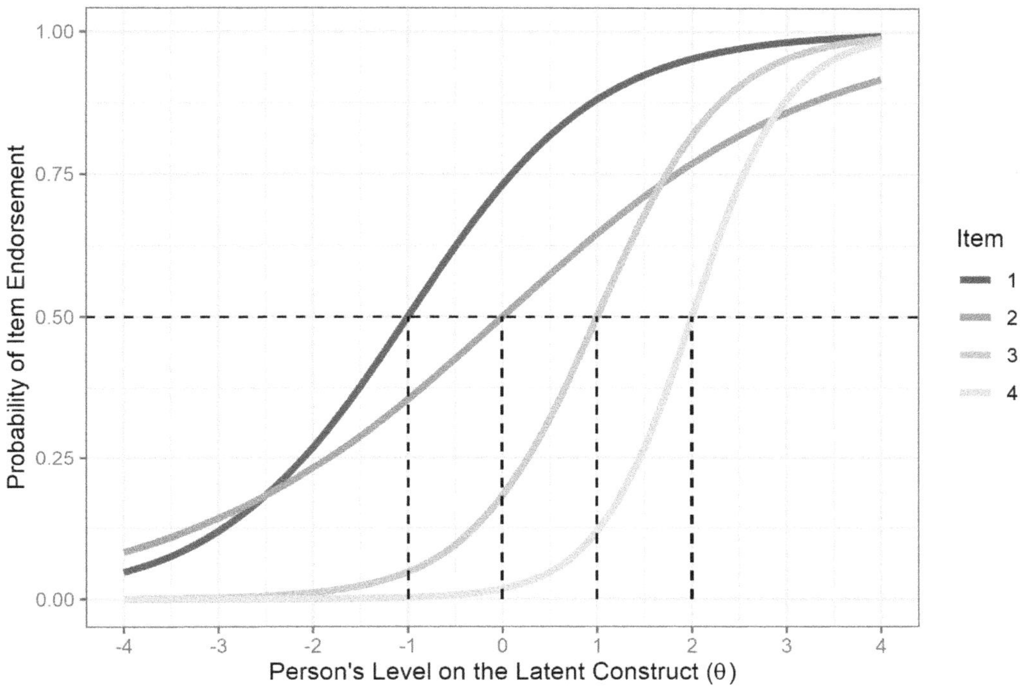

FIGURE 8.18 Item Characteristic Curves from Two-Parameter Logistic Model in Item Response Theory. The dashed horizontal line indicates a probability of item endorsement of .50. The dashed vertical line is the item difficulty, i.e., the person's level on the construct (the location on the x-axis) at the inflection point of the item characteristic curve. In a two-parameter logistic model, the inflection point corresponds to the probability of item endorsement is 50%. Thus, in a two-parameter logistic model, the difficulty of an item is the person's level on the construct where the probability of endorsing the item is 50%.

We can present the ICC in terms of an item information curve (see Figure 8.19). On the x-axis, the information peak is located at the difficulty/severity of the item. The higher the discrimination, the higher the information peak on the y-axis.

We can aggregate (sum) information across items to determine how much information the measure as a whole provides. This is called the test information curve (see Figure 8.20). Note that we get more information from likert/multiple response items compared to binary/dichotomous items. Having 10 items with a 5-level response scale yields as much information as 40 dichotomous items.

Based on test information, we can calculate the standard error of measurement (see Figure 8.21). Notice how the degree of (un)reliability differs at different construct levels.

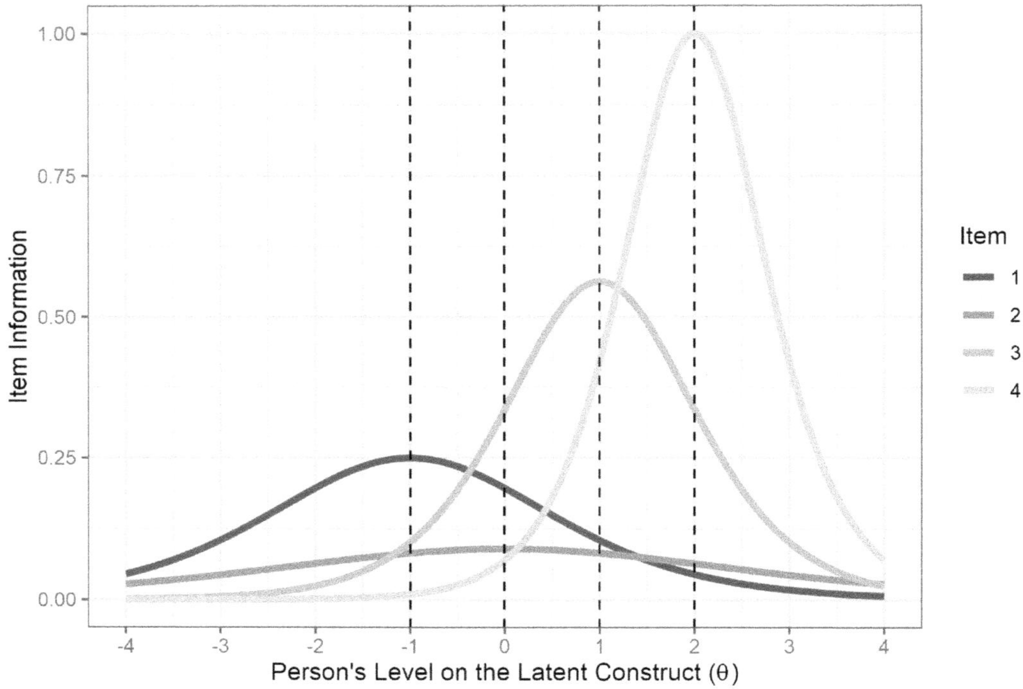

FIGURE 8.19 Item Information from Two-Parameter Logistic Model in Item Response Theory. The dashed vertical line is the item difficulty, which is located at the peak of the item information curve.

Based on test information, we can estimate the reliability (see Figure 8.22). Notice how the degree of (un)reliability differs at different construct levels.

8.1.7 Efficient Assessment

One of the benefits of IRT is for item selection to develop brief assessments. For instance, you could use two items to estimate where the person is on the construct: low, middle, or high (see Figure 8.23). If the responses to the two items do not meet expectations, for instance, the person passes the difficult item but fails the easy item, we would keep assessing additional items to determine their level on the construct. If two items perform similarly, that is, they have the same difficulty and discrimination, they are redundant, and we can sacrifice one of them. This leads to greater efficiency and better measurement in terms of reliability and validity. For more information on designing and evaluating short forms compared to their full-scale counterparts, see Smith et al. (2000).

IRT forms the basis of computerized adaptive testing, which is discussed in Chapter 20. As discussed earlier, briefer measures can increase reliability and validity of measurement if the items are tailored to the ability level of the participant. The idea of adaptive testing is that, instead of having a standard scale for all participants, the items adapt to each person. An example of a measure that has used computerized adaptive testing is the Graduate Record Examination (GRE).

With adaptive testing, it is important to develop a comprehensive item bank that spans

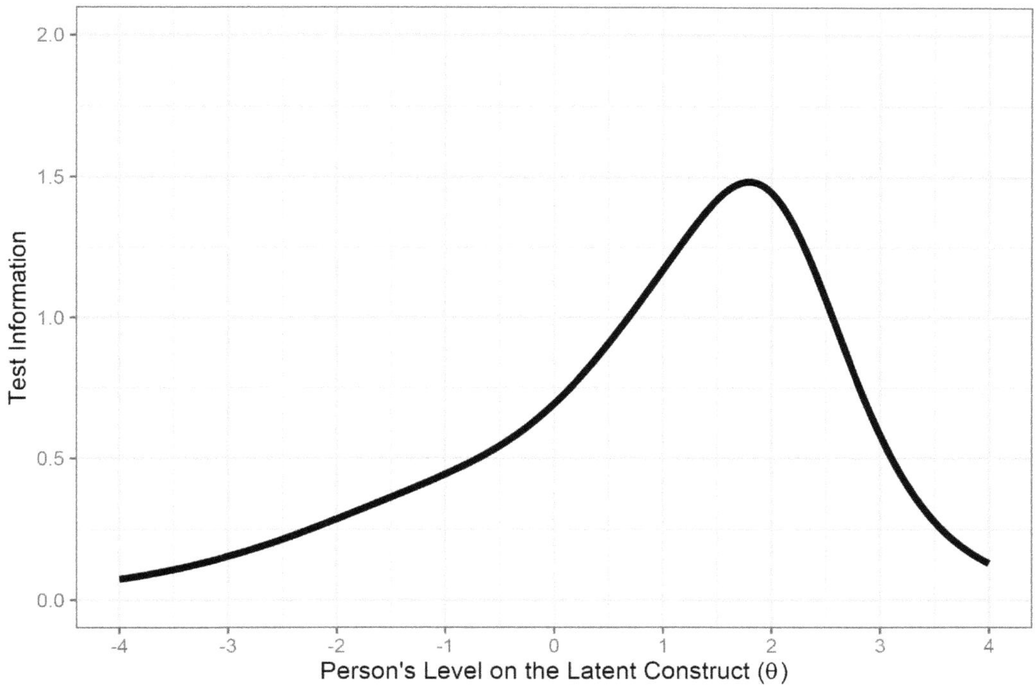

FIGURE 8.20 Test Information Curve from Two-Parameter Logistic Model in Item Response Theory.

the difficulty range of interest. The starting construct level is the 50th percentile. If the respondent gets the first item correct, it moves to the next item that would provide the most information for the person, based on a split of the remaining sample (e.g., 75th percentile). And so on... The goal of adaptive testing is to find the construct level where the respondent keeps getting items right and wrong 50% of the time. Adaptive testing is a promising approach that saves time because it tailors which items are administered to which person (based on their construct level) to get the most reliable estimate in the shortest time possible. However, it assumes that if you get a more difficult item correct, that you would have gotten easier items correct, which might not be true in all contexts (especially for constructs that are not unidimensional).

Although most uses of IRT have been in cognitive and educational testing, IRT may also benefit other domains of assessment including clinical assessment (Gibbons et al., 2016; Reise & Waller, 2009; Thomas, 2019).

8.1.7.1 A Good Measure

According to IRT, a good measure should:

1. fit your goals of the assessment, in terms of the range of interest regarding levels on the construct,
2. have good items that yield lots of information, and
3. have a good set of items that densely cover the construct within the range of interest, without redundancy.

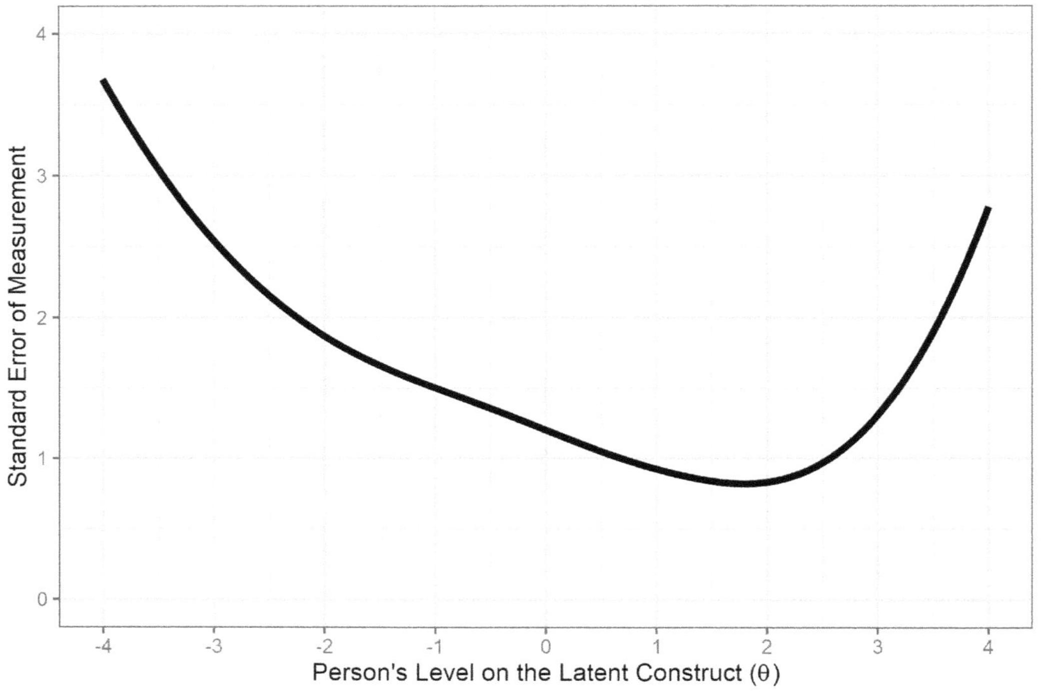

FIGURE 8.21 Test Standard Error of Measurement from Two-Parameter Logistic Model in Item Response Theory.

First, a good measure should fit your goals of the assessment, in terms of the "range of interest" or the "target range" of levels on the construct. For instance, if your goal is to perform diagnosis, you would only care about the high end of the construct (e.g., 1–3 standard deviations above the mean)—there is no use discriminating between "nothing", "almost nothing", and "a little bit." For secondary prevention, i.e., early identification of risk to prevent something from getting worse, you would be interested in finding people with elevated risk—e.g., you would need to know who is 1 or more standard deviations above the mean, but you would not need to discriminate beyond that. For assessing individual differences, you would want items that discriminate across the full range, including at the lower end. The items' difficulty should span the range of interest.

Second, a good measure should have good items that yield lots of information. For example, the items should have strong discrimination, that is, the items are strongly related to the construct. The items should have sufficient variability in responses. This can be achieved by having items with more response options (e.g., likert/multiple choice items, as opposed to binary items), items that differ in difficulty, and (at least some) items that are not too difficult or too easy (to avoid ceiling/floor effects).

Third, a good measure should have a good set of items that densely cover the construct within the range of interest, without redundancy. The items should not have the same difficulty or they would be considered redundant, and one of the redundant items could be dropped. The items' difficulty should densely cover the construct within the range of interest. For instance, if the construct range of interest is 1–2 standard deviations above the

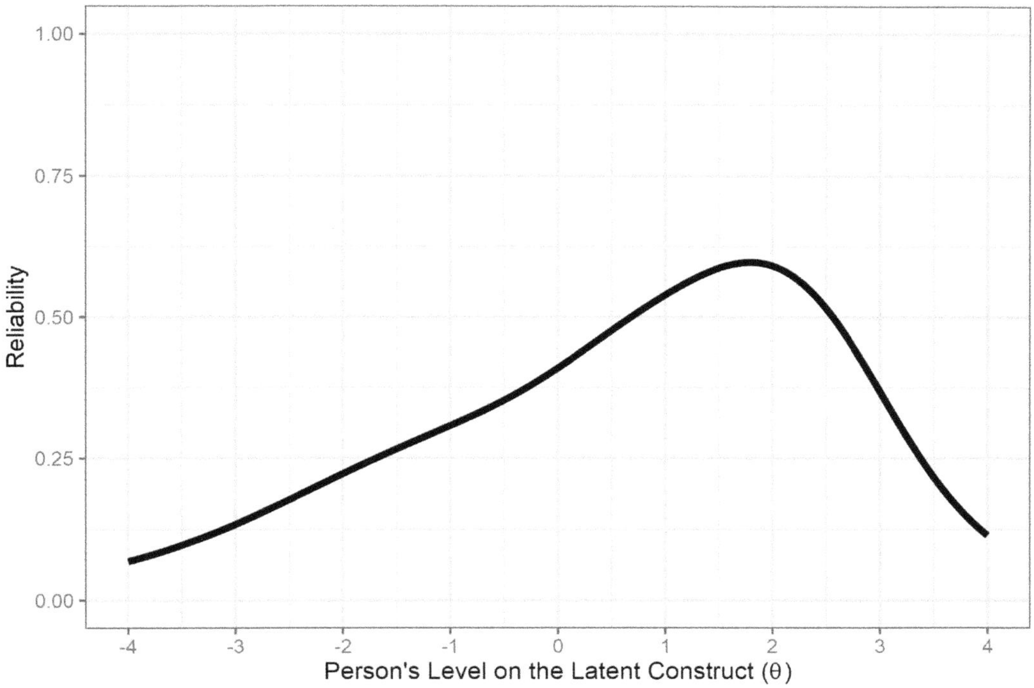

FIGURE 8.22 Test Reliability from Two-Parameter Logistic Model in Item Response Theory.

mean, the items should have difficulty that densely cover this range (e.g., 1.0, 1.05, 1.10, 1.15, 1.20, 1.25, 1.30, . . . , 2.0).

With items that (1) span the range of interest, (2) have high discrimination and information, and (3) densely cover the range of interest without redundancy, the measure should have a high information in the range of interest. This would allow it to efficiently and accurately assess the construct for the intended purpose.

An example of a bad measure for assessing the full range of individual differences is depicted in terms of ICCs in Figure 8.24 and in terms of test information in Figure 8.25. The measure performs poorly for the intended purpose, because its items do not (a) span the range of interest (-3 to 3 standard deviations from the mean of the latent construct), (b) have high discrimination and information, and (c) densely cover the range of interest without redundancy.

An example of a good measure for distinguishing clinical-range versus sub-clinical range is depicted in terms of ICCs in Figure 8.26 and in terms of test information in Figure 8.27. The measure is good for the intended purpose, in terms of having items that (a) span the range of interest (1–3 standard deviations above the mean of the latent construct), (b) have high discrimination and information, and (c) densely cover the range of interest without redundancy.

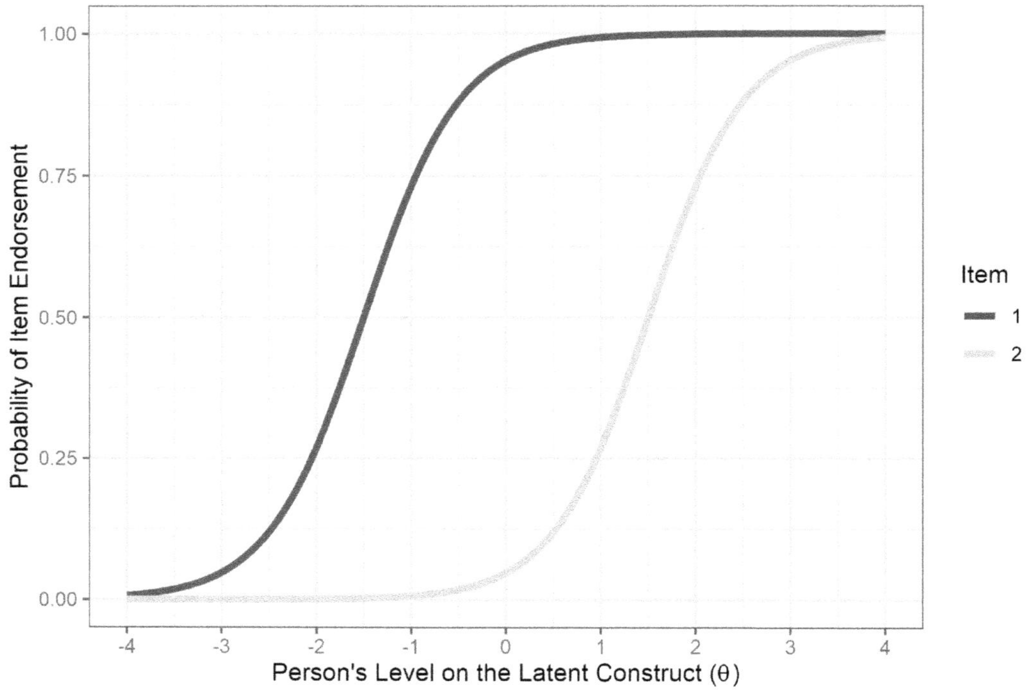

FIGURE 8.23 Visual Representation of an Efficient Assessment Based on Item Characteristic Curves from Two-Parameter Logistic Model in Item Response Theory.

8.2 Getting Started

8.2.1 Load Libraries

```
library("petersenlab")
library("mirt")
library("lavaan")
library("semTools")
library("semPlot")
library("lme4")
library("MOTE")
library("here")
library("tidyverse")
library("tinytex")
library("knitr")
library("kableExtra")
library("rmarkdown")
library("bookdown")
```

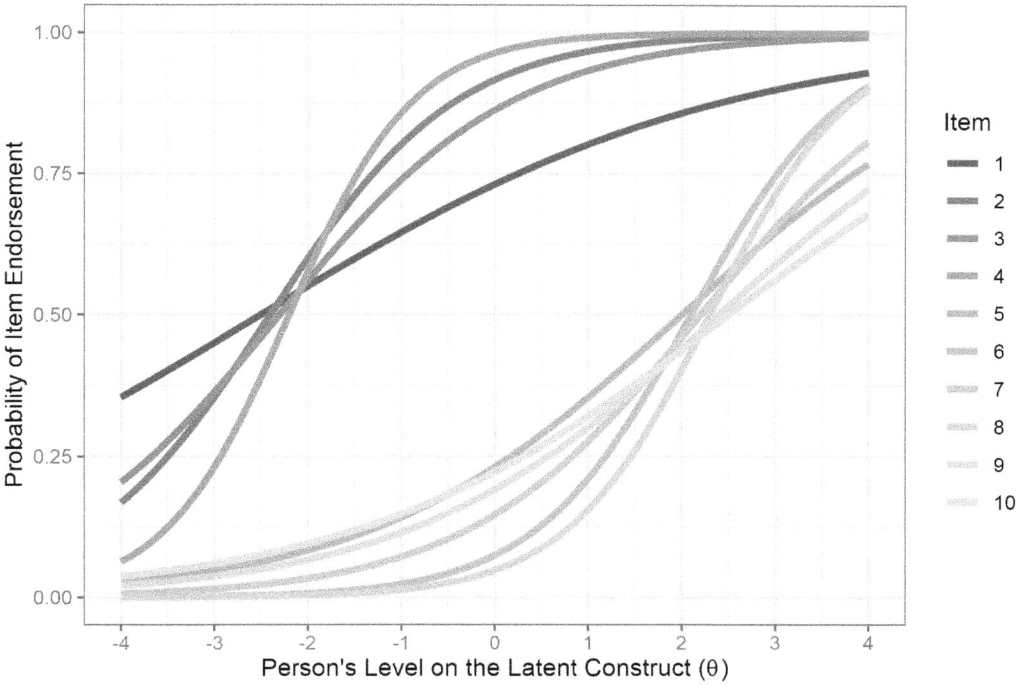

FIGURE 8.24 Visual Representation of a Bad Measure Based on Item Characteristic Curves of Items from a Bad Measure Estimated from Two-Parameter Logistic Model in Item Response Theory.

8.2.2 Load Data

`LSAT7` is a data set from the `mirt` package (Chalmers, 2020) that contains five items from the Law School Admissions Test.

```
mydataIRT <- expand.table(LSAT7)
```

8.2.3 Descriptive Statistics

```
itemstats(mydataIRT, ts.tables = TRUE)
```

```
$overall
    N mean_total.score sd_total.score ave.r  sd.r alpha
 1000            3.707          1.199 0.143 0.052 0.453

$itemstats
          N  mean    sd total.r total.r_if_rm alpha_if_rm
Item.1 1000 0.828 0.378   0.530         0.246       0.396
Item.2 1000 0.658 0.475   0.600         0.247       0.394
Item.3 1000 0.772 0.420   0.611         0.313       0.345
Item.4 1000 0.606 0.489   0.592         0.223       0.415
```

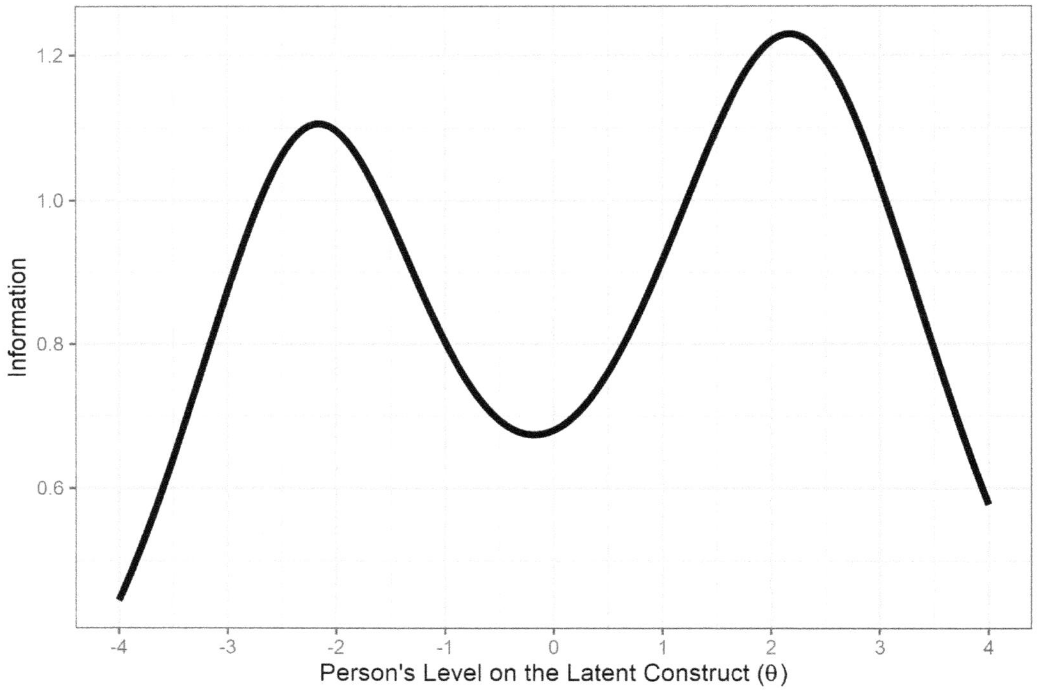

FIGURE 8.25 Visual Representation of a Bad Measure Based on the Test Information Curve.

```
Item.5 1000 0.843 0.364   0.461          0.175        0.438

$proportions
           0     1
Item.1 0.172 0.828
Item.2 0.342 0.658
Item.3 0.228 0.772
Item.4 0.394 0.606
Item.5 0.157 0.843

$total.score_frequency
      0  1   2   3   4   5
Freq 12 40 114 205 321 308

$total.score_means
           0     1
Item.1 2.314 3.996
Item.2 2.711 4.225
Item.3 2.360 4.105
Item.4 2.827 4.279
Item.5 2.427 3.945

$total.score_sds
```

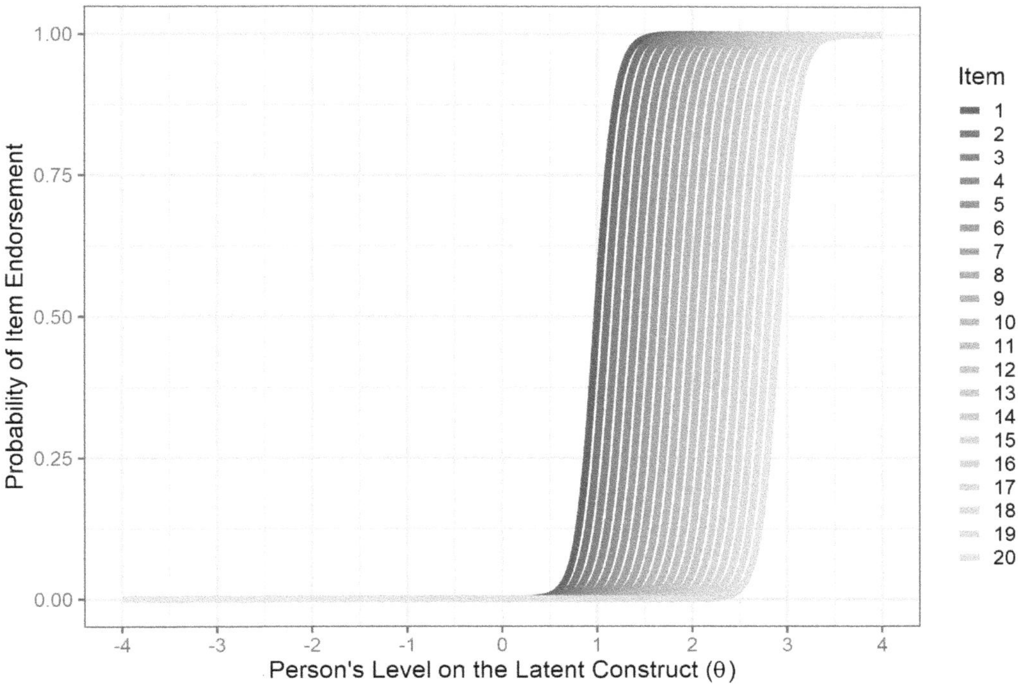

FIGURE 8.26 Visual Representation of a Good Measure Based on Item Characteristic Curves of Items from a Good Measure Estimated from Two-Parameter Logistic Model in Item Response Theory.

```
           0      1
Item.1 1.162 0.9841
Item.2 1.059 0.9038
Item.3 1.088 0.9043
Item.4 1.103 0.8661
Item.5 1.178 1.0416
```

8.3 Comparison of Scoring Approaches

A measure that is a raw symptom count (i.e., a count of how many symptoms a person endorses) is low in precision and has a high standard error of measurement. Some diagnostic measures provide an ordinal response scale for each symptom. For example, the Structured Clinical Interview of Mental Disorders (SCID) provides a response scale from 0 to 2, where 0 = the symptom is absent, 1 = the symptom is sub-threshold, and 2 = the symptom is present. If your measure was a raw symptom sum, as opposed to a count of how many symptoms were present, the measure would be slightly more precise and have a somewhat smaller standard error of measurement.

A weighted symptom sum is the classical test theory analog of IRT. In classical test theory, proportion correct (or endorsed) would correspond to item difficulty and the item–total

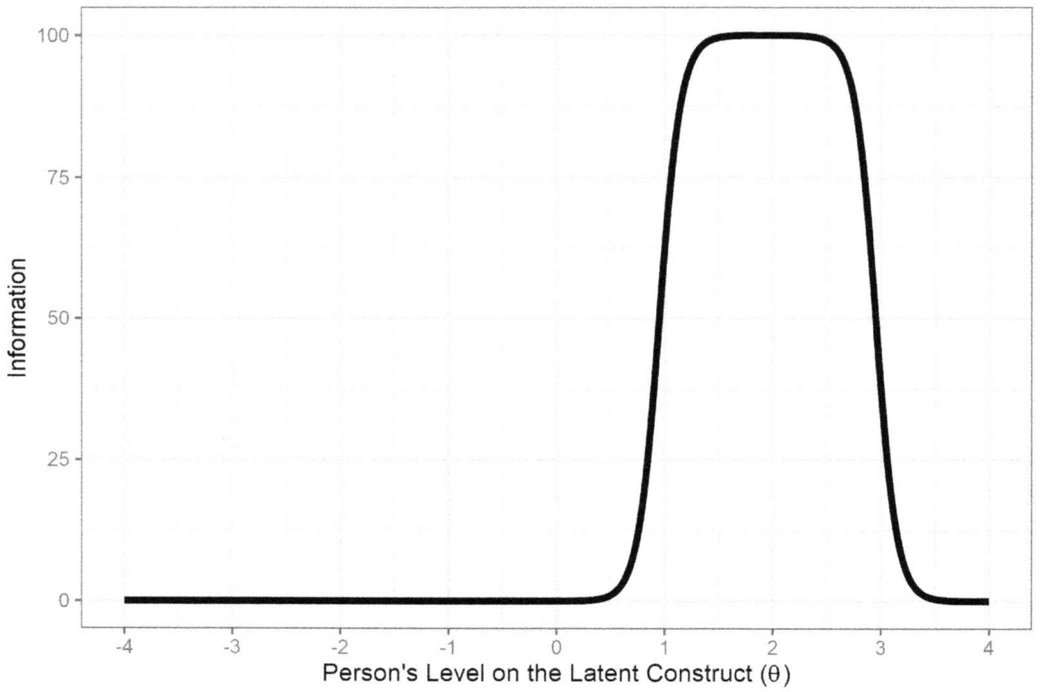

FIGURE 8.27 Visual Representation of a Good Measure (for Distinguishing Clinical-Range Versus Sub-clinical Range) Based on the Test Information Curve.

correlation (i.e., a point-biserial correlation) would correspond to item discrimination. If we were to compute a weighted sum of each item according to its strength of association with the construct (i.e., the item–total correlation), this measure would be somewhat more precise than the raw symptom sum, but it is not a latent variable method.

In IRT analysis, the weight for each item influences the estimate of a person's level on the construct. IRT down-weights the poorly discriminating items and up-weights the strongly discriminating items. This leads to greater precision and a lower standard error of measurement than non-latent scoring approaches.

According to Embretson (1996), many perspectives have changed because of IRT. First, according to classical test theory, longer tests are more reliable than shorter tests, as described in Section 3.5.5.4 in the chapter on reliability. However, according to IRT, shorter tests (i.e., tests with fewer items) can be more reliable than longer tests. Item selection using IRT can lead to briefer assessments that have greater reliability than longer scales. For example, adaptive tests that tailor the difficulty of the items to the ability level of the participant.

Second, in classical test theory, a score's meaning is tied to its location in a distribution (i.e., the norm-referenced standard). In IRT, however, the people and items are calibrated on a common scale. Based on a child's IRT-estimated ability level (i.e., level on the construct), we can have a better sense of what the child knows and does not know, because it indicates the difficulty level at which they would tend to get items correct 50% of the time; the person would likely fail items with a higher difficulty compared to this level, whereas the person would likely pass items with a lower difficulty compared to this level. Consider Binet's distribution of ability that arranges the items from easiest to most difficult. Based on the item difficulty and content of the items and the child's performance, we can have a better indication that a child can perform items successfully in a particular range (e.g., count to 10) but might not be able to perform more difficult items (e.g., tie their shoes). From an intervention perspective, this would allow working in the "window of opportunity" or the zone of proximal development. Thus, IRT can provide more meaningful understanding of a person's ability compared to traditional classical test theory interpretations such as the child being at the "63rd percentile" for a child of their age, which lacks conceptual meaning.

According to Cooper & Balsis (2009), our current diagnostic system relies heavily on how many symptoms a person endorses as an index of severity, but this assumes that all symptom endorsements have the same overall weight (severity). Using IRT, we can determine the relative severity of each item (symptom)—and it is clear that some symptoms indicate more severity than others. From this analysis, a respondent can endorse fewer, more severe items, and have overall more severe psychopathology than an individual who endorses more, less severe items. Basically, not all items are equally severe—know your items!

8.4 One-Parameter Logistic (Rasch) Model

A one-parameter logistic (1-PL) item response theory (IRT) model is a model fit to dichotomous data, which estimates a different difficulty (b) parameter for each item. Discrimination (a) is not estimated (i.e., it is fixed at the same value—one—across items). Rasch models were fit using the `mirt` package (Chalmers, 2020).

8.4.1 Fit Model

```
raschModel <- mirt(
  data = mydataIRT,
  model = 1,
  itemtype = "Rasch",
  SE = TRUE)
```

8.4.2 Model Summary

```
coef(raschModel, simplify = TRUE, IRTpars = TRUE)
```

```
$items
       a      b g u
Item.1 1 -1.868 0 1
Item.2 1 -0.791 0 1
Item.3 1 -1.461 0 1
Item.4 1 -0.521 0 1
Item.5 1 -1.993 0 1

$means
```

```
F1
 0


$cov
      F1
F1 1.022
```

8.4.3 Plots

8.4.3.1 Test Curves

The test curves suggest that the measure is most reliable (i.e., provides the most information has the smallest standard error of measurement) at lower levels of the construct.

8.4.3.1.1 Test characteristic curve

A test characteristic curve (TCC) plot of the expected total score as a function of a person's level on the latent construct (theta; θ) is in Figure 8.28.

```
plot(raschModel, type = "score")
```

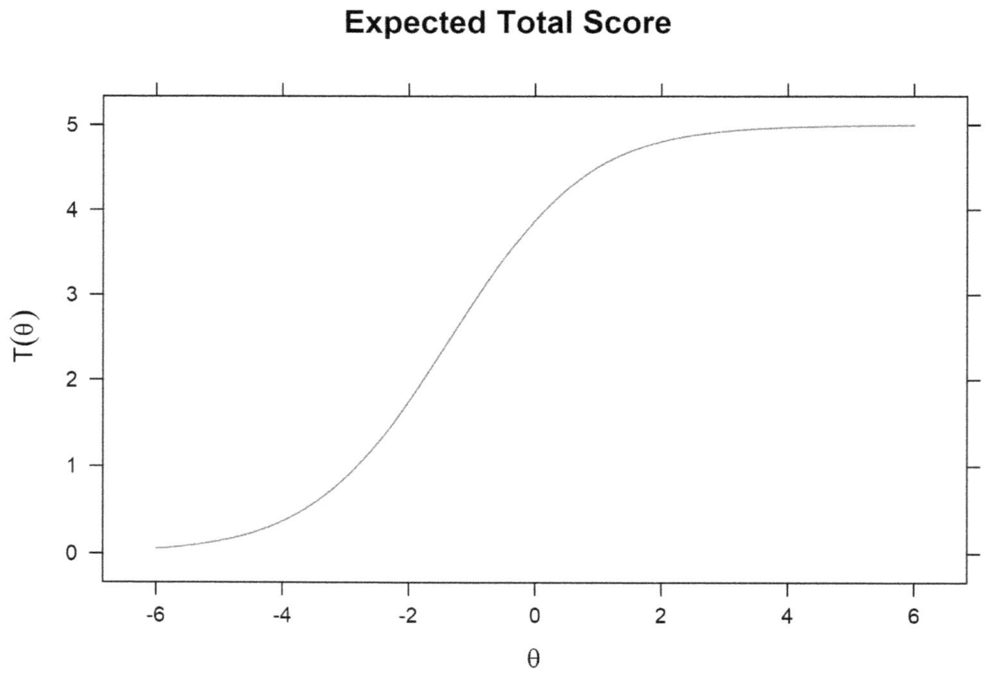

FIGURE 8.28 Test Characteristic Curve from Rasch Item Response Theory Model.

8.4.3.1.2 Test information curve

A plot of test information as a function of a person's level on the latent construct (theta; θ) is shown in Figure 8.29.

```
plot(raschModel, type = "info")
```

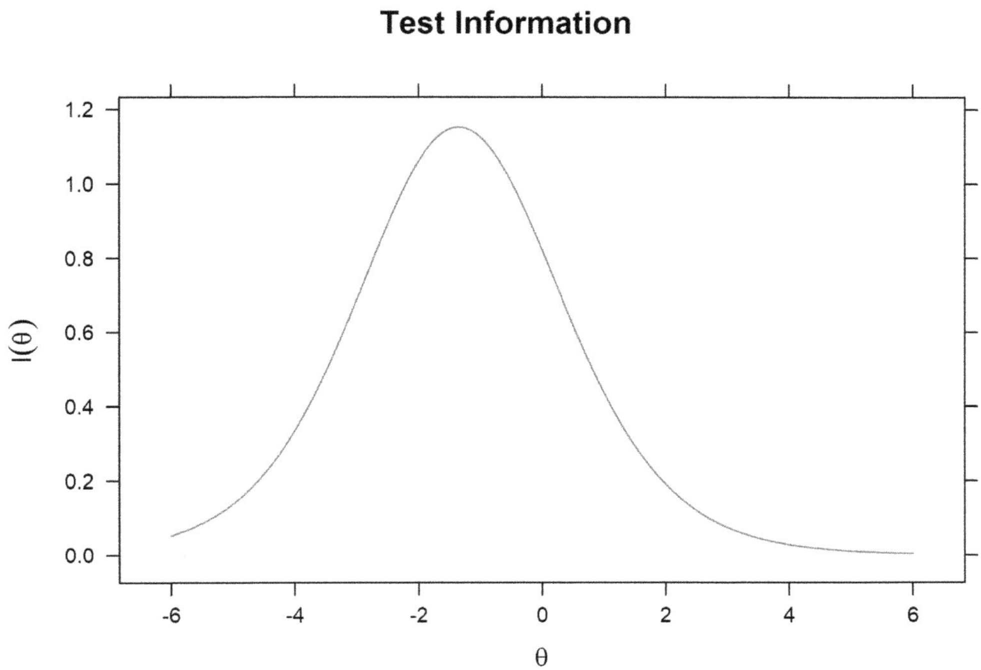

FIGURE 8.29 Test Information Curve from Rasch Item Response Theory Model.

8.4.3.1.3 Test reliability

The estimate of marginal reliability is below:

```
marginal_rxx(raschModel)
```

```
[1] 0.4206
```

A plot of test reliability as a function of a person's level on the latent construct (theta; θ) is depicted in Figure 8.30.

```
plot(raschModel, type = "rxx")
```

8.4.3.1.4 Test standard error of measurement

A plot of test standard error of measurement (SEM) as a function of a person's level on the latent construct (theta; θ) is shown in Figure 8.31.

```
plot(raschModel, type = "SE")
```

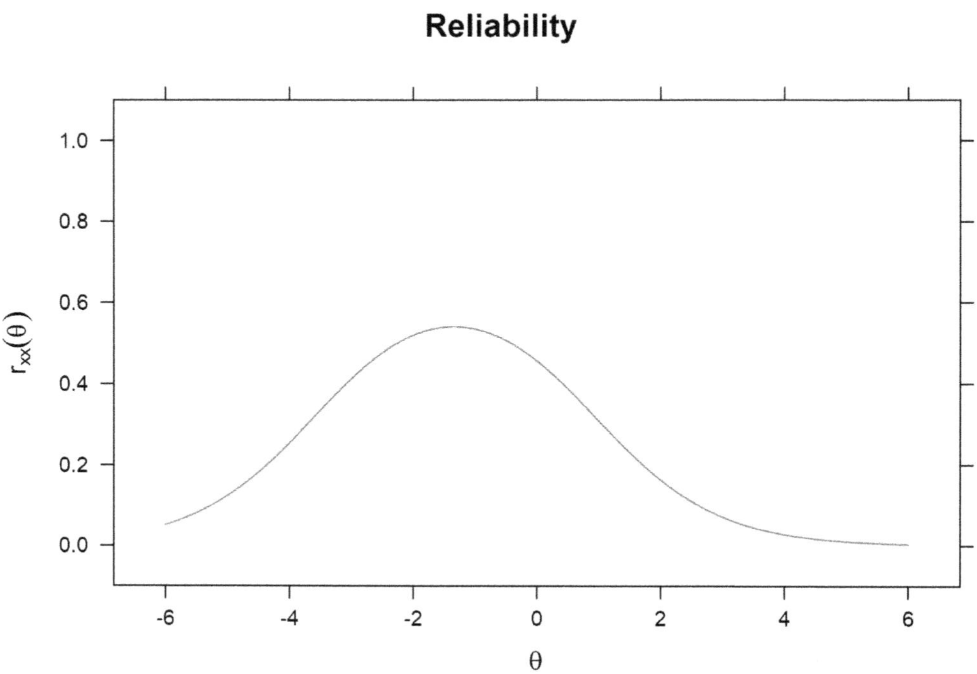

FIGURE 8.30 Test Reliability from Rasch Item Response Theory Model.

8.4.3.1.5 Test information curve and test standard error of measurement

A plot of test information and standard error of measurement (SEM) as a function of a person's level on the latent construct (theta; θ) is presented in Figure 8.32.

```
plot(
  raschModel,
  type = "infoSE")
```

8.4.3.2 Item Curves

8.4.3.2.1 Item characteristic curves

Item characteristic curve (ICC) plots of the probability of item endorsement (or getting the item correct) as a function of a person's level on the latent construct (theta; θ) are shown in Figure 8.33.

```
plot(
  raschModel,
  type = "itemscore",
  facet_items = FALSE)
```

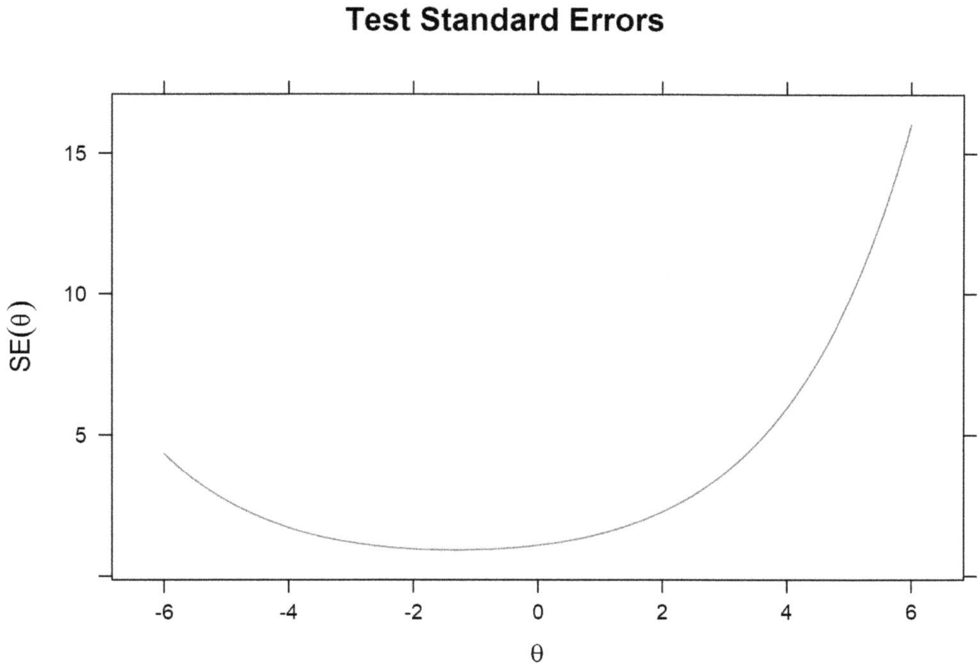

FIGURE 8.31 Test Standard Error of Measurement from Rasch Item Response Theory Model.

8.4.3.2.2 Item information curves

Plots of item information as a function of a person's level on the latent construct (theta; θ) are shown in Figure 8.34.

```
plot(
  raschModel,
  type = "infotrace",
  facet_items = FALSE)
```

8.4.4 CFA

A one-parameter logistic model can also be fit in a CFA framework, sometimes called item factor analysis. The item factor analysis models were fit in the `lavaan` package (Rosseel et al., 2022).

```
onePLModel_cfa <- '
# Factor Loadings (i.e., discrimination parameters)
latent =~ loading*Item.1 + loading*Item.2 + loading*Item.3 +
  loading*Item.4 + loading*Item.5

# Item Thresholds (i.e., difficulty parameters)
```

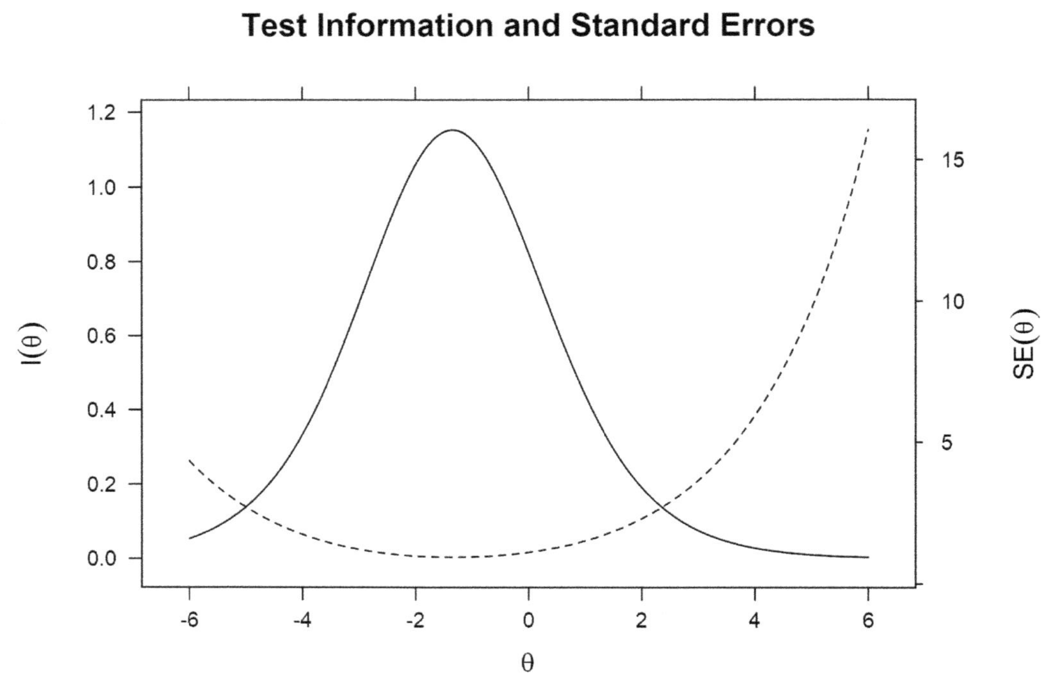

FIGURE 8.32 Test Information Curve and Standard Error of Measurement from Rasch Item Response Theory Model.

```
Item.1 | threshold1*t1
Item.2 | threshold2*t1
Item.3 | threshold3*t1
Item.4 | threshold4*t1
Item.5 | threshold5*t1
'

onePLModel_cfa_fit = sem(
  model = onePLModel_cfa,
  data = mydataIRT,
  ordered = c("Item.1", "Item.2", "Item.3", "Item.4","Item.5"),
  mimic = "Mplus",
  estimator = "WLSMV",
  std.lv = TRUE,
  parameterization = "theta")
```

8.4.5 Mixed Model

A Rasch model can also be fit in a mixed model framework. The Rasch model below was fit using the `lme4` package (Bates et al., 2022).

First, we convert the data from wide form to long form for the mixed model:

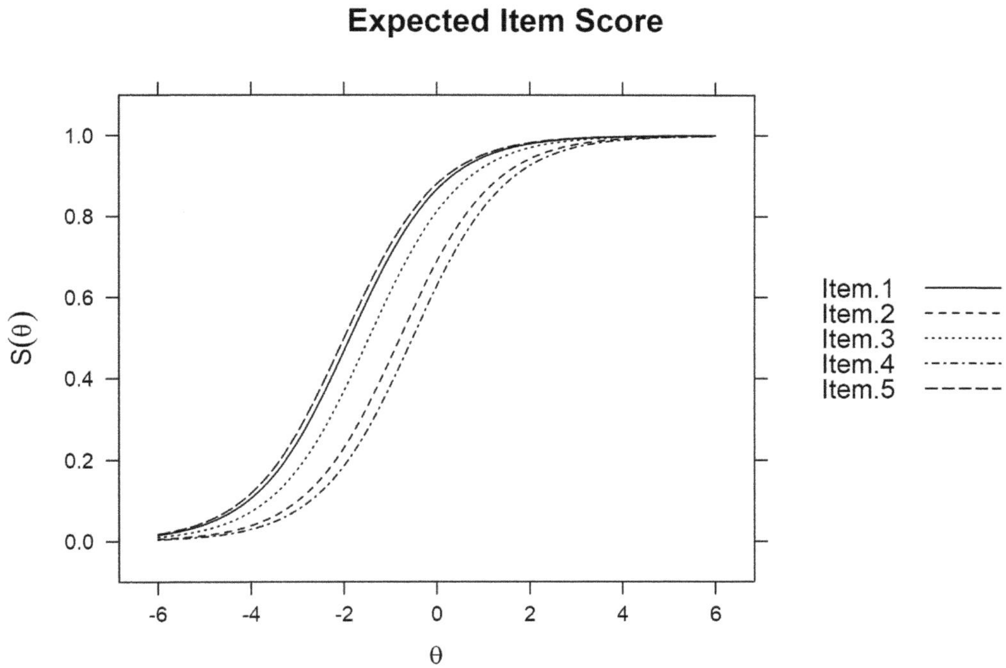

FIGURE 8.33 Item Characteristic Curves from Rasch Item Response Theory Model.

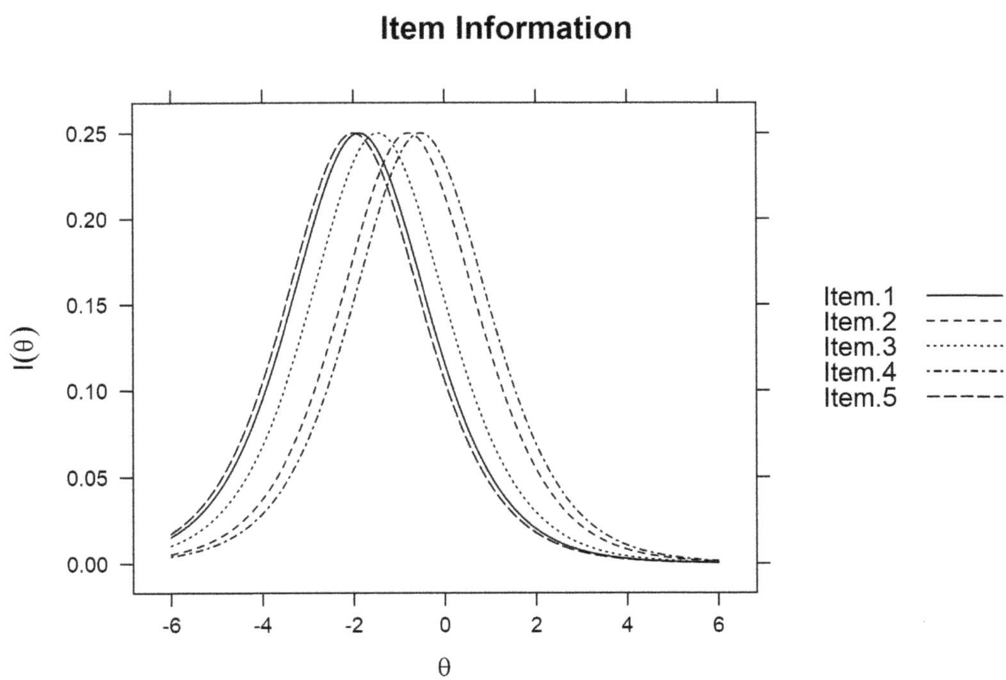

FIGURE 8.34 Item Information Curves from Rasch Item Response Theory Model.

```
mydataIRT_long <- mydataIRT %>%
  mutate(ID = 1:nrow(mydataIRT)) %>%
  pivot_longer(cols = Item.1:Item.5) %>%
  rename(
    item = name,
    response = value)
```

Then, we can estimate the Rasch model using a logit or probit link:

```
raschModel_mixed_logit <- glmer(
  response ~ -1 + item + (1|ID),
  mydataIRT_long,
  family = binomial(link = "logit"))

raschModel_mixed_probit <- glmer(
  response ~ -1 + item + (1|ID),
  mydataIRT_long,
  family = binomial(link = "probit"))
```

8.5 Two-Parameter Logistic Model

A two-parameter logistic (2-PL) IRT model is a model fit to dichotomous data, which estimates a different difficulty (b) and discrimination (a) parameter for each item. Two-parameter logistic models were fit using the `mirt` package (Chalmers, 2020).

8.5.1 Fit Model

```
twoPLModel <- mirt(
  data = mydataIRT,
  model = 1,
  itemtype = "2PL",
  SE = TRUE)
```

8.5.2 Convert Discrimination to Factor Loading

As described by Aiden Loe[1] (archived at https://perma.cc/H3QN-JAWW), one can convert a discrimination parameter to a standardized factor loading using Equation (8.14):

$$f = \frac{a}{\sqrt{1 + a^2}} \tag{8.14}$$

where a is equal to: discrimination/1.702.

[1]https://aidenloe.github.io/introToIRT.html#(alpha%7B%7D)_par_to_std_loading

The petersenlab package (Petersen, 2024) contains the discriminationToFactorLoading() function that converts discrimination parameters to standardized factor loadings.

```
discriminationParameters <- coef(
  twoPLModel,
  simplify = TRUE)$items[,1]

discriminationParameters
```

```
Item.1 Item.2 Item.3 Item.4 Item.5
0.9879 1.0809 1.7058 0.7652 0.7358
```

```
discriminationToFactorLoading(discriminationParameters)
```

```
Item.1 Item.2 Item.3 Item.4 Item.5
0.5020 0.5361 0.7079 0.4100 0.3968
```

8.5.3 CFA

A two-parameter logistic model can also be fit in a CFA framework, sometimes called item factor analysis. The item factor analysis models were fit in the lavaan package (Rosseel et al., 2022).

```
twoPLModel_cfa <- '
# Factor Loadings (i.e., discrimination parameters)
latent =~ loading1*Item.1 + loading2*Item.2 + loading3*Item.3 +
  loading4*Item.4 + loading5*Item.5

# Item Thresholds (i.e., difficulty parameters)
Item.1 | threshold1*t1
Item.2 | threshold2*t1
Item.3 | threshold3*t1
Item.4 | threshold4*t1
Item.5 | threshold5*t1
'

twoPLModel_cfa_fit = sem(
  model = twoPLModel_cfa,
  data = mydataIRT,
  ordered = c("Item.1", "Item.2", "Item.3", "Item.4","Item.5"),
  mimic = "Mplus",
  estimator = "WLSMV",
  std.lv = TRUE,
  parameterization = "theta")
```

8.6 Two-Parameter Multidimensional Logistic Model

A 2-PL multidimensional IRT model is a model that allows multiple dimensions (latent factors) and is fit to dichotomous data, which estimates a different difficulty (b) and discrimination (a) parameter for each item. Multidimensional IRT models were fit using the `mirt` package (Chalmers, 2020). In this example, we estimate a 2-PL multidimensional IRT model by estimating two factors.

8.6.1 Fit Model

```
twoPL2FactorModel <- mirt(
  data = mydataIRT,
  model = 2,
  itemtype = "2PL",
  SE = TRUE)
```

8.6.2 Model Summary

```
coef(twoPL2FactorModel, simplify = TRUE)
```

```
$items
           a1     a2     d g u
Item.1 -2.007  0.870 2.648 0 1
Item.2 -0.849 -0.522 0.788 0 1
Item.3 -2.153 -1.836 2.483 0 1
Item.4 -0.756 -0.028 0.485 0 1
Item.5 -0.757  0.000 1.864 0 1

$means
F1 F2
 0  0

$cov
   F1 F2
F1  1  0
F2  0  1
```

8.6.3 Compare Model Fit

The modified model with two factors and the original one-factor model are considered "nested" models. The original model is nested within the modified model because the modified model includes all of the terms of the original model along with additional terms. Model fit of nested models can be compared with a chi-square difference test.

```
anova(twoPLModel, twoPL2FactorModel)
```

```
                   AIC SABIC   HQ  BIC logLik     X2 df     p
twoPLModel        5338  5355 5356 5387  -2659
twoPL2FactorModel 5335  5359 5361 5404  -2654 10.571  4 0.032
```

Using a chi-square difference test to compare two nested models, the two-factor model fits significantly better than the one-factor model.

8.6.4 CFA

A two-parameter multidimensional model can also be fit in a CFA framework, sometimes called item factor analysis. The item factor analysis models were fit in the `lavaan` package (Rosseel et al., 2022).

```
twoPLModelMultidimensional_cfa <- '
# Factor Loadings (i.e., discrimination parameters)
latent1 =~ loading1*Item.1 + loading4*Item.4 + loading5*Item.5
latent2 =~ loading2*Item.2 + loading3*Item.3

# Item Thresholds (i.e., difficulty parameters)
Item.1 | threshold1*t1
Item.2 | threshold2*t1
Item.3 | threshold3*t1
Item.4 | threshold4*t1
Item.5 | threshold5*t1
'

twoPLModelMultidimensional_cfa_fit = sem(
  model = twoPLModelMultidimensional_cfa,
  data = mydataIRT,
  ordered = c("Item.1", "Item.2", "Item.3", "Item.4","Item.5"),
  mimic = "Mplus",
  estimator = "WLSMV",
  std.lv = TRUE,
  parameterization = "theta")
```

8.7 Three-Parameter Logistic Model

A three-parameter logistic (3-PL) IRT model is a model fit to dichotomous data, which estimates a different difficulty (b), discrimination (a), and guessing parameter for each item. Three-parameter logistic models were fit using the `mirt` package (Chalmers, 2020).

8.7.1 Fit Model

```
threePLModel <- mirt(
  data = mydataIRT,
  model = 1,
  itemtype = "3PL",
  SE = TRUE)
```

8.7.2 Model Summary

```
coef(threePLModel, simplify = TRUE, IRTpars = TRUE)
```

```
$items
           a      b     g u
Item.1 1.007 -1.853 0.000 1
Item.2 1.928 -0.049 0.295 1
Item.3 1.667 -1.068 0.000 1
Item.4 0.736 -0.655 0.000 1
Item.5 0.767 -2.436 0.000 1

$means
F1
 0

$cov
   F1
F1  1
```

8.8 Four-Parameter Logistic Model

A four-parameter logistic (4-PL) IRT model is a model fit to dichotomous data, which estimates a different difficulty (b), discrimination (a), guessing, and careless errors parameter for each item. Four-parameter logistic models were fit using the `mirt` package (Chalmers, 2020).

8.8.1 Fit Model

```
fourPLModel <- mirt(
  data = mydataIRT,
  model = 1,
  itemtype = "4PL",
  SE = TRUE,
  technical = list(NCYCLES = 2000))
```

8.8.2 Model Summary

```
coef(fourPLModel, simplify = TRUE, IRTpars = TRUE)
```

```
$items
           a      b     g     u
Item.1 2.570 -1.619 0.000 0.911
Item.2 8.490  0.093 0.370 0.992
Item.3 2.002 -0.646 0.271 0.999
Item.4 3.094 -1.224 0.000 0.708
Item.5 1.450 -2.166 0.002 0.920

$means
F1
 0

$cov
   F1
F1  1
```

8.9 Graded Response Model

A two-parameter graded response model (GRM) is an IRT model fit to polytomous data (in this case, 1–4 likert scale), which estimates a different difficulty (b) and discrimination (a) parameter for each item. It estimates four parameters for each item: difficulty [for each of three threshold transitions: 1–2 (b_1), 2–3 (b_2), and 3–4 (b_3)] and discrimination (a). GRM models were fit using the `mirt` package (Chalmers, 2020).

8.9.1 Fit Model

`Science` is a data set from the `mirt` package (Chalmers, 2020) that contains four items evaluating people's attitudes to science and technology on a 1–4 Likert scale. The data are from the Consumer Protection and Perceptions of Science and Technology section of the 1992 Euro-Barometer Survey of people in Great Britain.

```
gradedResponseModel <- mirt(
  data = Science,
   model = 1,
   itemtype = "graded",
   SE = TRUE)
```

8.9.2 Model Summary

```
coef(gradedResponseModel, simplify = TRUE, IRTpars = TRUE)
```

```
$items
            a     b1     b2    b3
Comfort 1.042 -4.669 -2.534 1.407
Work    1.226 -2.385 -0.735 1.849
Future  2.293 -2.282 -0.965 0.856
Benefit 1.095 -3.058 -0.906 1.542

$means
F1
 0

$cov
   F1
F1  1
```

8.9.3 Plots

8.9.3.1 Test Curves

The test curves suggest that the measure is most reliable (i.e., provides the most information and has the smallest standard error of measurement) across a wide range of construct. In general, this measure with polytomous (Likert-scale) items provides more information than the measure with binary items that were examined above. This is consistent with the idea that polytomous items tend to provide more information than binary/dichotomous items.

8.9.3.1.1 Test characteristic curve

A test characteristic curve (TCC) plot of the expected total score as a function of a person's level on the latent construct (theta; θ) is shown in Figure 8.35.

```
plot(gradedResponseModel, type = "score")
```

8.9.3.1.2 Test information curve

A plot of test information as a function of a person's level on the latent construct (theta; θ) is shown in Figure 8.36.

```
plot(gradedResponseModel, type = "info")
```

8.9.3.1.3 Test reliability

The estimate of marginal reliability is below:

```
marginal_rxx(gradedResponseModel)
```

```
[1] 0.6688
```

A plot of test reliability as a function of a person's level on the latent construct (theta; θ) is illustrated in Figure 8.37.

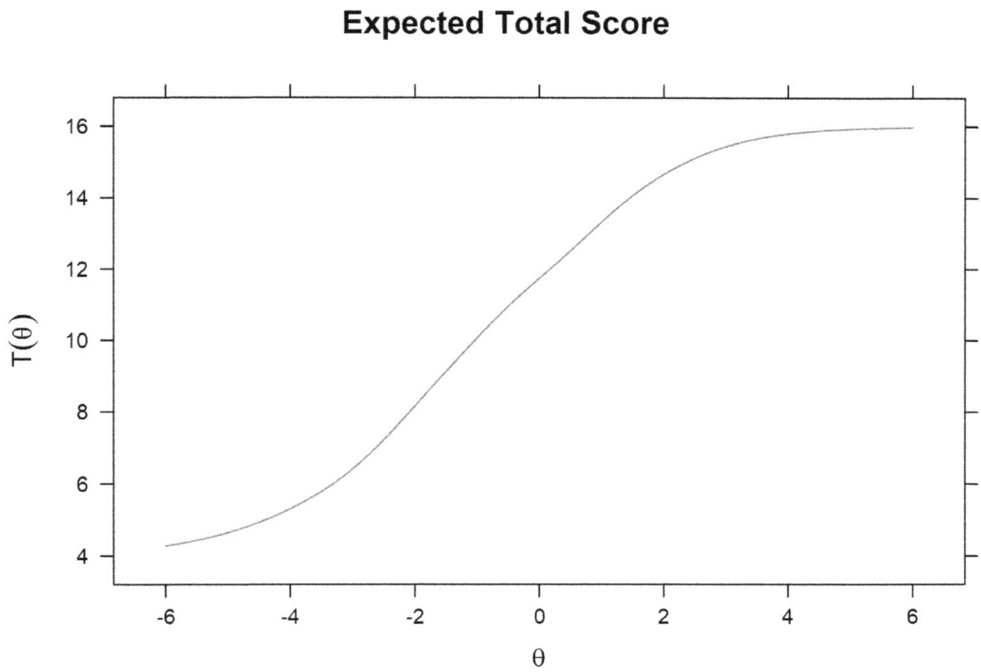

FIGURE 8.35 Test Characteristic Curve from Graded Response Model.

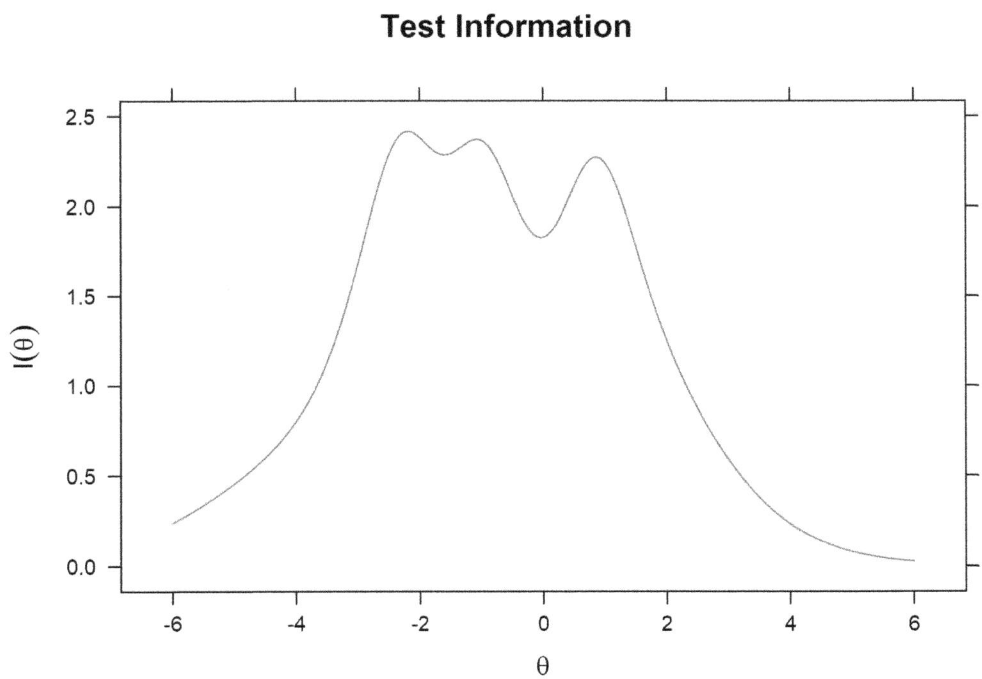

FIGURE 8.36 Test Information Curve from Graded Response Model.

```
plot(gradedResponseModel, type = "rxx")
```

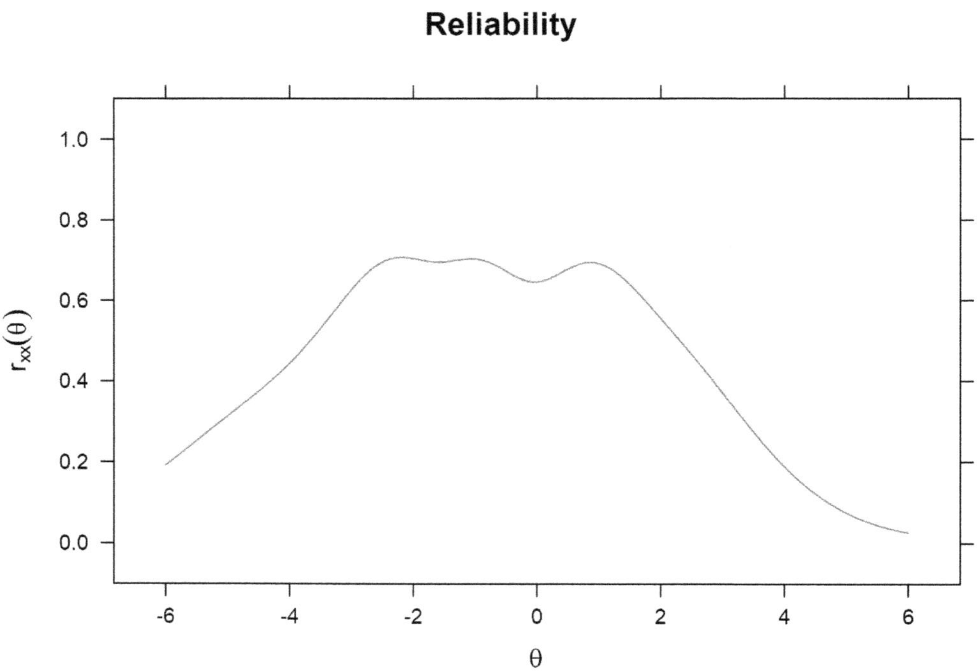

FIGURE 8.37 Test Reliability from Graded Response Model.

8.9.3.1.4 Test standard error of measurement

A plot of test standard error of measurement (SEM) as a function of a person's level on the latent construct (theta; θ) is depicted in Figure 8.38.

```
plot(gradedResponseModel, type = "SE")
```

8.9.3.1.5 Test information curve and standard errors

A plot of test information and standard error of measurement (SEM) as a function of a person's level on the latent construct (theta; θ) is shown in Figure 8.39.

```
plot(
  gradedResponseModel,
  type = "infoSE")
```

8.9.3.2 Item Curves

8.9.3.2.1 Item characteristic curves

Item characteristic curve (ICC) plots of the expected score on the item as a function of a person's level on the latent construct (theta; θ) are shown in Figure 8.40.

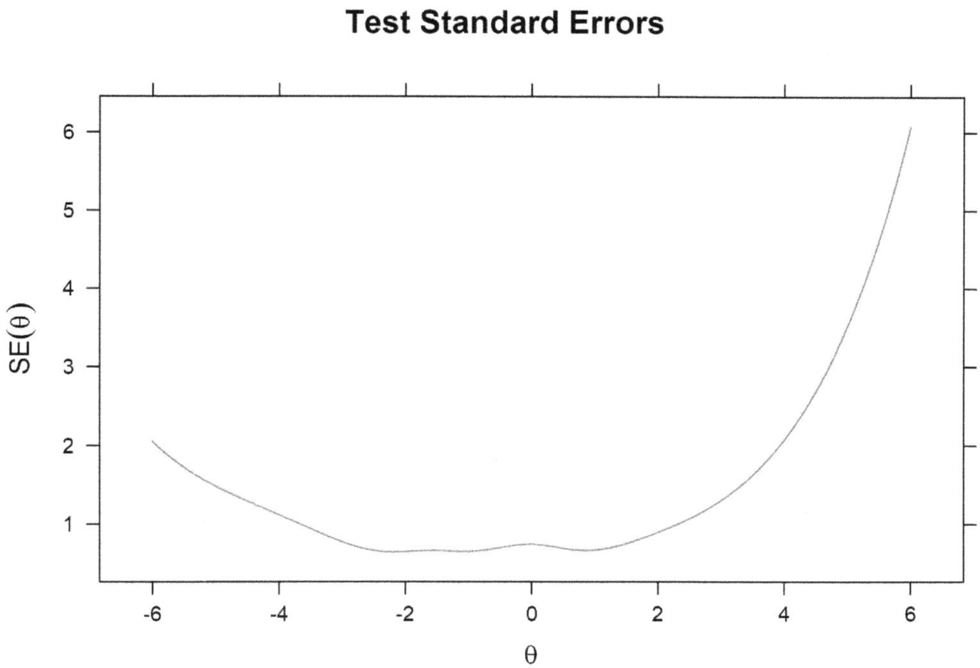

FIGURE 8.38 Test Standard Error of Measurement from Graded Response Model.

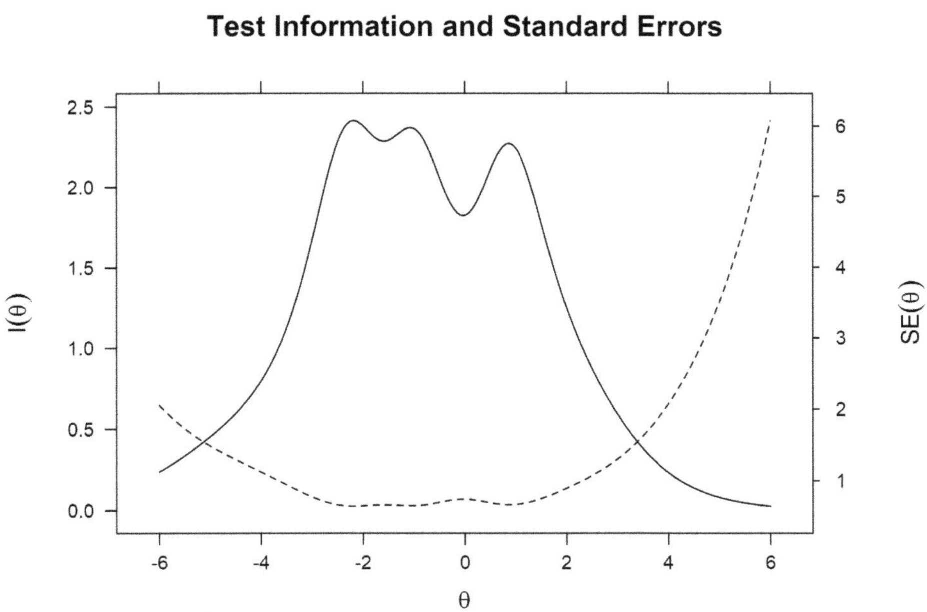

FIGURE 8.39 Test Information Curve and Standard Error of Measurement from Graded Response Model.

```
plot(
  gradedResponseModel,
  type = "itemscore",
  facet_items = FALSE)
```

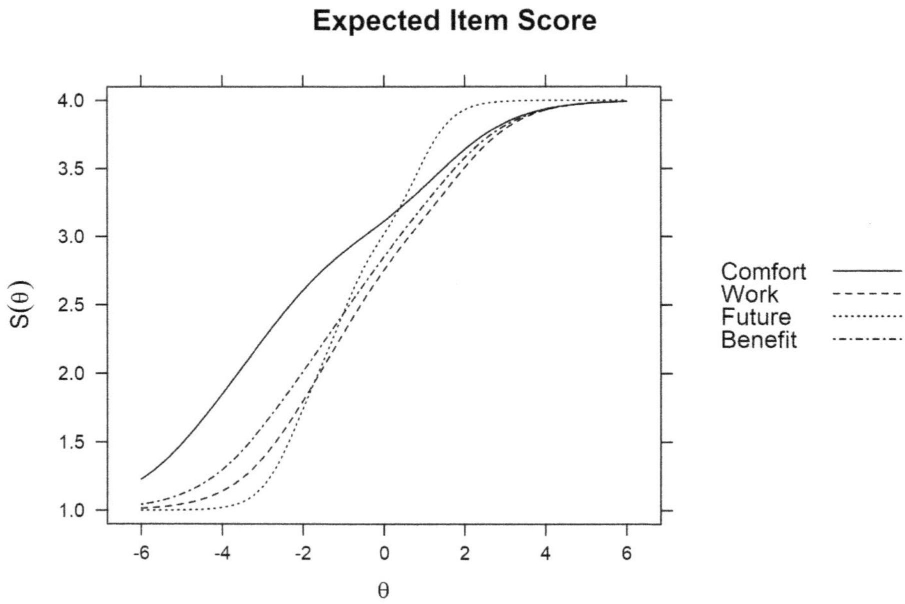

FIGURE 8.40 Item Characteristic Curves from Graded Response Model.

8.9.3.2.2 Item information curves

Plots of item information as a function of a person's level on the latent construct (theta; θ) are shown in Figure 8.41.

```
plot(
  gradedResponseModel,
  type = "infotrace",
  facet_items = FALSE)
```

8.9.3.2.3 Item response category characteristic curves

A plot of the probability of item threshold endorsement as a function of a person's level on the latent construct (theta; θ) is illustrated in Figure 8.42.

```
plot(
  gradedResponseModel,
  type = "trace")
```

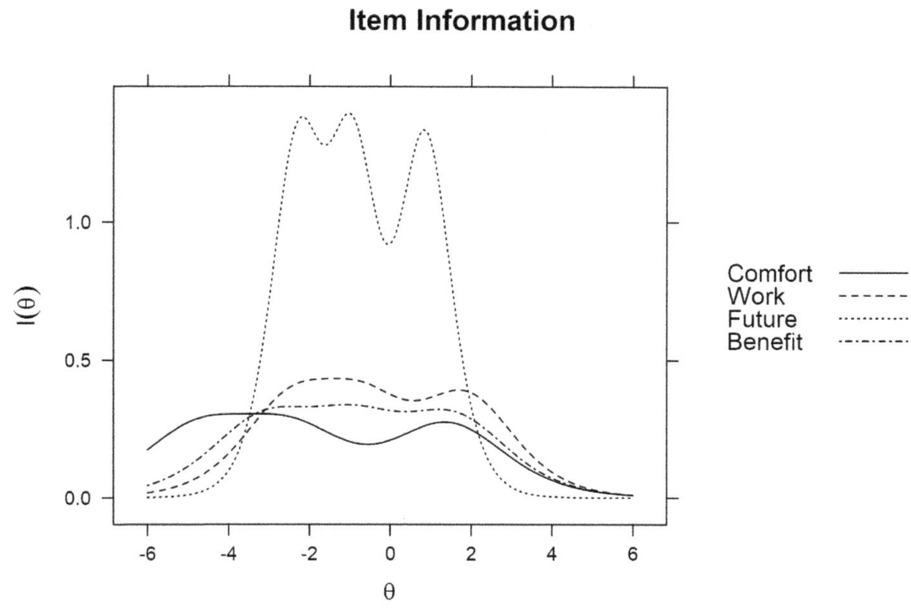

FIGURE 8.41 Item Information Curves from Graded Response Model.

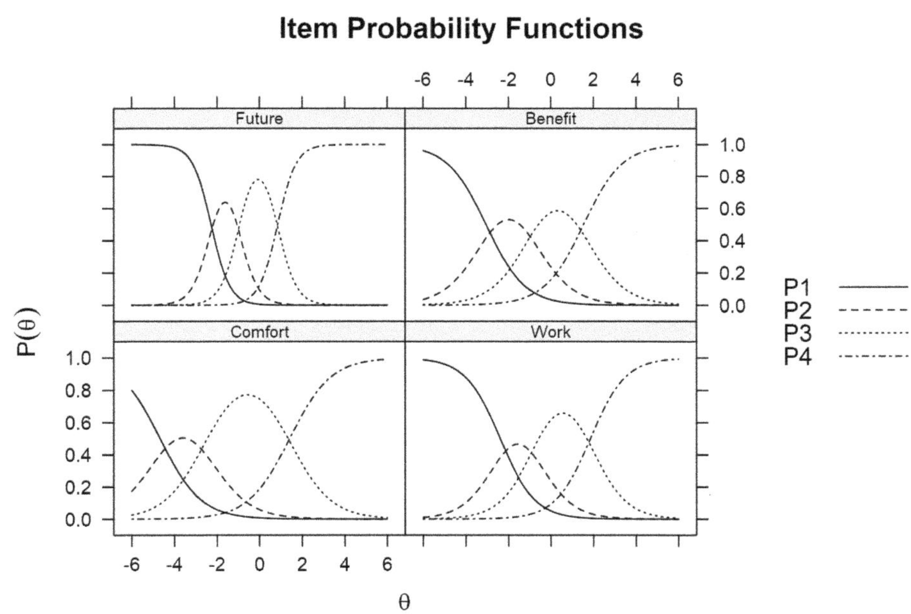

FIGURE 8.42 Item Response Category Characteristic Curves from Graded Response Model.

8.9.3.2.4 Item boundary characteristic curves (aka item operation characteristic curves)

A plot of item boundary characteristic curves is illustrated in Figure 8.43. The plot of item boundary characteristic curves was adapted from an example by Aiden Loe: https://aidenloe.github.io/irtplots.html (archived at https://perma.cc/D4YH-RV6N).

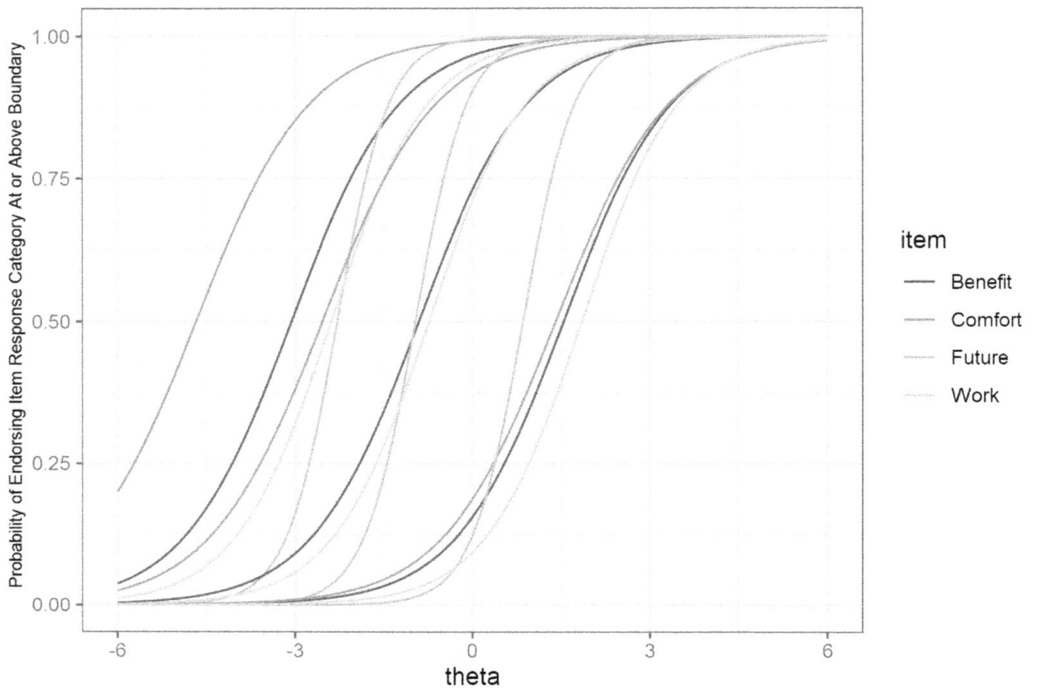

FIGURE 8.43 Item Boundary Category Characteristic Curves from Graded Response Model.

8.10 Conclusion

Item response theory is a measurement theory and advanced modeling approach that allows estimating latent variables as the common variance from multiple items, and it allows estimating how the items relate to the construct (latent variable). IRT holds promise to enable the development of briefer assessments, including short forms and adaptive assessments, that have strong reliability and validity.

8.11 Suggested Readings

If you are interested in learning more about IRT, we recommend the book by Embretson & Reise (2000).

9

Prediction

> It is very difficult to predict—especially the future.
>
> — Neils Bohr

9.1 Overview

In psychology, we are often interested in predicting behavior. Behavior is complex. The same behavior can occur for different reasons. Behavior is probabilistically influenced by many processes, including processes internal to the person in addition to external processes. Moreover, people's behavior occurs in the context of a dynamic system with nonlinear, probabilistic, and cascading influences that change across time. The ever-changing system makes behavior challenging to predict. And, similar to chaos theory, one small change in the system can lead to large differences later on.

Predictions can come in different types. Some predictions involve categorical data, whereas other predictions involve continuous data. When dealing with categorical data, we can evaluate predictions using a 2-by-2 table known as a confusion matrix (see Figure 9.4), or with logistic regression models. When dealing with continuous data, we can evaluate predictions using multiple regression or similar variants such as structural equation modeling and mixed models.

Let's consider a prediction example, assuming the following probabilities:

- The probability of contracting HIV is .3%
- The probability of a positive test for HIV is 1%
- The probability of a positive test if you have HIV is 95%

What is the probability of HIV if you have a positive test?

As we will see, the probability is: $\frac{95\% \times .3\%}{1\%} = 28.5\%$. So based on the above probabilities, if you have a positive test, the probability that you have HIV is 28.5%. Most people tend to vastly overestimate the likelihood that the person has HIV in this example. Why? Because they do not pay enough attention to the base rate (in this example, the base rate of HIV is .3%).

9.1.1 Issues Around Probability

9.1.1.1 Types of Probabilities

It is important to distinguish between different types of probabilities: marginal probabilities, joint probabilities, and conditional probabilities.

9.1.1.1.1 *Base rate (marginal probability)*

A *base rate* is the probability of an event. Base rates are marginal probabilities. A *marginal probability* is the probability of an event irrespective of the outcome of another variable. For instance, we can consider the following marginal probabilities:

$P(C_i)$ is the probability (i.e., base rate) of a classification, C, independent of other things. A base rate is often used as the "*prior probability*" in a Bayesian model. In our example above, $P(C_i)$ is the base rate (i.e., prevalence) of HIV in the population: $P(\text{HIV}) = .3\%$. $P(R_i)$ is the probability (base rate) of a response, R, independent of other things. In the example above, $P(R_i)$ is the base rate of a positive test for HIV: $P(\text{positive test}) = 1\%$. The base rate of a positive test is known as the *positivity rate* or *selection ratio*.

9.1.1.1.2 *Joint probability*

A *joint probability* is the probability of two (or more) events occurring simultaneously. For instance, the probability of events A and B both occurring together is $P(A, B)$. A joint probability can be calculated using the marginal probability of each event, as in Equation (9.1):

$$P(A, B) = P(A) \cdot P(B) \tag{9.1}$$

Conversely (and rearranging the terms for the calculation of conditional probability), a joint probability can also be calculated using the conditional probability and marginal probability, as in Equation (9.2):

$$P(A, B) = P(A|B) \cdot P(B) \tag{9.2}$$

9.1.1.1.3 *Conditional probability*

A *conditional probability* is the probability of one event occurring given the occurrence of another event. Conditional probabilities are written as: $P(A|B)$. This is read as the probability that event A occurs given that event B occurred. For instance, we can consider the following conditional probabilities:

$P(C|R)$ is the probability of a classification, C, given a response, R. In other words, $P(C|R)$ is the probability of having HIV given a positive test: $P(\text{HIV}|\text{positive test})$. $P(R|C)$ is the probability of a response, R, given a classification, C. In the example above, $P(R|C)$ is the probability of having a positive test given that a person has HIV: $P(\text{positive test}|\text{HIV}) = 95\%$.

A conditional probability can be calculated using the joint probability and marginal probability (base rate), as in Equation (9.3):

$$P(A|B) = \frac{P(A, B)}{P(B)} \tag{9.3}$$

9.1.1.2 Confusion of the Inverse

A conditional probability is not the same thing as its reverse (or inverse) conditional probability. Unless the base rate of the two events (C and R) are the same, $P(C|R) \neq P(R|C)$. However, people frequently make the mistake of thinking that two inverse conditional probabilities are the same. This mistake is known as the "confusion of the inverse", or the "inverse fallacy", or the "conditional probability fallacy". The confusion of inverse probabilities is the logical error of representative thinking that leads people to assume that the probability of C given R is the same as the probability of R given C, even though this is not true. As a few examples to demonstrate the logical fallacy, if 93% of breast cancers occur in high-risk women, this does not mean that 93% of high-risk women will eventually get breast cancer. As another example, if 77% of car accidents take place within 15 miles of a driver's home, this does not mean that you will get in an accident 77% of times you drive within 15 miles of your home.

Which car is the most frequently stolen? It is often the Honda Accord or Honda Civic—probably because they are among the most popular/commonly available cars. The probability that the car is a Honda Accord given that a car was stolen (p(Honda Accord | Stolen)) is what the media reports and what the police care about. However, that is not what buyers and car insurance companies should care about. Instead, they care about the probability that the car will be stolen given that it is a Honda Accord (p(Stolen | Honda Accord)).

9.1.1.3 Bayes' Theorem

An alternative way of calculating a conditional probability is using the inverse conditional probability (instead of the joint probability). This is known as Bayes' theorem. Bayes' theorem can help us calculate a conditional probability of some classification, C, given some response, R, if we know the inverse conditional probability and the base rate (marginal probability) of each. Bayes' theorem is in Equation (9.4):

$$P(C|R) = \frac{P(R|C) \cdot P(C_i)}{P(R_i)} \tag{9.4}$$

Or, equivalently (rearranging the terms):

$$\frac{P(C|R)}{P(R|C)} = \frac{P(C_i)}{P(R_i)} \tag{9.5}$$

Or, equivalently (rearranging the terms):

$$\frac{P(C|R)}{P(C_i)} = \frac{P(R|C)}{P(R_i)} \tag{9.6}$$

More generally, Bayes' theorem has been described as:

$$\begin{aligned} P(H|E) &= \frac{P(E|H) \cdot P(H)}{P(E)} \\ \text{posterior probability} &= \frac{\text{likelihood} \times \text{prior probability}}{\text{model evidence}} \end{aligned} \tag{9.7}$$

where H is the hypothesis, and E is the evidence—the new information that was not used in computing the prior probability.

In Bayesian terms, the *posterior probability* is the conditional probability of one event occurring given another event—it is the updated probability after the evidence is considered. In this case, the posterior probability is the probability of the classification occurring (C) given the response (R). The *likelihood* is the inverse conditional probability—the probability of the response (R) occurring given the classification (C). The *prior probability* is the marginal probability of the event (i.e., the classification) occurring, before we take into account any new information. The *model evidence* is the marginal probability of the other event occurring—i.e., the marginal probability of seeing the evidence.

In the HIV example above, we can calculate the conditional probability of HIV given a positive test using three terms: the conditional probability of a positive test given HIV (i.e., the sensitivity of the test), the base rate of HIV, and the base rate of a positive test for HIV. The conditional probability of HIV given a positive test is shown in Equation (9.8):

$$
\begin{aligned}
P(C|R) &= \frac{P(R|C) \cdot P(C_i)}{P(R_i)} \\
P(\text{HIV}|\text{positive test}) &= \frac{P(\text{positive test}|\text{HIV}) \cdot P(\text{HIV})}{P(\text{positive test})} \\
&= \frac{\text{sensitivity of test} \times \text{base rate of HIV}}{\text{base rate of positive test}} \\
&= \frac{95\% \times .3\%}{1\%} = \frac{.95 \times .003}{.01} \\
&= 28.5\%
\end{aligned} \tag{9.8}
$$

The `petersenlab` package (Petersen, 2024) contains the `pAgivenB()` function that estimates the probability of one event, A, given another event, B.

```
pAgivenB(pBgivenA = .95, pA = .003, pB = .01)
```

```
[1] 0.285
```

Thus, assuming the probabilities in the example above, the conditional probability of having HIV if a person has a positive test is 28.5%. Given a positive test, chances are higher than not that the person does not have HIV.

Bayes' theorem can be depicted visually (Ballesteros-Pérez et al., 2018). If we have 100,000 people in our population, we would be able to fill out a 2-by-2 confusion matrix, as depicted in Figure 9.1.

We know that .3% of the population contracts HIV, so 300 people in the population of 100,000 would contract HIV. Therefore, we put 300 in the marginal sum of those with HIV ($.003 \times 100,000 = 300$), i.e., the base rate of HIV. That means 99,700 people do not contract HIV ($100,000 - 300 = 99,700$). We know that 1% of the population tests positive for HIV, so we put 1,000 in the marginal sum of those who test positive $.01 \times 100,000 = 1,000$, i.e., the marginal probability of a positive test (the selection ratio). That means 99,000 people test negative for HIV ($100,000 - 1,000 = 99,000$). We also know that 95% of those who have HIV test positive for HIV. Three hundred people have HIV, so 95% of them (i.e., 285 people; $.95 \times 300 = 285$) tested positive for HIV (true positives). Because we know that 300 people

		Truth		Total Predicted	Selection Ratio
		HIV	No HIV		
Prediction	HIV	TP = 285 (.00285)	FP = 715 (.00715)	1,000	SR = .01
	No HIV	FN = 15 (.00015)	TN = 98,985 (.98985)	99,000	1 - SR = .99
Total Actual		300	99,700	*N* = 100,000	
Base Rate		BR = .003	1 - BR = .997		

FIGURE 9.1 Confusion Matrix: 2-by-2 Prediction Matrix. TP = true positives; TN = true negatives; FP = false positives; FN = false negatives; BR = base rate; SR = selection ratio.

have HIV and that 285 of those with HIV tested positive, that means that 15 people with HIV tested negative ($300 - 15 = 285$; false negatives). We know that 1,000 people tested positive for HIV, and 285 with HIV tested positive, so that means that 715 people without HIV tested positive ($1,000 - 285 = 715$; false positives). We know that 99,000 people tested negative for HIV, and 15 with HIV tested negative, so that means that 98,985 people without HIV tested negative ($99,000 - 15 = 98,985$; true negatives). So, to answer the question of what is the probability of having HIV if you have a positive test, we divide the number of people with HIV who had a positive test (285) by the total number of people who had a positive test (1000), which leads to a probability of 28.5%.

This can be depicted visually in Figures 9.2 and 9.3.[1]

Now let's see what happens if the person tests positive a second time. We would revise our "prior probability" for HIV from the general prevalence in the population (0.3%) to be the "posterior probability" of HIV given a first positive test (28.5%). This is known as *Bayesian updating*. We would also update the "evidence" to be the marginal probability of getting a second positive test.

If we do not know a marginal probability (i.e., base rate) of an event (e.g., getting a second positive test), we can calculate a marginal probability with the *law of total probability* using conditional probabilities and the marginal probability of another event (e.g., having HIV). According to the law of total probability, the probability of getting a positive test is the probability that a person with HIV gets a positive test (i.e., sensitivity) times the base rate of HIV plus the probability that a person without HIV gets a positive test (i.e., false positive rate) times the base rate of not having HIV, as in Equation (9.9):

$$
\begin{aligned}
P(\text{not } C_i) &= 1 - P(C_i) \\
P(R_i) &= P(R|C) \cdot P(C_i) + P(R|\text{not } C) \cdot P(\text{not } C_i) \\
1\% &= 95\% \times .3\% + P(R|\text{not } C) \times 99.7\%
\end{aligned}
\tag{9.9}
$$

In this case, we know the marginal probability ($P(R_i)$), and we can use that to solve for the unknown conditional probability that reflects the false positive rate ($P(R|\text{not } C)$), as in Equation (9.10):

[1] Please note that the areas in the figure are not drawn to scale; otherwise, some regions would be too small to include text.

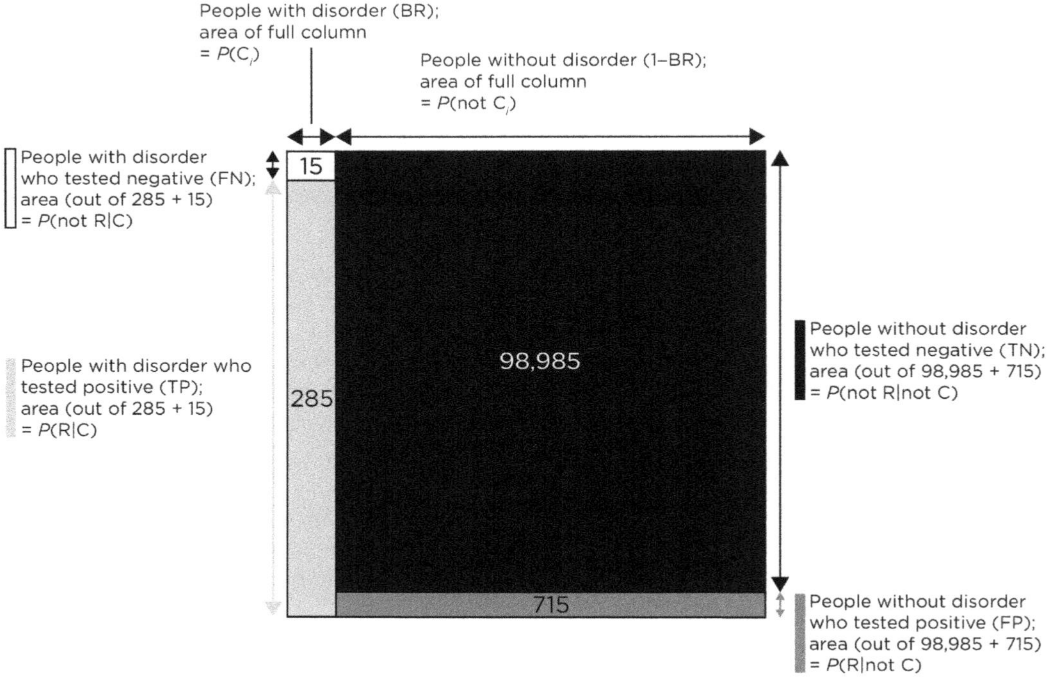

FIGURE 9.2 Bayes' Theorem (and Confusion Matrix) Depicted Visually, where the Marginal Probability is the Base Rate (BR). The four boxes represent the number of true positives (TP), true negatives (TN), false positives (FP), and false negatives (FN). Note: Boxes are not drawn to scale; otherwise, some regions would be too small to include text.

$$
\begin{aligned}
P(R_i) &= P(R|C) \cdot P(C_i) + P(R|\text{not } C) \cdot P(\text{not } C_i) \\
P(R_i) - [P(R|\text{not } C) \cdot P(\text{not } C_i)] &= P(R|C) \cdot P(C_i) && \text{Move } P(R|\text{not } C) \text{ to the left side} \\
-[P(R|\text{not } C) \cdot P(\text{not } C_i)] &= P(R|C) \cdot P(C_i) - P(R_i) && \text{Move } P(R_i) \text{ to the right side} \\
P(R|\text{not } C) \cdot P(\text{not } C_i) &= P(R_i) - [P(R|C) \cdot P(C_i)] && \text{Multiply by } -1 \\
P(R|\text{not } C) &= \frac{P(R_i) - [P(R|C) \cdot P(C_i)]}{P(\text{not } C_i)} && \text{Divide by } P(R|\text{not } C) \quad (9.10) \\
&= \frac{1\% - [95\% \times .3\%]}{99.7\%} = \frac{.01 - [.95 \times .003]}{.997} \\
&= .7171515\%
\end{aligned}
$$

The `petersenlab` package (Petersen, 2024) contains the `pBgivenNotA()` function that estimates the probability of one event, B, given that another event, A, did not occur.

```
pBgivenNotA(pBgivenA = .95, pA = .003, pB = .01)
```

```
[1] 0.007172
```

With this conditional probability ($P(R|\text{not } C)$), the updated marginal probability of having HIV ($P(C_i)$), and the updated marginal probability of not having HIV ($P(\text{not } C_i)$), we can now calculate an updated estimate of the marginal probability of getting a second positive test. The probability of getting a second positive test is the probability that a person with

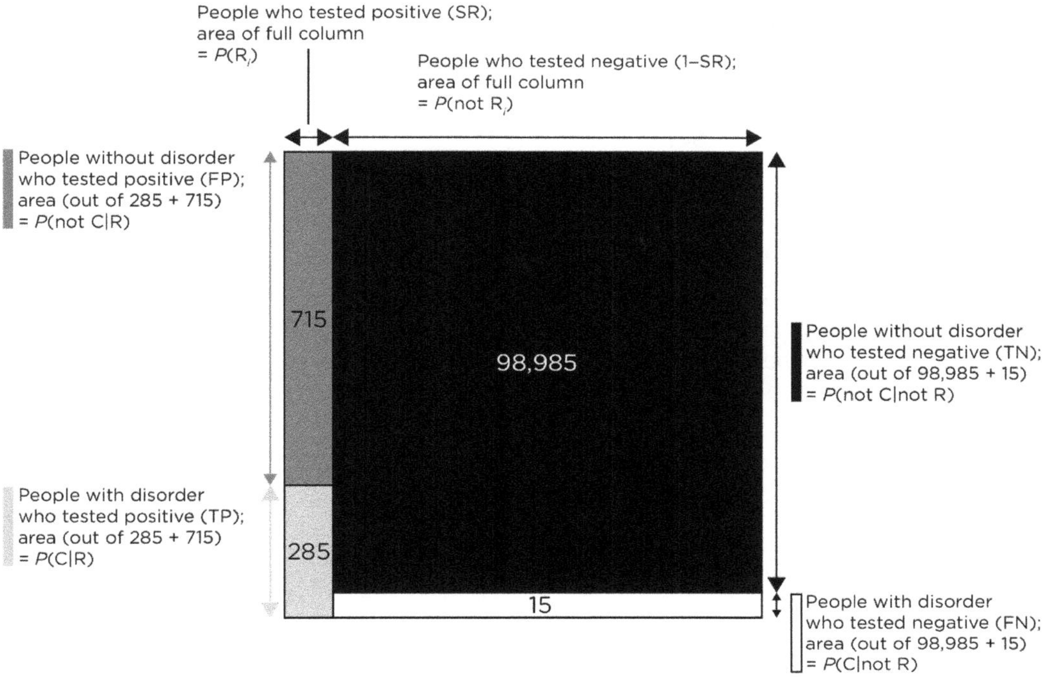

FIGURE 9.3 Bayes' Theorem (and Confusion Matrix) Depicted Visually, where the Marginal Probability is the Selection Ratio (SR). The four boxes represent the number of true positives (TP), true negatives (TN), false positives (FP), and false negatives (FN). Note: Boxes are not drawn to scale; otherwise, some regions would be too small to include text.

HIV gets a second positive test (i.e., sensitivity) times the updated probability of HIV plus the probability that a person without HIV gets a second positive test (i.e., false positive rate) times the updated probability of not having HIV, as in Equation (9.11):

$$\begin{aligned} P(R_i) &= P(R|C) \cdot P(C_i) + P(R|\text{not } C) \cdot P(\text{not } C_i) \\ &= 95\% \times 28.5\% + .7171515\% \times 71.5\% = .95 \times .285 + .007171515 \times .715 \\ &= 27.58776\% \end{aligned} \tag{9.11}$$

The `petersenlab` package (Petersen, 2024) contains the `pB()` function that estimates the marginal probability of one event, B.

```
pB(pBgivenA = .95, pA = .285, pBgivenNotA = .007171515)
```

```
[1] 0.2759
```

```
pB(
  pBgivenA = .95,
  pA = pAgivenB(
    pBgivenA = .95,
```

```
    pA = .003,
    pB = .01),
  pBgivenNotA = pBgivenNotA(
    pBgivenA = .95,
    pA = .003,
    pB = .01))
```

```
[1] 0.2759
```

We then substitute the updated marginal probability of HIV ($P(C_i)$) and the updated marginal probability of getting a second positive test ($P(R_i)$) into Bayes' theorem to get the probability that the person has HIV if they have a second positive test (assuming the errors of each test are independent, i.e., uncorrelated), as in Equation (9.12):

$$
\begin{aligned}
P(C|R) &= \frac{P(R|C) \cdot P(C_i)}{P(R_i)} \\
P(\text{HIV}|\text{a second positive test}) &= \frac{P(\text{a second positive test}|\text{HIV}) \cdot P(\text{HIV})}{P(\text{a second positive test})} \\
&= \frac{\text{sensitivity of test} \times \text{updated base rate of HIV}}{\text{updated base rate of positive test}} \\
&= \frac{95\% \times 28.5\%}{27.58776\%} \\
&= 98.14\%
\end{aligned}
\tag{9.12}
$$

```
pAgivenB(pBgivenA = .95, pA = .285, pB = .2758776)
```

```
[1] 0.9814
```

```
pAgivenB(
  pBgivenA = .95,
  pA = pAgivenB(
    pBgivenA = .95,
    pA = .003,
    pB = .01),
  pB = pB(
    pBgivenA = .95,
    pA = pAgivenB(
      pBgivenA = .95,
      pA = .003,
      pB = .01),
    pBgivenNotA = pBgivenNotA(
      pBgivenA = .95,
      pA = .003,
      pB = .01)))
```

```
[1] 0.9814
```

Thus, a second positive test greatly increases the posterior probability that the person has HIV from 28.5% to over 98%.

As seen in the rearranged formula in Equation (9.5), the ratio of the conditional probabilities is equal to the ratio of the base rates. Thus, it is important to consider base rates. People have a strong tendency to ignore (or give insufficient weight to) base rates when making predictions. The failure to consider the base rate when making predictions when given specific information about a case is a cognitive bias known as the base-rate fallacy or as base rate neglect. For example, people tend to say that the probability of a rare event is more likely than it actually is given specific information.

As seen in the rearranged formula in Equation (9.6), the inverse conditional probabilities ($P(C|R)$ and $P(R|C)$) are not equal unless the base rates of C and R are the same. If the base rates are not equal, we are making at least some prediction errors. If $P(C_i) > P(R_i)$, our predictions must include some false negatives. If $P(R_i) > P(C_i)$, our predictions must include some false positives.

Using the law of total probability, we can substitute the calculation of the marginal probability ($P(R_i)$) into Bayes' theorem to get an alternative formulation of Bayes' theorem, as in Equation (9.13):

$$\begin{aligned} P(C|R) &= \frac{P(R|C) \cdot P(C_i)}{P(R_i)} \\ &= \frac{P(R|C) \cdot P(C_i)}{P(R|C) \cdot P(C_i) + P(R|\text{not } C) \cdot P(\text{not } C_i)} \\ &= \frac{P(R|C) \cdot P(C_i)}{P(R|C) \cdot P(C_i) + P(R|\text{not } C) \cdot [1 - P(C_i)]} \end{aligned} \tag{9.13}$$

Instead of using marginal probability (base rate) of R, as in the original formulation of Bayes' theorem, it uses the conditional probability, $P(R|\text{not } C)$. Thus, it uses three terms: two conditional probabilities—$P(R|C)$ and $P(R|\text{not } C)$—and one marginal probability, $P(C_i)$. This alternative formulation of Bayes' theorem can be used to calculate positive predictive value, based on sensitivity, specificity, and the base rate, as presented in Equation (9.50).

Let us see how the alternative formulation of Bayes' theorem applies to the HIV example above. We can calculate the probability of HIV given a positive test using three terms: the conditional probability that a person with HIV gets a positive test (i.e., sensitivity), the conditional probability that a person without HIV gets a positive test (i.e., false positive rate), and the base rate of HIV. Using the $P(R|\text{not } C)$ calculated in Equation (9.10), the conditional probability of HIV given a single positive test is shown in Equation (9.14):

$$\begin{aligned} P(C|R) &= \frac{P(R|C) \cdot P(C_i)}{P(R|C) \cdot P(C_i) + P(R|\text{not } C) \cdot [1 - P(C_i)]} \\ &= \frac{\text{sensitivity of test} \times \text{base rate of HIV}}{\text{sensitivity of test} \times \text{base rate of HIV} + \text{false positive rate of test} \times (1 - \text{base rate of HIV})} \\ &= \frac{95\% \times .3\%}{95\% \times .3\% + .7171515\% \times (1 - .3\%)} = \frac{.95 \times .003}{.95 \times .003 + .007171515 \times (1 - .003)} \\ &= 28.5\% \end{aligned} \tag{9.14}$$

```
pAgivenB(pBgivenA = .95, pA = .003, pBgivenNotA = .007171515)
```

```
[1] 0.285
```

```
pAgivenB(
  pBgivenA = .95,
  pA = .003,
  pBgivenNotA = pBgivenNotA(
    pBgivenA = .95,
    pA = .003,
    pB = .01))
```

```
[1] 0.285
```

To calculate the conditional probability of HIV given a second positive test, we update our priors because the person has now tested positive for HIV. We update the prior probability of HIV ($P(C_i)$) based on the posterior probability of HIV after a positive test ($P(C|R)$) that we calculated above. We can calculate the conditional probability of HIV given a second positive test using three terms: the conditional probability that a person with HIV gets a positive test (i.e., sensitivity; which stays the same), the conditional probability that a person without HIV gets a positive test (i.e., false positive rate; which stays the same), and the updated marginal probability of HIV. The conditional probability of HIV given a second positive test is shown in Equation (9.15):

$$
\begin{aligned}
P(C|R) &= \frac{P(R|C) \cdot P(C_i)}{P(R|C) \cdot P(C_i) + P(R|\text{not } C) \cdot [1 - P(C_i)]} \\
&= \frac{\text{sensitivity of test} \times \text{updated base rate of HIV}}{\text{sensitivity of test} \times \text{updated base rate of HIV} + \text{false positive rate of test} \times (1 - \text{updated base rate of HIV})} \\
&= \frac{95\% \times 28.5\%}{95\% \times 28.5\% + .7171515\% \times (1 - 28.5\%)} = \frac{.95 \times .285}{.95 \times .285 + .007171515 \times (1 - .285)} \\
&= 98.14\%
\end{aligned}
\tag{9.15}
$$

```
pAgivenB(
  pBgivenA = .95,
  pA = .285,
  pBgivenNotA = .007171515)
```

```
[1] 0.9814
```

```
pAgivenB(
  pBgivenA = .95,
  pA = .285,
  pBgivenNotA = pBgivenNotA(
    pBgivenA = .95,
    pA = .003,
    pB = .01))
```

```
[1] 0.9814
```

If we want to compare the relative probability of two outcomes, we can use the odds form of Bayes' theorem, as in Equation (9.16):

$$\begin{aligned}
P(C|R) &= \frac{P(R|C) \cdot P(C_i)}{P(R_i)} \\
P(\text{not } C|R) &= \frac{P(R|\text{not } C) \cdot P(\text{not } C_i)}{P(R_i)} \\
\frac{P(C|R)}{P(\text{not } C|R)} &= \frac{\frac{P(R|C) \cdot P(C_i)}{P(R_i)}}{\frac{P(R|\text{not } C) \cdot P(\text{not } C_i)}{P(R_i)}} \\
&= \frac{P(R|C) \cdot P(C_i)}{P(R|\text{not } C) \cdot P(\text{not } C_i)} \\
&= \frac{P(C_i)}{P(\text{not } C_i)} \times \frac{P(R|C)}{P(R|\text{not } C)} \\
\text{posterior odds} &= \text{prior odds} \times \text{likelihood ratio}
\end{aligned} \tag{9.16}$$

In sum, the marginal probability, including the prior probability or base rate, should be weighed heavily in predictions unless there are sufficient data to indicate otherwise, i.e., to update the posterior probability based on new evidence. Bayes' theorem provides a powerful tool to anchor predictions to the base rate unless sufficient evidence changes the posterior probability (by updating the evidence and prior probability).

9.1.2 Prediction Accuracy

9.1.2.1 Decision Outcomes

To consider how we can evaluate the accuracy of predictions, consider an example adapted from Meehl & Rosen (1955). The military conducts a test of its prospective members to screen out applicants who would likely fail basic training. To evaluate the accuracy of our predictions using the test, we can examine a confusion matrix. A confusion matrix is a matrix that presents the predicted outcome on one dimension and the actual outcome (truth) on the other dimension. If the predictions and outcomes are dichotomous, the confusion matrix is a 2-by-2 matrix with two rows and two columns that represent four possible predicted-actual combinations (decision outcomes): true positives (TP), true negatives (TN), false positives (FP), and false negatives (FN).

When discussing the four decision outcomes, "true" means an accurate judgment, whereas "false" means an inaccurate judgment. "Positive" means that the judgment was that the person has the characteristic of interest, whereas "negative" means that the judgment was that the person does not have the characteristic of interest. A *true positive* is a correct judgment (or prediction) where the judgment was that the person has (or will have) the characteristic of interest, and, in truth, they actually have (or will have) the characteristic. A *true negative* is a correct judgment (or prediction) where the judgment was that the person does not have (or will not have) the characteristic of interest, and, in truth, they actually do not have (or will not have) the characteristic. A *false positive* is an incorrect judgment (or prediction) where the judgment was that the person has (or will have) the characteristic of interest, and, in truth, they actually do not have (or will not have) the characteristic. A *false negative* is an incorrect judgment (or prediction) where the judgment was that the person does not have (or will not have) the characteristic of interest, and, in truth, they actually do have (or will have) the characteristic.

An example of a confusion matrix is shown in Figure 9.4.

		Actual Adjustment	
		Poor	Good
Decision (Prediction)	Reject	TP = 86	FP = 422
	Retain	FN = 14	TN = 1,478

FIGURE 9.4 Confusion Matrix: 2-by-2 Prediction Matrix. TP = true positives; TN = true negatives; FP = false positives; FN = false negatives.

With the information in the confusion matrix, we can calculate the marginal sums and the proportion of people in each cell (in parentheses), as depicted in Figure 9.5.

		Actual Adjustment		Total Predicted
		Poor	Good	
Decision (Prediction)	Reject	TP = 86 (.043)	FP = 422 (.211)	508
	Retain	FN = 14 (.007)	TN = 1,478 (.739)	1,492
Total Actual		100	1,900	*N* = 2,000

FIGURE 9.5 Confusion Matrix: 2-by-2 Prediction Matrix with Marginal Sums. TP = true positives; TN = true negatives; FP = false positives; FN = false negatives.

That is, we can sum across the rows and columns to identify how many people actually showed poor adjustment ($n = 100$) versus good adjustment ($n = 1,900$), and how many people were selected to reject ($n = 508$) versus retain ($n = 1,492$). If we sum the column of predicted marginal sums ($508 + 1,492$) or the row of actual marginal sums ($100 + 1,900$), we get the total number of people ($N = 2,000$).

Based on the marginal sums, we can compute the marginal probabilities, as depicted in Figure 9.6.

		Actual Adjustment		Total Predicted	Selection Ratio
		Poor	Good		
Decision (Prediction)	Reject	TP = 86 (.043)	FP = 422 (.211)	508	SR = 0.254
	Retain	FN = 14 (.007)	TN = 1,478 (.739)	1,492	1 - SR = 0.746
Total Actual		100	1,900	*N* = 2,000	
Base Rate		BR = 0.05	1 - BR = 0.95		

FIGURE 9.6 Confusion Matrix: 2-by-2 Prediction Matrix with Marginal Sums and Marginal Probabilities. TP = true positives; TN = true negatives; FP = false positives; FN = false negatives; BR = base rate; SR = selection ratio.

The marginal probability of the person having the characteristic of interest (i.e., showing poor adjustment) is called the *base rate* (BR). That is, the base rate is the proportion of people who have the characteristic. It is calculated by dividing the number of people with poor adjustment ($n = 100$) by the total number of people ($N = 2,000$): $BR = \frac{FN+TP}{N}$. Here, the base rate reflects the prevalence of poor adjustment. In this case, the base rate is .05, so there is a 5% chance that an applicant will be poorly adjusted. The marginal probability of good adjustment is equal to 1 minus the base rate of poor adjustment.

The marginal probability of predicting that a person has the characteristic (i.e., rejecting a person) is called the *selection ratio* (SR). The selection ratio is the proportion of people who will be selected (in this case, rejected rather than retained); i.e., the proportion of people who are identified as having the characteristic. The selection ratio is calculated by dividing the number of people selected to reject ($n = 508$) by the total number of people ($N = 2,000$): $SR = \frac{TP+FP}{N}$. In this case, the selection ratio is .25, so 25% of people are rejected. The marginal probability of not selecting someone to reject (i.e., the marginal probability of retaining) is equal to 1 minus the selection ratio.

The selection ratio might be something that the test dictates according to its cutoff score. Or, the selection ratio might be imposed by external factors that place limits on how many people you can assign a positive test value. For instance, when deciding whether to treat a client, the selection ratio may depend on how many therapists are available and how many cases can be treated.

9.1.2.2 Percent Accuracy

Based on the confusion matrix, we can calculate the prediction accuracy based on the percent accuracy of the predictions. The percent accuracy is the number of correct predictions divided by the total number of predictions, and multiplied by 100. In the context of a confusion matrix, this is calculated as: $100\% \times \frac{\text{TP}+\text{TN}}{N}$. In this case, our percent accuracy was 78%—that is, 78% of our predictions were accurate, and 22% of our predictions were inaccurate.

9.1.2.3 Percent Accuracy by Chance

Seventy-eight percent sounds pretty accurate. And it is much higher than 50%, so we are doing a pretty good job, right? Well, it is important to compare our accuracy to what accuracy we would expect to get by chance alone, if predictions were made by a random process rather than using a test's scores. Our selection ratio was 25.4%. How accurate would we be if we randomly selected 25.4% of people to reject? To determine what accuracy we could get by chance alone given the selection ratio and the base rate, we can calculate the chance probability of true positives and the chance probability of true negatives. The probability of a given cell in the confusion matrix is a joint probability—the probability of two events occurring simultaneously. To calculate a joint probability, we multiply the probability of each event.

So, to get the chance expectancies of true positives, we would multiply the respective marginal probabilities, as in Equation (9.17):

$$\begin{aligned} P(TP) &= P(\text{Poor adjustment}) \times P(\text{Reject}) \\ &= BR \times SR \\ &= .05 \times .254 \\ &= .0127 \end{aligned} \tag{9.17}$$

To get the chance expectancies of true negatives, we would multiply the respective marginal probabilities, as in Equation (9.18):

$$\begin{aligned} P(TN) &= P(\text{Good adjustment}) \times P(\text{Retain}) \\ &= (1 - BR) \times (1 - SR) \\ &= .95 \times .746 \\ &= .7087 \end{aligned} \tag{9.18}$$

To get the percent accuracy by chance, we sum the chance expectancies for the correct predictions (TP and TN): $.0127 + .7087 = .7214$. Thus, the percent accuracy you can get by chance alone is 72%. This is because most of our predictions are to retain people, and the base rate of poor adjustment is quite low (.05). Our measure with 78% accuracy provides only a 6% increment in correct predictions. Thus, you cannot judge how good your judgment or prediction is until you know how you would do by random chance.

The chance expectancies for each cell of the confusion matrix are shown in Figure 9.7.

		Actual Adjustment		Selection Ratio
		Poor	Good	
Decision (Prediction)	Reject	.0127	.2413	SR = 0.254
	Retain	.0373	.7087	1 - SR = 0.746
Base Rate		BR = 0.05	1 - BR = 0.95	

FIGURE 9.7 Chance Expectancies in 2-by-2 Prediction Matrix. TP = true positives; TN = true negatives; FP = false positives; FN = false negatives; BR = base rate; SR = selection ratio.

9.1.2.4 Predicting from the Base Rate

Now, let us consider how well you would do if you were to predict from the base rate. Predicting from the base rate is also called "betting from the base rate", and it involves setting the selection ratio by taking advantage of the base rate so that you go with the most likely outcome in every prediction. Because the base rate is quite low (.05), we could predict from the base rate by selecting no one to reject (i.e., setting the selection ratio at zero). Our percent accuracy by chance if we predict from the base rate would be calculated by multiplying the marginal probabilities, as we did above, but with a new selection ratio, as in Equation (9.19):

$$\begin{aligned} P(TP) &= P(\text{Poor adjustment}) \times P(\text{Reject}) \\ &= BR \times SR \\ &= .05 \times 0 \\ &= 0 \\[2ex] P(TN) &= P(\text{Good adjustment}) \times P(\text{Retain}) \\ &= (1 - BR) \times (1 - SR) \\ &= .95 \times 1 \\ &= .95 \end{aligned} \tag{9.19}$$

We sum the chance expectancies for the correct predictions (TP and TN): $0 + .95 = .95$. Thus, our percent accuracy by predicting from the base rate is 95%. This is damning to our measure because it is a much higher accuracy than the accuracy of our measure. That is, we can be much more accurate than our measure simply by predicting from the base rate and selecting no one to reject.

Going with the most likely outcome in every prediction (predicting from the base rate) can be highly accurate (in terms of percent accuracy) as noted by Meehl & Rosen (1955), especially when the base rate is very low or very high. This should serve as an important reminder that we need to compare the accuracy of our measures to the accuracy by (1) random chance and (2) predicting from the base rate. There are several important implications of the impact of base rates on prediction accuracy. One implication is that using the same test in different settings with different base rates will markedly change the accuracy of the test. Oftentimes, using a test will actually *decrease* the predictive accuracy when the base rate deviates greatly from .50. But percent accuracy is not everything. Percent accuracy treats different kinds of errors as if they are equally important. However, the value we place on different kinds of errors may be different, as described next.

9.1.2.5 Different Kinds of Errors Have Different Costs

Some errors have a high cost, and some errors have a low cost. Among the four decision outcomes, there are two types of errors: false positives and false negatives. The extent to which false positives and false negatives are costly depends on the prediction problem. So, even though you can often be most accurate by going with the base rate, it may be advantageous to use a screening instrument despite lower overall accuracy because of the huge difference in costs of false positives versus false negatives in some cases.

Consider the example of a screening instrument for HIV. False positives would be cases where we said that someone is at high risk of HIV when they are not, whereas false negatives are cases where we said that someone is not at high risk when they actually are. The costs of false positives include a shortage of blood, some follow-up testing, and potentially some anxiety, but that is about it. The costs of false negatives may be people getting HIV. In this case, the costs of false negatives greatly outweigh the costs of false positives, so we use a screening instrument to try to identify the cases at high risk for HIV because of the important consequences of failing to do so, even though using the screening instrument will lower our overall accuracy level.

Another example is when the Central Intelligence Agency (CIA) used a screen for protective typists during wartime to try to detect spies. False positives would be cases where the CIA believes that a person is a spy when they are not, and the CIA does not hire them. False negatives would be cases where the CIA believes that a person is not a spy when they actually are, and the CIA hires them. In this case, a false positive would be fine, but a false negative would be really bad.

How you weigh the costs of different errors depends considerably on the domain and context. Possible costs of false positives to society include: unnecessary and costly treatment with side effects and sending an innocent person to jail (despite our presumption of innocence in the United States criminal justice system that a person is innocent until proven guilty). Possible costs of false negatives to society include: setting a guilty person free, failing to detect a bomb or tumor, and preventing someone from getting treatment who needs it.

The differential costs of different errors also depend on how much flexibility you have in the selection ratio in being able to set a stringent versus loose selection ratio. Consider if there is a high cost of getting rid of people during the selection process. For example, if you must hire 100 people and only 100 people apply for the position, you cannot lose people, so you need to hire even high-risk people. However, if you do not need to hire many people, then you can hire more conservatively.

Any time the selection ratio differs from the base rate, you will make errors. For example, if you reject 25% of applicants, and the base rate of poor adjustment is 5%, then you are making errors of over-rejecting (false positives). By contrast, if you reject 1% of applicants and the base rate of poor adjustment is 5%, then you are making errors of under-rejecting or over-accepting (false negatives).

A low base rate makes it harder to make predictions, and tends to lead to less accurate predictions. For instance, it is very challenging to predict low base rate behaviors, including suicide (Kessler et al., 2020). The difficulty in predicting events with a low base rate is apparent with the true score formula from classical test theory: $X = T + e$. As described in Equation (3.10), reliability is the ratio of true score variance to observed score variance. As true score variance increases, reliability increases. If the base rate is .05, the maximum variance of the true scores is .05. The lower true score variance makes the measure less reliable and hard to make accurate predictions.

9.1.2.6 Sensitivity, Specificity, PPV, and NPV

As described earlier, percent accuracy is not the only important aspect of accuracy. Percent accuracy can be misleading because it is highly influenced by base rates. You can have a high percent accuracy by predicting from the base rate and saying that no one has the condition (if the base rate is low) or that everyone has the condition (if the base rate is high). Thus, it is also important to consider other aspects of accuracy, including sensitivity (SN), specificity (SP), positive predictive value (PPV), and negative predictive value (NPV). We want our predictions to be sensitive to be able to detect the characteristic but also to be specific so that we classify only people actually with the characteristic as having the characteristic.

Let us return to the confusion matrix in Figure 9.8. If we know the frequency of each of the four predicted-actual combinations of the confusion matrix (TP, TN, FP, FN), we can calculate sensitivity, specificity, PPV, and NPV.

		Actual Adjustment		Total Predicted
		Poor	Good	
Decision (Prediction)	Reject	TP = 86	FP = 422	508
	Retain	FN = 14	TN = 1,478	1,492
Total Actual		100	1,900	*N* = 2,000

FIGURE 9.8 Confusion Matrix: 2-by-2 Prediction Matrix. TP = true positives; TN = true negatives; FP = false positives; FN = false negatives.

Sensitivity is the proportion of those with the characteristic (TP+FN) that we identified with our measure (TP): $\frac{\text{TP}}{\text{TP+FN}} = \frac{86}{86+14} = .86$. Specificity is the proportion of those who do not have the characteristic (TN + FP) that we correctly classify as not having the characteristic (TN): $\frac{\text{TN}}{\text{TN+FP}} = \frac{1{,}478}{1{,}478+422} = .78$. PPV is the proportion of those who we classify as having the characteristic (TP + FP) who actually have the characteristic (TP): $\frac{\text{TP}}{\text{TP+FP}} = \frac{86}{86+422} = .17$. NPV is the proportion of those we classify as not having the characteristic (TN + FN) who actually do not have the characteristic (TN): $\frac{\text{TN}}{\text{TN+FN}} = \frac{1{,}478}{1{,}478+14} = .99$.

Sensitivity, specificity, PPV, and NPV are proportions, and their values therefore range from 0 to 1, where higher values reflect greater accuracy. With sensitivity, specificity, PPV, and NPV, we have a good snapshot of how accurate the measure is at a given cutoff. In our case, our measure is good at finding whom to reject (high sensitivity), but it is rejecting too many people who do not need to be rejected (lower PPV due to many FPs). Most people whom we classify as having the characteristic do not actually have the characteristic. However, the fact that we are over-rejecting could be okay depending on our goals, for instance, if we do not care about over-dropping (i.e., the PPV being low).

9.1.2.6.1 Some accuracy estimates depend on the cutoff

Sensitivity, specificity, PPV, and NPV differ based on the cutoff (i.e., threshold) for classification. Consider the following example. Aliens visit Earth, and they develop a test to determine whether a berry is edible or inedible.

Figure 9.9 depicts the distributions of scores by berry type. Note how there are clearly two distinct distributions. However, the distributions overlap to some degree. Thus, any cutoff will have at least some inaccurate classifications. The extent of overlap of the distributions reflects the amount of measurement error of the measure with respect to the characteristic of interest.

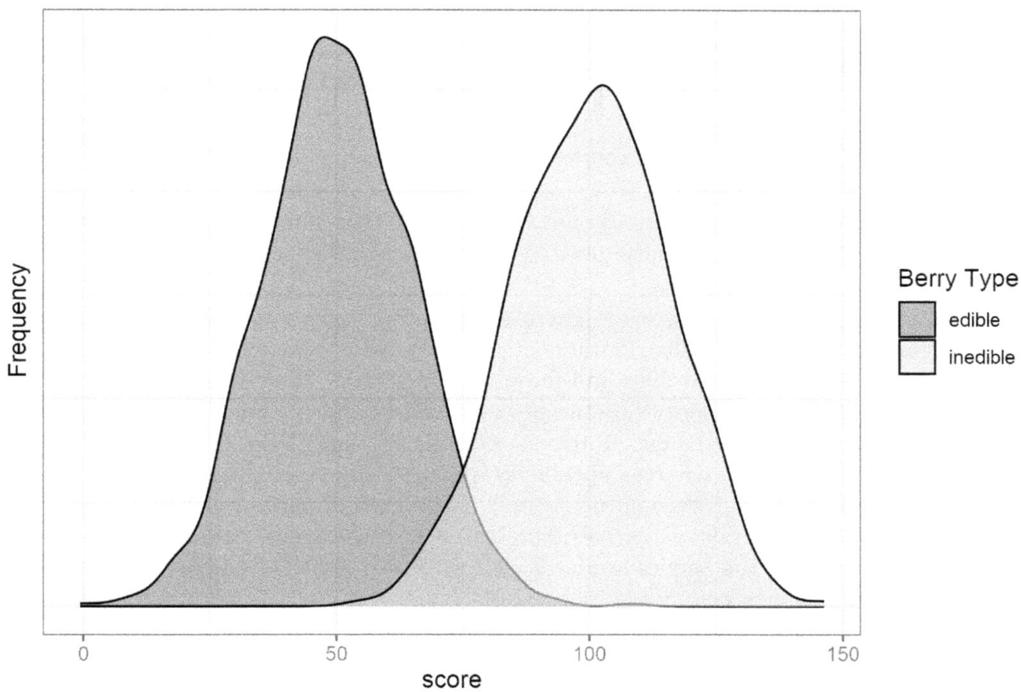

FIGURE 9.9 Distribution of Test Scores by Berry Type.

Figure 9.10 depicts the distributions of scores by berry type with a cutoff. The black line indicates the cutoff—the level above which berries are classified by the test as inedible. There are errors on each side of the cutoff. Below the cutoff, there are some false negatives: inedible berries that are inaccurately classified as edible. Above the cutoff, there are some false positives: edible berries that are inaccurately classified as inedible. Costs of false negatives could include sickness or death from eating the inedible berries. Costs of false positives could include taking longer to find food, finding insufficient food, and starvation.

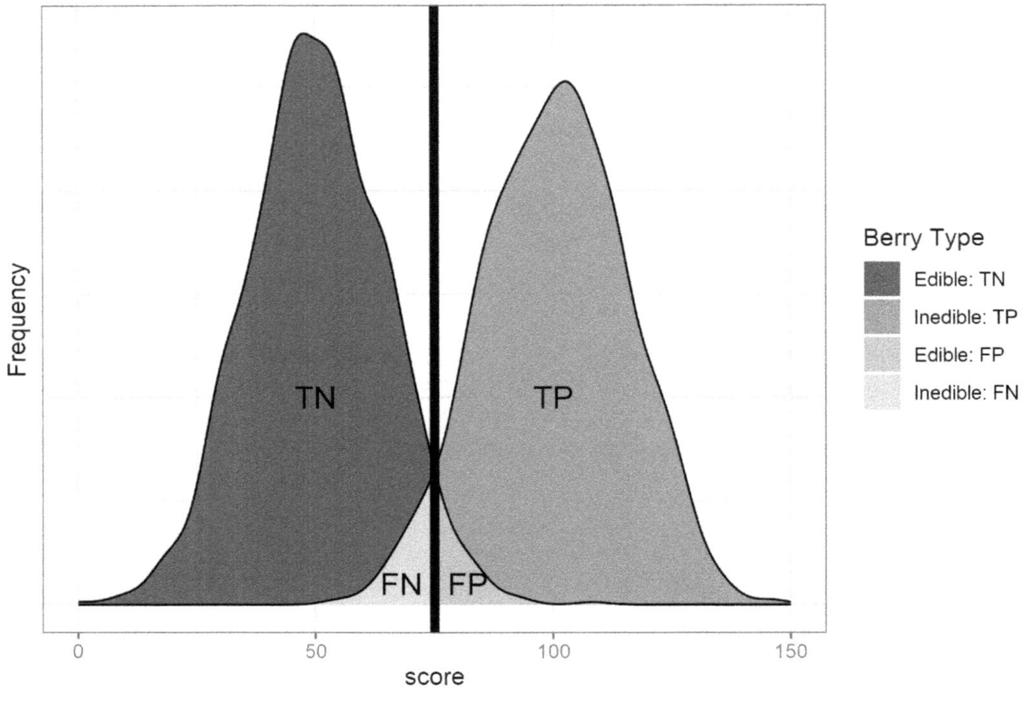

FIGURE 9.10 Classifications Based on a Cutoff. Note that some true negatives and true positives are hidden behind the false positives and false negatives.

Based on our assessment goals, we might use a different selection ratio by changing the cutoff. Figure 9.11 depicts the distributions of scores by berry type when we raise the cutoff. There are now more false negatives and fewer false positives. If we raise the cutoff (to be more conservative), the number of false negatives increases and the number of false positives decreases. Consequently, as the cutoff increases, sensitivity and NPV decrease (because we have more false negatives), whereas specificity and PPV increase (because we have fewer false positives). A higher cutoff could be optimal if the costs of false positives are considered greater than the costs of false negatives. For instance, if the aliens cannot risk eating the inedible berries because the berries are fatal, and there are sufficient edible berries that can be found to feed the alien colony.

Figure 9.12 depicts the distributions of scores by berry type when we lower the cutoff. There are now fewer false negatives and more false positives. If we lower the cutoff (to be more liberal), the number of false negatives decreases and the number of false positives increases. Consequently, as the cutoff decreases, sensitivity and NPV increase (because we have fewer false negatives), whereas specificity and PPV decrease (because we have more false positives). A lower cutoff could be optimal if the costs of false negatives are considered greater than the costs of false positives. For instance, if the aliens cannot risk missing edible berries because they are in short supply relative to the size of the alien colony, and eating the inedible berries would, at worst, lead to minor, temporary discomfort.

In sum, sensitivity and specificity differ based on the cutoff for classification. if we raise the cutoff, sensitivity and PPV increase (due to fewer false positives), whereas and sensitivity and NPV decrease (due to more false negatives). If we lower the cutoff, sensitivity and NPV increase (due to fewer false negatives), whereas specificity and PPV decrease (due to more

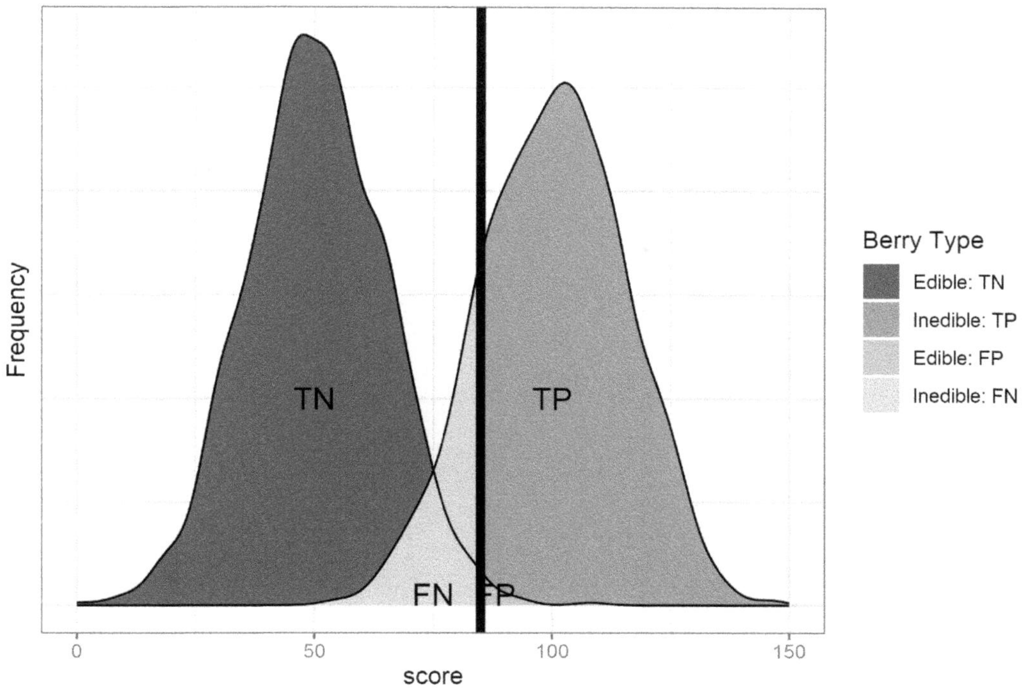

FIGURE 9.11 Classifications Based on Raising the Cutoff. Note that some true negatives and true positives are hidden behind the false positives and false negatives.

false positives). Thus, the optimal cutoff depends on how costly each type of error is: false negatives and false positives. If false negatives are more costly than false positives, we would set a low cutoff. If false positives are more costly than false negatives, we would set a high cutoff.

9.1.2.7 Signal Detection Theory

Signal detection theory (SDT) is a probability-based theory for the detection of a given stimulus (signal) from a stimulus set that includes non-target stimuli (noise). SDT arose through the development of radar (**RA**dio **D**etection **A**nd **R**anging) and sonar (**SO**und **N**avigation **A**nd **R**anging) in World War II based on research on sensory-perception research. The military wanted to determine which objects on radar/sonar were enemy aircraft/submarines, and which were noise (e.g., different object in the environment or even just the weather itself). SDT allowed determining how many errors operators made (how accurate they were) and decomposing errors into different kinds of errors. SDT distinguishes between sensitivity and bias. In SDT, *sensitivity* (or discriminability) is how well an assessment distinguishes between a target stimulus and non-target stimuli (i.e., how well the assessment detects the target stimulus amid non-target stimuli). *Bias* is the extent to which the probability of a selection decision from the assessment is higher or lower than the true rate of the target stimulus.

Some radar/sonar operators were not as sensitive to the differences between signal and noise, due to factors such as age, ability to distinguish gradations of a signal, etc. People who showed low sensitivity (i.e., who were not as successful at distinguishing between signal

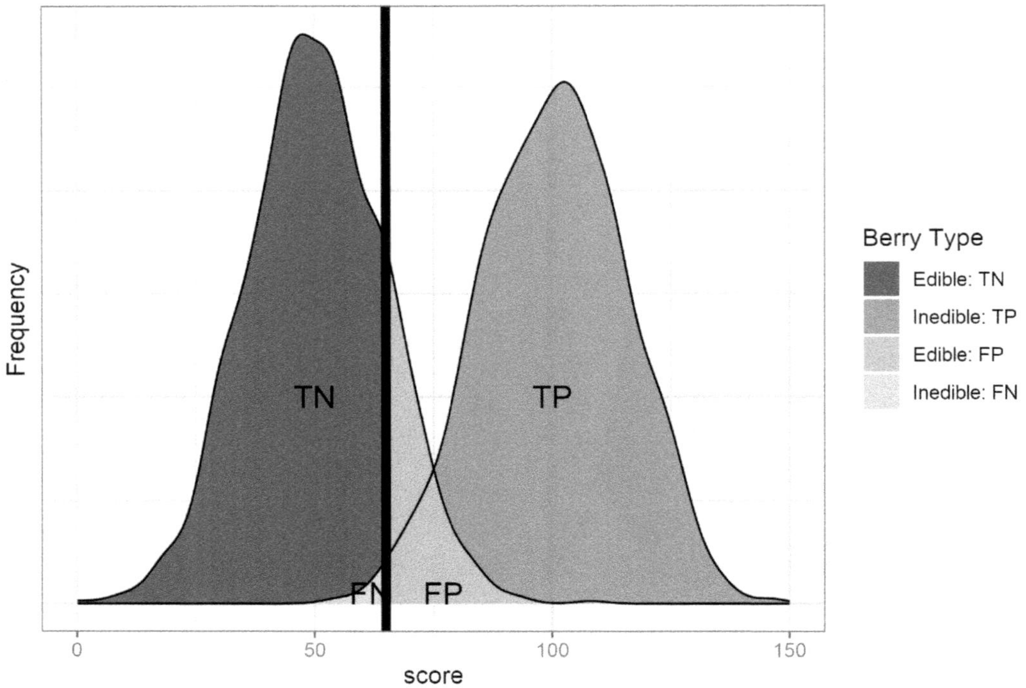

FIGURE 9.12 Classifications Based on Lowering the Cutoff. Note that some true negatives and true positives are hidden behind the false positives and false negatives.

and noise) were screened out because the military perceived sensitivity as a skill that was not easily taught. By contrast, other operators could distinguish signal from noise, but their threshold was too low or high—they could take in information, but their decisions tended to be wrong due to systematic bias or poor calibration. That is, they systematically over-rejected or under-rejected stimuli. Over-rejecting leads to many false negatives (i.e., saying that a stimulus is safe when it is not). Under-rejecting leads to many false positives (i.e., saying that a stimulus is harmful when it is not). A person who showed good sensitivity but systematic bias was considered more teach-able than a person who showed low sensitivity. Thus, radar and sonar operators were selected based on their sensitivity to distinguish signal from noise, and then were trained to improve the calibration so they reduce their systematic bias and do not systematically over- or under-reject.

Although SDT was originally developed for use in World War II, it now plays an important role in many areas of science and medicine. A medical application of SDT is tumor detection in radiology. SDT also plays an important role in psychology, especially cognitive psychology. For instance, research on social perception of sexual interest has shown that men tend to show lack of sensitivity to differences in women's affect—i.e., they have relative difficulties discriminating between friendliness and sexual interest (Farris et al., 2008). Men also tend to show systematic bias (poor calibration) such that they tend to overestimate women's sexual interest in them—i.e., men tend to have too low of a threshold for determining that a women is showing sexual interest in them (Farris et al., 2006).

SDT metrics of sensitivity include d' ("d-prime"), A (or A'), and the area under the receiver operating characteristic (ROC) curve. SDT metrics of bias include β (beta), c, and b.

9.1.2.7.1 Receiver operating characteristic curve

The x-axis of the receiver operating characteristic (ROC) curve is the false alarm rate or false positive rate (1− specificity). The y-axis is the hit rate or true positive rate (sensitivity). We can trace the ROC curve as the combination between sensitivity and specificity at every possible cutoff. At a cutoff of zero (top right of ROC curve), we calculate sensitivity (1.0) and specificity (0) and plot it. At a cutoff of zero, the assessment tells us to make an action for every stimulus (i.e., it is the most liberal). We then gradually increase the cutoff, and plot sensitivity and specificity at each cutoff. As the cutoff increases, sensitivity decreases and specificity increases. We end at the highest possible cutoff, where the sensitivity is 0 and the specificity is 1.0 (i.e., we never make an action; i.e., it is the most conservative). Each point on the ROC curve corresponds to a pair of hit and false alarm rates (sensitivity and specificity) resulting from a specific cutoff value. Then, we can draw lines or a curve to connect the points.

Figure 9.13 depicts an empirical ROC plot where lines are drawn to connect the hit and false alarm rates.

Figure 9.14 depicts an ROC curve where a smoothed and fitted curve is drawn to connect the hit and false alarm rates.

9.1.2.7.1.1 Area under the ROC curve

ROC methods can be used to compare and compute the discriminative power of measurement devices free from the influence of selection ratios, base rates, and costs and benefits. An ROC analysis yields a quantitative index of how well an index predicts a signal of interest or can discriminate between different signals. ROC analysis can help tell us how often our assessment would be correct. If we randomly pick two observations, and we were right once and wrong once, we were 50% accurate. But this would be a useless measure because it reflects chance responding.

The geometrical area under the ROC curve reflects the discriminative accuracy of the measure. The index is called the **a**rea **u**nder the **c**urve (AUC) of an ROC curve. AUC quantifies the discriminative power of an assessment. AUC is the probability that a randomly selected target and a randomly selected non-target is ranked correctly by the assessment method. AUC values range from 0.0 to 1.0, where chance accuracy is 0.5 as indicated by diagonal line in the ROC curve. That is, a measure can be useful to the extent that its ROC curve is above the diagonal line (i.e., its discriminative accuracy is above chance).

As an example, given an AUC of .75, this says that the overall score of an individual who has the characteristic in question will be higher 75% of the time than the overall score of an individual who does not have the characteristic. In lay terms, AUC provides the probability that we will classify correctly based on our instrument if we were to randomly pick one good and one bad outcome. AUC is a stronger index of accuracy than percent accuracy, because you can have high percent accuracy just by going with the base rate. AUC tells us how much better than chance a measure is at discriminating outcomes. AUC is useful as a measure of general discriminative accuracy, and it tells us how accurate a measure is at all possible cutoffs. Knowing the accuracy of a measure at all possible cutoffs can be helpful for selecting the optimal cutoff, given the goals of the assessment. In reality, however, we may not be interested in all cutoffs because not all errors are equal in their costs.

If we lower the base rate, we would need a larger sample to get enough people to classify into each group. SDT/ROC methods are traditionally about dichotomous decisions (yes/no),

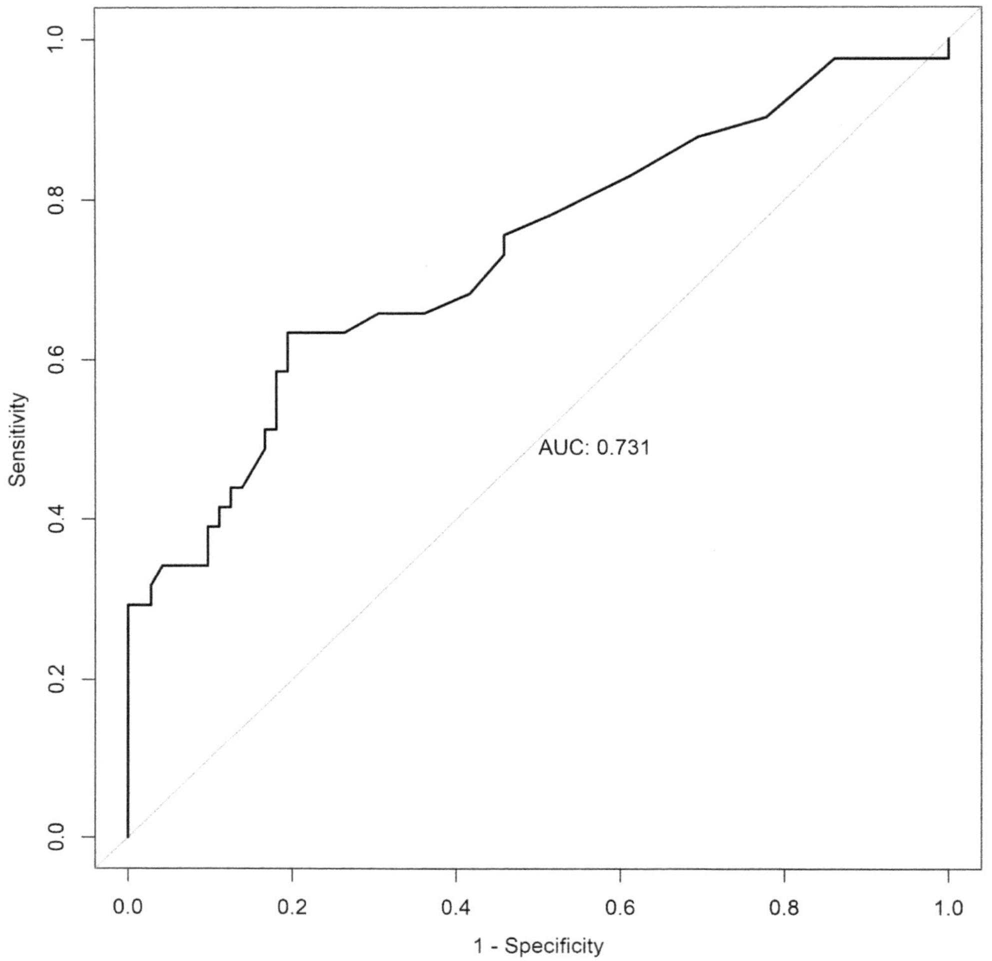

FIGURE 9.13 Empirical Receiver Operating Characteristic Curve. AUC = Area under the receiver operating characteristic curve.

not graded judgments. SDT/ROC methods can get messy with ordinal data that are more graded because you would have an AUC curve for each ordinal grouping.

9.2 Getting Started

9.2.1 Load Libraries

```
library("petersenlab")
library("pROC")
```

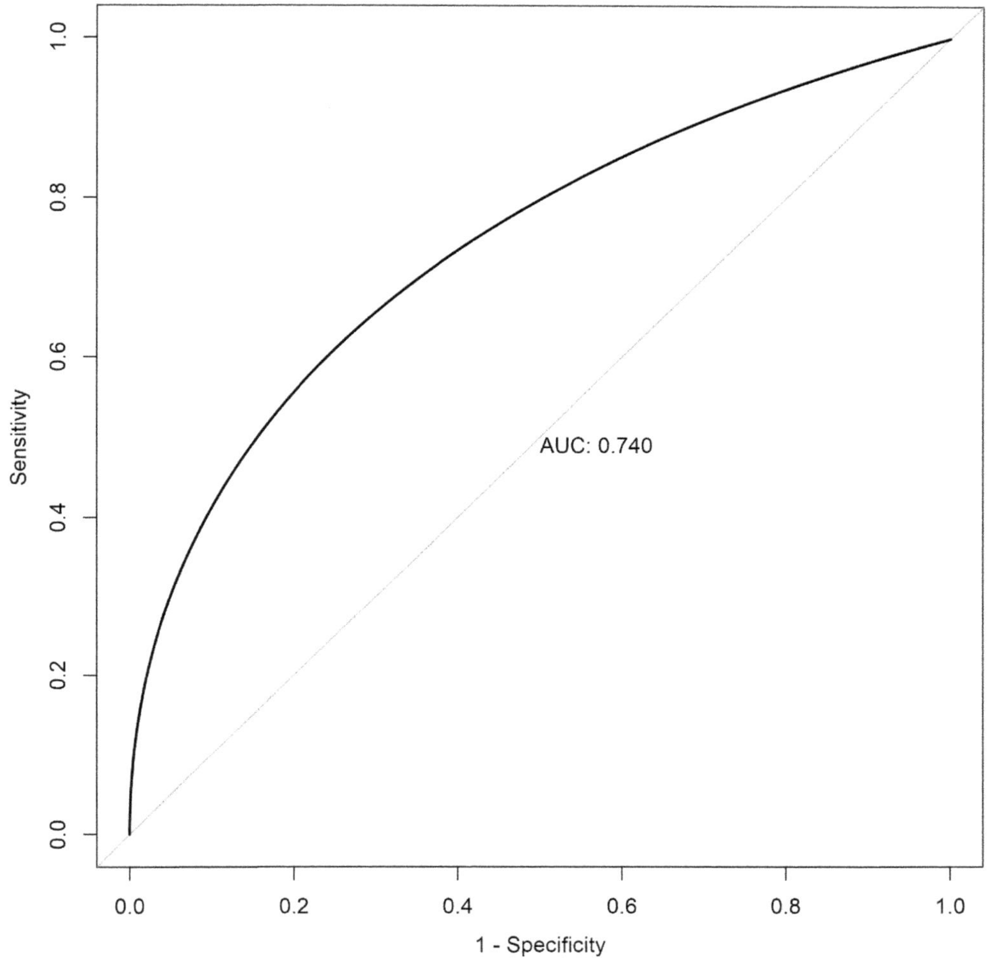

FIGURE 9.14 Smooth Receiver Operating Characteristic Curve. AUC = Area under the receiver operating characteristic curve.

```
library("ROCR")
library("rms")
library("ResourceSelection")
library("PredictABEL")
library("uroc")
library("rms")
library("gridExtra")
library("grid")
library("ggpubr")
library("msir")
library("car")
library("viridis")
```

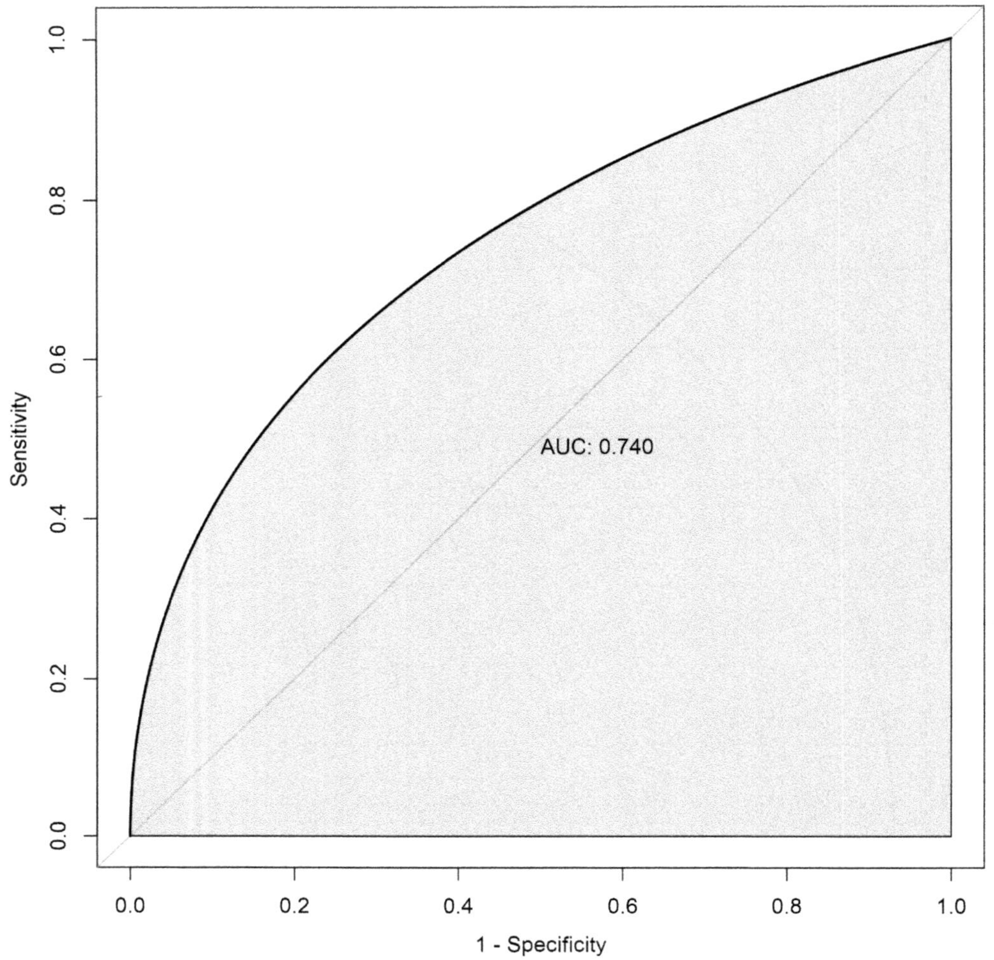

FIGURE 9.15 Area under the Receiver Operating Characteristic Curve (AUC).

```
library("ggrepel")
library("MOTE")
library("here")
library("tidyverse")
library("tinytex")
library("knitr")
library("kableExtra")
library("rmarkdown")
library("bookdown")
```

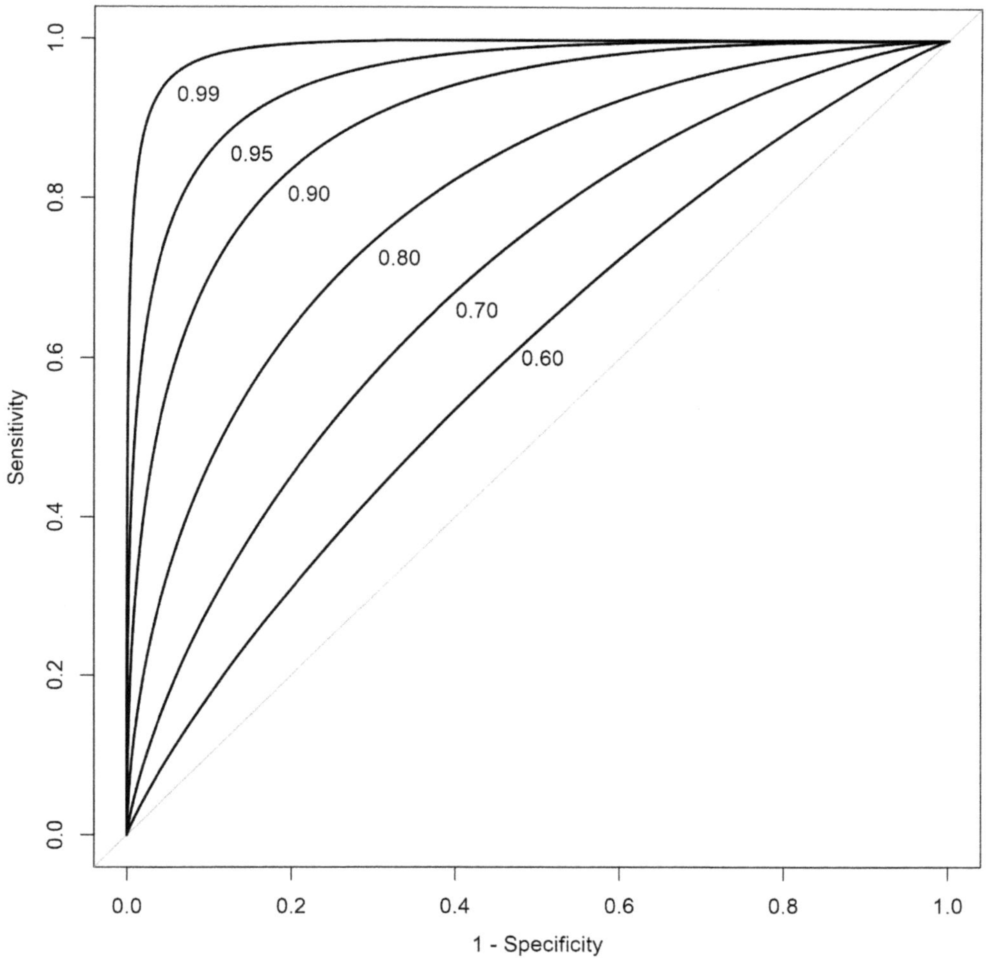

FIGURE 9.16 Receiver Operating Characteristic (ROC) Curves for Various Levels of Area under the ROC Curve (AUC) for Various Measures.

9.2.2 Prepare Data

9.2.2.1 Load Data

`aSAH` is a data set from the `pROC` package (Robin et al., 2021) that contains test scores (`s100b`) and clinical outcomes (`outcome`) for patients.

```
data(aSAH)
mydataSDT <- aSAH
```

9.2.2.2 Simulate Data

```
set.seed(52242)

mydataSDT$testScore <- mydataSDT$s100b
mydataSDT <- mydataSDT %>%
  mutate(testScoreSimple = ntile(testScore, 10))

mydataSDT$predictedProbability <-
  (mydataSDT$s100b - min(mydataSDT$s100b, na.rm = TRUE)) /
  (max(mydataSDT$s100b, na.rm = TRUE) -
     min(mydataSDT$s100b, na.rm = TRUE))
mydataSDT$continuousOutcome <- mydataSDT$testScore +
  rnorm(nrow(mydataSDT), mean = 0.20, sd = 0.20)
mydataSDT$disorder <- NA
mydataSDT$disorder[mydataSDT$outcome == "Good"] <- 0
mydataSDT$disorder[mydataSDT$outcome == "Poor"] <- 1
```

9.2.2.3 Add Missing Data

Adding missing data to dataframes helps make examples more realistic to real-life data and helps you get in the habit of programming to account for missing data.

```
mydataSDT$testScore[c(5,10)] <- NA
mydataSDT$disorder[c(10,15)] <- NA
```

9.3 Receiver Operating Characteristic Curve

The receiver operating characteristic (ROC) curve shows the combination of hit rate (sensitivity) and false alarm rate (1 − specificity) at every possible cutoff. It depicts that, as the cutoff increases (i.e., becomes more conservative), sensitivity decreases and specificity increases. It also depicts that, as the cutoff decreases (i.e., becomes more liberal), sensitivity increases and specificity decreases.

Receiver operating characteristic (ROC) curves were generated using the `pROC` package (Robin et al., 2021). The examples depict ROC curves that demonstrate that the measure is moderately accurate—the measure is more accurate than chance but there remains considerable room for improvement in predictive accuracy.

9.3.1 Empirical ROC Curve

The syntax used to generate an empirical ROC plot is below, and the plot is shown in Figure 9.13.

```
rocCurve <- roc(
  data = mydataSDT,
```

```
  response = disorder,
  predictor = testScore,
  smooth = FALSE)
```

```
plot(rocCurve, legacy.axes = TRUE, print.auc = TRUE)
```

An empirical ROC plot with cutoffs overlaid is shown in Figure 9.17.

```
pred <- prediction(na.omit(mydataSDT[,c(
  "testScoreSimple","disorder")])$testScoreSimple,
  na.omit(mydataSDT[,c("testScoreSimple","disorder")])$disorder)
perf <- performance(pred, "tpr", "fpr")
plot(
  perf,
  print.cutoffs.at = 1:11,
  text.adj = c(1, -1),
  ylim = c(0, 1.05))
abline(coef = c(0,1))
```

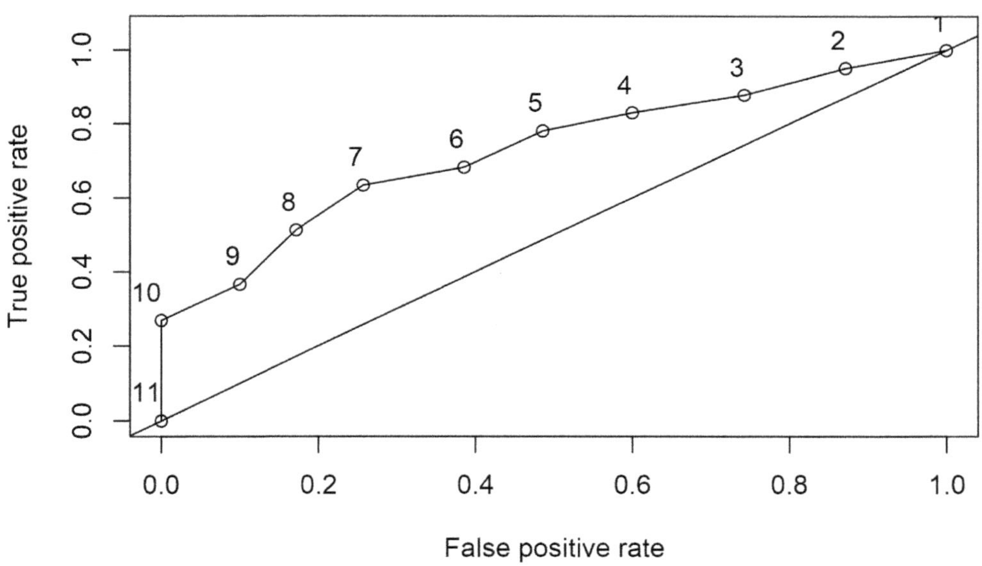

FIGURE 9.17 Empirical Receiver Operating Characteristic Curve with Cutoffs Overlaid.

9.3.2 Smooth ROC Curve

The syntax used to generate a smooth ROC plot is below, and the plot is shown in Figure 9.14.

```
rocCurveSmooth <- roc(
  data = mydataSDT,
  response = disorder,
  predictor = testScore,
  smooth = TRUE)

plot(rocCurveSmooth, legacy.axes = TRUE, print.auc = TRUE)
```

9.3.3 Youden's J Statistic

The threshold at the Youden's J statistic is the threshold where the test has the maximum combination (i.e., sum) of sensitivity and specificity: $\max(\text{sensitivity} + \text{specificity} - 1)$

```
youdenJ <- coords(
  rocCurve,
  x = "best",
  best.method = "youden")

youdenJ
```

```
  threshold specificity sensitivity
1     0.205         0.8        0.65
```

For this test, the Youden's J Statistic is at a threshold of 0.205, where sensitivity is 0.65 and specificity is 0.8.

9.3.4 The Point Closest to the Top Left of the ROC Curve

The point closest to the top-left part of the ROC plot with perfect sensitivity and specificity: $\min[(1 - \text{sensitivity})^2 + (1 - \text{specificity})^2]$

```
closestTopLeft <- coords(
  rocCurve,
  x = "best",
  best.method = "closest.topleft")

closestTopLeft
```

```
  threshold specificity sensitivity
1     0.205         0.8        0.65
```

For this test, the combination of sensitivity and specificity is closest to the top left of the ROC plot at a threshold of 0.205, where sensitivity is 0.65 and specificity is 0.8.

TABLE 9.1 Estimates of Prediction Accuracy Across Cutoffs.

ME	−0.11
MAE	0.34
MSE	0.21
RMSE	0.46
MPE	59.62
MAPE	64.97
sMAPE	82.46
MASE	0.74
RMSLE	0.30
rsquared	0.18
rsquaredAdj	0.17
rsquaredPredictive	0.12

9.4 Prediction Accuracy Across Cutoffs

There are two primary dimensions of accuracy: (1) discrimination (e.g., sensitivity, specificity, area under the ROC curve) and (2) calibration. Some general indexes of accuracy combine discrimination and calibration, as described in Section 9.4.1. This section (9.4) describes indexes of accuracy that span all possible cutoffs. That is, each index of accuracy described in this section provides a single numerical index of accuracy that aggregates the accuracy across all possible cutoffs. Aspects of accuracy at a particular cutoff are described in Section 9.5.

The `petersenlab` package (Petersen, 2024) contains the `accuracyOverall()` function that estimates the prediction accuracy across cutoffs. Estimates of prediction accuracy across cutoffs are presented in Table 9.1.

```
accuracyEstimates <- accuracyOverall(
  predicted = mydataSDT$testScore,
  actual = mydataSDT$disorder,
  dropUndefined = TRUE)
```

9.4.1 General Prediction Accuracy

There are many metrics of general prediction accuracy. When thinking about which metric(s) may be best for a given problem, it is important to consider the purpose of the assessment. The estimates of general prediction accuracy are separated below into scale-dependent and scale-independent accuracy estimates.

9.4.1.1 Scale-Dependent Accuracy Estimates

The estimates of prediction accuracy described in this section are scale-dependent. These accuracy estimates depend on the unit of measurement and therefore cannot be compared across measures with different scales or across data sets.

9.4.1.1.1 Mean error

Here, "error" (e) is the difference between the predicted and observed value for a given individual (i). Mean error (ME; also known as bias, see Section 3.5.1.3.2) is the mean difference between the predicted and observed values across individuals (i), that is, the mean of the errors across individuals (e_i). Values closer to zero reflect greater accuracy. If mean error is above zero, it indicates that predicted values are, on average, greater than observed values (i.e., overestimating errors). If mean error is below zero, it indicates that predicted values are, on average, less than observed values (i.e., underestimating errors). If both overestimating and underestimating errors are present, however, they can cancel each other out. As a result, even with a mean error of zero, there can still be considerable error present. Thus, although mean error can be helpful for examining whether predictions systematically under- or overestimate the actual scores, other forms of accuracy are necessary to examine the *extent* of error. The formula for mean error is shown in Equation (9.20):

$$\begin{aligned}\text{mean error} &= \frac{\sum\limits_{i=1}^{n}(\text{predicted}_i - \text{observed}_i)}{n} \\ &= \text{mean}(e_i)\end{aligned} \tag{9.20}$$

9.4.1.1.2 Mean absolute error

Mean absolute error (MAE) is the mean of the absolute value of differences between the predicted and observed values across individuals, that is, the mean of the absolute value of errors. Smaller MAE values (closer to zero) reflect greater accuracy. MAE is preferred over root mean squared error (RMSE) when you want to give equal weight to all errors and when the outliers have considerable impact. The formula for MAE is shown in Equation (9.21):

$$\begin{aligned}\text{mean absolute error (MAE)} &= \frac{\sum\limits_{i=1}^{n}|\text{predicted}_i - \text{observed}_i|}{n} \\ &= \text{mean}(|e_i|)\end{aligned} \tag{9.21}$$

9.4.1.1.3 Mean squared error

Mean squared error (MSE) is the mean of the square of the differences between the predicted and observed values across individuals, that is, the mean of the squared value of errors. Smaller MSE values (closer to zero) reflect greater accuracy. MSE penalizes larger errors more heavily than smaller errors (unlike MAE). However, MSE is sensitive to outliers and can be impacted if the errors are skewed. The formula for MSE is shown in Equation (9.22):

$$\begin{aligned}\text{mean squared error (MSE)} &= \frac{\sum\limits_{i=1}^{n}(\text{predicted}_i - \text{observed}_i)^2}{n} \\ &= \text{mean}(e_i^2)\end{aligned} \tag{9.22}$$

9.4.1.1.4 Root mean squared error

Root mean squared error (RMSE) is the square root of the mean of the square of the differences between the predicted and observed values across individuals, that is, the root mean squared value of errors. Smaller RMSE values (closer to zero) reflect greater accuracy. RMSE penalizes larger errors more heavily than smaller errors (unlike MAE). However, RMSE is sensitive to outliers and can be impacted if the errors are skewed. The formula for RMSE is shown in Equation (9.23):

$$\begin{aligned}\text{root mean squared error (RMSE)} &= \sqrt{\frac{\sum\limits_{i=1}^{n}(\text{predicted}_i - \text{observed}_i)^2}{n}} \\ &= \sqrt{\text{mean}(e_i^2)}\end{aligned} \tag{9.23}$$

9.4.1.2 Scale-Independent Accuracy Estimates

The estimates of prediction accuracy described in this section are intended to be scale-*independent* (unit-free) so the accuracy estimates can be compared across measures with different scales or across data sets (Hyndman & Athanasopoulos, 2018).

9.4.1.2.1 Mean percentage error

Mean percentage error (MPE) values closer to zero reflect greater accuracy. The formula for percentage error is shown in Equation (9.24):

$$\text{percentage error } (p_i) = \frac{100\% \times (\text{observed}_i - \text{predicted}_i)}{\text{observed}_i} \tag{9.24}$$

We then take the mean of the percentage errors to get MPE. The formula for MPE is in Equation (9.25):

$$\begin{aligned}\text{mean percentage error (MPE)} &= \frac{100\%}{n}\sum_{i=1}^{n}\frac{\text{observed}_i - \text{predicted}_i}{\text{observed}_i} \\ &= \text{mean(percentage error)} \\ &= \text{mean}(p_i)\end{aligned} \tag{9.25}$$

9.4.1.2.2 Mean absolute percentage error

Smaller mean absolute percentage error (MAPE) values (closer to zero) reflect greater accuracy. The formula for MAPE is shown in Equation (9.26): MAPE is asymmetric because it overweights underestimates and underweights overestimates. MAPE can be preferable to symmetric mean absolute percentage error (sMAPE) if there are no observed values of zero and if you want to emphasize the importance of underestimates (relative to overestimates).

$$\begin{aligned}\text{mean absolute percentage error (MAPE)} &= \frac{100\%}{n}\sum_{i=1}^{n}\left|\frac{\text{observed}_i - \text{predicted}_i}{\text{observed}_i}\right| \\ &= \text{mean(|percentage error|)} \\ &= \text{mean}(|p_i|)\end{aligned} \tag{9.26}$$

9.4.1.2.3 Symmetric mean absolute percentage error

Unlike MAPE, symmetric mean absolute percentage error (sMAPE) is symmetric because it equally weights underestimates and overestimates. Smaller sMAPE values (closer to zero) reflect greater accuracy. The formula for sMAPE is shown in Equation (9.27):

$$\text{symmetric mean absolute percentage error (sMAPE)} = \frac{100\%}{n} \sum_{i=1}^{n} \frac{|\text{predicted}_i - \text{observed}_i|}{|\text{predicted}_i| + |\text{observed}_i|} \tag{9.27}$$

9.4.1.2.4 Mean absolute scaled error

Mean absolute scaled error (MASE) is described by (Hyndman & Athanasopoulos, 2018). Values closer to zero reflect greater accuracy.

The adapted formula for MASE with non-time series data is described here: https://stats.stackexchange.com/a/108963/20338 (archived at https://perma.cc/G469-8NAJ). Scaled errors are calculated using Equation (9.28):

$$\begin{aligned} \text{scaled error}(q_i) &= \frac{\text{observed}_i - \text{predicted}_i}{\text{scaling factor}} \\ &= \frac{\text{observed}_i - \text{predicted}_i}{\frac{1}{n}\sum\limits_{i=1}^{n} |\text{observed}_i - \overline{\text{observed}}|} \end{aligned} \tag{9.28}$$

Then, we calculate the mean of the absolute value of the scaled errors to get MASE, as in Equation (9.29):

$$\begin{aligned} \text{mean absolute scaled error (MASE)} &= \frac{1}{n}\sum_{i=1}^{n} |q_i| \\ &= \text{mean}(|\text{scaled error}|) \\ &= \text{mean}(|q_i|) \end{aligned} \tag{9.29}$$

9.4.1.2.5 Root mean squared log error

The squared log of the accuracy ratio is described by Tofallis (2015). The accuracy ratio is shown in Equation (9.30):

$$\text{accuracy ratio} = \frac{\text{predicted}_i}{\text{observed}_i} \tag{9.30}$$

However, the accuracy ratio is undefined with observed or predicted values of zero, so it is common to modify it by adding 1 to the predictor and denominator, as in Equation (9.31):

$$\text{accuracy ratio} = \frac{\text{predicted}_i + 1}{\text{observed}_i + 1} \tag{9.31}$$

Squaring the log values keeps the values positive, such that smaller values (values closer to zero) reflect greater accuracy. Then we take the mean of the squared log values, which keeps the values positive, and calculate the square root of the mean squared log values to put them back on the (pre-squared) log metric. This is known as the root mean squared log error (RMSLE). Division inside the log is equal to subtraction outside the log. So, the formula can be reformulated with the subtraction of two logs, as in Equation (9.32):

$$\begin{aligned}
\text{root mean squared log error (RMSLE)} &= \sqrt{\sum_{i=1}^{n} log\left(\frac{\text{predicted}_i + 1}{\text{observed}_i + 1}\right)^2} \\
&= \sqrt{\text{mean}\left[log\left(\frac{\text{predicted}_i + 1}{\text{observed}_i + 1}\right)^2\right]} \\
&= \sqrt{\text{mean}\left[log(\text{accuracy ratio})^2\right]} \\
&= \sqrt{\text{mean}\left\{\left[log(\text{predicted}_i + 1) - log(\text{actual}_i + 1)\right]^2\right\}}
\end{aligned} \tag{9.32}$$

RMSLE can be preferable when the scores have a wide range of values and are skewed. RMSLE can help to reduce the impact of outliers. RMSLE gives more weight to smaller errors in the prediction of small observed values, while also penalizing larger errors in the prediction of larger observed values. It overweights underestimates and underweights overestimates.

There are other variations of prediction accuracy metrics that use the log of the accuracy ratio. One variation makes it similar to median symmetric percentage error (Morley et al., 2018).

9.4.1.2.6 Coefficient of Determination (R^2)

The coefficient of determination (R^2) is a general index of accuracy that combines both discrimination and calibration. It reflects the proportion of variance in the outcome (dependent) variable that is explained by the model predictions: $R^2 = \frac{\text{variance explained in } Y}{\text{total variance in } Y}$. Larger values indicate greater accuracy.

R^2 is commonly estimated in multiple regression, in which multiple predictors are allowed to predict one outcome. Multiple regression can be conceptualized with overlapping circles in what is called a Ballantine graph[2] (archived at https://perma.cc/C7CU-KFVG). R^2 in multiple regression is depicted conceptually with a Ballantine graph in Figure 9.18.

R^2:

```
summary(lm(
  disorder ~ testScore,
  data = mydataSDT))$r.squared
```

```
[1] 0.1779
```

The predictor (`testScore`) explains 17.79% of the variance ($R^2 = .1779$) in the outcome (`disorder` status).

[2] https://www.andrewheiss.com/blog/2021/08/21/r2-euler

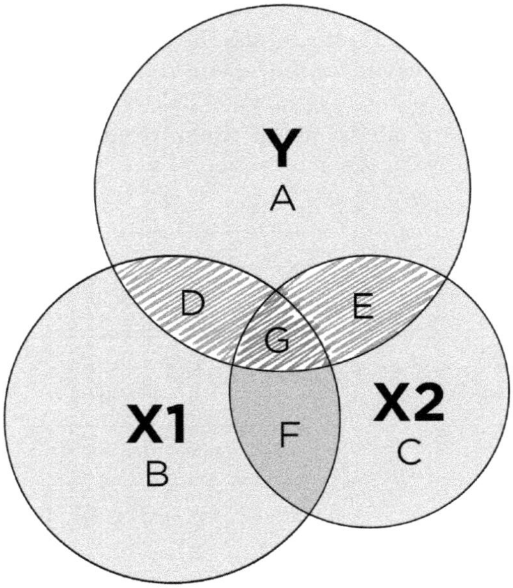

$$R^2 = \frac{\mathrm{D} + \mathrm{E} + \mathrm{G}}{\mathrm{A} + \mathrm{D} + \mathrm{E} + \mathrm{G}}$$

FIGURE 9.18 Conceptual Depiction of Proportion of Variance Explained (R^2) in an Outcome Variable (Y) by Multiple Predictors ($X1$ and $X2$) in Multiple Regression. The size of each circle represents the variable's variance. The proportion of variance in Y that is explained by the predictors is depicted by the areas covered in scribbled lines. The space with the dark scribbled lines (G) is where multiple predictors explain overlapping variance in the outcome. Overlapping variance that is explained in the outcome (G) will not be recovered in the regression coefficients when both predictors are included in the regression model.

9.4.1.2.6.1 Adjusted R^2 (R^2_{adj})

Adjusted R^2 is similar to the coefficient of determination, but it accounts for the number of predictors included in the regression model to penalize overfitting. Adjusted R^2 reflects the proportion of variance in the outcome (dependent) variable that is explained by the model predictions over and above what would be expected to be accounted for by chance, given the number of predictors in the model. Larger values indicate greater accuracy. The formula for adjusted R^2 is shown in Equation (9.33):

$$R^2_{adj} = 1 - (1 - R^2)\frac{n - 1}{n - p - 1} \tag{9.33}$$

where p is the number of predictors in the model, and n is the sample size.

```
summary(lm(
```

```
  disorder ~ testScore,
  data = mydataSDT))$adj.r.squared
```

```
[1] 0.1703
```

Adjusted R^2 is described further in Section 9.9.

9.4.1.2.6.2 Predictive R^2

Predictive R^2 is described here: https://tomhopper.me/2014/05/16/can-we-do-better-than-r-squared/ (archived at https://perma.cc/BK8J-HFUK). Predictive R^2 penalizes overfitting, unlike traditional R^2. Larger values indicate greater accuracy.

Predictive R^2 can be estimated using the `accuracyOverall()` function of the `petersenlab` package (Petersen, 2024).

9.4.2 Discrimination

When dealing with a categorical outcome, discrimination is the ability to separate events from non-events. When dealing with a continuous outcome, discrimination is the strength of the association between the predictor and the outcome. Aspects of discrimination at a particular cutoff (e.g., sensitivity, specificity) are described in Section 9.5.

9.4.2.1 Area Under the ROC Curve

The area under the ROC curve (AUC) is a general index of discrimination accuracy for a categorical outcome. It is also called the concordance (c) statistic. Larger values reflect greater discrimination accuracy. AUC was estimated using the `pROC` package (Robin et al., 2021).

```
rocCurve$auc
```

```
Area under the curve: 0.731
```

9.4.2.2 Coefficient of Predictive Ability

The coefficient of predictive ability (CPA) is a generalization of AUC to handle non-binary outcomes including ordinal and continuous outcomes (Gneiting & Walz, 2021). Larger values reflect greater accuracy. It was calculated using the `uroc` package (Gneiting & Walz, 2021).

```
cpaNoMissing <- na.omit(
  mydataSDT[,c("testScore","continuousOutcome")])

cpa(
  response = cpaNoMissing$continuousOutcome,
  predictor = cpaNoMissing$testScore)
```

```
[1] 0.8381
```

9.4.2.3 Spearman's Rho (ρ) Rank Correlation

When the coefficient of predictive ability is applied to an ordinal or continuous outcome, it is linearly related to Spearman's rho (ρ) rank correlation (Gneiting & Walz, 2021). Larger values reflect greater accuracy.

```
cor(
  x = mydataSDT$testScore,
  y = mydataSDT$continuousOutcome,
  use = "pairwise.complete.obs",
  method = "spearman")
```

```
[1] 0.6769
```

9.4.2.4 Somers' D_{xy} Rank Correlation

Somers D_{xy} is an index of discrimination for an ordinal outcome (Harrell, 2015). Larger values reflect greater accuracy. Somers' D_{xy} was estimated in the `rms` package (Harrell, Jr., 2021).

```
lrm(
  continuousOutcome ~ testScore,
  data = mydataSDT)$stats["Dxy"]
```

```
   Dxy
0.4978
```

9.4.2.5 Kendall's Tau-a (τ_A) Rank Correlation

Kendall's tau-a (τ_A) is an index of the discrimination for an ordinal outcome (Harrell, 2015). Larger values reflect greater accuracy. Kendall's tau-a was estimated in the `rms` package (Harrell, Jr., 2021).

```
lrm(continuousOutcome ~ testScore,
    data = mydataSDT)$stats["Tau-a"]
```

```
 Tau-a
0.4978
```

9.4.2.6 c Index

The c index, also called the concordance probability, is a generalization of the area under the ROC curve that applies to a continuous outcome (Harrell, 2015). The c index is the proportion of all pairs of predicted-actual values whose actual value can be ordered such that the pair with the higher predicted value is the one who had the higher actual value. Larger values reflect greater accuracy. The Brown–Hollander–Korwar non-parametric test of association was estimated in the `rms` package (Harrell, Jr., 2021).

```
lrm(
  continuousOutcome ~ testScore,
  data = mydataSDT)$stats["C"]
```

```
     C
0.7489
```

9.4.2.7 Effect Size (β) of Regression

The effect size of a predictor, i.e., the standardized regression coefficient is called a beta (β) coefficient, is a general index of discrimination accuracy for a continuous outcome. Larger values reflect greater accuracy. We can obtain standardized regression coefficients by standardizing the predictors and outcome using the `scale()` function in R.

β:

```
lm(
  scale(continuousOutcome) ~ scale(testScore),
  data = mydataSDT)$coef["scale(testScore)"]
```

```
scale(testScore)
          0.8285
```

9.4.3 Calibration

When dealing with a categorical outcome, calibration is the degree to which a probabilistic estimate of an event reflects the true underlying probability of the event. When dealing with a continuous outcome, calibration is the degree to which the predicted values are close in value to the outcome values. The importance of examining calibration (in addition to discrimination) is described by Lindhiem et al. (2020).

Calibration came to be considered a central aspect of weather forecast accuracy. For instance, on the days that the meteorologist says there is a 60% chance of rain, it should rain about 60% of the time. Through improvements in scientific understanding of weather systems, rain forecasts have become more accurate. For instance, rain forecasts from the National Weather Service are well calibrated (see Figure 9.20, reprinted from Charba & Klein, 1980). However, forecasts of rain may be exaggerated by local TV meteorologists to boost ratings (Silver, 2012). Interestingly, rain forecasts from The Weather Channel are somewhat miscalibrated under certain conditions. For instance, on days when they forecast a 20% chance of rain, the actual chance of rain is around 5% (see Figure 9.19, Bickel & Kim, 2008). However, this miscalibration is deliberate. People tend to be more angry when the meteorologist says it will not rain when it actually does (false negative) compared to when the meteorologist says it will rain when it actually does not (false positive). As Silver (2012) notes, "If it rains when it isn't supposed to, [people] curse the weatherman for ruining their picnic, whereas an unexpectedly sunny day is taken as a serendipitous bonus. It isn't good science, but as Dr. Rose at The Weather Channel acknowledged to [Mr. Silver]: 'If the forecast was objective, if it has zero bias in precipitation, we'd probably be in trouble.' " (p. 135).

Calibration is not just important for weather forecasts. It is also important for psychological assessment. Calibration can be examined in several ways, including Brier Scores (see Section 9.4.3.2), the Hosler-Lemeshow test (see Section 9.4.3.3), Spiegelhalter's z (see Section 9.4.3.4), and the mean difference between predicted and observed values at different binned thresholds as depicted graphically with a calibration plot (see Figure 9.22).

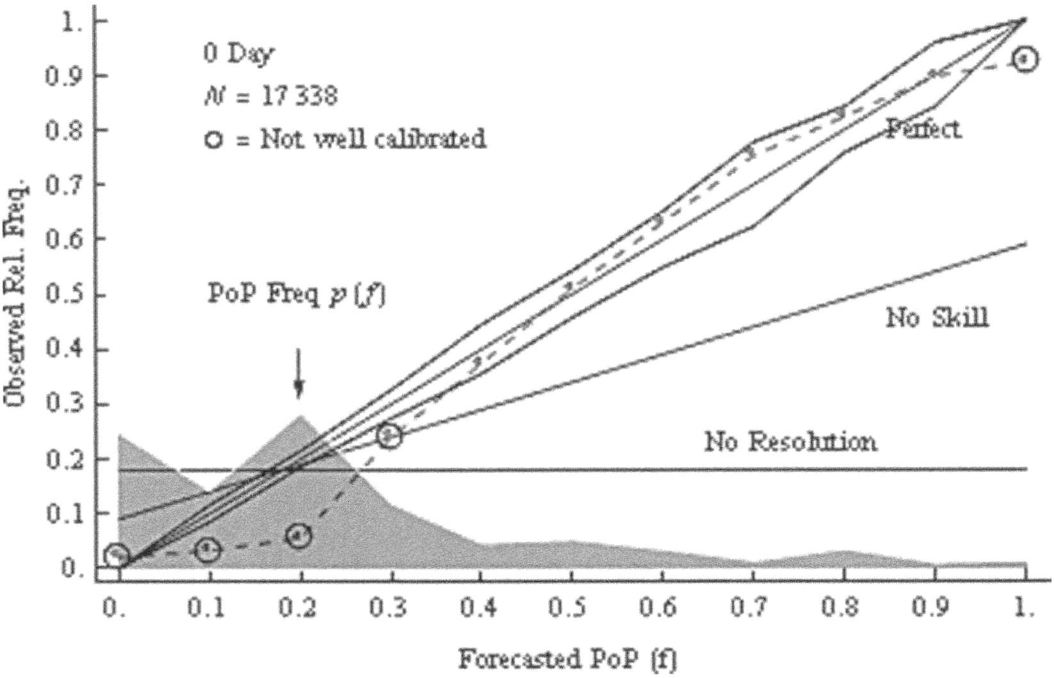

FIGURE 9.19 Calibration Plot of Same-Day Probability of Precipitation (PoP) Forecasts from The Weather Channel. The plot depicts that the rain forecasts are generally well calibrated, but shows some miscalibration. For instance, the forecasted probability of rain is lower than the actual probability of rain when the forecasted probability of rain is 20%. (Figure reprinted from Bickel & Kim (2008), figure 2, p. 4872. Bickel, J. E., & Kim, S. D. (2008). Verification of The Weather Channel probability of precipitation forecasts. *Monthly Weather Review*, *136*(12), 4867–4881. doi: https://doi.org/10.1175/2008MWR2547.1 Copyright ©American Meteorological Society. Used with permission.)

9.4.3.1 Calibration Plot

Calibration plots can be helpful for identifying miscalibration. A calibration plot depicts the predicted probability of an event on the x-axis, and the actual (observed) probability of the event on the y-axis. The predictions are binned into a certain number of groups (commonly 10). The diagonal line reflects predictions that are perfectly calibrated. To the extent that predictions deviate from the diagonal line, the predictions are miscalibrated. There are four general patterns of miscalibration: overextremity, underextremity, overprediction, and underprediction (see Figure 9.21). *Overextremity* exists when the predicted probabilites are too close to the extremes (zero or one). *Underextremity* exists when the predicted probabilities are too far away from the extremes. *Overprediction* exists when the predicted probabilities are consistently greater than the observed probabilities. *Underprediction* exists when the predicted probabilities are consistently less than the observed probabilities. For a more thorough description of these types of miscalibration, see Lindhiem et al. (2020).

A calibration plot was generated using the `PredictABEL` package (Kundu et al., 2020), and is depicted in Figure 9.22.

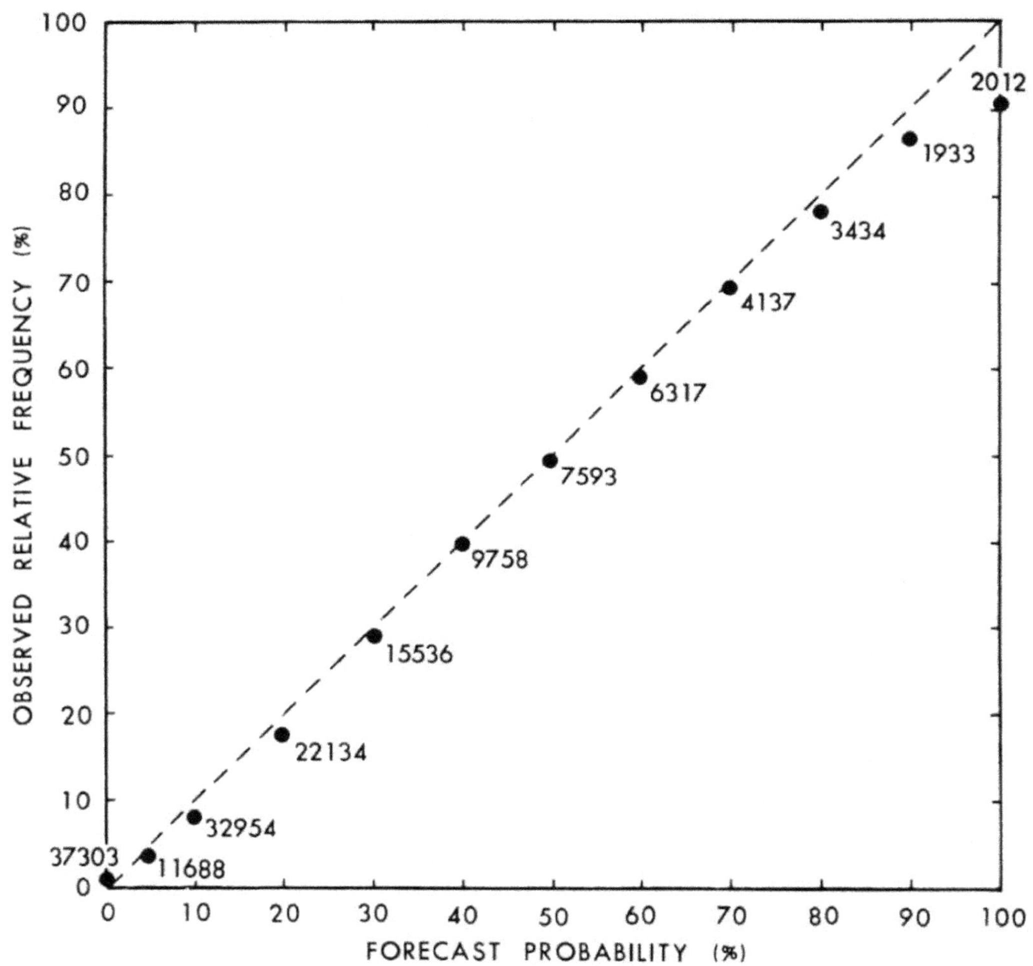

FIGURE 9.20 Calibration Plot of Local Probability of Precipitation (PoP) Forecasts for 87 Stations from the United States National Weather Service. Numbers next to the plotted points are the sample sizes. (Figure reprinted from Charba & Klein (1980), figure 6, p. 1550. Charba, J. P., & Klein, W. H. (1980). Skill in precipitation forecasting in the National Weather Service. *Bulletin of the American Meteorological Society, 61*(12), 1546–1555. https://doi.org/10.1175/1520-0477(1980)061%3C1546:SIPFIT%3E2.0.CO;2. Copyright ©American Meteorological Society. Used with permission.)

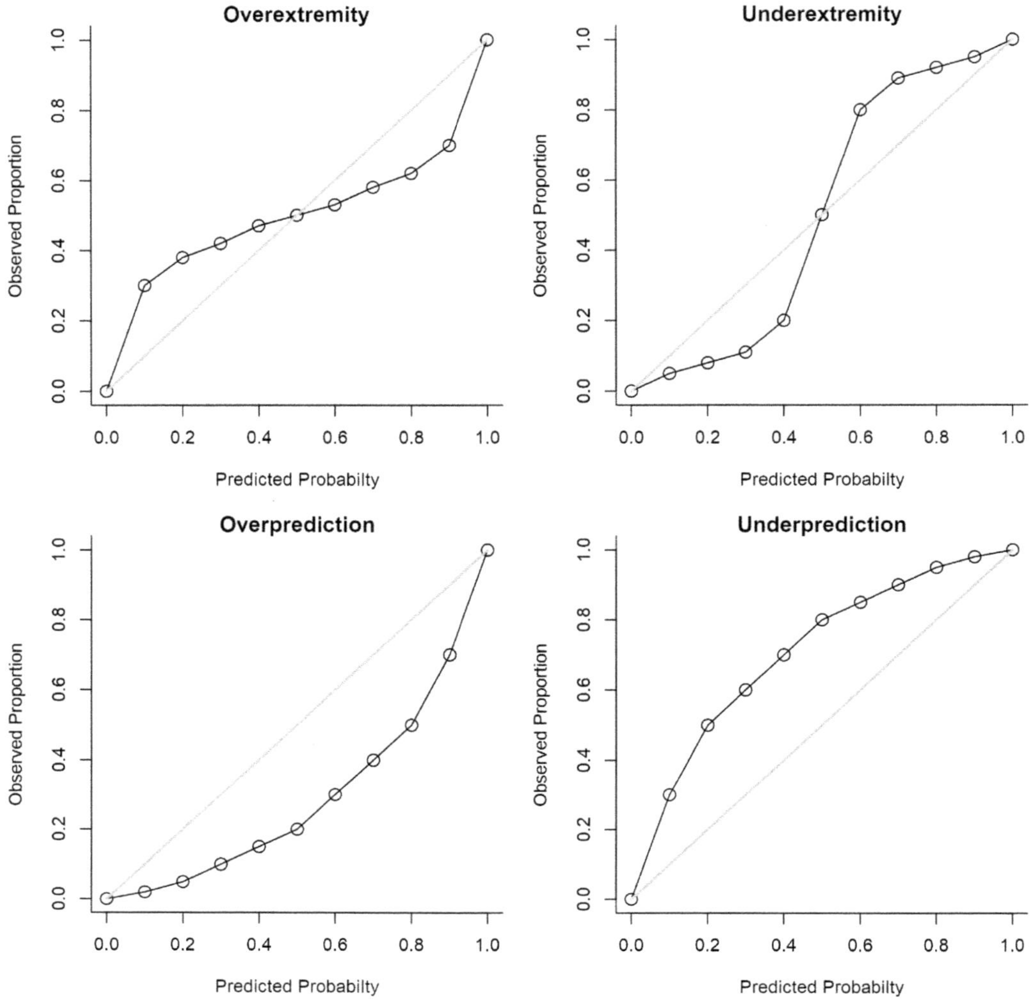

FIGURE 9.21 Types of Miscalibration.

```
colNumberOutcome <- which(names(mydataSDT) == "disorder")
myDataNoMissing <- na.omit(mydataSDT)
```

```
plotCalibration(
  data = na.omit(myDataNoMissing),
  cOutcome = colNumberOutcome,
  predRisk = myDataNoMissing$predictedProbability,
  groups = 10)
```

```
$Table_HLtest
                total meanpred meanobs predicted observed
[0.0000,0.0245)    19    0.013   0.211      0.25        4
```

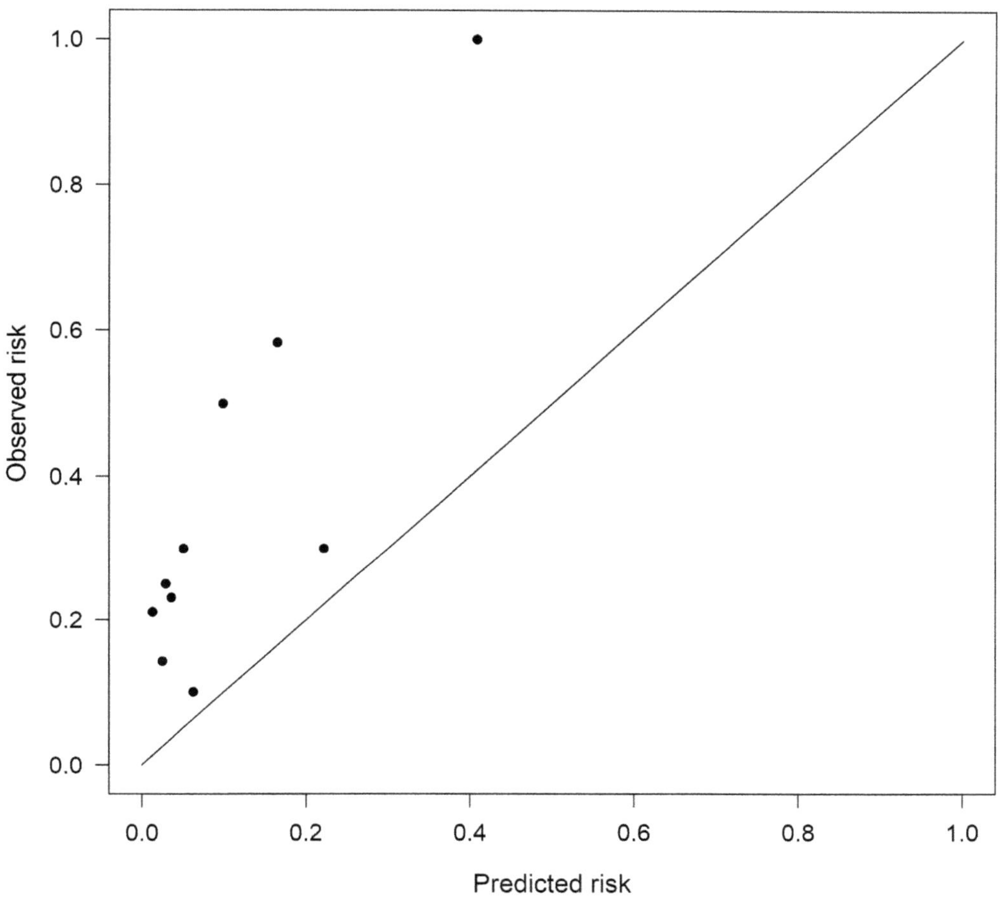

FIGURE 9.22 Example Calibration Plot.

```
0.0245                 7    0.025   0.143       0.17         1
0.0294                 8    0.029   0.250       0.24         2
[0.0343,0.0441)       13    0.036   0.231       0.47         3
[0.0441,0.0588)       10    0.051   0.300       0.51         3
[0.0588,0.0735)       10    0.063   0.100       0.63         1
[0.0735,0.1324)       10    0.099   0.500       0.99         5
[0.1324,0.2059)       12    0.165   0.583       1.98         7
[0.2059,0.2598)       10    0.222   0.300       2.22         3
[0.2598,1.0000]       11    0.408   1.000       4.49        11

$Chi_square
[1] 152.3

$df
```

```
[1] 8

$p_value
[1] 0
```

9.4.3.2 Brier Scores

Brier scores were calculated using the `rms` package (Harrell, Jr., 2021). Smaller values reflect greater calibration accuracy.

```
val.prob(
  mydataSDT$predictedProbability,
  mydataSDT$disorder, pl = FALSE)["Brier"]
```

```
 Brier
0.2659
```

9.4.3.3 Hosler-Lemeshow Test

The Hosler-Lemeshow goodness of fit (GOF) test evaluates the null hypothesis that there is no difference between the predicted versus observed frequencies of an event. The test requires specifying how many groups/bins (g) to use to calculate quantiles. Smaller χ^2 values (and larger p-values) reflect greater calibration accuracy. A statistically significant χ^2 ($p < .05$) indicates a significant degree of miscalibration. The Hosler-Lemeshow GOF test was calculated using the `ResourceSelection` package (Lele et al., 2019). The table of predicted versus observed frequencies was generated using the `PredictABEL` package (Kundu et al., 2020).

For the number of bins ($g = 10$) specified below, the predictions show statistically significant miscalibration.

```
gValue <- 10

hoslem.test(
  mydataSDT$disorder,
  mydataSDT$predictedProbability,
  g = gValue)
```

```

	Hosmer and Lemeshow goodness of fit (GOF) test

data:  mydataSDT$disorder, mydataSDT$predictedProbability
X-squared = 154, df = 8, p-value <2e-16
```

9.4.3.4 Spiegelhalter's z

Spiegelhalter's z was calculated using the `rms` package (Harrell, Jr., 2021). Smaller z values (and larger associated p-values) reflect greater calibration accuracy. A statistically significant Spiegelhalter's z ($p < .05$) indicates a significant degree of miscalibration.

In this case, the predictions show statistically significant miscalibration.

```
val.prob(
  mydataSDT$predictedProbability,
  mydataSDT$disorder,
  pl = FALSE)["S:z"]
```

```
  S:z
10.53
```

```
val.prob(
  mydataSDT$predictedProbability,
  mydataSDT$disorder,
  pl = FALSE)["S:p"]
```

```
      S:p
6.513e-26
```

9.4.3.5 Calibration for Predicting a Continuous Outcome

When predicting a continuous outcome, calibration of the predicted values in relation to the outcome values can be examined in multiple ways including:

- in a calibration plot, the extent to which the intercept is near zero and the slope is near one
- in a calibration plot, the extent to which the 95% confidence interval of the observed value, across all values of the predicted values, includes the diagonal reference line with an intercept of zero and a slope of one.
- mean error
- mean absolute error
- mean squared error
- root mean squared error

With a plot of the predictions on the x-axis, and the outcomes on the y-axis (i.e., a calibration plot), calibration can be examined graphically as the extent to which the best-fit regression line has an intercept (alpha) close to zero and a slope (beta) close to one (Stevens & Poppe, 2020; Steyerberg & Vergouwe, 2014). The intercept is also called "calibration-in-the-large", whereas "calibration-in-the-small" refers to the extent to which the predicted values match the observed values at a specific predicted value (e.g., when the weather forecaster says that there is a 10% chance of rain, does it actually rain 10% of the time?). For predictions to be well calibrated, the intercept should be close to zero and the slope should be close to one. If the slope is close to one but the intercept is not close to zero (or the intercept is close to zero but the slope is not close to one), the predictions would not be considered well calibrated. The 95% confidence interval of the observed value, across all values of the predicted values, should include the diagonal reference line whose intercept is zero and whose slope is one.

For instance, based on the intercept and slope of the calibration plot in Figure 9.23, the predictions are not well calibrated, despite having a slope near one, because the 95% confidence interval of the intercept does not include zero. The best-fit line is the white line. The intercept from the best-fit line is positive, as shown in the regression equation. This is a case of underprediction, where the predicted values are consistently less than the observed values. The confidence interval of the observed value (i.e., the gray band) is the interval within which we have 95% confidence that the true observed value would lie for a given predicted value, based on the model. The 95% prediction interval of the observed value (i.e., the dashed lines) is the interval within which we would expect that 95% of future observations would lie for a given predicted value. The black diagonal line indicates the reference line with an intercept of zero and a slope of one. The predictions would be significantly miscalibrated at a given level of the predicted values if the 95% confidence interval of the observed value does not include the reference line at that level of the predicted value. In this case, the 95% confidence interval of the observed value does not include the reference line (i.e., the actual observed value) at lower levels of the predicted values, so the predictions are miscalibrated lower levels of the predicted values.

Gold-standard recommendations include examining the predicted values in relation to the observed values using locally estimated scatterplot smoothing (LOESS) (Austin & Steyerberg, 2014), such as in Figure 9.24. We can examine whether the LOESS-based 95% confidence interval of the observed value at every level of the predicted values includes the diagonal reference line (i.e., the actual observed value). In this case, the 95% confidence interval of the observed value does not include the reference line at lower levels of the predicted values, so the predictions are miscalibrated at lower levels of the predicted values.

9.5 Prediction Accuracy at a Given Cutoff

9.5.1 Set a Cutoff

Here, we set a cutoff at the Youden's J Statistic to calculate the accuracy statistics at that cutoff:

```
cutoff <- 0.205

mydataSDT$diagnosis <- NA
mydataSDT$diagnosis[mydataSDT$testScore < cutoff] <- 0
mydataSDT$diagnosis[mydataSDT$testScore >= cutoff] <- 1

mydataSDT$diagnosisFactor <- factor(
  mydataSDT$diagnosis,
  levels = c(1, 0),
  labels = c("Decision: Diagnosis", "Decision: No Diagnosis"))

mydataSDT$disorderFactor <- factor(
  mydataSDT$disorder,
  levels = c(1, 0),
  labels = c("Truth: Disorder", "Truth: No Disorder"))
```

9.5.2 Accuracy at a Given Cutoff

The `petersenlab` package (Petersen, 2024) contains the `accuracyAtCutoff()` function that estimates the prediction accuracy at a given cutoff. Estimates of prediction accuracy at a given cutoff are in Table 9.2.

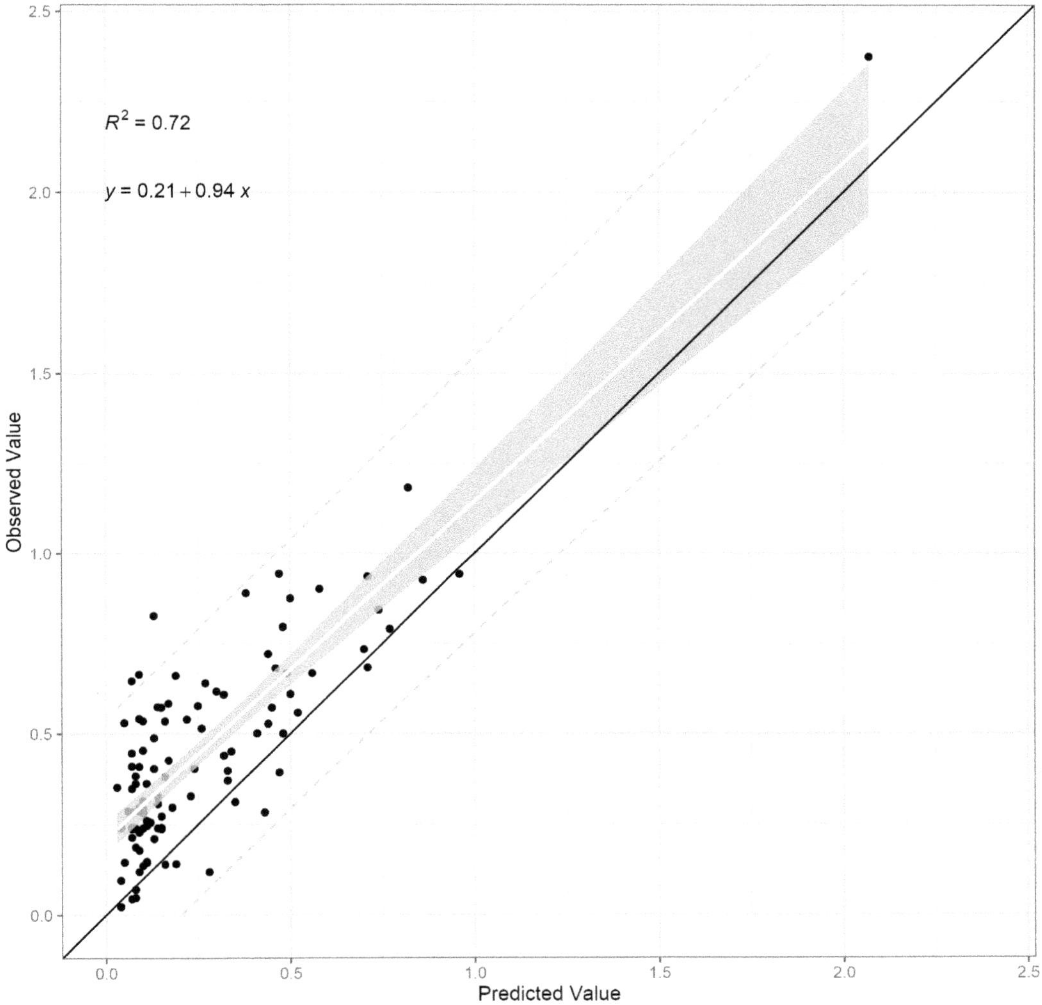

FIGURE 9.23 Calibration Plot for Predictions of a Continuous Outcome, with Best-Fit Line. The black diagonal line indicates the reference line with an intercept of zero and a slope of one. The white line is the best-fit line. The gray band is the 95% confidence interval of the observed value. The dashed black lines are the 95% prediction interval of the observed value. The predictions are not well calibrated because the 95% confidence interval of the intercept does not include zero (even though the 95% confidence interval of the slope includes one). The intercept from the best-fit line is positive, as shown in the regression equation. This is a case of underprediction, where the predicted values are consistently less than the observed values. The 95% confidence interval of the observed value does not include the reference line (i.e., the actual observed value) at lower levels of the predicted values, so the predictions are miscalibrated at lower levels of the predicted values.

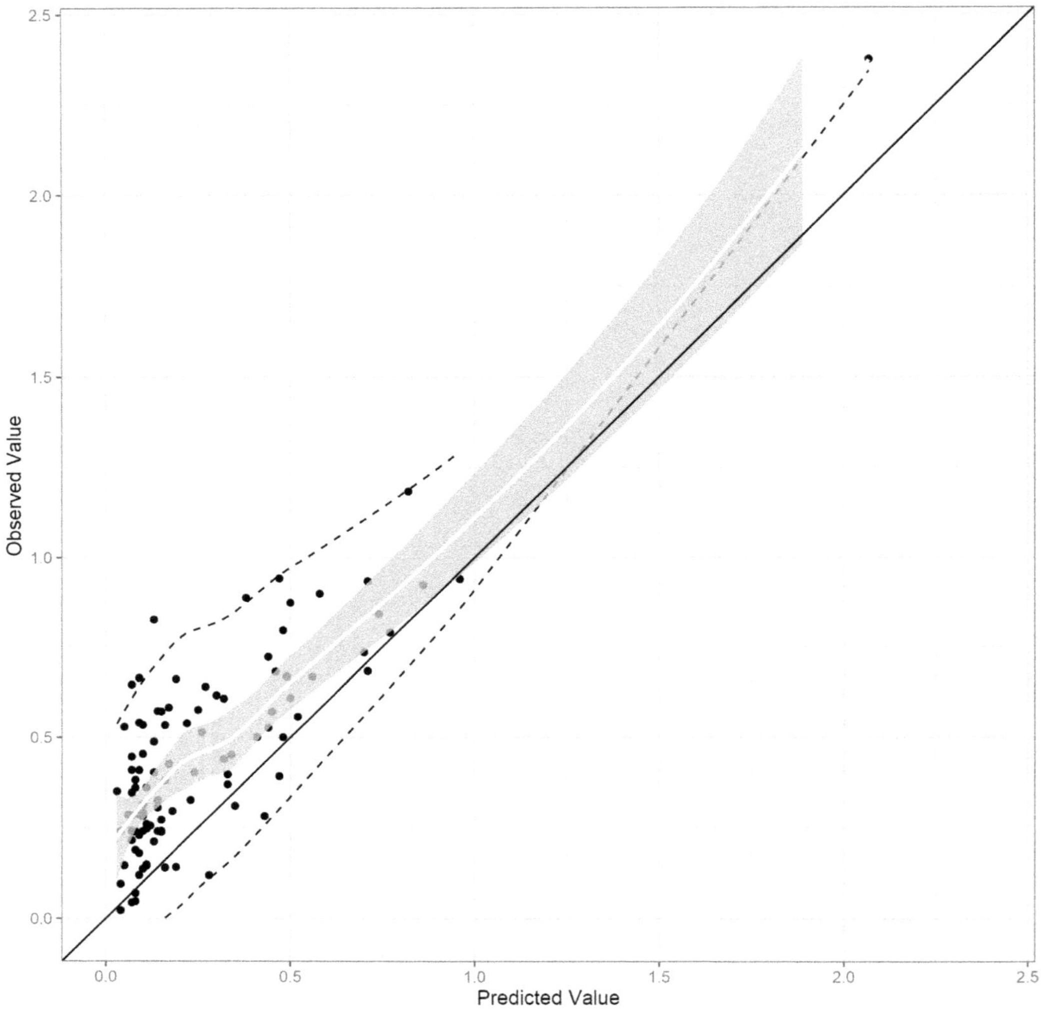

FIGURE 9.24 Calibration Plot for Predictions of a Continuous Outcome, with LOESS Best-Fit Line. The white line is the best-fit line based on LOESS. The gray band is the 95% confidence interval of the observed value. The dashed black lines are the 95% prediction interval of the observed value. The 95% confidence interval of the observed value does not include the reference line (i.e., the actual observed value) at lower levels of the predicted values, so the predictions are miscalibrated at lower levels of the predicted values.

```
accuracyEstimatesAtCutoff <- accuracyAtCutoff(
  predicted = mydataSDT$testScore,
  actual = mydataSDT$disorder,
  cutoff = cutoff)
```

9.5.3 Confusion Matrix

A confusion matrix (aka 2-by-2 accuracy table, cross-tabulation table, or contingency table) is a matrix for categorical data that presents the predicted outcome on one dimension and the actual outcome (truth) on the other dimension. If the predictions and outcomes are dichotomous, the confusion matrix is a 2-by-2 matrix with two rows and two columns that represent four possible predicted-actual combinations (decision outcomes). In such a case, the confusion matrix provides a tabular count of each type of accurate cases (true positives and true negatives) versus the number of each type of error (false positives and false negatives), as shown in Figure 9.25. An example of a confusion matrix is given in Figure 9.4.

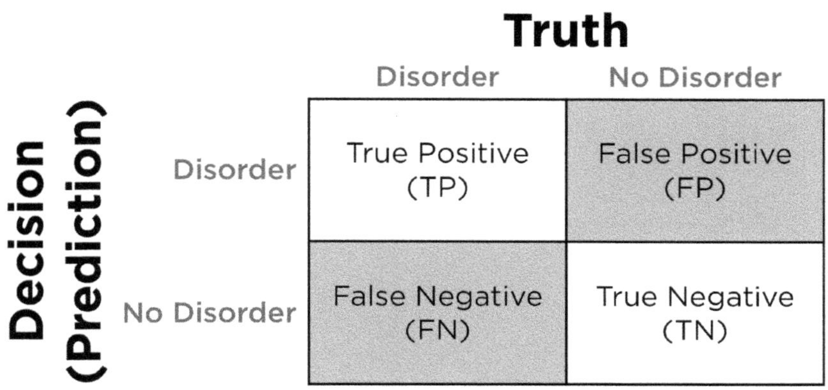

FIGURE 9.25 Confusion Matrix.

9.5.3.1 Number

```
table(mydataSDT$diagnosisFactor, mydataSDT$disorderFactor)
```

```
                        Truth: Disorder Truth: No Disorder
  Decision: Diagnosis                26                 14
  Decision: No Diagnosis             14                 56
```

9.5.3.2 Number with Margins Added

```
addmargins(table(mydataSDT$diagnosisFactor, mydataSDT$disorderFactor))
```

```
                        Truth: Disorder Truth: No Disorder Sum
  Decision: Diagnosis                26                 14  40
```

TABLE 9.2 Estimates of Prediction Accuracy at a Given Cutoff.

Index	Value
cutoff	0.20
True Positives	26.00
True Negatives	56.00
False Positives	14.00
False Negatives	14.00
Selection Rate	0.36
Base Rate	0.36
Percent Accuracy	74.55
Percent Accuracy by Chance	53.72
Percent Accuracy Predicting from the Base Rate	63.64
Relative Improvement over Chance	0.45
Relative Improvement over Predicting from the Base Rate	0.15
Sensitivity	0.65
Specificity	0.80
True Positive Rate	0.65
True Negative Rate	0.80
False Negative Rate	0.35
False Positive Rate	0.20
Hit Rate	0.65
False Alarm Rate	0.20
Positive Predictive Value	0.65
Negative Predictive Rate	0.80
False Discovery Rate	0.35
False Omission Rate	0.20
Youden's J index	0.45
Balanced Accuracy	0.73
F-1 score	0.65
Matthews Correlation Coefficient	0.45
Diagnostic Odds Ratio	7.43
Positive Likelihood Ratio	3.25
Negative Likelihood Ratio	0.44
d-Prime from SDT	1.23
Beta from SDT	1.32
c from SDT	0.23
a from SDT	0.79
b from SDT	1.33
Difference Between Predicted and Observed Value	−0.27
Information Gain	0.15

```
Decision: No Diagnosis              14                  56  70
Sum                                 40                  70 110
```

9.5.3.3 Proportions

```
prop.table(table(mydataSDT$diagnosisFactor, mydataSDT$disorderFactor))
```

```
                         Truth: Disorder Truth: No Disorder
  Decision: Diagnosis             0.2364             0.1273
  Decision: No Diagnosis          0.1273             0.5091
```

9.5.3.4 Proportions with Margins Added

```
addmargins(prop.table(table(
  mydataSDT$diagnosisFactor,
  mydataSDT$disorderFactor)))
```

```
                         Truth: Disorder Truth: No Disorder    Sum
  Decision: Diagnosis             0.2364             0.1273 0.3636
  Decision: No Diagnosis          0.1273             0.5091 0.6364
  Sum                             0.3636             0.6364 1.0000
```

9.5.4 True Positives

True positives (TPs) are instances in which a positive classification (e.g., a disorder present) is correct—that is, the test says that a classification is present, and the classification is present. True positives are also called valid positives (VPs) or hits. Higher values (relative to the same sample size) reflect greater accuracy. The formula for true positives is shown in Equation (9.34):

$$\mathrm{TP} = \mathrm{BR} \times \mathrm{SR} \times N \tag{9.34}$$

```
TPvalue <- length(which(
  mydataSDT$diagnosis == 1 & mydataSDT$disorder == 1))

TPvalue
```

```
[1] 26
```

9.5.5 True Negatives

True negatives (TNs) are instances in which a negative classification (e.g., absence of a disorder) is correct—that is, the test says that a classification is not present, and the classification is actually not present. True negatives are also called valid negatives (VNs) or correct rejections. Higher values (relative to the same sample size) reflect greater accuracy. The formula for true negatives is given in Equation (9.35):

$$\mathrm{TN} = (1 - \mathrm{BR}) \times (1 - \mathrm{SR}) \times N \tag{9.35}$$

```
TNvalue <- length(which(
  mydataSDT$diagnosis == 0 & mydataSDT$disorder == 0))

TNvalue
```

```
[1] 56
```

9.5.6 False Positives

False positives (FPs) are instances in which a positive classification (e.g., a disorder present) is incorrect—that is, the test says that a classification is present, and the classification is not present. False positives are also called false alarms (FAs). Lower values (relative to the same sample size) reflect greater accuracy. The formula for false positives is given in Equation (9.36):

$$\mathrm{FP} = (1 - \mathrm{BR}) \times \mathrm{SR} \times N \tag{9.36}$$

```
FPvalue <- length(which(
  mydataSDT$diagnosis == 1 & mydataSDT$disorder == 0))

FPvalue
```

```
[1] 14
```

9.5.7 False Negatives

False negatives (FNs) are instances in which a negative classification (e.g., absence of a disorder) is incorrect—that is, the test says that a classification is not present, and the classification is present. False negatives are also called misses. Lower values (relative to the same sample size) reflect greater accuracy. The formula for false negatives is shown in Equation (9.37):

$$\mathrm{FN} = \mathrm{BR} \times (1 - \mathrm{SR}) \times N \tag{9.37}$$

```
FNvalue <- length(which(
  mydataSDT$diagnosis == 0 & mydataSDT$disorder == 1))

FNvalue
```

```
[1] 14
```

9.5.8 Sample Size (N)

$$N = \text{TP} + \text{TN} + \text{FP} + \text{FN} \tag{9.38}$$

9.5.9 Selection Ratio

The selection ratio (SR) is the marginal probability of selection, independent of other things: $P(R_i)$. In clinical psychology, the selection ratio is the proportion of people who test positive for the disorder, as in Equation (9.39):

$$\begin{aligned} \text{SR} &= P(R_i) \\ &= \frac{\text{TP} + \text{FP}}{N} \end{aligned} \tag{9.39}$$

9.5.10 Base Rate

The base rate (BR) of a classification is its marginal probability, independent of other things: $P(C_i)$. In clinical psychology, the base rate of a disorder is its prevalence in the population, as in Equation (9.40). Without additional information, the base rate is used as the initial *pretest probability*.

$$\begin{aligned} \text{BR} &= P(C_i) \\ &= \frac{\text{TP} + \text{FN}}{N} \end{aligned} \tag{9.40}$$

9.5.11 Pretest Odds

The pretest odds of a classification can be estimated using the pretest probability (i.e., base rate). To convert a probability to odds, divide the probability by one minus that probability, as in Equation (9.41).

$$\text{pretest odds} = \frac{\text{pretest probability}}{1 - \text{pretest probability}} \tag{9.41}$$

9.5.12 Percent Accuracy

Percent Accuracy is also called overall accuracy. Higher values reflect greater accuracy. The formula for percent accuracy is given in Equation (9.42). Percent accuracy has several problems. First, it treats all errors (FP and FN) as equally important. However, in practice, it is rarely the case that false positives and false negatives are equally important. Second, percent accuracy can be misleading because it is highly influenced by base rates. You can have a high percent accuracy by predicting from the base rate and saying that no one has the characteristic (if the base rate is low) or that everyone has the characteristic (if the base rate is high). Thus, it is also important to consider other aspects of accuracy.

$$\text{Percent Accuracy} = 100\% \times \frac{\text{TP} + \text{TN}}{N} \tag{9.42}$$

9.5.13 Percent Accuracy by Chance

The formula for calculating percent accuracy by chance is given in Equation (9.43).

$$\begin{aligned}\text{Percent Accuracy by Chance} &= 100\% \times [P(\text{TP}) + P(\text{TN})] \\ &= 100\% \times \{(\text{BR} \times \text{SR}) + [(1 - \text{BR}) \times (1 - \text{SR})]\}\end{aligned} \tag{9.43}$$

9.5.14 Percent Accuracy Predicting from the Base Rate

Predicting from the base rate is going with the most likely outcome in every prediction. It is also called "betting from the base rate". If the base rate is less than .50, it would involve predicting that the condition is absent for every case. If the base rate is .50 or above, it would involve predicting that the condition is present for every case. Predicting from the base rate is a special case of percent accuracy by chance when the selection ratio is set to either one (if the base rate $\geq .5$) or zero (if the base rate $< .5$).

9.5.15 Relative Improvement Over Chance

Relative improvement over chance (RIOC) is a prediction's improvement over chance as a proportion of the maximum possible improvement over chance, as described by (Farrington & Loeber, 1989). Higher values reflect greater accuracy. The formula for calculating RIOC is given in Equation (9.44).

$$\begin{aligned}&\text{relative improvement over chance (RIOC)} = \\ &\frac{\text{total correct} - \text{chance correct}}{\text{maximum correct} - \text{chance correct}}\end{aligned} \tag{9.44}$$

9.5.16 Relative Improvement Over Predicting from the Base Rate

Relative improvement over predicting from the base rate is a prediction's improvement over predicting from the base rate as a proportion of the maximum possible improvement over predicting from the base rate. Higher values reflect greater accuracy. The formula for calculating relative improvement over predicting from the base rate is in Equation (9.45).

$$\begin{aligned}&\text{relative improvement over predicting from base rate} = \\ &\frac{\text{total correct} - \text{correct by predicting from base rate}}{\text{maximum correct} - \text{correct by predicting from base rate}}\end{aligned} \tag{9.45}$$

9.5.17 Sensitivity

Sensitivity (SN) is also called true positive rate (TPR), hit rate (HR), or recall. Sensitivity is the conditional probability of a positive test given that the person has the condition: $P(R|C)$. Higher values reflect greater accuracy. The formula for calculating sensitivity is given in Equation (9.46). As described in Section 9.1.2.6.1 and as depicted in Figure 9.26, as the cutoff increases (becomes more conservative), sensitivity decreases. As the cutoff decreases, sensitivity increases.

$$\text{sensitivity (SN)} = P(R|C) = \frac{\text{TP}}{\text{TP} + \text{FN}} = \frac{\text{TP}}{N \times \text{BR}} = 1 - \text{FNR} \quad (9.46)$$

Below, we present sensitivity and specificity at every possible cutoff.

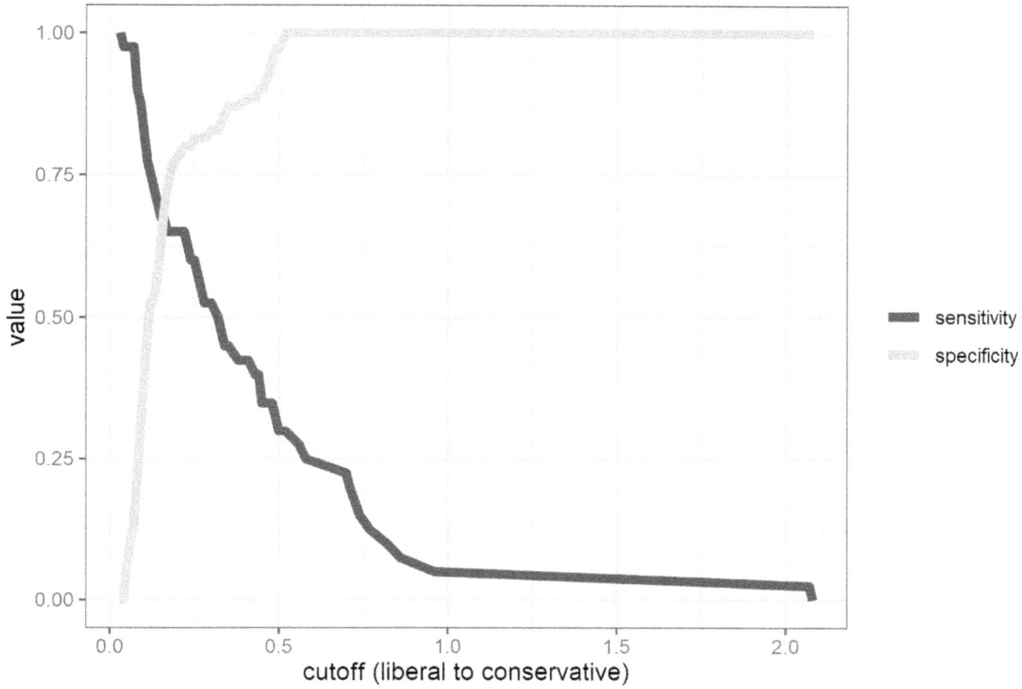

FIGURE 9.26 Sensitivity and Specificity as a Function of the Cutoff.

9.5.18 Specificity

Specificity is also called true negative rate (TNR) or selectivity. Specificity is the conditional probability of a negative test given that the person does not have the condition: $P(\text{not } R|\text{not } C)$. Higher values reflect greater accuracy. The formula for calculating specificity is given in Equation (9.47). As described in Section 9.1.2.6.1 and as depicted in Figure 9.26, as the cutoff increases (becomes more conservative), specificity increases. As the cutoff decreases, specificity decreases.

$$\text{specificity (SP)} = P(\text{not } R|\text{not } C) = \frac{\text{TN}}{\text{TN} + \text{FP}} = \frac{\text{TN}}{N(1 - \text{BR})} = 1 - \text{FPR} \quad (9.47)$$

9.5.19 False Negative Rate

The false negative rate (FNR) is also called the miss rate. The false negative rate is the conditional probability of a negative test given that the person has the condition: $P(\text{not } R|C)$.

Lower values reflect greater accuracy. The formula for calculating false negative rate is given in Equation (9.48).

$$\begin{aligned}\text{false negative rate (FNR)} &= P(\text{not } R|C) \\ &= \frac{\text{FN}}{\text{FN} + \text{TP}} = \frac{\text{FN}}{N \times \text{BR}} = 1 - \text{TPR}\end{aligned} \tag{9.48}$$

9.5.20 False Positive Rate

The false positive rate (FPR) is also called the false alarm rate (FAR) or fall-out. The false positive rate is the conditional probability of a positive test given that the person does not have the condition: $P(R|\text{not } C)$. Lower values reflect greater accuracy. The formula for calculating false positive rate is given in Equation (9.49).

$$\begin{aligned}\text{false positive rate (FPR)} &= P(R|\text{not } C) \\ &= \frac{\text{FP}}{\text{FP} + \text{TN}} = \frac{\text{FP}}{N(1 - \text{BR})} = 1 - \text{TNR}\end{aligned} \tag{9.49}$$

9.5.21 Positive Predictive Value

The positive predictive value (PPV) is also called the positive predictive power (PPP) or precision. Many people confuse sensitivity ($P(R|C)$) with its inverse conditional probability, PPV ($P(C|R)$). PPV is the conditional probability of having the condition given a positive test: $P(C|R)$. Higher values reflect greater accuracy. The formula for calculating positive predictive value is given in Equation (9.50).

PPV can be low even when sensitivity is high because it depends not only on sensitivity, but also on specificity and the base rate. Because PPV depends on the base rate, PPV is not an intrinsic property of a measure. The same measure will have a different PPV in different contexts with different base rates (Treat & Viken, 2023). As described in Section 9.1.2.6.1 and as depicted in Figure 9.27, as the base rate increases, PPV increases. As the base rate decreases, PPV decreases. PPV also differs as a function of the cutoff. As described in Section 9.1.2.6.1 and as depicted in Figure 9.28, as the cutoff increases (becomes more conservative), PPV increases. As the cutoff decreases (becomes more liberal), PPV decreases.

$$\begin{aligned}\text{positive predictive value (PPV)} &= P(C|R) \\ &= \frac{\text{TP}}{\text{TP} + \text{FP}} = \frac{\text{TP}}{N \times \text{SR}} \\ &= \frac{\text{sensitivity} \times \text{BR}}{\text{sensitivity} \times \text{BR} + [(1 - \text{specificity}) \times (1 - \text{BR})]}\end{aligned} \tag{9.50}$$

Below, we present PPV and NPV at every possible base rate given the sensitivity and specificity at the current cutoff.

In the section below, we present PPV and NPV at every possible cutoff.

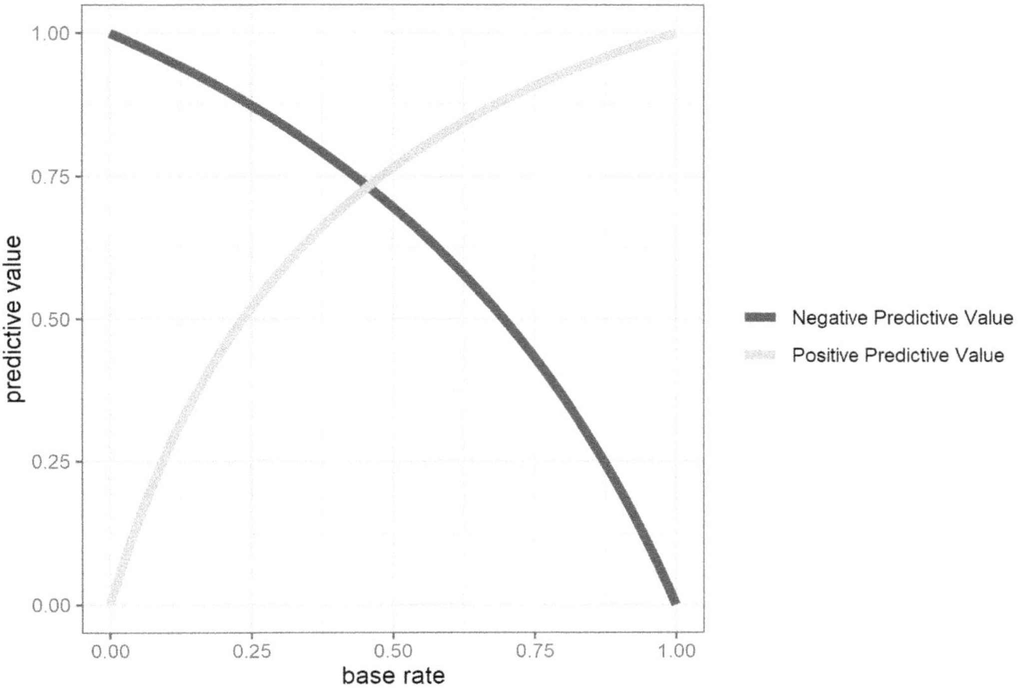

FIGURE 9.27 Positive Predictive Value and Negative Predictive Value as a Function of the Base Rate.

9.5.22 Negative Predictive Value

The negative predictive value (NPV) is also called the negative predictive power (NPP). Many people confuse specificity ($P(\text{not } R|\text{not } C)$) with its inverse conditional probability, NPV ($P(\text{not } C|\text{not } R)$). NPV is the conditional probability of not having the condition given a negative test: $P(\text{not } C|\text{not } R)$. Higher values reflect greater accuracy. The formula for calculating negative predictive value is given in Equation (9.51).

NPV can be low even when specificity is high because it depends not only on specificity, but also on sensitivity and the base rate. Because NPV depends on the base rate, NPV is not an intrinsic property of a measure. The same measure will have a different NPV in different contexts with different base rates (Treat & Viken, 2023). As described in Section 9.1.2.6.1 and as depicted in Figure 9.27, as the base rate increases, NPV decreases. As the base rate decreases, NPV increases. NPV also differs as a function of the cutoff. As described in Section 9.1.2.6.1 and as depicted in Figure 9.28, as the cutoff increases (becomes more conservative), NPV decreases. As the cutoff decreases (becomes more liberal), NPV decreases.

$$
\begin{aligned}
\text{negative predictive value (NPV)} &= P(\text{not } C|\text{not } R) \\
&= \frac{\text{TN}}{\text{TN} + \text{FN}} = \frac{\text{TN}}{N(1 \text{ - SR})} \\
&= \frac{\text{specificity} \times (1 - \text{BR})}{\text{specificity} \times (1 - \text{BR}) + [(1 - \text{sensitivity}) \times \text{BR}]}
\end{aligned}
\tag{9.51}
$$

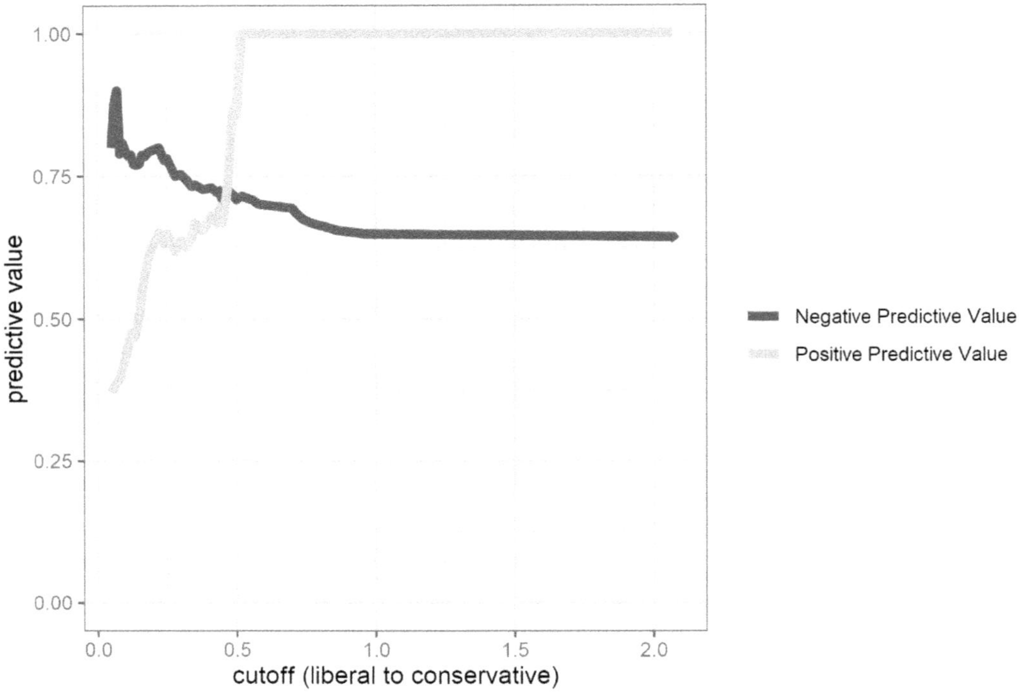

FIGURE 9.28 Positive Predictive Value and Negative Predictive Value as a Function of the Cutoff.

9.5.23 False Discovery Rate

Many people confuse the false positive rate ($P(R|\text{not } C)$) with its inverse conditional probability, the false discovery rate (FDR) ($P(\text{not } C|R)$). The false discovery rate is the conditional probability of not having the condition given a positive test: $P(\text{not } C|R)$. Lower values reflect greater accuracy. The formula for calculating false discovery rate is given in Equation (9.52).

$$\begin{aligned}\text{false discovery rate (FDR)} &= P(\text{not } C|R) \\ &= \frac{\text{FP}}{\text{FP} + \text{TP}} = 1 - \text{PPV}\end{aligned} \tag{9.52}$$

9.5.24 False Omission Rate

Many people confuse the false negative rate ($P(\text{not } R|C)$) with its inverse conditional probability, the false omission rate (FOR) ($P(C|\text{not } R)$). The false omission rate is the conditional probability of having the condition given a negative test: $P(C|\text{not } R)$. Lower values reflect greater accuracy. The formula for calculating false omission rate is given in Equation (9.53).

$$\text{false omission rate (FOR)} = P(C|\text{not } R)$$
$$= \frac{\text{FN}}{\text{FN} + \text{TN}} = 1 - \text{NPV} \tag{9.53}$$

9.5.25 Youden's J Statistic

Youden's J statistic is also called Youden's Index or informedness. Youden's J statistic is the sum of sensitivity and specificity (and subtracting one). Higher values reflect greater accuracy. The formula for calculating Youden's J statistic is given in Equation (9.54).

$$\text{Youden's J statistic} = \text{sensitivity} + \text{specificity} - 1 \tag{9.54}$$

9.5.26 Balanced Accuracy

Balanced accuracy is the average of sensitivity and specificity. Higher values reflect greater accuracy. The formula for calculating balanced accuracy is given in Equation (9.55).

$$\text{balanced accuracy} = \frac{\text{sensitivity} + \text{specificity}}{2} \tag{9.55}$$

9.5.27 F-Score

The F-score combines precision (positive predictive value) and recall (sensitivity), where β indicates how many times more important sensitivity is than the positive predictive value. If sensitivity and the positive predictive value are equally important, $\beta = 1$, and the F-score is called the F_1 score. Higher values reflect greater accuracy. The formula for calculating the F-score is given in Equation (9.56).

$$\begin{aligned} F_\beta &= (1 + \beta^2) \cdot \frac{\text{positive predictive value} \cdot \text{sensitivity}}{(\beta^2 \cdot \text{positive predictive value}) + \text{sensitivity}} \\ &= \frac{(1 + \beta^2) \cdot \text{TP}}{(1 + \beta^2) \cdot \text{TP} + \beta^2 \cdot \text{FN} + \text{FP}} \end{aligned} \tag{9.56}$$

The formula for calculating the F_1 score is given in Equation (9.57).

$$\begin{aligned} F_1 &= \frac{2 \cdot \text{positive predictive value} \cdot \text{sensitivity}}{(\text{positive predictive value}) + \text{sensitivity}} \\ &= \frac{2 \cdot \text{TP}}{2 \cdot \text{TP} + \text{FN} + \text{FP}} \end{aligned} \tag{9.57}$$

9.5.28 Matthews Correlation Coefficient

The Matthews correlation coefficient (MCC) is also called the phi coefficient. It is a correlation coefficient between predicted and observed values from a binary classification. Higher values reflect greater accuracy. The formula for calculating the MCC is given in Equation (9.58).

$$\text{MCC} = \frac{\text{TP} \times \text{TN} - \text{FP} \times \text{FN}}{\sqrt{(\text{TP} + \text{FP})(\text{TP} + \text{FN})(\text{TN} + \text{FP})(\text{TN} + \text{FN})}} \tag{9.58}$$

9.5.29 Diagnostic Odds Ratio

The diagnostic odds ratio is the odds of a positive test among people with the condition relative to the odds of a positive test among people without the condition. Higher values reflect greater accuracy. The formula for calculating the diagnostic odds ratio is given in Equation (9.59).

$$\begin{aligned} \text{diagnostic odds ratio} &= \frac{\text{TP} \times \text{TN}}{\text{FP} \times \text{FN}} \\ &= \frac{\text{sensitivity} \times \text{specificity}}{(1 - \text{sensitivity}) \times (1 - \text{specificity})} \\ &= \frac{\text{PPV} \times \text{NPV}}{(1 - \text{PPV}) \times (1 - \text{NPV})} \\ &= \frac{\text{LR}+}{\text{LR}-} \end{aligned} \tag{9.59}$$

If the predictor is bad, the diagnostic odds ratio could be less than one, and values can go up from there. If the diagnostic odds ratio is greater than 2, we take the odds ratio seriously because we are twice as likely to predict accurately than inaccurately. However, the diagnostic odds ratio ignores/hides base rates. When interpreting the diagnostic odds ratio, it is important to keep in mind the clinical significance, because otherwise it is not very meaningful. Consider a risk factor that has a diagnostic odds ratio of 3 for tuberculosis, i.e., it puts you at 3 times as likely to develop tuberculosis. The prevalence of tuberculosis is relatively low. Assuming the prevalence of tuberculosis is less than 1/10th of 1%, your risk of developing tuberculosis is still very low even if the risk factor (with a diagnostic odds ratio of 3) is present.

9.5.30 Diagnostic Likelihood Ratio

A likelihood ratio is the ratio of two probabilities. It can be used to compare the likelihood of two possibilities. The diagnostic likelihood ratio is an index of the predictive validity of an instrument: it is the ratio of the probability that a test result is correct to the probability that the test result is incorrect. The diagnostic likelihood ratio is also called the risk ratio. There are two types of diagnostic likelihood ratios: the positive likelihood ratio and the negative likelihood ratio.

9.5.30.1 Positive Likelihood Ratio

The positive likelihood ratio (LR+) compares the true positive rate to the false positive rate. Higher values reflect greater accuracy, because it indicates the degree to which a true positive is more likely than a false positive. The formula for calculating the positive likelihood ratio is given in Equation (9.60).

$$\begin{aligned}\text{positive likelihood ratio (LR+)} &= \frac{\text{TPR}}{\text{FPR}} \\ &= \frac{P(R|C)}{P(R|\text{not } C)} \\ &= \frac{P(R|C)}{1 - P(\text{not } R|\text{not } C)} \\ &= \frac{\text{sensitivity}}{1 - \text{specificity}}\end{aligned} \tag{9.60}$$

9.5.30.2 Negative Likelihood Ratio

The negative likelihood ratio (LR-) compares the false negative rate to the true negative rate. Smaller values reflect greater accuracy, because it indicates that a false negative is less likely than a true negative. The formula for calculating the negative likelihood ratio is given in Equation (9.61).

$$\begin{aligned}\text{negative likelihood ratio (LR}-) &= \frac{\text{FNR}}{\text{TNR}} \\ &= \frac{P(\text{not } R|C)}{P(\text{not } R|\text{not } C)} \\ &= \frac{1 - P(R|C)}{P(\text{not } R|\text{not } C)} \\ &= \frac{1 - \text{sensitivity}}{\text{specificity}}\end{aligned} \tag{9.61}$$

9.5.31 Posttest Odds

As presented in Equation (9.16), the posttest (or posterior) odds are equal to the pretest odds multiplied by the likelihood ratio. The posttest odds and posttest probability can be useful to calculate when the pretest probability is different from the pretest probability (or prevalence) of the classification. For instance, you might use a different pretest probability if a test result is already known and you want to know the updated posttest probability after conducting a second test. The formula for calculating posttest odds is given in Equation (9.62).

$$\text{posttest odds} = \text{pretest odds} \times \text{likelihood ratio} \tag{9.62}$$

For calculating the posttest odds of a true positive compared to a false positive, we use the positive likelihood ratio, described later. We would use the negative likelihood ratio if we wanted to calculate the posttest odds of a false negative compared to a true negative.

9.5.32 Posttest Probability

The posttest probability is the probability of having the disorder given a test result. When the base rate is used as the pretest probability, the posttest probability given a positive test is equal to positive predictive value. To convert odds to a probability, divide the odds by one plus the odds, as is shown in Equation (9.63).

$$\text{posttest probability} = \frac{\text{posttest odds}}{1 + \text{posttest odds}} \tag{9.63}$$

```
posttestProbability <- function(
    TP, TN, FP, FN, pretestProb = NULL, SN = NULL, SP = NULL,
    likelihoodRatio = NULL){
  if(!is.null(pretestProb) & !is.null(SN) & !is.null(SP)){
    pretestProbability <- pretestProb
    pretestOdds <- pretestProbability / (1 - pretestProbability)

    likelihoodRatio <- SN/(1 - SP)
  }  else if(!is.null(pretestProb) & !is.null(likelihoodRatio)){
    pretestProbability <- pretestProb
    pretestOdds <- pretestProbability / (1 - pretestProbability)

    likelihoodRatio <- likelihoodRatio
  } else {
    N <- TP + TN + FP + FN
    pretestProbability <- (TP + FN)/N
    pretestOdds <- pretestProbability / (1 - pretestProbability)

    SN <- TP/(TP + FN)
    SP <- TN/(TN + FP)
    likelihoodRatio <- SN/(1 - SP)
  }

  posttestOdds <- pretestOdds * likelihoodRatio
  value <- posttestOdds / (1 + posttestOdds)

  return(value)
}
```

Consider the following example: Assume the base rate of the condition is .03%. We have two tests. Test A has a sensitivity of .95 and a specificity of .80. Test B has a sensitivity of .70 and a specificity of .90. What is the probability of having the condition if a person has a positive test on Test A? Assuming the errors of the two tests are independent, what is the probability of having the condition if the person has a positive test on Test B after having a positive test on Test A?

```
probGivenTestA <- posttestProbability(
  pretestProb = .003,
  SN = .95,
  SP = .80)

probGivenTestAthenB <- posttestProbability(
```

```
  pretestProb = probGivenTestA,
  SN = .70,
  SP = .90)
```

```
probGivenTestA
```

```
[1] 0.01409
```

```
probGivenTestAthenB
```

```
[1] 0.09095
```

The probability of having the condition if a person has a positive test on Test A is 1.4%. The probability of having the condition if the person has a positive test on Test B after having a positive test on Test A is 9.1%.

9.5.33 d' Sensitivity from Signal Detection Theory

d' (d prime) is an index of sensitivity from signal detection theory, as described by Stanislaw & Todorov (1999). Higher values reflect greater accuracy. The formula for calculating d' is given in Equation (9.64).

$$d' = z(\text{hit rate}) - z(\text{false alarm rate}) \tag{9.64}$$

9.5.34 A (Non-Parametric) Sensitivity from Signal Detection Theory

A is a non-parametric index of sensitivity from signal detection theory, as described by Zhang & Mueller (2005). Higher values reflect greater accuracy. The formula for calculating A is given in Equation (9.65).

$$A = \begin{cases} \frac{3}{4} + \frac{H-F}{4} - F(1-H) & \text{if } F \leq 0.5 \leq H; \\ \frac{3}{4} + \frac{H-F}{4} - \frac{F}{4H} & \text{if } F \leq H \leq 0.5; \\ \frac{3}{4} + \frac{H-F}{4} - \frac{1-H}{4(1-F)} & \text{if } 0.5 \leq F \leq H. \end{cases} \tag{9.65}$$

where H is the hit rate and F is the false alarm rate.

9.5.35 β Bias from Signal Detection Theory

β is an index of bias from signal detection theory, as described by Stanislaw & Todorov (1999). Smaller values reflect greater accuracy. The formula for calculating β is given in Equation (9.66).

$$\beta = e^{\left\{\frac{\left[\phi^{-1}(F)\right]^2 - \left[\phi^{-1}(H)\right]}{2}\right\}^2} \tag{9.66}$$

where H is the hit rate, F is the false alarm rate, and ϕ (phi) is a mathematical function that converts a z score to a probability by determining the portion of the normal distribution that lies to the left of the z score.

9.5.36 c Bias from Signal Detection Theory

c is an index of bias from signal detection theory, as described by Stanislaw & Todorov (1999). Smaller values reflect greater accuracy. The formula for calculating c is given in Equation (9.67).

$$c = -\frac{\phi^{-1}(H) + \phi^{-1}(F)}{2} \tag{9.67}$$

where H is the hit rate, F is the false alarm rate, and ϕ (phi) is a mathematical function that converts a z score to a probability by determining the portion of the normal distribution that lies to the left of the z score.

9.5.37 b (Non-Parametric) Bias from Signal Detection Theory

b is a non-parametric index of bias from signal detection theory, as described by Zhang & Mueller (2005). Smaller values reflect greater accuracy. The formula for calculating b is given in Equation (9.68).

$$b = \begin{cases} \frac{5-4H}{1+4F} & \text{if } F \leq 0.5 \leq H; \\ \frac{H^2+H}{H^2+F} & \text{if } F \leq H \leq 0.5; \\ \frac{(1-F)^2+(1-H)}{(1-F)^2+(1-F)} & \text{if } 0.5 \leq F \leq H. \end{cases} \tag{9.68}$$

9.5.38 Mean Difference between Predicted Versus Observed Values

The mean difference between predicted values versus observed values at a given cutoff is an index of miscalibration of predictions at that cutoff. It is called "calibration-in-the-small" (as opposed to calibration-in-the-large, which spans all cutoffs). Values closer to zero reflect greater accuracy. Values above zero indicate that the predicted values are, on average, greater than the observed values. Values below zero indicate that the observed values are, on average, greater than the predicted values.

9.6 Optimal Cutoff Specification

There are two ways to improve diagnostic performance (Swets et al., 2000). One way is to increase the diagnostic accuracy of the assessment. The second way is to increase the utility of the diagnostic decisions that are made, based on where we set the cutoff. The optimal cutoff depends on the differential costs of false positives versus false negatives, as applied in decision theory. When differential costs of false positives versus false negatives cannot be specified, an alternative approach to specifying the optimal cutoff is to use information theory.

9.6.1 Decision Theory

According to the decision theory approach to picking the optimal cutoff, the optimal cutoff depends on the value/importance placed on each of the four decision outcomes [(true positives, true negatives, false positives, false negatives); Treat & Viken (2023)]. Utility is the relative value placed on a specific decision-making outcome (i.e., user-perceived benefit or cost): utilities typically range between zero and one, where a value of zero represents the least desired outcome, and a value of one indicates the most desired outcome. According to the decision theory approach, the optimal cutoff is the cutoff with the highest overall utility.

9.6.1.1 Overall Utility of a Specific Cutoff Value

The overall utility of a specific cutoff value is a utilities-weighted sum of the probabilities of the four decision-making outcomes (hits, misses, correct rejections, false alarms). That is, overall utility is the sum of the product of the probability of a particular outcome (e.g., BR × TP rate) and the utility of that outcome (e.g., how much we value TPs relative to other outcomes). Higher values reflect greater utility, so you would pick the cutoff with the highest overall utility. The formula for calculating overall utility is in Equation (9.69):

$$\begin{aligned} U_{\text{overall}} = {} & (\text{BR})(\text{HR})(U_{\text{H}}) \\ & + (\text{BR})(1 - \text{HR})(U_{\text{M}}) \\ & + (1 - \text{BR})(\text{FAR})(U_{\text{FA}}) \\ & + (1 - \text{BR})(1 - \text{FAR})(U_{\text{CR}}) \end{aligned} \tag{9.69}$$

where BR = base rate, HR = hit rate (true positive rate), FAR = false alarm rate (false positive rate), U_{H} = utility of hits (true positives), U_{M} = utility of misses (false negatives), U_{FA} = utility of false alarms (false positives), U_{CR} = utility of correct rejections (true negatives).

9.6.1.2 Utility Ratio

The utility ratio is the user-perceived relative importance of decisions about negative versus positive cases. If the utility ratio value is one, it indicates that identifying negative cases and positive cases is equally important. Values above one indicate greater relative importance of identifying negative cases than positive cases. Values below one indicate greater relative importance of identifying positive cases than negative cases. Values of one indicate that you are maximizing percent accuracy. The formula for calculating the utility ratio is given in Equation (9.70):

$$\text{Utility Ratio} = \frac{U_{\text{CR}} - U_{\text{FA}}}{U_{\text{H}} - U_{\text{M}}} \tag{9.70}$$

where U_{H} = utility of hits (true positives), U_{M} = utility of misses (false negatives), U_{FA} = utility of false alarms (false positives), U_{CR} = utility of correct rejections (true negatives).

Decision theory has key advantages, because it identifies the cutoff that would help you best achieve the goals/purpose of the assessment. However, it can be challenging to specify the relative costs of errors. If you cannot decide values for outcomes (relative importance between FP and FN), you can use information theory to identify the optimal cutoff.

9.6.2 Information Theory

When the user does not differentially weigh the value/importance of the four decision-making outcomes (hits, misses, correct rejections, false alarms), the information theory approach can be useful for specifying the optimal cutoff. According to the information theory approach, the optimal cutoff is the cutoff that provides the greatest information gain (Treat & Viken, 2023).

9.6.2.1 Information Gain

Information gain (I_{gain}) is the reduction of uncertainty about the true classification of a case that results from administering an assessment or prediction measure (Treat & Viken, 2023). Greater values reflect greater reduction of uncertainty, so the optimal cutoff can be specified as the cutoff with the highest information gain.

The formula from Treat & Viken (2023) for calculating information gain is given in Equation (9.71):

$$
\begin{aligned}
I_{\text{gain}} = {} & (\text{BR})(\text{HR})\left[\log_2\left(\frac{\text{HR}}{G}\right)\right] \\
& + (\text{BR})(1-\text{HR})\left[\log_2\left(\frac{1-\text{HR}}{1-G}\right)\right] \\
& + (1-\text{BR})(\text{FAR})\left[\log_2\left(\frac{\text{FAR}}{G}\right)\right] \\
& + (1-\text{BR})(1-FAR)\left[\log_2\left(\frac{1-\text{FAR}}{1-G}\right)\right]
\end{aligned}
\tag{9.71}
$$

where BR = base rate, HR = hit rate (true positive rate), FAR = false alarm rate (false positive rate), G = selection ratio = BR(HR) + (1 − BR)(FAR), as reported in Somoza et al. (1989) (see below).

9.6.2.1.1 Effect of base rate

Information gain depends on the base rate (Treat & Viken, 2023), as depicted in Figure 9.29. The maximum reduction of uncertainty (i.e., greatest information) occurs when the base rate is 0.5. A base rate tells us little a priori about the condition if the probability of the condition is 50/50, so the measure can provide more benefit. If the base rate is 0.3 or 0.7, we can do better than going with the base rate. If the base rate is 0.9 or 0.1, it is difficult for our measure to do better than going with the base rate. If the base rate is 0.05 of 0.95 (or more extreme), it is likely that our measure will do almost nothing in terms of information gain.

9.7 Accuracy at Every Possible Cutoff

9.7.1 Specify Utility of Each Outcome

```
utilityHits <- 1
utilityMisses <- 0
utilityCorrectRejections <- 0.75
utilityFalseAlarms <- 0.25
```

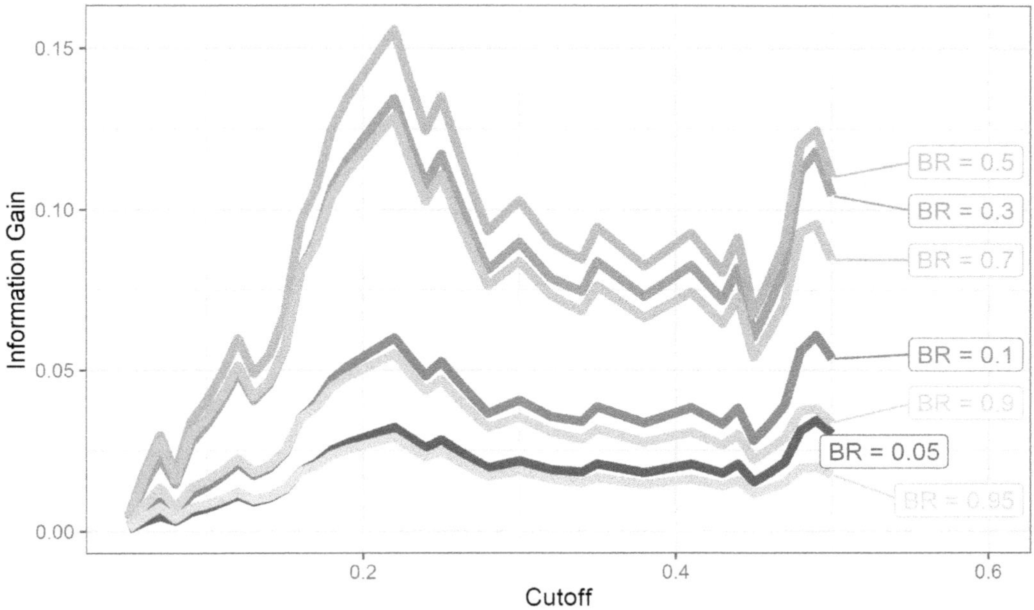

FIGURE 9.29 Information Gain as a Function of the Base Rate (BR).

9.7.2 Calculate Accuracy

The `petersenlab` package (Petersen, 2024) contains an R function that estimates the prediction accuracy at every possible cutoff.

```
accuracyAtEachCutoff(
  predicted = mydataSDT$testScore,
  actual = mydataSDT$disorder,
  UH = utilityHits,
  UM = utilityMisses,
  UCR = utilityCorrectRejections,
  UFA = utilityFalseAlarms)
```

9.7.3 Cutoff That Optimizes Each of Various Accuracy Estimates

The `petersenlab` package (Petersen, 2024) contains an R function that identifies the cutoff that optimizes each of various accuracy estimates.

```
optimalCutoff(
  predicted = mydataSDT$testScore,
  actual = mydataSDT$disorder,
  UH = utilityHits,
  UM = utilityMisses,
  UCR = utilityCorrectRejections,
  UFA = utilityFalseAlarms)
```

TABLE 9.3 Example Data of Predictor (x1) and Outcome (y) Used for Regression Model.

y	x1
7	1
13	2
29	7
10	2

TABLE 9.4 Example Data of Predictors (x1 and x2) and Outcome (y) Used for Regression Model.

y	x1	x2
7	1	3
13	2	5
29	7	1
10	2	2

9.8 Regression for Prediction of Continuous Outcomes

When predicting a continuous outcome, regression is particularly relevant (or multiple regression, when dealing with multiple predictors). Regression takes the general form in Equation (9.72):

$$y = b_0 + b_1 \cdot x_1 + e \tag{9.72}$$

where y is the outcome, b_0 is the intercept, b_1 is the slope of the association between the predictor (x_1) and outcome, and e is the error term.

9.9 Pseudo-Prediction

Consider the following example where you have one predictor and one outcome, as shown in Table 9.3.

Using the data, the best fitting regression model is: $y = 3.98 + 3.59 \cdot x_1$. In this example, the R^2 is 0.98. The equation is not a perfect prediction, but with a single predictor, it captures the majority of the variance in the outcome.

Now consider the following example where you add a second predictor to the data above, as shown in Table 9.4.

With the second predictor, the best fitting regression model is: $y = 0.00 + 4.00 \cdot x_1 + 1.00 \cdot x_2$. In this example, the R^2 is 1.00. The equation with the second predictor provides a perfect prediction of the outcome.

TABLE 9.5 Example Data of Predictors (x1 and x2) and Outcome (y) Used for Regression Model.

y	x1	x2
9	2.0	4
11	3.0	6
17	4.0	8
3	1.0	2
21	5.0	10
13	3.5	7

Providing perfect prediction with the right set of predictors is the dream of multiple regression. So, in psychology, we often add predictors to incrementally improve prediction. Knowing how much variance would be accounted for by random chance follows Equation (9.73):

$$E(R^2) = \frac{K}{n-1} \tag{9.73}$$

where $E(R^2)$ is the expected value of R^2 (the proportion of variance explained), K is the number of predictors, and n is the sample size. The formula demonstrates that the more predictors in the regression model, the more variance will be accounted for by chance. With many predictors and a small sample, you can account for a large share of the variance merely by chance—this would be an example of pseudo-prediction.

As an example, consider that we have 13 predictors to predict behavior problems for 43 children. Assume that, with 13 predictors, we explain 38% of the variance ($R^2 = .38; r = .62$). Explaining more than 20–30% of the variance can be a big deal in psychology. We explained a lot of the variance in the outcome, but it is important to consider how much variance could have been explained by random chance: $E(R^2) = \frac{K}{n-1} = \frac{13}{43-1} = .31$. We expect to explain 31% of the variance, by chance, in the outcome. So, 82% of the variance explained was likely spurious. As the sample size increases, the spuriousness decreases. Adjusted R^2 accounts for the number of predictors in the model, based on how much would be expected to be accounted for by chance. But adjusted R^2 also has its problems.

9.9.1 Multicollinearity

Multicollinearity occurs when two or more predictors in a regression model are highly correlated. The problem is that it makes it challenging to estimate the regression coefficients accurately.

Multicollinearity in multiple regression is depicted conceptually in Figure 9.30.

Consider the following example where you have two predictors and one outcome, as shown in Table 9.5.

The second measure is not very good—it is exactly twice the value of the first measure. This means that there are different prediction equation possibilities that are equally good—see Equations in (9.74):

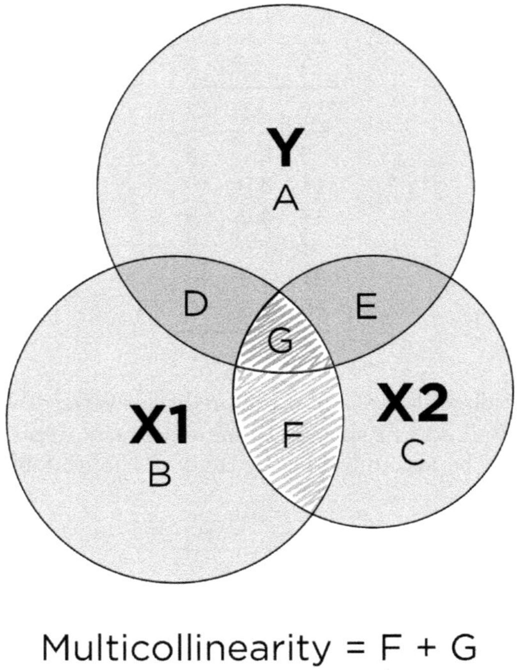

FIGURE 9.30 Conceptual Depiction of Multicollinearity in Multiple Regression.

$$\begin{aligned} 2x_2 &= y \\ 0x_1 + 2x_2 &= y \\ 4x_1 &= y \\ 4x_1 + 0x_2 &= y \\ 2x_1 + 1x_2 &= y \\ 5x_1 - 0.5x_2 &= y \\ ... &= y \end{aligned} \tag{9.74}$$

Then, what are the regression coefficients? We do not know, and we could come up with arbitrary estimates with an enormous standard error around each estimate. Any predictors that have a correlation above $\sim r = .30$ with each other could have an impact on the confidence interval of the regression coefficient. As the correlations among the predictors increase, the chance of getting an arbitrary answer increases, sometimes called "bouncing betas." So, it is important to examine a correlation matrix of the predictors before putting them in the same regression model. You can also examine indices such as variance inflation factor (VIF).

Generalized VIF (GVIF) values are estimated below using the `car` package (Fox et al., 2022) and are shown in Table 9.6.

```
set.seed(52242)
mydataSDT$collinearPredictor <- mydataSDT$ndka +
```

TABLE 9.6 Generalized VIF (GVIF) Estimates.

	GVIF	Df	GVIF^(1/(2*Df))
ndka	6.300	1	2.510
gender	1.150	1	1.072
age	1.128	1	1.062
wfns	1.208	4	1.024
collinearPredictor	6.405	1	2.531

```
rnorm(nrow(mydataSDT), sd = 20)

collinearRegression_model <- lm(
  s100b ~ ndka + gender + age + wfns + collinearPredictor,
  data = mydataSDT)
```

```
vif(collinearRegression_model)
```

To address multicollinearity, you can drop a redundant predictor or you can also use principal component analysis or factor analysis of the predictors to reduce the predictors down to a smaller number of meaningful predictors. For a meaningful answer in a regression framework that is precise and confident, you need a low level of intercorrelation among predictors, unless you have a very large sample size.

However, multicollinearity does not bias parameter estimates (i.e., multicollinearity does not lead to mean error). Instead, multicollinearity increases the uncertainty (i.e., standard errors) around the parameter estimates[3], which makes it more challenging to detect an effect as statistically significant. Some forms of multicollinearity are ignorable[4], including when the multicollinearity is among (a) the control variables rather than the variables of interest, (b) the powers (e.g., quadratic term) or products (e.g., interaction term) of other variables, or (c) dummy-coded categories. Ultimately, it is important to examine the question of interest, even if that means inclusion of predictors that are inter-correlated in a regression model. However, it would not make sense to include two predictors that are perfectly correlated, because they are redundant.

9.10 Ways to Improve Prediction Accuracy

On the whole, experts' predictions are inaccurate. Experts' predictions from many different domains tend to be inaccurate, including political scientists (Tetlock, 2017), physicians (Koehler et al., 2002), clinical psychologists (Oskamp, 1965), stock market traders and corporate financial officers (Skala, 2008), seismologists' predictions of earthquakes (Hough, 2016), economists' predictions about the economy (Makridakis et al., 2009), lawyers (Koehler et al., 2002), and business managers (Russo & Schoemaker, 1992). The most common pattern of experts' predictions is that they show overextremity, that is, their predictions

[3]https://janhove.github.io/analysis/2019/09/11/collinearity archived at https://perma.cc/DJ7L-TCUK
[4]https://statisticalhorizons.com/multicollinearity/ archived at https://perma.cc/2JV5-2QEZ

have probability judgments that tend to be too extreme, as described in Section 9.4.3. Overextremity of experts' predictions likely reflects over-confidence. The degree of confidence of a person's predictions is often not a good indicator of the accuracy of their predictions [and confidence and prediction accuracy are sometimes inversely associated; Silver (2012)]. Cognitive biases including the anchoring bias (Tversky & Kahneman, 1974), the confirmation bias (Hoch, 1985; Koriat et al., 1980), and base rate neglect (Eddy, 1982; Koehler et al., 2002) could contribute to over-confidence of predictions. Poorly calibrated predictions are especially likely when the base rate is very low (e.g., suicide), as is often the case in clinical psychology, or when the base rate is very high (Koehler et al., 2002).

Nevertheless, there are some domains that have shown greater predictive accuracy, from which we may learn what practices may lead to greater accuracy. For instance, experts have shown stronger predictive accuracy in weather forecasting (Murphy & Winkler, 1984), horse race betting (Johnson & Bruce, 2001), and playing the card game of bridge (Keren, 1987), but see Koehler et al. (2002) for exceptions.

Here are some potential ways to improve the accuracy (and honesty) of predictions and judgments:

- Provide appropriate anchoring of your predictions to the base rate of the phenomenon you are predicting. To the extent that the base rate of the event you are predicting is low, more extreme evidence should be necessary to consistently and accurately predict that the event will occur. Applying Bayes' theorem and Bayesian approaches can help you appropriately weigh base rate and evidence.
- Include multiple predictors, ideally from different measures and measurement methods. Include the predictors with the strongest validity based on theory of the causal process and based on criterion-related validity.
- When possible, aggregate multiple perspectives of predictions, especially predictions made independently (from different people/methods/etc.). The "wisdom of the crowd" is often more accurate than individuals' predictions, including predictions by so-called "experts" (Silver, 2012).
- A goal of prediction is to capture as much signal as possible and as little noise (error) as possible (Silver, 2012). Parsimony (i.e., not having too many predictors) can help reduce the amount of error variance captured by the prediction model. However, to accurately model complex systems like human behavior, the brain, etc., complex models may be necessary. Nevertheless, strong theory of the causal processes and dynamics may be necessary to develop accurate complex models.
- Although incorporating theory can be helpful, provide more weight to empiricism than to theory, until our theories and measures are stronger. Ideally, we would use theory to design a model that mirrors the causal system, with accurate measures of each process in the system, so we could make accurate predictions. However, as described in Section 4.3.1.3.3, our psychological theories of the causal processes that influence outcomes are not yet very strong. Until we have stronger theories that specify the causal process for a given outcome, and until we have accurate measures of those causal processes, actuarial approaches are likely to be most accurate, as discussed in Chapter 10. At the same time, keep in mind that measures in psychology, and their resulting data, are often noisy. As a result, theoretically (conceptually) informed empirical approaches may lead to more accuracy than empiricism alone.
- Use an empirically validated and cross-validated statistical algorithm to combine information from the predictors in a formalized way. Give each predictor appropriate weight in the statistical algorithm, according to its strength of association with the outcome. Use measures with strong reliability and validity for assessing these processes to be used in the

algorithm. Cross-validation will help reduce the likelihood that your model is fitting to noise and will maximize the likelihood that the model predicts accurately when applied to new data (i.e., the model's predictions accurately generalize), as described in Section 10.4.

- When presenting your predictions, acknowledge what you do not know.
- Express your predictions in terms of probabilistic estimates and present the uncertainty in your predictions with confidence intervals [even though bolder, more extreme predictions tend to receive stronger television ratings; Silver (2012)].
- Qualify your predictions by identifying and noting counter-examples that would not be well fit by your prediction model, such as extreme cases, edge cases, and "broken leg" (Meehl, 1957) cases.
- Provide clear, consistent, and timely feedback on the outcomes of the predictions to the people making the predictions (Bolger & Önkal-Atay, 2004).
- Be self-critical about your predictions. Update your judgments based on their accuracy, rather than trying to confirm your beliefs (Atanasov et al., 2020).
- In addition to considering the accuracy of the prediction, consider the quality of the prediction *process*, especially when random chance is involved to a degree (such as in poker) (Silver, 2012).
- Work to identify and mitigate potential blindspots; be aware of cognitive biases, such as confirmation bias and base rate neglect.

9.11 Conclusion

Human behavior is challenging to predict. People commonly make cognitive pseudo-prediction errors, such as the confusion of inverse probabilities. People also tend to ignore base rates when making predictions. When the base rate of a behavior is very low or very high, you can be highly accurate in predicting the behavior by predicting from the base rate. Thus, you cannot judge how accurate your prediction is until you know how accurate your predictions would be by random chance. Moreover, maximizing percent accuracy may not be the ultimate goal because different errors have different costs. Though there are many types of accuracy, there are two broad types: discrimination and calibration—and they are orthogonal. Discrimination accuracy is frequently evaluated with the area under the receiver operating characteristic curve, or with sensitivity and specificity, or standardized regression coefficients. Calibration accuracy is frequently evaluated graphically and with various indices. Sensitivity and specificity depend on the cutoff. Therefore, the optimal cutoff depends on the purposes of the assessment and how much one weights the various costs of the different types of errors: false negatives and false positives. It is important to evaluate both discrimination and calibration when evaluating prediction accuracy.

9.12 Suggested Readings

Steyerberg et al. (2010); Meehl & Rosen (1955); Treat & Viken (2023); Wiggins (1973)

10

Clinical Judgment Versus Algorithmic Prediction

10.1 Approaches to Prediction

There are two primary approaches to prediction: human (i.e., clinical) judgment and the actuarial (i.e., statistical) method.

10.1.1 Human/Clinical Judgment

Using the clinical judgment method of prediction, all gathered information is collected and formulated into a diagnosis or prediction in the clinician's mind. The clinician selects, measures, and combines risk factors and produces risk estimate solely according to clinical experience and judgment.

10.1.2 Actuarial/Statistical Method

In the actuarial or statistical method of prediction (i.e., statistical prediction rules), information is gathered and combined systematically in an evidence-based statistical prediction formula, and established cutoffs are used. The method is based on equations and data, so both are needed.

An example of a statistical method of prediction is the Violence Risk Appraisal Guide (Rice et al., 2013). The Violence Risk Appraisal Guide is used in an attempt to predict violence and is used for parole decisions. For instance, the equation might be something like Equation (10.1):

$$\text{Violence risk} = \beta \cdot \text{conduct disorder} + \beta \cdot \text{substance use} + \beta \cdot \text{suspended from school} + \beta \cdot \text{childhood aggression} + \ldots \tag{10.1}$$

Then, based on their score and the established cutoffs, a person is given a "low risk", "medium risk", or "high risk" designation.

10.1.3 Combining Human Judgment and Statistical Algorithms

There are numerous ways in which humans and statistical algorithms could be involved. On one extreme, humans make all judgments (consistent with the clinical judgment approach). On the other extreme, although humans may be involved in data collection, a statistical formula makes all decisions based on the input data, consistent with an actuarial approach. However, the clinical judgment and actuarial approaches can be combined in a hybrid way (J. Dana & Thomas, 2006). For example, to save time and money, a clinician might use an actuarial approach in all cases, but might only use a clinical approach when the actuarial approach gives a "positive" test. Or, the clinician might use both human judgment and an actuarial approach independently to see whether they agree. That is, the clinician may make a prediction based on their judgment and might also generate a prediction from an actuarial approach.

The challenge is what to do when the human and the algorithm disagree. Hypothetically, humans reviewing and adjusting the results from the statistical algorithm could lead to more accurate predictions. However, human input also could lead to the possibility or exacerbation of biased predictions. In general, with very few exceptions, actuarial approaches are as accurate or more accurate than clinical judgment (Ægisdóttir et al., 2006; Baird & Wagner, 2000; Dawes et al., 1989; Grove et al., 2000; Grove & Meehl, 1996). Moreover, the superiority of actuarial approaches to clinical judgment tends to hold even when the clinician is given more information than the actuarial approach (Dawes et al., 1989). Allowing clinicians to override actuarial predictions consistently leads to lower predictive accuracy (Garb & Wood, 2019).

In general, validity tends to increase with greater structure (e.g., structured or semi-structured interviews as opposed to free-flowing, unstructured interviews), in terms of administration, responses, scoring, interpretation, etc. Unstructured interviews are susceptible to confirmatory bias, such as exploring only the diagnoses that confirm the clinician's hypotheses rather than attempting to explore diagnoses that disconfirm the clinician's hypotheses, which leads to fewer diagnoses. Unstructured interviews are also susceptible to bias relating to race, gender, class, etc. (Garb, 1997, 2005).

There is sometimes a misconception that formulas cannot account for qualitative information. However, that is not true. Qualitative information can be scored or coded to be quantified so that it can be included in statistical formulas. That said, the quality of predictions rests on the quality and relevance of the assessment information for the particular prediction/judgment decision. If the assessment data are lousy, it is unlikely that a statistical algorithm (or a human for that matter) will make an accurate prediction: "Garbage in, garbage out". A statistical formula cannot rescue inaccurate assessment data.

10.2 Errors in Clinical Judgment

Clinical judgment is naturally subject to errors. Below, we describe a few errors to which clinical judgment seems particularly prone.

When operating freely, clinicians tend to overestimate exceptions to the established rules (i.e., the broken leg syndrome). Meehl (1957) acknowledged that there may be some situations where it is glaringly obvious that the statistical formula would be incorrect because it fails to account for an important factor. He called these special cases "broken leg" cases, in which the human should deviate from the formula (i.e., broken leg countervailing). The example goes like this:

> If a sociologist were predicting whether Professor X would go to the movies on a certain night, he might have an equation involving age, academic specialty, and introversion score. The equation might yield a probability of .90 that Professor X goes to the movie tonight. But if the family doctor announced that Professor X had just broken his leg, no sensible sociologist would stick

> with the equation. Why didn't the factor of 'broken leg' appear in the formula? Because broken legs are very rare, and in the sociologist's entire sample of 500 criterion cases plus 250 cross-validating cases, he did not come upon a single instance of it. He uses the broken leg datum confidently, because 'broken leg' is a subclass of a larger class we may crudely denote as 'relatively immobilizing illness or injury,' and movie-attending is a subclass of a larger class of 'actions requiring moderate mobility'. (Meehl, 1957, pp. 269–270)

However, people too often think that cases where they disagree with the statistical algorithm are broken leg cases. People too often think their case is an exception to the rule. As a result, they too often change the result of the statistical algorithm and are more likely to be wrong than right in doing so. Because actuarial methods are based on actual population levels (i.e., base rates), unique exceptions are not overestimated.

Actuarial predictions are perfectly reliable—they will always return the same conclusion given an identical set of data. The human judge is likely to both disagree with others and with themselves given the same set of symptoms.

A clinician's decision is likely to be influenced by past experiences, and given the sample of humanity that the clinician is exposed to, the clinician is likely (based on prior experience) to overestimate the likelihood of occurrence of infrequent phenomena. Actuarial methods are based on objective algorithms, and past personal experience and personal biases do not factor into any decisions. Clinicians give weight to less relevant information, and often give too much weight to singular variables (e.g., Graduate Record Examination scores). Actuarial formulas do a better job of focusing on relevant variables. Computers are good at factoring in base rates, inverse conditional probabilities, etc. Humans ignore base rates (base rate neglect), and tend to show confusion of the inverse.

Computers are better at accurately weighing risk factors and calculating unbiased risk estimates. In an actuarial formula, the relevant risk factors are weighted according to their predictive power. This stands in contrast to the Diagnostic and Statistical Manual of Mental Disorders (DSM), in which each symptom is equally weighted.

Humans are typically given no feedback on their judgments. To improve accuracy of judgments, it is important for feedback to be clear, consistent, and timely. It is especially unlikely for feedback in clinical psychology to be timely because we will have to wait a long time to see the outcomes of predictions.

Clinicians are susceptible to representative schema biases (Dawes, 1986). Clinicians are exposed to a skewed sample of humanity, and they make judgments based on a prototype from their (biased) experiences. This is known as the representativeness heuristic. Different clinicians may have different prototypes, leading to lower inter-rater reliability.

10.3 Humans Versus Computers

10.3.1 Advantages of Computers

Here are some advantages of computers over humans:

- Computers can process lots of information simultaneously. So can humans. But computers can do that to an even greater degree.
- Computers are faster at making calculations.
- Computations by computers are error-free (as long as the computations are programmed correctly).
- Computers' judgments will not be biased by fatigue or emotional responses.
- Computers' judgments will tend not to be biased in the way that humans' cognitive biases are, such as with anchoring bias, representativeness bias, confirmation bias, or recency bias. Computers are less likely to be over-confident in their judgments.
- Computers can more accurately weight the set of predictors based on large data sets. Humans tend to give too much weight to singular predictors.

10.3.2 Advantages of Humans

Computers are bad at some things too. Here are some advantages of humans over computers (as of now):

- Humans can be better at identifying patterns in data (but also can mistakenly identify patterns where there are none).
- Humans can be flexible and take a different approach if a given approach is not working.
- Humans are better at tasks requiring creativity and imagination, such as developing theories that explain phenomena.
- Humans have the ability to reason, which is especially important when dealing with complex, abstract, or open-ended problems, or problems that have not been faced before (or for which we have insufficient data).
- Humans are better able to learn.
- Humans are better at holistic, gestalt processing, including facial and linguistic processing.

There *may* be situations in which a clinical judgment would do better than an actuarial judgment. One situation where clinical judgment would be important is when no actuarial method exists for the judgment or prediction. For instance, when no actuarial method exists for the diagnosis or disorder (e.g., suicide), it is up to the clinical judge. However, we could collect data on the outcomes or on clinicians' judgments to develop an actuarial method that will be more reliable than the clinicians' judgments. That is, an actuarial method developed based on clinicians' judgments will be more accurate than clinicians' judgments. In other words, we do not necessarily need clients' outcome data to develop an actuarial method. We could use the client's data as predictors of the clinicians' judgments to develop a structured approach to prediction that weighs factors similarly to clinicians, but with more reliable predictions.

Another situation in which clinical judgment could outperform a statistical algorithm is in true "broken leg" cases, e.g., important and rare events (edge cases) that are not yet accounted for by the algorithm.

Another situation in which clinical judgment could be preferable is if advanced, complex theories exist. Computers have a difficult time adhering to complex theories, so clinicians may be better suited. However, we do not have any of these complex theories in psychology that are accurate. We would need strong theory informed by data regarding causal influences, and accurate measures to assess them. If theories alone were true and could explain everything, the psychoanalytic tradition would give us all the answers, as depicted in Figure 10.1. However, no theories in psychology are that good. Nevertheless, predictive accuracy can be improved when considering theory (Garb & Wood, 2019; Silver, 2012).

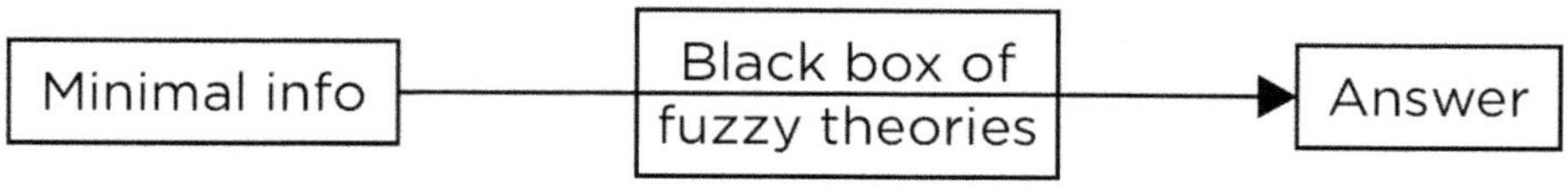

FIGURE 10.1 Conceptual Depiction of the Psychoanalytic Tradition.

If the diagnosis/prediction requires complex configural relations that a computer will have a difficult time replicating, a clinician's judgment may be preferred. Although the likelihood that the clinician can accurately work through these complex relations is theoretically possible, it is highly unlikely. Holistic pattern recognition (such as language and faces) tends to be better by humans than computers. But computers are getting better with holistic pattern recognition through machine learning. An example of a simple decision (as opposed to a complex decision) would be whether to provide treatment A (e.g., cognitive behavior therapy) or treatment B (e.g., medication) for someone who shows melancholy.

In sum, the clinician seeks to integrate all information to make a decision, but is biased.

10.3.3 Comparison of Evidence

Hundreds of studies have examined clinical versus actuarial prediction methods across many disciplines. Findings consistently show that actuarial methods are as accurate or more accurate than clinical prediction methods. "There is no controversy in social science that shows such a large body of qualitatively diverse studies coming out so uniformly... as this one" (Meehl, 1986, pp. 373–374).

Actuarial methods are particularly valuable for criterion-referenced assessment tasks, in which the aim is to predict specific events or outcomes (Garb & Wood, 2019). For instance, actuarial methods have shown promise in predicting violence, criminal recidivism, psychosis onset, course of mental disorders, treatment selection, treatment failure, suicide attempts, and suicide (Garb & Wood, 2019). Psychometric methods of scale construction such as factor analysis may be preferred to statistical prediction rules for norm-referenced assessment tasks such as describing personality and psychopathology (Garb & Wood, 2019).

Moreover, actuarial methods are explicit; they can be transparent and lead to informed scientific criticism to improve them. By contrast, clinical judgment methods are not typically transparent; clinical judgment relies on mental processes that are often difficult to specify.

10.4 Accuracy of Different Statistical Models

It is important to evaluate the accuracy of different types of statistical models to provide guidance on which types of models may be most accurate for a given prediction problem. Simpler statistical formulas are more likely to generalize to new samples than complex statistical models due to model *over-fitting*. As described in Section 4.3.1.3.3.3, over-fitting occurs when the statistical model accounts for error variance (an overly specific prediction), which will not generalize to future samples.

Youngstrom et al. (2018) discussed the benefits of the probability nomogram. The probability nomogram combines the risk ratio with the base rate (according to Bayes' theorem) to generate a prediction. The risk ratio (diagnostic likelihood ratio) is an index of the predictive validity of an instrument: it is the ratio of the probability that a test result is correct to the probability that the test result is incorrect. There are two types of diagnostic likelihood ratios: the positive likelihood ratio and the negative likelihood ratio. As described in Equation (9.60), the positive likelihood ratio is the probability that a person with the disease tested positive for the disease (true positive rate) divided by the probability that a person without the disease tested positive for the disease (false positive rate). As described in Equation (9.61), the negative likelihood ratio is the probability that a person with the disease tested negative for the disease (false negative rate) divided by the probability that a person without the disease tested negative for the disease (true negative rate). Using a probability nomogram, you start with the base rate, then plot the diagnostic likelihood ratio corresponding to a second source of information (e.g., positive test), then connect the base rate (pretest probability) to the posttest probability through the likelihood ratio. These approaches are described in greater detail in Section 12.5.

Youngstrom et al. (2018) ordered actuarial approaches to diagnostic classification from less to more complex:

- Predicting from the base rate
- Take the best
- The probability nomogram
- Naïve Bayesian algorithms
- Logistic regression with one predictor
- Logistic regression with multiple predictors
- Least absolute shrinkage and selection option (LASSO)

As described in Section 9.1.2.4, predicting from the base rate is selecting the most likely outcome in every case. "Take the best" refers to focusing on the single variable with the largest validity coefficient, and making a decision based on it (based on some threshold). The probability nomogram combines the base rate (prior probability) with the information offered by an assessment finding to revise the probability. Naïve Bayesian algorithms use the probability nomogram with multiple assessment findings. Basically, you continue to calculate a new posttest probability based on each assessment finding, revising the pretest probability for the next assessment finding based on the posttest probability of the last assessment finding. However, this approach assumes that all predictors are uncorrelated, which is probably not true in practice.

Logistic regression is useful for classification problems because it deals with a dichotomous dependent variable, but one could extrapolate it to a continuous dependent variable with multiple regression. The effect size from logistic regression is equivalent to receiver operating characteristic (ROC) curve analysis. Logistic regression with multiple predictors combines multiple predictors into one regression model. Including multiple predictors in the same model optimizes the weights of multiple predictors, but it is important for predictors not to be collinear.

LASSO is a form of regression that can handle multiple predictors (like multiple regression). However, it can handle more predictors than multiple regression. For instance, LASSO can accommodate situations where there are more predictors than there are participants. Moreover, unlike multiple regression, it can handle collinear predictors. LASSO uses internal cross-validation to avoid over-fitting.

Youngstrom et al. (2018) found that model complexity improves accuracy but only to a point; some of the simpler models (Naïve Bayesian and Logistic regression) did just as well and in some cases better than LASSO models in classifying bipolar disorder. Although LASSO models showed the highest discrimination accuracy in the internal sample, they showed the largest shrinkage in the external sample. Moreover, the LASSO models showed poor calibration in the internal sample; they over-diagnosed bipolar disorder. By contrast, simpler models showed better calibration in the internal sample. The probability nomogram with one or multiple assessment findings showed better calibration than LASSO models because they accounted for the original base rate, so they did not over-diagnose bipolar disorder.

In summary, the best models are those that are relatively simple (parsimonious), that can account for one or several of the most important predictors and their optimal weightings, and that account for the base rate of the phenomenon. Even unit-weighted formulas (formulas whose predictors are equally weighted with a weight of one) can sometimes generalize better to other samples than complex weightings (Garb & Wood, 2019). Differential weightings sometimes capture random variance and over-fit the model, thus leading to predictive accuracy shrinkage in cross-validation samples (Garb & Wood, 2019), as described below. The choice of predictive variables often matters more than their weighting.

In general, there is often shrinkage of estimates from training data set to a test data set. *Shrinkage* is when variables with stronger predictive power in the original data set tend to show somewhat smaller predictive power (smaller validity coefficients) when applied to new groups. Shrinkage reflects a model over-fitting (i.e., fitting to error by capitalizing on chance). Shrinkage is especially likely when the original sample is small and/or unrepresentative and the number of variables considered for inclusion is large. Cross-validation with large, representative samples can help evaluate the amount of shrinkage of estimates, particularly for more complex models such as machine learning models (Ursenbach et al., 2019). Ideally, cross-validation would be conducted with a separate sample (external cross-validation) to see the generalizability of estimates. However, you can also do internal cross-validation. For example, you can perform k-fold cross-validation, where you:

- split the data set into k groups
- for each unique group:
    - take the group as a hold-out data set (also called a test data set)
    - take the remaining groups as a training data set
    - fit a model on the training data set and evaluate it on the test data set
    - after all k-folds have been used as the test data set, and all models have been fit, you average the estimates across the models, which presumably yields more robust, generalizable estimates

An emerging technique that holds promise for increasing predictive accuracy of actuarial methods is machine learning (Garb & Wood, 2019). However, one challenge of some machine learning techniques is that they are like a "black box" and are not transparent, which raises ethical issues (Garb & Wood, 2019). Machine learning may be most valuable when the data available are complex and there are many predictive variables (Garb & Wood, 2019).

10.5 Getting Started

10.5.1 Load Libraries

```
library("petersenlab")
library("pROC")
```

```
library("caret")
library("MASS")
library("randomForest")
library("e1071")
library("ranger")
library("ordinalForest")
library("elasticnet")
library("LiblineaR")
library("glmnet")
library("viridis")
library("MOTE")
library("here")
library("tidyverse")
library("tinytex")
library("knitr")
library("kableExtra")
library("rmarkdown")
library("bookdown")
```

10.5.2 Prepare Data

10.5.2.1 Load Data

`aSAH` is a data set from the `pROC` package (Robin et al., 2021) that contains test scores (`s100b`) and clinical outcomes (`outcome`) for patients.

```
data(aSAH)
mydataActuarial <- aSAH

mydataActuarial$disorder <- NA
mydataActuarial$disorder[which(
  mydataActuarial$outcome == "Poor")] <- 1
mydataActuarial$disorder[which(
  mydataActuarial$outcome == "Good")] <- 0
```

10.5.2.2 Simulate Data

```
set.seed(52242)

mydataActuarial$ordinal <- sample(
  0:2,
  nrow(mydataActuarial),
  replace = TRUE)

mydataActuarial$ordinalFactor <-
  factor(mydataActuarial$ordinal, ordered = TRUE)
```

10.6 Fitting the Statistical Models

10.6.1 Regression with One Predictor

Dichotomous Outcome:

```
summary(
  glm(disorder ~ s100b,
  data = mydataActuarial))
```

Ordinal Outcome:

```
summary(
  polr(ordinalFactor ~ s100b,
  data = mydataActuarial))

lrm(
  ordinal ~ s100b,
  data = mydataActuarial,
  x = TRUE,
  y = TRUE)

ordinalModel <- train(
  ordinalFactor ~ s100b,
  data = mydataActuarial,
  method = "polr")
```

Continuous Outcome:

```
summary(
  lm(s100b ~ ndka,
  data = mydataActuarial))
```

10.6.2 Regression with Multiple Predictors

Dichotomous Outcome:

```
summary(
  glm(disorder ~ s100b + ndka + gender + age + wfns,
  data = mydataActuarial))
```

Ordinal Outcome:

```
summary(
  polr(ordinalFactor ~ s100b + ndka + gender + age + wfns,
  data = mydataActuarial))
```

```
lrm(
  ordinal ~ s100b + ndka + gender + age + wfns,
  data = mydataActuarial,
  x = TRUE,
  y = TRUE)

ordinalModelPredictors <- train(
  ordinalFactor ~ s100b + ndka + gender + age + wfns,
  data = mydataActuarial,
  method = "polr")
```

Continuous Outcome:

```
summary(
  lm(s100b ~ ndka + gender + age + wfns,
  data = mydataActuarial))
```

10.6.3 Least Absolute Shrinkage and Selection Option

The least absolute shrinkage and selection option (LASSO) models were fit in the `caret` package (Kuhn, 2022).

Continuous Outcome:

```
lassoModelContinuous <- train(
  s100b ~ ndka + gender + age + wfns,
  data = mydataActuarial,
  method = "lasso")
```

10.6.4 Ridge Regression

The ridge regression models were fit in the `caret` package (Kuhn, 2022).

Continuous Outcome:

```
ridgeModelContinuous <- train(
  s100b ~ ndka + gender + age + wfns,
  data = mydataActuarial,
  method = "ridge")
```

10.6.5 Random Forest Machine Learning

The random forest models were fit in the `caret` package (Kuhn, 2022).

Dichotomous Outcome:

```
rfModelDichotomous <- train(
  outcome ~ s100b + ndka + gender + age + wfns,
  data = mydataActuarial,
  method = "rf")
```

Ordinal Outcome:

```
rfModelOrdinal <- train(
  ordinalFactor ~ s100b + ndka + gender + age + wfns,
  data = mydataActuarial,
  method = "ordinalRF")
```

Continuous Outcome:

```
rfModelContinuous <- train(
  s100b ~ ndka + gender + age + wfns,
  data = mydataActuarial,
  method = "rf")
```

10.6.6 *k*-Fold Cross-Validation

The k-fold cross-validation models were fit in the `caret` package (Kuhn, 2022).

```
kFolds <- 10

train.control <- trainControl(
  method = "cv",
  number = kFolds)
```

Dichotomous Outcome:

```
cvModelDichotomous <- train(
  outcome ~ s100b + ndka + gender + age + wfns,
  data = mydataActuarial,
  method = "glm",
  trControl = train.control)
```

Continuous Outcome:

```
cvModelContinuous <- train(
  s100b ~ ndka + gender + age + wfns,
  data = mydataActuarial,
  method = "lm",
  trControl = train.control)
```

10.6.7 Leave-One-Out Cross-Validation

The leave-one-out (LOO) cross-validation models were fit in the `caret` package (Kuhn, 2022).

```
train.control <- trainControl(
  method = "LOOCV")
```

Dichotomous Outcome:

```
loocvModelDichotomous <- train(
  outcome ~ s100b + ndka + gender + age + wfns,
  data = mydataActuarial,
  method = "glm",
  trControl = train.control)
```

Continuous Outcome:

```
loocvModelContinuous <- train(
  s100b ~ ndka + gender + age + wfns,
  data = mydataActuarial,
  method = "lm",
  trControl = train.control)
```

10.7 Why Clinical Judgment Is More Widely Used Than Statistical Formulas

Despite actuarial methods being generally more accurate than clinical judgment, clinical judgment is much more widely used. There are several reasons why actuarial methods have not caught on; one reason is professional traditions. Experts in any field do not like to think that a computer could outperform them. Some practitioners argue that judgment/prediction is an "art form" and that using a statistical formula is treating people like a number. However, using an approach (i.e., clinical judgment) that systematically leads to less accurate decisions and predictions is an ethical problem.

Some clinicians do not think that group averages (e.g., in terms of which treatment is most effective) apply to an individual client. This invokes the distinction between nomothetic (group-level) inferences and idiographic (individual-level) inferences. However, the scientific evidence and probability theory strongly favor the nomothetic approach to clinical prediction—it is better to generalize from group-level evidence than throwing out all the evidence and taking the approach of "anything goes." Clinicians frequently believe the broken leg fallacy, i.e., thinking that your client is an exception to the algorithmic prediction. In most cases, deviating from the statistical formula will result in less accurate predictions. People tend to overestimate the probability of low base rate conditions and events.

Another reason why actuarial methods have not caught on is the belief that receiving a treatment is the only thing that matters. But it is an empirical question which treatment is most effective for whom. What if we could do better? For example, we could potentially use a formula to identify the most effective treatment for a client. Some treatments are no better than placebo; other treatments are actually harmful (Lilienfeld, 2007; Williams et al., 2021).

Another reason why clinical methods are more widely used than actuarial methods is the over-confidence in clinicians' predictions—clinicians think they are more accurate than they actually are. We see this when examining their calibration; their predictions tend to be mis-calibrated. For example, things they report with 80% confidence occur less than 80% of the time. Clinicians will sometimes be correct by chance, and they tend to mis-attribute that to their assessment; clinicians tend to remember the successes and forget the failures. Note, however, that it is not just clinicians who are over-confident; humans in general tend to be over-confident in their predictions.

Another argument against using actuarial methods is that "no methods exist". In some cases, that is true—actuarial methods do not yet exist for some prediction problems. However, one can always create an algorithm of the clinicians' judgments, even if one does not have access to the clients' outcome information. A model of clinicians' responses tends to be more accurate than clinicians' judgments themselves because the model gives the same outcome with the same input data—i.e., it is perfectly reliable.

Another argument from some clinicians is that, "My job is to understand, not to predict". But what kind of understanding does not involve predictions? Accurate predictions help in understanding. Knowing how people would perform in different conditions is the same thing as good understanding.

10.8 Conclusion

In general, it is better to develop and use structured, actuarial approaches than informal approaches that rely on human or clinical judgment. Actuarial approaches to prediction tend to be as accurate or more accurate than clinical judgment. Nevertheless, clinical judgment tends to be much more widely used than actuarial approaches, which is a major ethical problem.

10.9 Suggested Readings

Dawes et al. (1989); Garb & Wood (2019); Grove et al. (2000)

11

General Issues in Clinical Assessment

11.1 Historical Perspectives on Clinical Assessment

Historically, assessment has played a key role in clinical psychology. A history of clinical psychology is provided by Benjamin (2005). Many would consider assessment—especially the assessment of intelligence—the beginning of clinical psychology, and the role that distinguished clinical psychology from other fields. Intelligence testing has been one of the real successes of clinical psychology and assessment. For example, several early measures were developed to assess intelligence, including James Cattell's measure and the Binet-Simon Intelligence scale. Lewis Terman at Stanford extended the Binet-Simon Intelligence scale to study gifted people, which became known as the Stanford-Binet Intelligence Scales.

During World War I, instruments were used to select people for various military occupations (e.g., pilot versus submariner). Intellectual assessment, including the Army Alpha and Beta Tests, was used to decide who was psychologically unfit to serve. Then came the development of personality assessments, such as assessment of "shell shock", which would eventually become known as post-traumatic stress disorder (PTSD). The military conducted personality assessments to identify people who would be susceptible to shell shock, which would be labeled today as a measure of "neuroticism".

Intellectual assessment and personality assessment became the two principal tools for clinical psychologists. Initially, psychologists were primarily psychometricians. They developed assessment devices and helped score and interpret them. Early on, clinical psychologists did not play a large role in making diagnoses or in treatment—instead, psychiatrists did. However, that changed after World War I. Between World War I and World War II, assessment was the dominant role of practicing clinical psychologists, especially projective personality testing—such as word-association tests, the Rorschach Inkblot Test, and the Thematic Apperception Test—and more objective personality testing. The Rorschach (1921) gave clinical psychologists a "voice at the table" with psychiatrists, even though doubts arose about its accuracy. Projective testing dominated personality assessment through the 1940s. The Minnesota Multiphasic Personality Inventory (MMPI), which became a popular objective personality test, was published in 1943.

During World War II, many of the modern psychology departments, clinical psychology programs, and VA-funded clinical psychology internships were created, not by the psychology community, but by the federal government to address wartime and post-wartime needs. Likewise, many measures were developed as a need to meet wartime needs. One of the origins of the psychometric movement in psychology was spurred by historical pressures to create tests to classify people during wartime, such as with the Army Alpha and Beta Tests.

11.2 Contemporary Trends

There has been a general decline in the frequency with which clinical assessment (and psychotherapy) is conducted by clinical psychologists. Assessment and measurement are crucial to research but are declining in treatment. This is in great part due to managed care, in which a primary goal is cost containment of mental health services. Managed care has resulted in greatly reduced patient access to mental health services, a dramatic reduction in insurance funds for reimbursement of services, more clinician time spent on paperwork and less time seeing clients, having less time for assessment because fewer sessions are reimbursed, tendencies to administer less frequent or less comprehensive assessments, and increased provision of psychological services from master's degree-level providers because they are less expensive than doctoral providers.

Nevertheless, there are contexts in which clinical assessment is more common. There is still considerable assessment in the Department of Veterans Affairs (VA) system, including testing and integrated reports. In addition to the VA, there is still considerable neuropsychological and aptitude testing. What is the future of assessment for treatment? Our hope is that it will be evidence-based assessment (along with evidence-based treatment).

11.3 Terminology

Several terms are relevant for clinical assessment. *Prevalence* is the proportion of the population that has the condition at a given point in time, whereas *incidence* is the rate of occurrence of new cases. Incidence indicates the risk of developing or contracting the condition, whereas prevalence indicates how widespread the condition is. *Point prevalence* is the proportion of the population that has the condition at a single point in time. *Lifetime prevalence* is the proportion of the population that will ever have a condition at any point in their lifetime.

The *positivity rate* is the proportion of tests that are positive (the marginal probability or base rate of positive tests; i.e., the selection ratio). The *case fatality rate* is the proportion of people with a condition who die as a result of that condition.

11.3.1 The Three S's: Signs, Symptoms, and Syndromes

The Three S's of assessment in clinical psychology are signs, symptoms, and syndromes. *Signs* are observable features (or manifestations) of a disorder (Lilienfeld et al., 2015). Therefore, signs can be perceived by a clinician. By contrast, *symptoms* are unobservable manifestations of a disorder that can only be perceived by the client (Lilienfeld et al., 2015). The term "sign" has a connotation of being somewhat more objective than symptom because a symptom is based on the client's perceptions, but at least in clinical psychology (and also in many medical fields), both signs and symptoms have considerable elements of subjectivity. A *syndrome* is a collection of signs and symptoms that co-occur and may reflect a particular disorder.

11.4 Errors of Pseudo-Prediction

There are many errors of pseudo-prediction that are relevant to clinical assessment. One error of pseudo-prediction is the confusion of inverse probabilities, as described in Section 9.1.1.2. Another error of pseudo-prediction involves, when predicting a low base-rate phenomenon, only capitalizing on chance occurrences.

Another form of pseudo-prediction is constructing predictions that seem compelling but that have no basis, for instance using the date and place of birth to predict one's personality. Several techniques are used by people to make their predictions seem more compelling: make it true, make it positive, make it ambiguous, and make it mysterious or intimidating. Making it "true" means surrounding predictions with true statements, and using Barnum statements. Barnum statements are statements that are true for most people, such as: "You have a tendency to be critical of yourself." Including, in your prediction, outcomes that are a common occurrence for 80% of respondents (blanket statements) may make it more likely that people believe the prediction. Most of the statements are correct, so people tend to think the whole thing is correct. Making it "positive" means making the statement positive about the person. People tend to believe positive things about the self. However, if the statement is about a third person, people tend to believe it more if the statement is partially negative. Making it "ambiguous" means using vague language such as "it has not been unusual," "sometimes," "at times," "you tend to be," etc. Making it mysterious or intimidating could involve making the prediction from some organization or process with authority. An example of making statement mysterious is the PaTE report ("Psychodynamic and Therapeutic Evaluation") (Kriegman & Kriegman, 1965).

Unsupported fad treatments are another form of pseudo-prediction. There is unfortunately a large gap between science and practice. Many of the treatments known to work are not commonly implemented in practice; instead, many treatments implemented in practice have been shown not to be helpful (compared to placebo), or have been shown to be harmful (Lilienfeld, 2007), or have insufficient evidence supporting their use. Selecting a given treatment is a prediction by the therapist that the treatment will lead to the most positive outcomes for the client than the alternatives. There are likely a multitude of reasons for the disparity between practice and research. For instance, some practitioners feel that research is useless. Other practitioners are unaware that there are more effective treatments. Others may not have the time or money to learn new treatments on top of their already-busy schedules. Yet other therapists are greedy. In other cases, it is difficult to determine which treatments work due to a variety of effects.

For instance, some ineffective treatments may appear to "work" because of placebo effects, whereby merely receiving a treatment and expecting to improve yields positive benefits—not because of the specific treatment per se. In addition to client expectancy effects, there can also be therapist expectancy effects. There can also be demand effects, where participants form an interpretation of the study's purpose and subconsciously change their behavior to fit that interpretation. In addition, ineffective treatments can appear to work due to maturational effects, especially with children and long treatments. Ineffective treatments can appear to work due to differential dropout or attrition, where the people who are improving are the most likely to stay in treatment.

In addition, there are regression effects that can make an ineffective treatment appear to work. As a reminder, the true score formula in classical test theory is: $X = T + e$. There are random fluctuations in an observed score; part of the observed score is stable true score and part of it is random error. As an example, consider that we will use Norwegian acupuncture. We will select clients who are at the extremes in terms of high pain. They will ultimately converge or regress to their mean (i.e., their true score). So, on average, their pain will be lower the next time. In therapy, clients tend to come in at their worst, so they are bound to improve. The clients would have tended (on average) to get better, even without treatment. This is known as regression to the mean. For these reasons, it is important to include a control group to compare how clients would have done had they received no treatment, a placebo, or some other treatment. For example, in experiments that test the efficacy of cognitive behavioral therapy (CBT), it is important to include a control group, such as no treatment control, waitlist control, treatment as usual, or best available treatment.

Violating the extension rule (the conjunction fallacy) is another form of pseudo-prediction. The extension rule states that a special outcome cannot be more probable than a general one of which it is part. But in spite of this, we tend to assign high probabilities to prototypical combinations of characteristics, events, or sequences, and irrationally low probabilities to atypical single characteristics, events, or sequences. Here's an example from Dawes (1986):

> Linda is 31 years old, single, outspoken, and very bright. She majored in philosophy. As a student, she was deeply concerned with issues of discrimination and social justice, and also participated in anti-nuclear demonstrations." Which is more probable?
>
> A) Linda is a bank teller.
>
> B) Linda is a bank teller and is active in the feminist movement.

The probability that a woman is a bank teller and feminist is less likely than the probability that she is a bank teller. However, people tend to say that B is more probable. People tend to make judgments based on the representativeness heuristic—how similar to the prototypes the cases are.

Another form of pseudo-prediction is imposing structure (non-randomness) on a pattern where there are none. In addition, expecting alternation, known as the "belief in the law of small numbers", is a form of pseudo-prediction. Expecting alternation is believing that even small sequences should be representative of populations, even though that is false. For instance, it might involve expecting that one will get three heads if flipping a coin six times.

Spurious correlations are another form of pseudo-prediction. The expected value of R^2 is $\frac{K}{n-1}$, where K is the number of predictors. The more predictors in the model, the more variance is accounted for in the outcome. Thus, with many predictors and a small sample, there is pseudo-prediction, as described in Section 9.9. However, as the sample size increases, spurious correlations decrease.

Multicollinearity is also a form of pseudo-prediction. As the correlation among the predictors increase, the chance of getting an arbitrary answer increases.

Another form of pseudo-prediction is the hot hand fallacy. The hot hand fallacy in basketball is believing that making a shot makes it more likely that you will make the next shot. Most research suggests that there is no such thing as a "hot hand" (Avugos et al., 2013; Bar-Eli et al., 2006; Gilovich et al., 1985). Some recent research, however, has suggested that there may be a small hot hand effect in some contexts (Bocskocsky et al., 2014; J. B. Miller & Sanjurjo, 2014).

Capitalizing on regression effects is pseudo-prediction. When underestimating regression effects, a person can capitalize on regression effects by predicting an extremity in one variable (e.g., amount of improvement over time) due to an extremity in another variable (e.g., pain severity), when in fact, regression to the mean is most likely.

11.5 Conclusion

Many of the origins of assessment came from attempts to address wartime needs. Since the 1980s, there has been a general decline in the frequency with which clinical assessments (and psychotherapy) are conducted by clinical psychologists, due to managed care and cost containment. Many errors of pseudo-prediction are relevant to clinical assessment.

11.6 Suggested Readings

Wood et al. (2002)

12

Evidence-Based Assessment

This whole book is about doing assessment in the strongest, most scientifically supported (i.e., evidence-based) ways. This chapter summarizes many of the important considerations in ensuring our assessments are strong for their intended uses, especially in clinical psychology, and to discuss the value of some cutting-edge (and some not-so-cutting-edge) techniques to maximize the validity of inferences. A case study in evidence-based assessment is provided by Antony & Rowa (2005).

12.1 Considerations

In general, we need to use assessment devices that are:

- clinically relevant (if used in a clinical domain): they inform decision-making processes
- culturally sensitive: they are relevant to individuals from various backgrounds, especially the backgrounds in the population of interest
- scientifically sound: strong psychometrics (reliability and validity)

12.2 Clinically Relevant

Effective treatment depends on accurate assessment. Thus, it is important to consider the treatment utility of assessment to determine whether the assessment has value. Several study methods were designed to examine the treatment utility of assessment, including manipulated assessment (compares assessment versus no assessment) and manipulated use (compares use versus no use of data from the assessment for treatment matching).

It is also important to consider the ease of dissemination of an assessment: is it time- and money-efficient, especially in terms of its cost–benefit ratio? Brief assessments, computerized testing, and adaptive testing can help assessments be clinically practical. It should be straightforward to score and interpret. And it should provide incremental validity, i.e., additional useful information above and beyond what is gained by other assessment devices.

We have already discussed how assessments can yield more effective outcomes indirectly through matching the right treatment approach to the client. It is also worth noting, however, that assessments can also lead *directly* to improved treatment outcomes. Conducting an assessment is an intervention—it can have carryover effects, and can result in self-reflection, self-awareness, and reactivity, i.e., change due to observing it.

Assessment is also an important component of measurement-based care. Measurement-based care is the approach of treatment monitoring and modifying treatment accordingly (Lutz et al., 2022). Assessment does not stop at the beginning of the treatment—it is continuous and ongoing. So, ongoing measurement is recommended throughout treatment so that the clinician can modify the treatment in response to measurements. Assessment of treatment progress needs to be sensitive to change, i.e., the assessment needs to show treatment sensitivity, and it needs to be actionable, i.e., it needs to have utility.

In clinical psychological assessment, it is important for assessments to:

- consider co-occurrence of multiple issues (comorbidity) and differential diagnosis
- accurately assess conditions that frequently co-occur or co-vary (e.g., depression and anxiety), and to
- differentiate between multiple possibilities for what may explain the client's difficulties.

In addition, it is valuable to:

- pose alternative or competing hypotheses and test them to rule out other potential explanations
- look for disconfirming evidence, not just evidence that confirms one's suspicions
- consider assessments from multiple informants (e.g., parents, teachers, peers) and multiple levels of analysis, including biological, psychological, and social-contextual factors
- consider functional impairment and not just diagnostic status, and to
- consider the context of the client's difficulties, including the onset, duration, and course of the problem, the client's treatment history, family history, familial and cultural context, and medical conditions.

12.3 Culturally Sensitive

It is important to mitigate cultural bias of instruments. It is also important for the measure to be useful across the population of interest. To accomplish this, one may have to modify an assessment approach to account for clinically significant moderating variables. We discuss culturally sensitive assessment more in Chapter 24, and we discuss test bias in Chapter 15.

12.4 Scientifically Sound

The development and selection of measures should be based on scientifically supported theories in psychopathology and basic psychological science. Measures should be standardized, with similar procedures across participants, clients, and examiners.

Reliability and validity of measures' scores are specific to a particular use of the test, and are specific for a given population and context. So, it is important to clearly specify the purpose of the assessment. As just a few examples, the purpose of the assessment could be screening for early identification of risk, for diagnosis, for treatment monitoring, for treatment evaluation, or for measuring a phenomenon of interest in research. In general, the purposes of an assessment can be summarized into the 3 Ps (Youngstrom et al., 2017): predict, prescribe, and process. The purpose of an assessment is to predict if the purpose is to relate an assessment to a criterion at a later point in time. An assessment is used to prescribe if it informs decision-making about the participant or client—for example, a decision about which treatment to give, identifying moderators of treatment effectiveness, or specifying potential confounds or alternative explanations that would warrant a different treatment. An assessment is used to understand process if it informs understanding of the participant or client—for example, identifying mediators of treatment effectiveness or tracking treatment progress.

Whichever the purpose of the assessment, it is important to test and evaluate the psychometrics of the assessment device for that particular purpose. Only use the assessment device in a test battery if it advances that purpose. Youngstrom et al. (2017) describe the different core psychometric features that are especially relevant for each purpose. For instance, predictive and discriminative validity are crucial for prediction, whereas inter-rater reliability is crucial for prescription, and treatment sensitivity—a form of criterion-related validity—is crucial for understanding process.

12.4.1 Standard for Excellent Tests

Additionally, when making norm-referenced judgments, it is important that the assessment has appropriate norms and evidence of accuracy for any cut-scores (e.g., diagnostic thresholds). Per Youngstrom et al. (2017), below are the norms and psychometric standards for excellent tests:

- If the assessment has norms, the norms provide a mean and standard deviation for the total score (and any subscores) that were determined from multiple, large samples that are representative of the populations to which it is intended for the test to be administered.
- Internal consistency: Greater than .90 based on Cronbach's alpha or (better yet) omega.
- Inter-rater reliability: Cohen's kappa $\geq .85$; intraclass correlation $\geq .90$.
- Test–retest reliability: If the construct is stable, the measure shows stability of individual differences and repeatability. However, note that not all constructs are expected to be stable. For stable constructs, the measure should show stability of individual differences (i.e., relative or rank-order stability): $rs \geq .70$ over a year or longer. For stable constructs, the measure should also show repeatability, i.e., absolute stability in level: A Bland–Altman plot and corresponding regression shows no significant bias or trends, and the repeatability coefficient (also known as Smallest Real Difference, SRD, or limits of agreement, LOA) is small.
- Content validity: The test developers clearly defined the domain and ensured representation of the entire set of facets. All elements of the assessment are evaluated by quantitative ratings by multiple groups of judges.
- Construct validity: The assessment has evidence in support of construct validity, including concurrent, predictive, convergent, and discriminant validity, that has been replicated by independent researchers.
- Incremental validity: The assessment shows incremental utility above other measures.
- Discriminative validity: For diagnostic assessment, the measure should have an area under the receiver operating characteristic curve (AUC) of .75 to .90 under clinically realistic conditions. AUC is the single best index of discrimination accuracy, but it is also helpful to know the sensitivity, specificity, positive predictive value, and negative predictive value at particular cutoffs of interest to determine whether the assessment is aligned with its purpose.
- Prescriptive validity: An assessment that has strong prescriptive validity regarding which diagnosis to give would have good inter-rater reliability (kappa) for diagnosis in more than one sample. An assessment that has strong prescriptive validity regarding which treatment

to give would have a moderate effect size (or larger) for treatment moderation—i.e., there is evidence for treatment matching based on the characteristic.

- Validity generalization: The bulk of the evidence supports use of the assessment with more than one demographic group (if it is to be used with more than one group) and in multiple settings.
- Sensitivity to change and treatment sensitivity: Replications from independent researchers show evidence that the assessment detects (i.e., is sensitive to) change over time, change over the course of treatment, and differences as a function of different types of treatment.
- Clinical utility: After practical considerations, including costs, respondent burden, ease of administration and scoring, replication from independent researchers shows that the assessment data are likely to be clinically actionable and confer clinical benefits, such as better outcomes, lower attrition, and greater satisfaction in areas that are important to the stakeholders.

The whole assessment process should be empirically evaluated, including the selection, administration, scoring, and interpretation of an instrument, the integration of multiple sources of assessment data, and the decision-making process. When possible, it is valuable to evaluate the accuracy of the decision-making, ideally against some gold standard, for quality control improvement.

In general, it is better to include a wide range of assessment tools than a single strong measure. For instance, assessment tools could include self- and informant-report questionnaires, interviews, self-monitoring diaries, behavioral observation, performance-based techniques, and psychophysiological techniques. Then, each measure can be weighted according to its diagnostic likelihood ratio—i.e., its concurrent/predictive validity in the form of the positive likelihood ratio.

One challenge is how to handle a situation where different instruments yield different answers. For instance, if the results from parent report versus teacher report conflict with each other. To address potential discrepancies, one can weight the different instruments or informant sources according to their predictive accuracy. For instance, you might give more weight to youths' self-report for assessing anxiety but might give more weight to parent report for assessing ADHD. One way to handle informant discrepancies when there is not a clear primary informant who is best-positioned to rate the person most accurately is to count a symptom as present if it is endorsed by any of the informants (Hinshaw & Nigg, 1999).

12.5 Bayesian Updating

As presented in Equation (9.16), the posttest (or posterior) odds are equal to the pretest odds multiplied by the likelihood ratio. Bayes' theorem is discussed in Section 9.1.1.3. Using this formula, and converting odds to probabilities, we can use a Fagan probability nomogram to determine the posttest probability following a test result. The calculation of posttest probability is described in Section 9.5.32. A *probability nomogram* is a way of visually applying Bayes' theorem to determine the posttest probability of having a condition based on the pretest (or prior) probability and likelihood ratio, as depicted in Figure 12.1. To use a probability nomogram, connect the dots from the starting probability (left line) with the likelihood ratio (middle line) to see the updated probability. The updated (posttest) probability is where the connecting line crosses the third, right line.

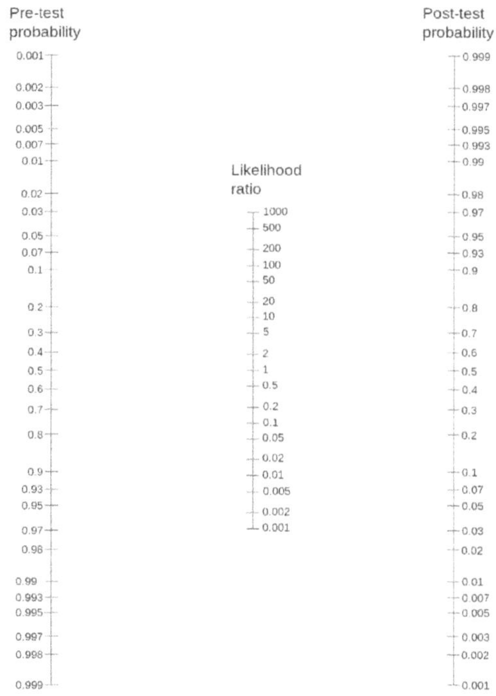

FIGURE 12.1 Probability Nomogram. (Figure retrieved from https://upload.wikimedia.org/wikipedia/commons/thumb/6/66/Fagan_nomogram.svg/945px-Fagan_nomogram.svg.png).

For instance, if the starting probability is .5% and the likelihood ratio is 10 (e.g., sensitivity = .90, specificity = .91: likelihood ratio = $\frac{\text{sensitivity}}{1-\text{specificity}} = \frac{.9}{1-.91} = 10$), the updated probability is less than 5%, as depicted in Figure 12.2. The formula and function for computing posttest probability are provided in Section 9.5.32.

```
posttestProbability(
  pretestProb = .005,
  likelihoodRatio = 10)
```

```
[1] 0.04785
```

A probability nomogram calculator can be found at the following link: http://araw.mede.uic.edu/cgi-bin/testcalc.pl (archived at https://perma.cc/X8TF-7YBX).

12.6 Dimensional Approaches to Psychopathology

The Diagnostic and Statistical Manual of Mental Disorders (DSM) takes primarily a categorical approach to psychopathology—it classifies mental disorders as discrete categories. That is, anxiety is classified as a distinct disorder from depression in the DSM, despite their strong covariation and co-occurrence. Moreover, disorders are generally classified in the DSM in a binary fashion—according to the DSM, you either "have" the disorder or "do not have"

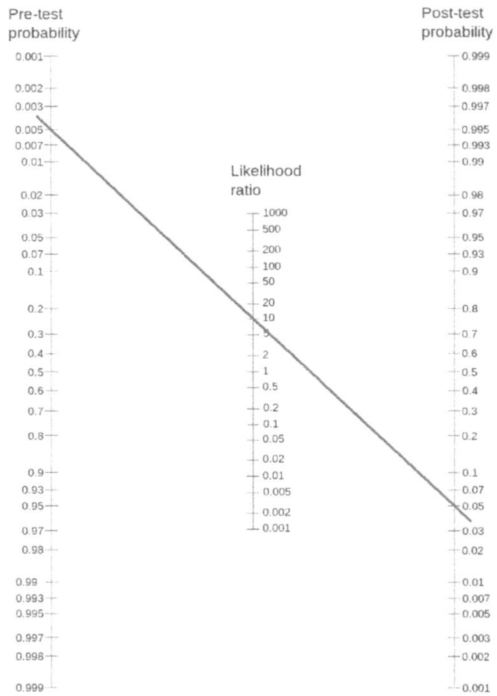

FIGURE 12.2 Probability Nomogram Example. (Figure adapted from https://upload.wikimedia.org/wikipedia/commons/thumb/6/66/Fagan_nomogram.svg/945px-Fagan_nomogram.svg.png)

the disorder—there is no middle ground, and there is not a finer differentiation among those who are given the disorder.

Despite the categorical approach of the DSM, most disorders seem to be more accurately conceptualized as dimensional than categorical (Markon et al., 2011). As described in Section 16.5.2, DSM disorders are fictive categories. They do not carve nature at its joints. Many disorders show high comorbidity with other disorders. Transdiagnostic dimensions can better account for the heterogeneity within and across disorders—and more parsimoniously—than DSM categories. For instance, depression and anxiety may share an underlying construct of negative emotionality. A dimensional approach considers a person's level on each dimension, even if the person is sub-threshold. Moreover a transdiagnostic approach may afford greater flexibility in treatment across disorders by focusing on dimensions of difficulties that may cut across traditional diagnostic boundaries. For instance, the Unified Protocol is a form of psychotherapy designed to address a range of emotional disorders, not just depression or anxiety (Ellard et al., 2010).

12.6.1 Multi-Stage Approach to Assessment

Another way in which a dimensional approach to psychopathology can provide greater treatment flexibility than a categorical approach is in applying a multi-stage approach to assessment. Youngstrom & Van Meter (2016) described a multi-stage approach to assessment in which the treatment provider calculates the posterior probability of disorder based on an instrument score, the extent of risk factors present, and the base rate of the disorder. Based on the posterior probability of disorder, the treatment provider places the client into one of three graded strata: the Green zone, Yellow zone, or Red zone (depicted with the left, middle, and right sections, respectively, of Figure 12.3).

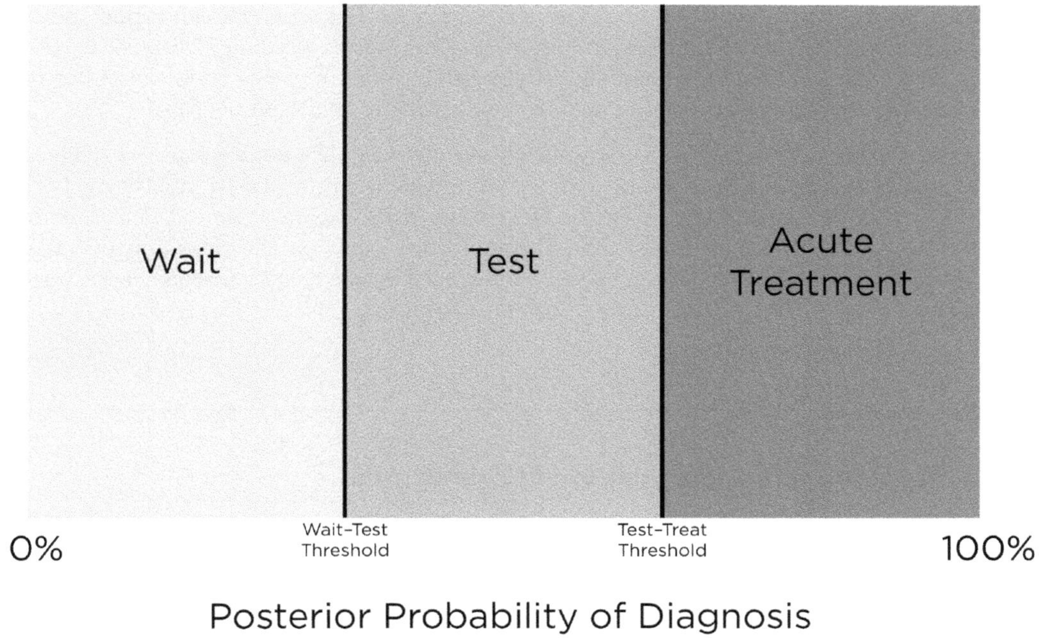

FIGURE 12.3 Multi-Stage Approach to Assessment.

The Green zone is the "Low Probability/Wait Zone". If the client is in the Green zone, the course of action would be to either do nothing or to engage the client in primary prevention techniques that are safe and inexpensive. The threshold between the Green zone and Yellow zone is the "wait–test" threshold. If the client exceeds the wait–test threshold, they move to the Yellow zone.

The Yellow zone is the "Moderate Probability/Assessment Zone". If the client is in the Yellow zone, secondary intervention would be indicated, including targeted intervention efforts, or nonspecific and low-risk treatment, such as skills-oriented psychotherapies. More assessment would be indicated until the posterior probability rises into the treatment zone (Red zone) or falls into the wait zone (Green zone). The threshold between the Yellow zone and Red zone is the "test–treat" threshold. If the client exceeds the test–treat threshold, they move to the Red zone.

The Red zone is the "High Probability/Acute Treatment Zone". If the client is in the Red zone, tertiary intervention would be indicated. The locations of the wait–test threshold and the test–treat threshold depend on the risks and benefits and the client's preferences.

To conduct a multi-stage approach to assessment, Youngstrom & Van Meter (2016) recommend starting with an instrument with high sensitivity, such as tests with broad content coverage. Low scores on a measure with high sensitivity rule out diagnosis (i.e., the client is in the Green zone), but high scores are ambiguous (i.e., the client is in the Yellow zone) because the measure does not have high specificity. The mnemonic device that can be helpful for remembering the utility of sensitivity and specificity is "SNout" and "SPin". Low (i.e., negative) scores on a test with high sensitivity rule OUT a diagnosis, whereas high (i.e., positive) scores on a test with high specificity rule IN a diagnosis. If a person scores high on the test with high sensitivity and goes to the Yellow zone, follow up with tests that have higher specificity, including more focused tests, to reduce the number of false positives. Ideally, use multiple tests that have incremental validity and do not have high inter-correlation ($r < .3$) so that they are not redundant (e.g., not all self-report) and so they meaningfully update the posterior probability. To avoid redundancy with rating scales, you can "take the best"—i.e., include only the most valid rating scale from each informant to test each hypothesis to avoid high inter-correlations and multicollinearity.

To integrate the results of multiple assessments, use a probability nomogram or a diagnostic test calculator (http://araw.mede.uic.edu/cgi-bin/testcalc.pl; archived at https://perma.cc/X8TF-7YBX) to update the posterior probability after each assessment. The locations of the wait–test threshold and test–treat threshold are based on the risks and benefits of diagnosis and treatment, and they can also be influenced by the client's preference for various approaches.

12.7 Reporting Guidelines for Publications

When publishing papers, it is important to report effect sizes, including the AUC, diagnostic likelihood ratios, and correlations between test scores and the criterion. Do not just rely on statistical significance. The effect size is important for determining the practical or clinical significance of the effects. Guidelines for reporting about and evaluating assessments in research reports are provided by Kazdin (1995).

It is also important to report aspects of reliability and validity, both in the current sample and from prior studies. Describe the current sample in adequate detail to understand the population to whom the findings from the study may best generalize. Describe how many items were included in the assessment, the item content (or a description of the content, if proprietary), how the assessment was scored, how scores were aggregated (e.g., sum or mean), the range of possible values, the mean and standard deviation of scores, and what higher values represent.

12.8 Many Measures Are Available

Assessment in psychology is similar to the Wild West. There are many different measures available. Many measures in psychology do not have evidence of strong psychometrics (reliability/validity) and are not based on research in basic psychological science including cognitive psychology, social psychology, etc. Measures in clinical psychology often focus on complex syndromes and conditions rather than basic states or processes, unlike most tests in medicine.

Because there are so many measures, it can be challenging to know which ones to use. To learn about good tests or the strengths and weaknesses of assessment devices in psychology, there are resources that provide reviews of measures, including the Buros Mental Measurements Yearbook (Buros Center for Testing, 2021), which is published by the Buros Center for

Testing, and the Handbook of Psychiatric Measures (Rush et al., 2009), which is published by the American Psychiatric Association.

12.9 Conclusion

Evidence-based assessment involves using assessment devices that are clinically relevant, culturally sensitive, and scientifically sound. Standards are available for excellent tests. Bayesian updating is a key technique for evidence-based assessment. For assessing psychopathology, evidence-based techniques include dimensional and multi-stage assessment approaches. There are many measures available for assessment; the Buros *Mental Measurements Yearbook* (Buros Center for Testing, 2021) and the *Handbook of Psychiatric Measures* (Rush et al., 2009) provide reviews of measures.

12.10 Suggested Readings

Hunsley & Mash (2007); Youngstrom et al. (2017)

13

Ethical Issues in Assessment

Ethics are relevant to all of our domains as psychologists, including (but not limited to) research, teaching, assessment, intervention, and supervision.

13.1 Belmont Report

The Belmont Report informs professional ethics. The principles from the Belmont Report include: respect for persons, beneficence, and justice.

13.1.1 Respect for Persons

A key component of respect for persons is informed consent. It also involves special considerations to protect the welfare of vulnerable people, including children, prisoners, pregnant women, people with intellectual disability, and people who are economically or educationally disadvantaged. It is important to get full informed consent from clients or participants before taking actions that will affect them.

13.1.2 Beneficence

The principle of beneficence is about maximizing benefit and minimizing harm, similar to the aphorism, "First, do no harm". Clients and participants have the prerogative to make choices about whether to receive a procedure, so they need to know the benefits and harm of each procedure. Just having the intent to help is not enough—you also need to be using a helpful technique and to have the knowledge of how to implement the technique.

13.1.3 Justice

Justice goes beyond the interaction with the individual client or participant; it deals with broader, societal concerns. For instance, justice involves ensuring that the people taking the risk will also benefit. For example, if a study to test the effectiveness of a medication enrolls primarily homeless people, the participant population may be taking the risk of trying the drug but not ultimately benefiting from the knowledge gained.

13.2 Our Ethical Advice

Our ethical advice is summarized in the following:

1. Don't do stupid things
2. Don't do bad things

13.2.1 Don't Do Stupid Things

First, don't do stupid things. With respect to assesement, for instance, do not use weak assessment instruments. The assessment techniques you use should be reliable and valid for the tasks and population of interest. They should be based on scientific research, not by professional judgment. Reliability and validity have many facets and all facets must be used in evaluating assessment techniques. Reliability and validity are characteristics of *uses* of tests, not the tests themselves. So, identify what is important, for example test–retest reliability versus internal consistency. Reliability and validity may differ for populations that vary in characteristics (e.g., age, gender, education, ethnicity).

13.2.2 Don't Do Bad Things

Second, don't do bad things. For instance, do not administer services without first getting the person's consent. Informed consent for an assessment includes multiple components. Ensure that the person being assessed is informed about important aspects of the testing situation. Say what services will be administered (i.e., the nature of testing), why the testing will be administered (i.e., the purpose of testing), what the evidence is for the assessment devices, the costs and potential side effects of the assessment and the tests, the pros and cons of underdoing the assessment, and other options available. Describe the type of information that the client will receive. Describe any third-party involvement (e.g., insurance companies, schools, employers, court) in accessing the assessment information. Describe the limits of confidentiality, which typically would include when someone is in danger, as defined by unreported child abuse or neglect, elder abuse, or imminent suicidality or homicidality. If the assessment is court-ordered or the results of the assessment are subpoenaed by a court of law, the limits of confidentiality change. It is also important to describe the psychologist's role relative to the client. Be transparent about what services are experimental; do not pretend to know more than you know. Do not make false or misleading claims or promises.

Honor the agreement implied by the explanation provided in the informed consent. For an example of a document that we use with clients that describes the pros and cons of an intervention technique (parent management training) and other options available, see here: https://osf.io/qmnu6.

It is also important to maintain the integrity of assessment techniques. Do not teach people how to raise their scores. There has to be integrity to begin assessment.

13.2.3 Consult, Consult, Consult

If you are unsure how to handle an ethical dilemma, CONSULT, CONSULT, CONSULT! In notes and reports, provide documentation of the rationale for decisions made. Professional ethics boards want to know that you are acting in good faith of the client's best interests.

13.3 APA Ethics Code

The American Psychological Association (APA) publishes ethics guidelines in its document entitled, *Ethical Principles of Psychologists and Code of Conduct* (hereafter referred to as the "APA Ethics Code") (American Psychological Association, 2017). The latest version of the APA Ethics Code is available here: https://www.apa.org/ethics/code (archived at https://perma.cc/6F4Z-WQ57).

Here, we emphasize a few of the guidelines from the APA Ethics Code with respect to assessment. However, you should read and follow the entire APA Ethics Code. That said, the APA Ethics Code is not up to date for clinical science. But there are many important components. Case illustrations of ethical guidelines from the APA Ethics Code are provided by L. Campbell et al. (2010). Ethical issues in psychological assessment are also discussed by Bersoff et al. (2012) and Nagy (2011).

13.3.1 Competence

Section 2 of the APA Ethics Code notes that you should only act withing the boundaries of your competence. It is also important to be aware of and report conflicts of interest.

13.3.2 Bases for Assessments

Section 9 of the APA Ethics Code describes ethics guidelines for assessment. Section 9.01 describes ethics guidelines regarding the bases for assessments. Use techniques that are sufficient to substantiate the findings, based on strong psychometrics. In a professional context, sit down face to face and evaluate the individual, as opposed to just relying on automated reports. If using computerized assessments, you should have the expertise to consider the appropriateness of the interpretations. Work to reduce or eliminate bias. If using record review, explain the sources of information used for conclusions and recommendations. Maintain a high standard when recording assessment information. Psychologists have responsibility for maintenance and retention of their records. Records should describe the nature, delivery, progress, and results of services, and related fees. Take reasonable steps to maintain confidentiality of records. When a client might want to know how records will be maintained, disclose record-keeping procedures in the informed consent. The duration that full records should be kept depends on whether they are adults or children. For adults, keep full records for 7 years after the last date of service. For children, keep full records for 7 years after the last date of service, or for 3 years after they become adults, whichever is later. The latest version of the APA record-keeping guidelines is available here: https://www.apa.org/practice/guidelines/record-keeping (archived at https://perma.cc/S37L-5VNX).

13.3.3 Use of Assessments

Section 9.02 describes ethics guidelines regarding the use of assessments. It notes to use assessments "in light of research or evidence". But how would research and evidence not go together? This phrase from the APA Ethics Code suggests that some forms of non-research-based evidence have equal footing with research in terms of deciding what assessments to use. We would argue that assessments should be selected based on the best available scientific evidence. And if scientific evidence does not yet exist to use an assessment device for a particular purpose with a particular population, the assessment device should be studied and evaluated before it is used to make important decisions.

The assessment should be reliable and valid for the population **and** purpose. When the reliability and validity has not been established, describe the strengths and weaknesses. Use language and competence level that is appropriate for the participant/client. Consider the potential social consequences of testing. High stakes decisions probably should not be made on the basis of the results of a single test.

13.3.4 Informed Consent in Assessments

Section 9.03 describes ethics guidelines regarding informed consent in assessments. Informed consent should be obtained unless:

- the assessment is government mandated (which changes things a bit),
- it is implied because it is considered voluntary (e.g., when applying for a job), or
- evaluating decisional capacity and the person is not capable of providing consent; in these cases, you should still inform them of what testing will include and the purpose of assessment.

13.3.5 Release of Test Data

Section 9.04 describes ethics guidelines regarding release of test data. "Test data" include raw and scaled scores, a client's responses to questions or stimuli, and the psychologist's notes about the participant. You are expected to release test data if the client provides a signed release, unless it would cause substantial harm or would be a misrepresentation of the data or test. You may also have to release test data if there is a law or court order, but you may be able to fight these.

13.3.6 Other Guidelines

Section 9.07 notes that you should not promote the use of assessment techniques by unqualified people. Section 9.08 notes that you should not use obsolete tests and outdated results.

13.3.7 Maintain Test Security (Integrity)

Section 9.11 describes ethics guidelines regarding maintaining test security (integrity). Maintaining test integrity involves protecting test instruments, protocols, questions or stimuli, and manuals from unauthorized access. If releasing test data, take care to release only the scores of copyrighted tests; do not release the copyrighted tests themselves. For example, if performing intellectual testing, try to release the subscale scores and summary scores (e.g., T scores) without releasing test stimuli. Also, do not coach people on how to perform better on questions, and do not let them take tests home.

13.4 Clinical Report Writing

Write every report as if it will be used in a court of law. You want it to be able to stand up in court. Always identify the source of each inference (e.g., "Per the client's report, ..."). Do not write a self-reported statement as if it were a factual statement. Instead of writing, "The client cut herself", write "The client reported that she cut herself". Do not overstate findings. Information from reports can be used to make decisions that significantly impact people's lives, so it is important not to misrepresent information. Recognize factors, such as language, culture, and the situation, that could have impacted the results, and note them in the report. Recognize limitations in the recommendations.

13.5 Open Science

There has been a replication crisis in psychology and social science, in which the findings from many studies have failed to replicate when independent researchers attempt to replicate the studies' findings (Open Science Collaboration, 2015). Due to the replication crisis, there has been a movement toward open, transparent science where researchers pre-register their methods, and share their data and analysis scripts. Open practices reduce threats to replicability and increase the public accessibility of science. The movement to open practices in science is known as the open science movement.

The open science movement seeks to increase the replicability and accessibility of science through three primary methods. First, the open science movement seeks to improve transparency, i.e., what researchers are actually doing in their studies and analyses. Second, especially when researchers have confirmatory hypotheses, the open science movement seeks to restrict researcher degrees of freedom so that the researchers do what they said they would do rather than contingent analysis decisions to get a desired result. Similar to a garden of forking paths (see Figure 1), there are so many decision points in a study, and different decisions can lead to drastically different results. Third, the open science movement seeks to prevent ethically questionable research practices. Ethically questionable research practices may include (John et al., 2012):

- not reporting all dependent variables
- deciding to collect more data after looking at the data to see whether the results were significant
- not reporting all of a study's conditions
- stopping collecting data earlier than planned because the expected result is detected
- rounding down a p-value
- selectively reporting studies that worked
- deciding whether to exclude data after looking at the impact of doing so on the results
- reporting an unexpected finding as having been predicted from the start (known as HARK-ing: **h**ypothesizing **a**fter the **r**esults are **k**nown)
- claiming that results are unaffected by demographic variables when one is actually unsure
- falsifying data
- p-Hacking: multiple testing, selective reporting, and misreporting of the true effect size

To advance reproducibility and replicability in science, researchers are encouraged to provide greater transparency and sharing of their research. For instance, one way to provide greater transparency and to limit the researcher's degrees of freedom is to (pre-)register a study. There is a continuum of study registration that includes pre-registration, co-registration, and post-registration, depending on when the registration occurs relative to data collection and analysis (Benning et al., 2019). Study pre-registration involves publicly posting a study's design, hypotheses, methods, materials, and data analysis plan prior to data collection. Co-registration occurs after data collection starts but before data analysis begins. Post-registration occurs after data analysis has begun.

Although pre-registration is most commonly used with confirmatory research in which you have a directional hypothesis, you can also pre-register exploratory research in which you have no directional hypothesis. Pre-registration helps to make it more explicit what tests are confirmatory (based on a priori directional hypotheses) and which are exploratory. It is important to interpret the results of confirmatory and exploratory tests differently, because you are more likely to get false positive results if conducting lots of exploratory tests. You can also pre-register decision trees that allow flexibility for multiple approaches depending on the data.

Some journals see the value of pre-registered studies and publish registered reports. A registered report is a study that is evaluated based on the pre-registered methods, hypotheses, and data analysis plan, and if the pre-registered study is accepted, the eventual paper will be accepted (as long as the researchers followed the pre-registered plan) regardless of whether the findings supported the hypotheses. Registered reports of exploratory analyses are sometimes called exploratory reports.

There are many tools that aim to advance the open science movement. A key tool is the Open Science Framework (OSF; https://osf.io). The OSF is a free, open source platform that supports the transparency of scientific research. There are numerous ways that researchers can make use of the OSF to advance the aims of open science. Here is a template for a pre-registration of a study on the OSF: https://osf.io/2hrfy. Researchers can (pre-)register their study on the OSF by posting their hypotheses, study methods, and data analysis plan. In addition, researchers can use the OSF to post manuals, protocols, lab notebooks, data, data processing syntax, statistical analysis code, detailed results, computational notebooks, and paper preprints (Tackett, Brandes, & Reardon, 2019). A computational notebook (e.g., Jupyter notebook, R Markdown, Quarto) is a document in which the analysis code, output, and text are weaved together, so the reader can see how each statistical result was obtained for reproducibility. An example of an R Markdown computational notebook is on the book's page on the OSF: https://osf.io/nkyve (the associated `.Rmd` file that generated the html is here: https://osf.io/fxrzm). An example of a Quarto computational notebook is also on the book's page on the OSF: https://osf.io/8ybtk (the associated `.qmd` file that generated the html is here: https://osf.io/zbruf).

After pre-registration, you can share a preprint of your paper on a preprint server like arXiv[1], PsyArXiv[2], bioRxiv[3], SocArXiv[4], EdArXiv[5], MetaArXiv[6], or medRxiv[7]. For an example of a preprint, see here: https://psyarxiv.com/gtsvw. Posting a preprint disseminates the paper without waiting for peer review and the publishing process. It also provides free access to papers that might otherwise be hidden behind journals' paywalls. Also, it helps establishes who was first to perform work on a topic.

There are now journals dedicated to publishing replication studies, including *ReScienceX* (http://rescience.org/x) and to publishing null findings, including the *Journal of Articles in Support of the Null Hypothesis* (https://www.jasnh.com).

Nevertheless, open science does not provide a one-size-fits-all solution to the vast diversity of scientific methods. For instance, there may be important ways needed to adapt open science and pre-registration practices to longitudinal research (Petersen et al., in press).

[1]https://arxiv.org
[2]https://psyarxiv.com
[3]https://www.biorxiv.org
[4]http://socarxiv.org
[5]https://osf.io/preprints/edarxiv
[6]https://osf.io/preprints/metaarxiv
[7]https://www.medrxiv.org

13.6 Conclusion

According to the Belmont Report, professional ethics includes respect for persons, beneficence, and justice. It is also important to follow the APA Ethics Code (American Psychological Association, 2017) and AERA guidelines (American Educational Research Association et al. (2014)). It is also important to produce a replicable science, which requires better science, including use of measures with strong psychometrics (reliability and validity), in addition to not engaging in questionable research practices. The open science movement, including pre-registrations, sharing data, preprints, and research materials may help improve the replicability of science.

13.7 Suggested Readings

American Psychological Association (2017); American Educational Research Association et al. (2014); Bersoff et al. (2012); Nagy (2011); L. Campbell et al. (2010)

14

Intellectual Assessment

14.1 Defining Intelligence

Definitions for intelligence are many. Some define intelligence as problem-solving abilities and the capacity for learning, where general intelligence is called "g" and reflects the ability to use this capacity. We can also consider emotional aspects of intelligence. For instance, social cognition reflects adaptive functioning. We can consider intelligence to be what reflects adaptive functioning. We can also consider whatever we value to be intelligence. For example, you might hear about a player's "basketball IQ". Some conceptualizations of intelligence emphasize it as a brain thing that involves speed of processing, processing capacity, and connectedness. From this perspective, intelligence includes components such as working memory, processing speed, visual and auditory perception, etc. We could also consider the products of these skills and components in interaction with the world. This is the goal of behavioral measures that are thought to reflect the underlying neural mechanism of general intelligence ("g").

14.2 History of Intelligence Research

A history of intelligence research is described in Sechrest et al. (1998). The assessment of intelligence is considered one of the key successes in psychology. Intelligence is one of the most widely assessed constructs in research and practice. Information from intelligence tests has important uses. Many people have contributed in important ways to the assessment of intelligence. Here, we outline just a few key figures as a way to introduce different models of intelligence. Please note that our discussion of the history of intelligence and key figures is no endorsement of their views. For instance, historically, some of the researchers on intelligence were proponents of eugenics.

14.2.1 Sir Francis Galton (1822–1911)

Sir Francis Galton was known for his work on lots of topics, including correlation, regression, twin studies, heredity, individual differences, the fax machine, and the telegraph. His work discovered the importance of reaction time, and conceptualized it as reflecting an underlying construct. He examined individual differences in many domains: vision, hearing, reaction time, other sensorimotor functions, and physical characteristics. Many of these individual differences would fall into the construct of "intelligence" now.

14.2.2 James Cattell (1860–1944)

James Cattell was Wihelm Wundt's first American student. Cattell measured sensory acuity and psychophysical characteristics. Cattell's work followed Galton's, and he examined whether reaction time might shed light on consciousness. Cattell used factor analysis to formally approach Galton's questions about why scores correlated—why people who tended to be good at one thing also tended to be good at lots of other things. He was credited with initiating the individual differences movement and with the first published reference to a mental test in the psychological literature.

14.2.3 Alfred Binet (1857–1911)

Alfred Binet was a French psychologist, and his work was more applied than the work by Galton and Cattell. He tried to apply principles of psychology to ameliorate mental problems. In France, he was forward-thinking at the time: he sought to identify children with an intellectual disability so that they could receive training and live a productive life. He and his colleague, Théodore Simon, asked who is trainable and when. And with their work, so begins clinical assessment.

In 1905, Binet and Simon developed the Binet–Simon Intelligence Scale for children. It was developed from a government commission to study the education of children with an intellectual disability (called mentally retarded or "arriéré" at the time). Items on the scales were administered from easiest to hardest, until the participant could not do three-quarters of the items. This approach is similar to modern-day item response theory approaches to adaptive testing. Items were selected for inclusion in the scales if they showed criterion-related validity in relation to two criteria:

- age—discriminative validity (i.e., age differentiation); items were identified for which older children performed better than younger children, and
- performance in school; items were selected that differentiated children who showed success versus failure in school.

This approach of using ceiling criteria to establish stop points in testing is still widely used today. The Binet–Simon Intelligence Scale included subtests that are still widely used today involving:

- Naming objects in pictures (similar to the Peabody Picture Vocabulary Test): phone, squash, etc.
- Digit span and reverse digit span: having a respondent repeat numbers of a progressively longer and longer length, then having respondents repeat numbers in the reverse number; examines how much information a person can store in working memory and their underlying capacity.
- A vocabulary test: asking children to define words to show they know the meaning of words; a concrete measure reflective of ability to learn words.
- Similarities: examines abstraction and understanding.
- Block design: having the respondent manipulate blocks to make different designs; examines visuospatial reasoning.
- Comprehension questions: how much the person has learned information about life and culture because of their capacity.

Binet and Simon assessed performance of typically developing children and children with intellectual disability. They quantified children's performance on the tests with what they called "mental age" (as opposed to chronological age). The child's mental age was estimated by correcting for the expected (median) score at that age. For instance, if a child has a mental age of a 7-year-old, that means that the child's performance is the same as the average (50th percentile) 7-year-old.

The Binet–Simon Intelligence Scale was validated with the opinions of teachers of children's academic functioning. Teachers' reports used to show stronger criterion-related validity compared to intelligence tests. Now, intelligence tests are the gold standard; they show stronger criterion-related validity compared to teacher reports.

14.2.4 Lewis Terman (1877–1956)

Lewis Terman at Stanford University revised the Binet–Simon Intelligence Scale, and the revised test became known as the Stanford–Binet Intelligence Scales. After the release of the Stanford–Binet, academics became excited about intelligence testing.

14.2.5 William Stern (1871–1938)

A key challenge that intelligence researchers had was how to quantify children's performance on the tests. Binet had introduced the concept of the mental age—the typical age for participants with that score. Mental age had a generalizable notion that was informative. It provided meaning compared to saying that someone received a score of 8 on the measure. Mental age conceptualizes intelligence as a measure of current functioning to inform how to improve their functioning to efficiently use resources.

However, performance does not increase across all domains with age through adulthood. That is, the same level of performance could have multiple mental ages. Therefore, William Stern changed the scoring to a trait measure by developing the Intelligence Quotient (IQ) that Terman used in the Stanford–Binet. IQ was calculated using Equation (14.1):

$$\text{Intelligence Quotient (IQ)} = \frac{\text{mental age}}{\text{chronological age}} \times 100 \tag{14.1}$$

This helped keep IQ to be a more stable as a characteristic of the person. IQ was more trait-like and stable than mental age, and it does not change as much with age because it accounts for age.

Today, this index is known as the "Ratio IQ". It involves taking a ratio of two numbers, but it is not a ratio measure because it does not have a meaningful zero, and the gaps between the scores might not be equidistant.

Stern was a German psychologist who moved to America and promoted Binet's ideas. Compared to England where you became what your parents were, in America, your future was thought to be determined by your underlying ability. This was based on the idea that "everyone who is able could become successful". Therefore, intelligence took hold with the idea that individual abilities determine success. Intelligence took hold, then World War I occurred.

14.2.6 Robert Yerkes (1876–1956)

World War I involved using lots of technology. In 1917, under the lead of Robert Yerkes and others, the United States Army developed the Army Alpha and Beta Test, a precursor to the eventual Armed Services Vocational Aptitude Battery (ASVAB). The U.S. Army sought to improve the army by classifying people in rank and tasks according to their capabilities—it is important to have the best army possible or you will lose the war.

The content was similar to the Binet scales, but it was changed from a clinical test to a multiple-choice, paper-and-pencil test that a clerk could give to large groups. The Alpha Test included words and letters for literate recruits. The Beta Test was a picture-based intelligence test without words for illiterate recruits or recent immigrants. For instance, the Beta Test involved having recruits code digits with symbols, which is still part of the Wechsler Adult Intelligence Scales today.

The Army Alpha and Beta Tests are among the first examples of affirmative action because anybody could get picked based on their test performance compared to only doing what one's parents did. However, the Army Alpha and Beta Tests turned out to be biased against rural, non-whites because they were less experienced with standardized setting. The Army Alpha and Beta Tests were the precursors to much of the modern psychometric movement in psychology, and to the development of more advanced intelligence tests.

14.2.7 Charles Spearman (1863–1945)

Charles Spearman found that performance on many tasks was highly correlated. Using factor analysis, he proposed that an underlying "force" ("g") drove performance on all tests. However, he found that "g" could not explain all variance in tasks. He proposed a two factor-theory. According to Spearman two-factor theory, the variation between people on all cognitive tasks is a function of two factors: general intelligence ("g") and test-specific variance ("s"), as depicted in Figure 14.1.

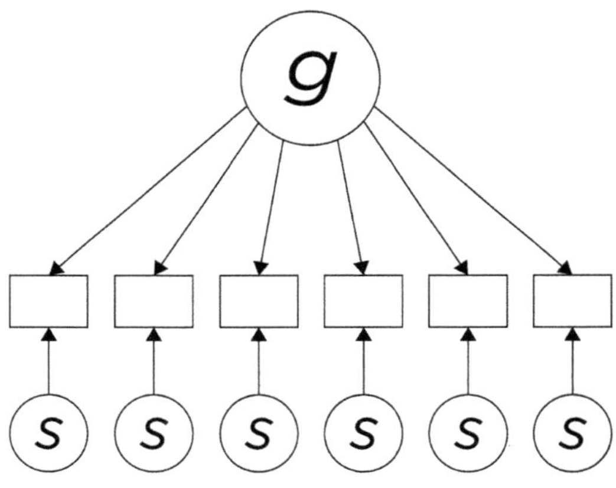

FIGURE 14.1 Spearman's Two-Factor Theory of Intelligence.

14.2.8 Louis Leon Thurstone (1887–1955)

Louis Leon Thurstone had restricted range in his samples and observed lower correlations among the skills than Charles Spearman observed. Thurstone hypothesized that the tests tapped specific abilities or faculties, not just a general factor. Thus, he argued that intelligence was not one thing—it was many things. He argued that the intelligences consisted of independent, lower-order processes, such as memory, verbal skills, and spatial skills, with a clearer psychological meaning than "g" or test-specific skills, and that these lower-order processes might better explain the pattern of correlations among cognitive tests than a general factor. Examples of independent abilities are depicted in Figure 14.2.

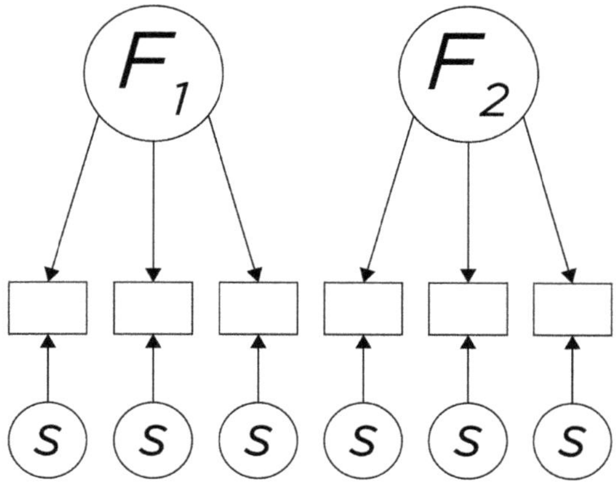

FIGURE 14.2 Thurstone's Theory of Intelligence (with Only Two Factors Depicted for Simplicity).

14.2.9 Raymond Cattell (1905–1998)

Raymond Cattell proposed splitting "g" into two factors: fluid intelligence (G_f) and crystallized intelligence (G_c), as depicted in Figure 14.3. Fluid intelligence (G_f) was considered to be the capacity to respond adaptively in novel situations. It was thought to be based on neural integrity (versus noise), neural connectedness, processing speed, memory size, spatial processing, abstract reasoning, and one's capacity for novel learning. Crystallized intelligence (G_c) was considered to be preserved with age and was based on life experience (e.g., quality of schools, number of words spoken to child, etc.), history, learned skills, cultural knowledge, verbal skills, and vocabulary. Crystallized intelligence could be further sub-divided into historical G_c and current G_c. Historical G_c was considered what a person had learned prior to receiving specialized training or practice. Current G_c was considered the domains of expert knowledge and skills. Most assessment tests assess historical G_c rather than current G_c. Tests include both G_f and G_c, but we do not know how much.

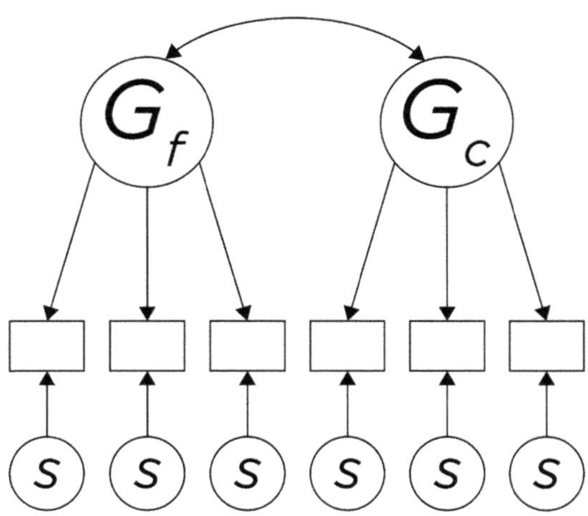

FIGURE 14.3 Cattell's G_f-G_c Theory of Intelligence. G_f = fluid intelligence; G_c = crystallized intelligence.

Fluid intelligence was hypothesized by Cattell to be one's inborn and physiologically based cognitive processing capacity which develops rapidly in childhood and is then invested in developing crystallized skills. Fluid intelligence was thought to be necessary for acquiring knowledge that becomes crystallized intelligence. Fluid intelligence increases with age from childhood to adulthood, peaks in the early 20s, and decreases in middle and older age. Fluid intelligence is more likely to be impaired (compared to crystallized intelligence) following brain trauma.

Crystallized intelligence is theoretically expected to continue expanding with age, but historical G_c does seem to peak around late 30s. Given extensive age-related changes in intelligence (including fluid and crystallized intelligence), performance needs to be compared to same-aged peers.

14.2.10 John Horn (1926–2006)

John Horn extended Cattell's G_f-G_c model to include 10 broad abilities, including:

- G_f: fluid reasoning (fluid intelligence)
- G_c: comprehension-knowledge (crystallized intelligence)
- G_a: auditory processing
- G_{lr}: long-term storage and retrieval
- G_q: quantitative knowledge
- G_{rw}: reading and writing ability
- G_s: processing speed
- G_{sm}: short-term memory
- G_t: reaction time/decision speed
- G_v: visual processing

14.2.11 John Carroll (1916–2003)

John Carroll proposed a three-stratum hierarchical model that included narrow abilities (stratum 1), broad abilities (stratum 2), and general abilities (stratum 3), as depicted in Figure 14.4.

This model of intelligence became known as the Cattell-Horn-Carroll (CHC) model, which is now the most prominent contemporary theory of intelligence.

14.2.12 David Wechsler (1896–1981)

David Wechsler developed the Wechsler Adult Intelligence Scale (WAIS) and Wechsler Intelligence Scale for Children (WISC), which are among the most widely used intelligence tests. These tests sub-divide intelligence into verbal IQ and performance IQ, along with more narrowly defined abilities.

14.3 Alternative Conceptualizations of Intelligence

As noted earlier, the CHC model (Figure 14.4) is the most prominent contemporary theory of intelligence. However, there are alternative conceptualizations of intelligence. One alternative conceptualization of intelligence is the bifactor model, which is depicted in Figure 14.5. In a

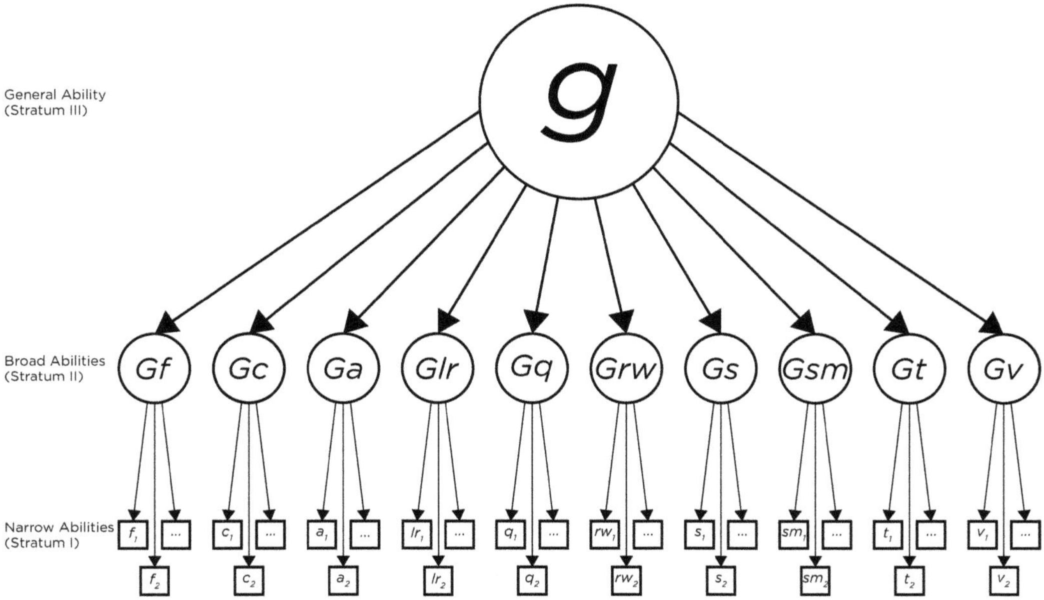

FIGURE 14.4 Cattell-Horn-Carroll Hierarhical Theory of Intelligence.

bifactor model, "g" is modeled in a non-hierarchical fashion where it is extracted first, and the primary factors are extracted separately from the remaining common variance among the tests. In this model, the resulting factors are independent of variance due to "g". Variation in performance on subtests can be due to g and/or to primary factors, which are independent. Evidence has provided support for the bifactor model of intelligence when fit to several intelligence measures, though the structure often depends on the measure used (Dombrowski et al., 2021).

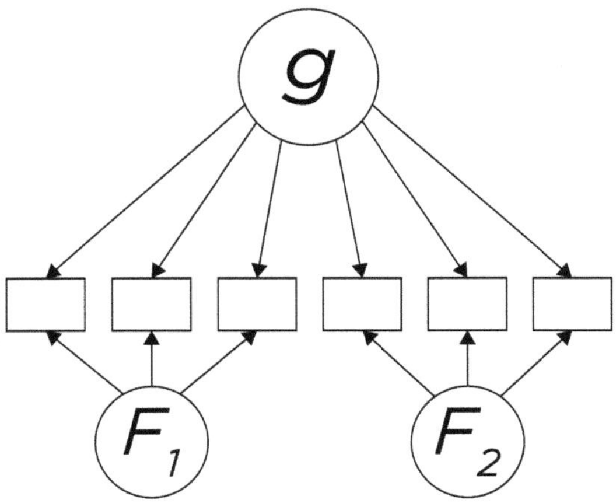

FIGURE 14.5 Bifactor Model of Intelligence.

14.4 Purposes of Intelligence Tests

Intelligence tests have multiple purposes, though these uses are limited. Scores on intelligence tests have been shown to predict future academic achievement. They can also be helpful for characterizing functional impairment. For instance, they can be helpful for academic planning—i.e., whether a person is gifted or in need of remediation. Intelligence tests can also be helpful for identifying change in functioning over time, for example that may be related to dementia or brain injury.

Scores on intelligence tests can also influence approaches to clinical assessment. Many assessment strategies assume average intelligence for question comprehension. A clinician might use assessments with more basic instructions or nonverbal assessments for those with poorer intelligence. Moreover, intelligence scores can influence the approaches to treatment, including the vocabulary used by the clinician, the extent of use of written material, and the clinician's expectations that the client engages in abstract reasoning. For example, a clinician might not focus on the cognitive side of therapy in cognitive-behavior therapy; instead, they might focus more on the behavioral side of cognitive-behavior therapy: exposure therapy for anxiety and behavioral activation for depression.

14.5 Intelligence Versus Achievement Versus Aptitude

In theory, intelligence is what you "have" (in terms of ability), whereas achievement is "what you do with it". Aptitude is what you will be able to do with maximum training and opportunity.

Tests that are intended to assess intelligence include the Wechsler Adult Intelligence Scale (WAIS), Wechsler Intelligence Scale for Children (WISC), Wechsler Abbreviated Scale of Intelligence (WASI), Wechsler Preschool and Primary Scale of Intelligence (WPPSI), Woodcock-Johnson Tests of Cognitive Abilities, Stanford–Binet Intelligence Scale, Differential Ability Scales (DAS), and Kaufman Brief Intelligence Test (KBIT).

Tests that are intended to assess achievement include the Wechsler Individual Achievement Test (WIAT), Wide Range Achievement Test (WRAT), and Woodcock-Johnson Tests of Achievement.

Tests that are intended to assess aptitude include the Graduate Record Examination (GRE), Scholastic Aptitude Test (SAT), American College Testing (ACT), Graduate Management Admission Test (GMAT), and Law School Admission Test (LSAT).

Achievement presumably depends on both intelligence and aptitude, as well as motivation and effort. In reality, these constructs are difficult to differentiate at a measurement level. Assessment instruments that are intended to assess one of these likely assess elements of all of these.

14.6 Theory Influences Intepretation of Scores

Despite the considerable research on intelligence, it is still difficult to define intelligence. What is intelligence? According to the 1994 academic workgroup, "Mainstream Science on Intelligence", intelligence "involves the ability to reason, plan, solve problems, think abstractly, comprehend complex ideas, learn quickly, and learn from experience" (Arvey et al., 1994; L. S. Gottfredson, 1997). Some of the most widely used assessments of intelligence lack a clear theoretical foundation. They are more based on psychometrics than theory. Thus, it has been argued that "intelligence is what intelligence tests measure" (Boring, 1923).

Theory plays an important role in interpretation of scores from tests. With the Iowa Tests of Basic Skills (ITBS) and other tests, they have divergent goals from traditional intelligence tests: evaluating schools as opposed to evaluating children. For example, some stakeholders may be more interested in how much learning occurs in particular schools rather than merely a person's level of ability. Thus, the content that comprises "intelligence" differs depending on the purpose of assessment. You would also prioritize different predictive criteria depending on the goal, with items and subtests selected accordingly. For example, predictive criteria could focus on school performance versus job performance versus life skills.

14.7 Time-Related Influences

Individual differences in intelligence scores tend to be relatively stable as people age, despite changes in absolute performance. Nevertheless, there are time-related influences on intelligence scores. One time-related influence on intelligence scores is called the Flynn effect. The Flynn effect is the phenomenon that there are age cohort differences in IQ scores such that IQ scores rise around 3 points every decade; younger generations perform better on intelligence tests than older generations, when they were at the same age. So your children's generation is likely to be more intelligent than your generation, at least as assessed with the currently available instruments.

14.8 Concerns with Intelligence Tests

Despite the utility of intelligence tests, there are numerous concerns with intelligence tests. For instance, there are concerns about the content validity of intelligence tests. That is, there are concerns that intelligence tests do not assess all important aspects of the construct of intelligence. Intelligence tests typically do not assess creativity, emotional intelligence, empathy, etc.

Another concern is that intelligence tests encourage participants to put forth maximum mental effort. However, the *typical* mental effort needed to solve problems may be more important for many assessment questions than what someone can answer with maximum mental effort. Fluid intelligence is most likely to be affected by effort and attention.

Another concern is that scores can be influenced by factors other than intelligence. For instance, IQ scores may be affected, at least indirectly, by socioeconomic status and educational background. IQ scores are moderately associated with socioeconomic status and level of education. IQ scores might also be influenced by cultural background (due to the potential for intelligence tests to have cultural biases), motivation, intimidation or anxiety, and the physical testing conditions.

There are also concerns about the predictive utility of intelligence tests. Scores from intelligence tests have been shown to predict some aspects of functioning, but only in limited ways. For instance, IQ scores have been shown to predict grades in K–12 school, number of school years completed, academic performance through freshman year of college, and whether someone obtains a job. However, there are limits to what IQ scores can predict and the (weak) magnitude in which they predict these phenomena. Moreover, IQ scores do not appear to predict how successfully one performs in their job, the quality of their interpersonal relationships, or their happiness.

14.9 Aptitude Testing

The primary origin of considerations of the predictive utility of aptitude testing was World War I. Robert Ladd Thorndike (1910–1990) developed a test to assess aptitude for becoming a pilot. The tests examined individual differences in keeping track of all things to predict who will be a good pilot—including skills involving stress, vision, attention, reaction time, working memory, navigation, being upside down, etc. Intelligence and aptitude testing took off from there.

McClelland (1973; 1994) examined the data on aptitude predicting outcomes. He examined the question of whether grades and intelligence tests predict life and occupation success. He says no—or at least, intelligence does not influence life and occupation success, but rather intelligence opens up access to education, which serves as an important credential for access to good jobs. That is, McClelland argued that there is criterion contamination in the evaluation of criterion-related validity of intelligence tests.

He argued that intelligence and aptitude tests are culturally and socioeconomically biased. That is, the associations between intelligence test scores and job scores that have been observed in prior research may be an artifact given that socioeconomic status (SES) influences both. Others argue that IQ scores do predict later life and occupation success, and that they have shown validity across groups and SES levels—i.e., that the association is not an artifact of SES. Moreover, others have argued that the observed associations are weaker than true associations because of restriction of range. For example, students with lowest SAT/GRE scores are typically not admitted, so one cannot examine their outcomes in association with the full range of SAT/GRE scores because we do not have access to outcomes for the people who are not admitted.

McClelland argues that, instead of performing aptitude tests, we should look at life characteristics and job-related competencies. To understand McClelland's position, it can be helpful to distinguish between signs and samples. Signs are instances where human behavior is viewed as a sign of some underlying characteristic. For instance, the Rorschach Inkblot Test is all sign and no sample. Psychodynamic theorists view responses as signs of underlying personality dynamics. By contrast, samples focus on operations (behaviors). Samples come from a behavioral perspective in which behaviors are just what they are; no underlying causes are inferred—i.e., there is less inference for samples than for signs. Examples of a sample for an occupation as a pilot could involve evaluating how well the person flies an airplane. A sample from a driving test would be to literally sample driving behavior. These are examples of *criterion sampling*. Criterion sampling involves sampling of the behavior in the area of interest to use as the criterion. For example, criterion sampling could involve assessing a sample of abilities relevant for a position (i.e., competency testing) based on a job analysis of the duties and responsibilities of a particular job and the skills and abilities necessary to perform the job well. McClelland's goal is to use the criterion sample to reduce bias for minorities. However, using a criterion sample actually increased bias.

McClelland was interested in shifting the field from using signs to using samples. McClelland argued that use of intelligence tests for job selection involves too much inference about an underlying ability—i.e., the test is used as a sign rather than as a sample. McClelland would argue that, instead, employers should do testing for competencies such as communication skills, goal setting, ego development, and patience. However, he does not say how to assess these skills. He would argue that it is important to sample multiple aspects of the construct of interest; a wider array of talents—not just academic performance. For a relevant criterion sample of competencies for a particular job or position, you need strong theory. However, criterion sampling is very difficult.

Consider tests for selection of firefighters. Evaluative tests for selecting firefighters include fitness tests, among other tests. Fitness tests may include activities like running with heavy objects, climbing ladders, and willingness to go into burning buildings—skills which translate to the activities that many firefighters perform on the job. However, these fitness tests have been shown to lead to adverse impact toward women—i.e., they result in lower selection rates of women than men. The fitness tests are also biased in favor of people who had practiced, and who had previous training. Criterion sampling without pre-training makes things worse. You could lead bootcamps of pre-training to level the playing field for job applicants and then conduct testing. However, pre-training takes time and money, and many organizations may not be willing to do that.

Range restriction leads to artifactually lower validity estimates of intelligence/aptitude tests with school and job performance. After accounting for range restriction, predictive validity coefficients are around .5 with school and job performance. Thus, many intelligence/aptitude tests tend to show some predictive validity for academic/job performance. However, it is also important to consider whether test bias exists. We discuss test bias in the next chapter.

14.10 Scales

IQ has had various scales.

14.10.1 Ratio IQ

Ratio IQ is mental age divided by chronological age, known as the intelligence quotient (see Equation (14.1)). Ratio IQ changes with age, and it is not widely used today. Deviation IQ is more widely used today.

14.10.2 Deviation IQ

Deviation IQ (also called Standard Scores) is a standardized norm-referenced score with a mean of 100 and a standard deviation of 15. Deviation IQ was developed by David Wechsler. Scores are norm-referenced to same-aged peers. It has no reference to mental age. Using Deviation IQ scores, intellectual disability is defined as a score of 70 or below (along with functional impairment) because the score represents two standard deviations below the mean. However, this cutoff is based on an arbitrary statistical decision and tradition. Giftedness is defined as a score of 130 or above, which is two standard deviations above the mean.

14.10.3 Nominal, Ordinal, Interval, or Ratio?

Intelligence scores are ordinal or interval, not ratio. You cannot talk about someone as being twice as intelligent as someone else because we do not know what zero intelligence is or what the maximum intelligence is.

14.11 Conclusion

Intelligence has been defined in many ways, and intelligence assessment has a long history. The assessment of intelligence is considered one of the key successes in psychology. The most prominent contemporary theory of intelligence is the CHC model, which is a three-stratum hierarchical model that includes narrow abilities (stratum 1), broad abilities (stratum 2), and general abilities (stratum 3). Assessments of intelligence have utility for various purposes, including predicting future academic achievement, characterizing functional impairment, and identifying change in functioning over time. However, there are many things that intelligence does not predict well, such as how successfully one will perform in their job, the quality of their interpersonal relationships, or their happiness. Moreover, there are potential weaknesses of intelligence tests, including content validity because they do not assess creativity or emotional aspects of intelligence such as empathy.

14.12 Suggested Readings

Ackerman (2013)

15

Test Bias

15.1 Overview

There are multiple definitions of the term "bias" depending on the context. In general, bias is a systematic error (Reynolds & Suzuki, 2012). Mean error is an example of systematic error, and is sometimes called bias. Cognitive biases are systematic errors in thinking, including confirmation bias and hindsight bias. Method biases are a form of systematic error that involve the influence of measurement on a person's score that is not due to the person's level on the construct. Method biases include response biases or response styles, including acquiescence and social desirability bias. Attentional bias refers to the tendency to process some types of stimuli more than others.

Sometimes bias is used to refer in particular to systematic error (in measurement, prediction, etc.) as a function of group membership, where test bias refers to the same score having different meaning for different groups. Under this meaning, a test is unbiased if a given test score has the same meaning regardless of group membership. For example, a test is biased if there is differential validity of test scores for groups (e.g., age, education, culture, race, sex). Test bias would exist, for instance, if a test is a less valid predictor for racial minorities or linguistic minorities. Test bias would also exist if scores on the Scholastic Aptitude Test (SAT) underestimate women's grades in college, for instance.

There are some known instances of test bias, as described in Section 15.3. Research has not produced much empirical evidence of test bias (Brown et al., 1999; Hall et al., 1999; Jensen, 1980; Kuncel & Hezlett, 2010; Reynolds et al., 2021; Reynolds & Suzuki, 2012; Sackett et al., 2008; Sackett & Wilk, 1994), though some item-level bias is not uncommon. Moreover, where test bias has been observed, it is often small, unclear, and does not always generalize (N. S. Cole, 1981). However, just because there is not much empirical evidence of test bias does not mean that test bias does not exist. Moreover, just because a test does not show bias does not mean that it should be used.

It is also worth pointing out that group differences in scores do not necessarily indicate bias. Group differences in scores could reflect true group differences in the construct. For instance, women have better verbal abilities, on average, compared to men. So, if women's scores on a verbal ability test are higher on average than men's scores, this would not be sufficient evidence for bias.

There are two broad categories of test bias:

1. predictive bias
2. test structure bias

Predictive bias refers to differences between groups in the relation between the test and criterion. As with all criterion-related validity tests, the findings depend on the strength and quality of the criterion. Test structure bias refers to differences in the internal test characteristics across groups.

15.2 Ways to Investigate/Detect Test Bias

15.2.1 Predictive Bias

Predictive bias exists when differences emerge between groups in terms of predictive validity to a criterion. It is assessed by using a regression line looking at the association between test score and job performance. For instance, consider a 2-by-2 confusion matrix used for the standard prediction problem. A confusion matrix for whom to select for a job is depicted in Figure 15.1.

		Predicted Job Performance ("Test")	
		Bad	Good
Actual Job Performance ("Truth")	Good	FN	TP
	Bad	TN	FP

FIGURE 15.1 2-by-2 Confusion Matrix for Job Selection. TP = true positive; TN = true negative; FP = false positive; FN = false negative.

We can also visualize the confusion matrix in terms of a scatterplot of the test scores (i.e., predicted job performance) and the "truth" scores (i.e., actual job performance), as depicted in Figure 15.2. The predictor (test score) is on the x-axis. The criterion (job performance) is on the y-axis. The quadrants reflect the cutoffs (i.e., thresholds) imposed from the 2-by-2 confusion matrix. The vertical line reflects the cutoff for selecting someone for a job. The horizontal line reflects the cutoff for good job performance (i.e., people who should have been selected for the job).

The data points in the top right quadrant are true positives: people who the test predicted would do a good job and who did a good job. The data points in the bottom left quadrant are true negatives: people who the test predicted would do a poor job and who would have done a poor job. The data points in the bottom right quadrant are false positives: people who the test predicted would do a good job and who did a poor job. The data points in the top left quadrant are false negatives: people who the test predicted would do a poor job and who would have done a good job.

Figure 15.3 depicts a strong predictor. The best-fit regression line has a steep slope where there are lots of data points that are true positives and true negatives, with relatively few false positives and false negatives.

Figure 15.4 depicts a poor predictor. The best-fit regression line has a shallow slope where there are just as many data points that are in the false cells (false positives and false negatives) as there are in the true cells (true positives and true negatives). In general, the steeper the slope, the better the predictor.

We can evaluate predictive bias using a best-fit regression line between the predictor and criterion for each group.

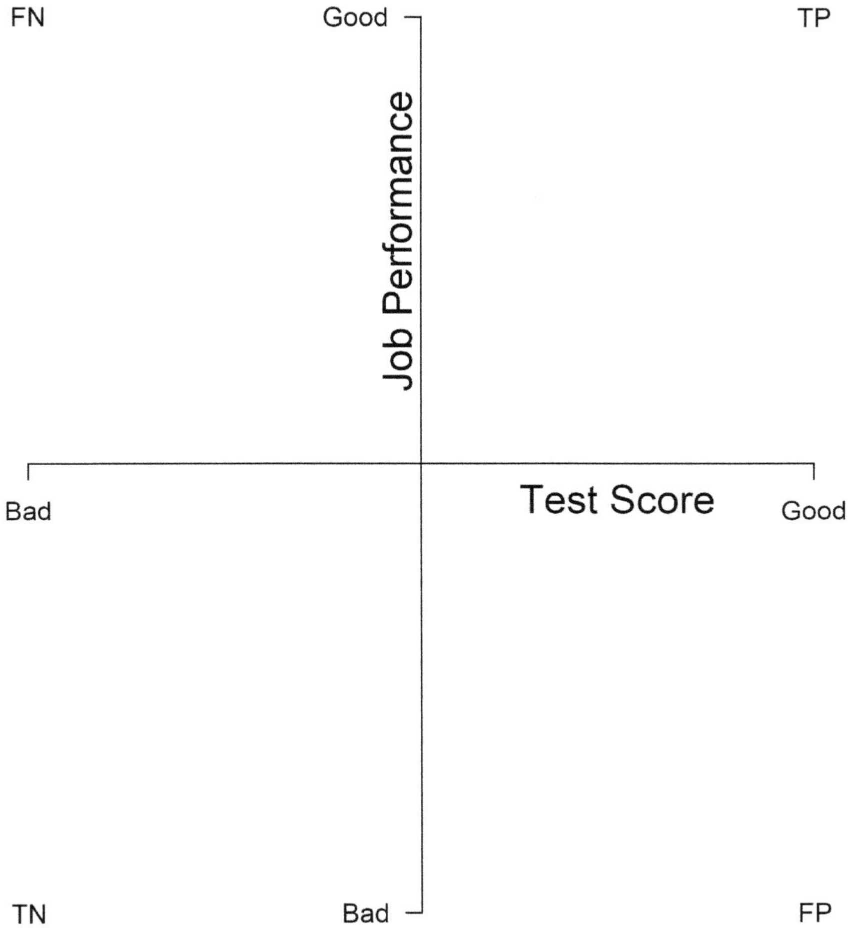

FIGURE 15.2 2-by-2 Confusion Matrix for Job Selection in the Form of a Graph with Predicted Performance on the x-Axis and Actual Job Performance on the y-Axis. TP = true positive; TN = true negative; FP = false positive; FN = false negative.

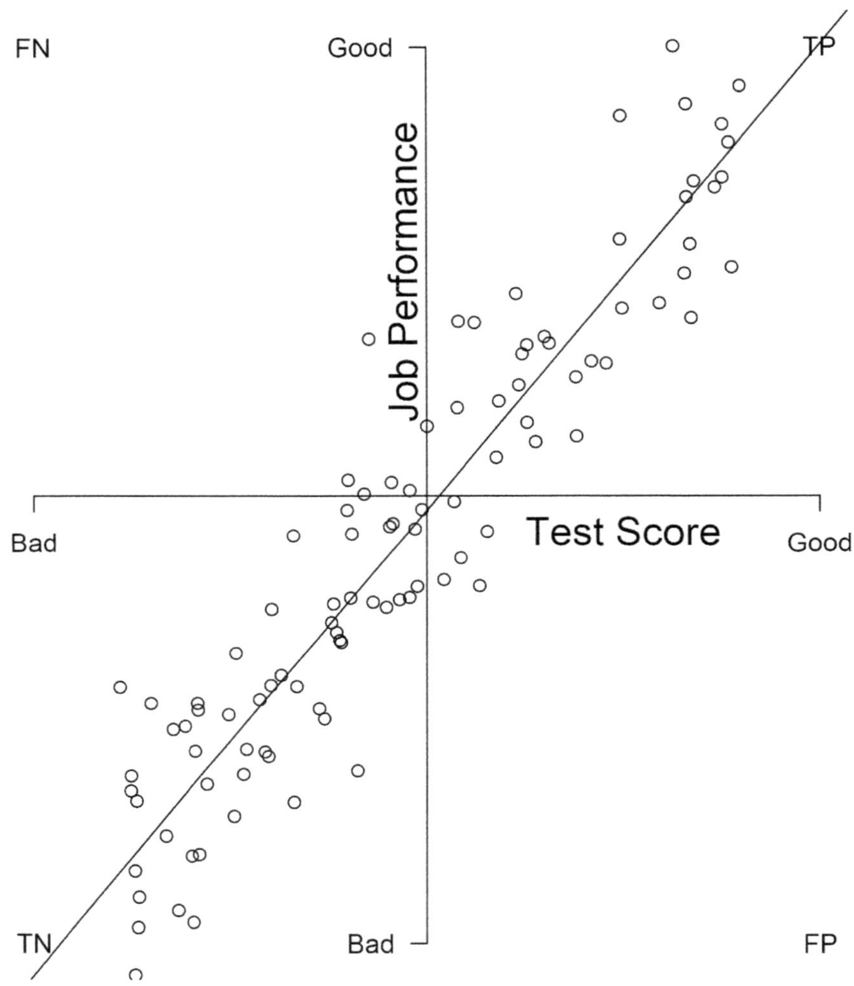

FIGURE 15.3 Example of a Strong Predictor. TP = true positive; TN = true negative; FP = false positive; FN = false negative.

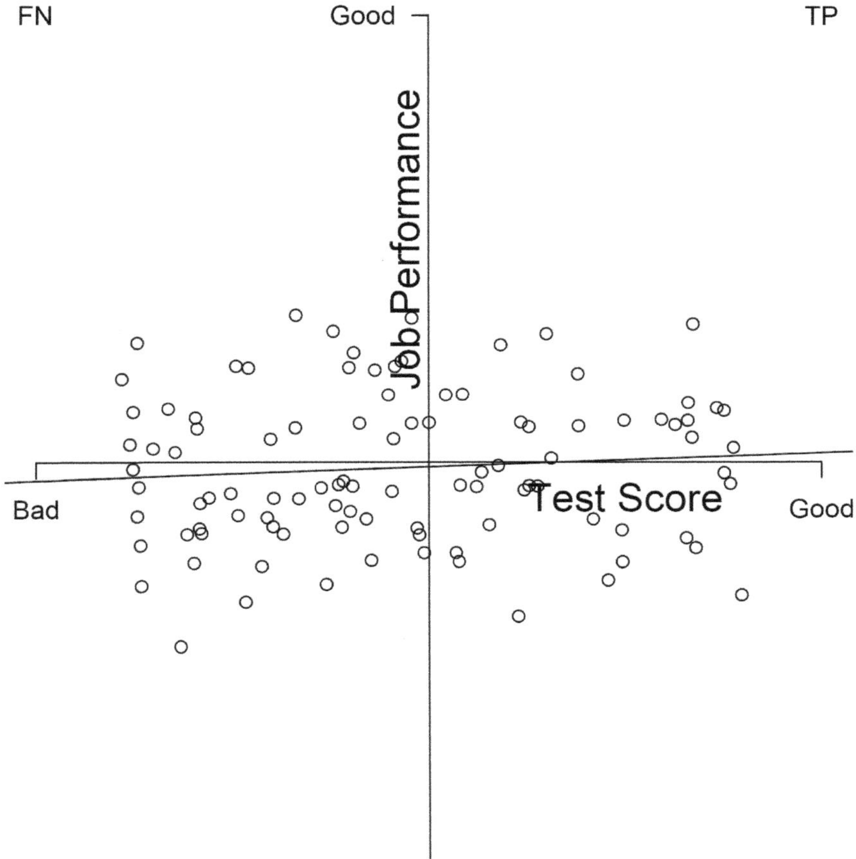

FIGURE 15.4 Example of a Poor Predictor. TP = true positive; TN = true negative; FP = false positive; FN = false negative.

15.2.1.1 Types of Predictive Bias

There are three types of predictive bias:

1. Different slopes
2. Different intercepts
3. Different intercepts and slopes

The slope of the regression line is the steepness of the line. The intercept of the regression line is the y-value of the point where the line crosses the y-axis (i.e., when $x = 0$). If a measure shows predictive test bias, when looking at the regression line for each group, the groups' regression lines differ in either slopes and/or intercepts.

15.2.1.1.1 Different slopes

Predictive bias in terms of different slopes exists when there are differences in the slope of the regression line between minority and majority groups. The slope describes the *direction* and *steepness* of the regression line. The slope of a regression line is the amount of change in y for every unit change in x (i.e., rise over run). Differing slopes indicate differential predictive validity, in which the test is a more effective predictor of performance in one group over the other. Different slopes predictive bias is depicted in Figure 15.5. In the figure, the predictor performs well in the majority group. However, the slope is close to zero in the minority group, indicating that there is no association between the predictor and the criterion for the minority group.

Different slopes can especially occur if we develop our measure and criterion based on the normative majority group. Not much evidence has found empirical evidence of different slopes across groups. However, samples often do not have the power to detect differing slopes (Aguinis et al., 2010). Theoretically, to fix biases related to different slopes, you should find another measure that is more predictive for the minority group. If the predictor is a strong predictor in both groups but shows slight differences in the slope, within-group norming could be used.

15.2.1.1.2 Different intercepts

Predictive bias in terms of different intercepts exists when there are differences in the intercept of the regression line between minority and majority groups. The y-intercept describes the point on the y-axis that the line intersects with the y-axis (when $x = 0$). When the distributions have similar slopes, intercept differences suggest that the measure systematically under- or overestimates group performance relative to the person's ability. The same test score leads to systematically different predictions for the majority and minority groups. In other words, minority group members get different tests scores than majority group members with the same ability. Different intercepts predictive bias is depicted in Figure 15.6.

A higher intercept (relative to zero) indicates that the measure *under*-estimates a person's ability (at that test score)—i.e., the person's job performance is better than what the test score would suggest. A lower intercept (relative to zero) indicates that the measure *over*-estimates a person's ability (at that test score)—i.e., the person's job performance is worse than what the test score would suggest. Figure 15.6 indicates that the measure systematically underestimates the job performance of the minority group.

Performance among members of a minority group could be under- or overestimated. For example, historically, women's grades in math and engineering classes tended to be underes-

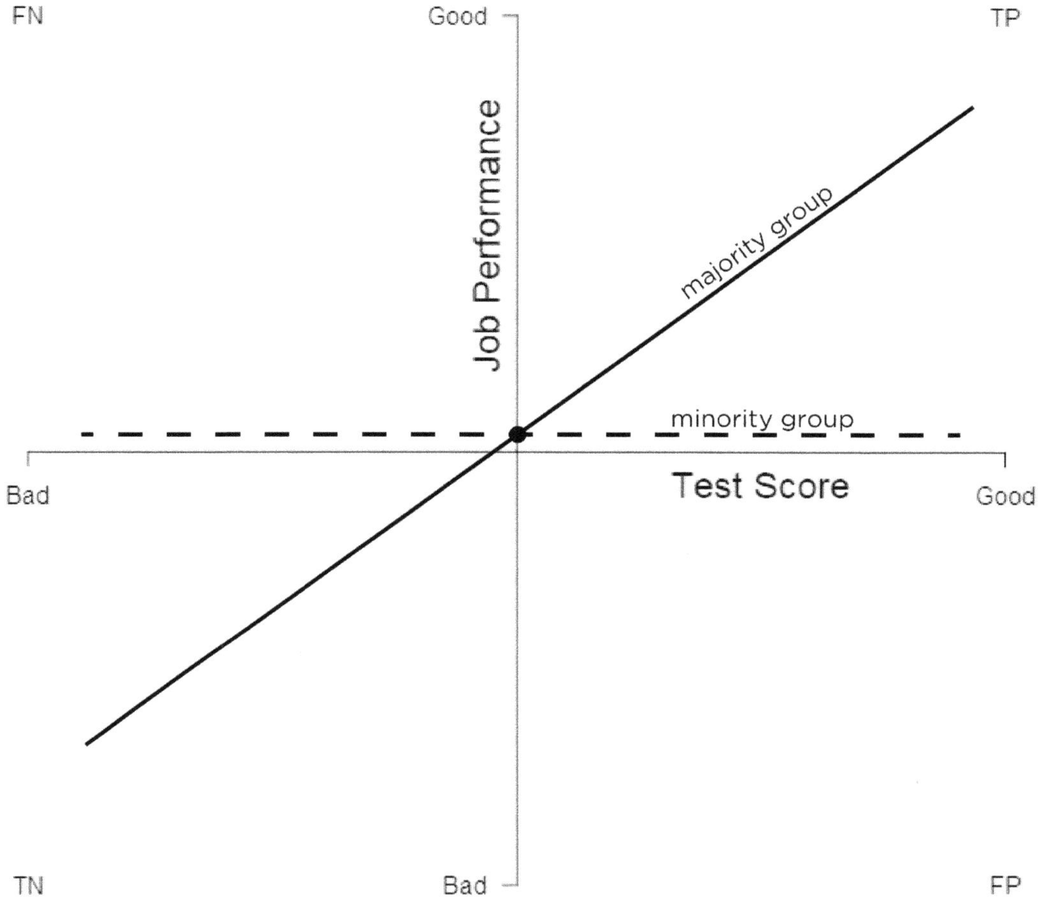

FIGURE 15.5 Test Bias: Different Slopes. TP = true positive; TN = true negative; FP = false positive; FN = false negative.

timated by the Scholastic Aptitude Test [(SAT); M. J. Clark & Grandy (1984)]. However, where intercept differences have been observed, measures often show small *over*estimation of school and job performance among minority groups (Reynolds & Suzuki, 2012). For example, women's physical strength and endurance is overestimated based on physical ability tests (Sackett & Wilk, 1994). In addition, overestimation of African Americans' and Hispanics' school and job performance has been observed based on cognitive ability tests (N. S. Cole, 1981; Reynolds & Suzuki, 2012; Sackett et al., 2008; Sackett & Wilk, 1994). At the same time, the Black–White difference in job performance is less than the Black–White difference in test performance.

The over-prediction of lower-scoring groups is likely mostly an artifact of measurement error (L. S. Gottfredson, 1994). The overestimation of African Americans' and Hispanics' school and job performance may be due to measurement error in the tests. Moreover, test scores explain only a portion of the variation in job performance. Black people are far less disadvantaged on the noncognitive determinants of job performance than on the cognitive ones. Nevertheless, the overestimation that has been often observed is *on average*—the performance is not overestimated for all individuals of the groups even if there is an average

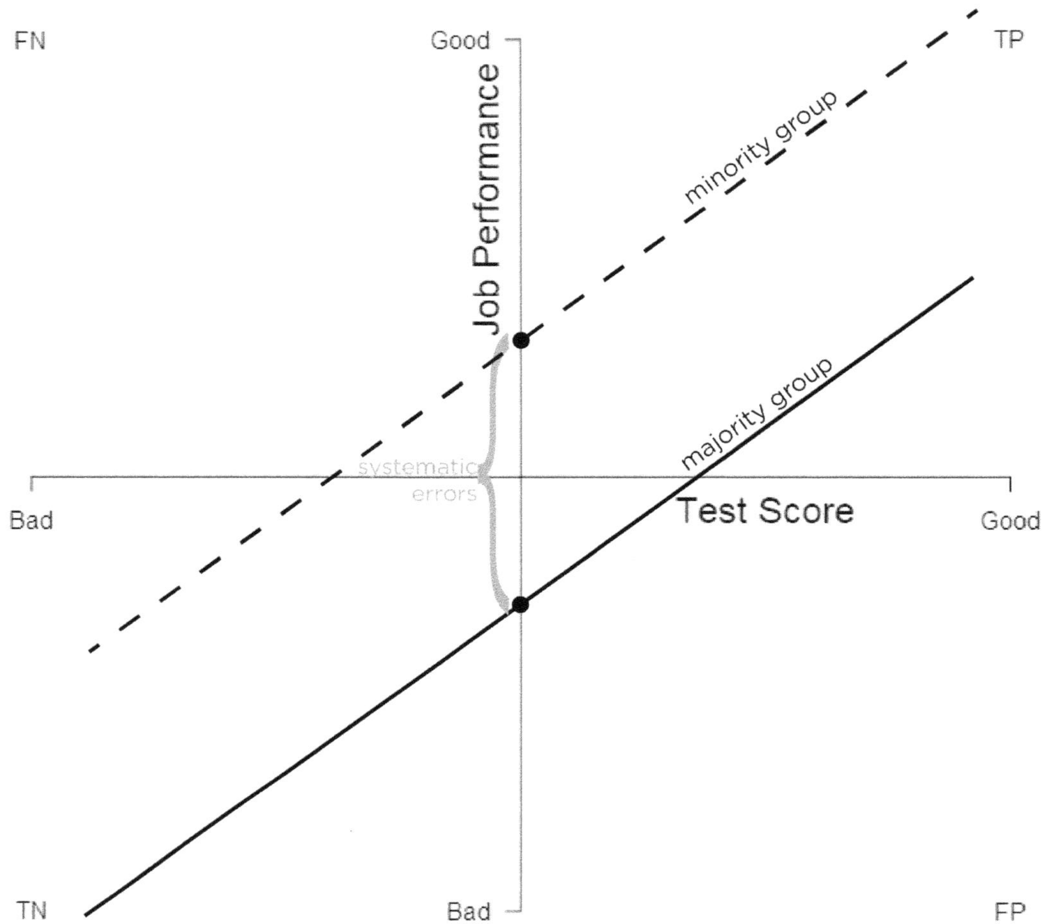

FIGURE 15.6 Test Bias: Different Intercepts. TP = true positive; TN = true negative; FP = false positive; FN = false negative.

overestimation effect. In addition, simulation findings indicate that lower intercepts (i.e., overestimation) among minority groups compared to majority groups could be observed if there are different slopes but not different intercepts in the population, because different slopes are likely to go undetected due to low power (Aguinis et al., 2010). That is, if a test shows weaker validity for a minority group than the majority group, it could appear as different intercepts that favor the minority group when, in fact, it reflects shallower slopes of the minority group that go undetected.

Predictive biases in intercepts could especially occur if we develop tests that are based on the majority group, and the items assess constructs other than the construct of interest which are systematically biased in favor of the majority group or against the minority group. Arguments about reduced power to detect differences are less relevant for intercepts and means than for slopes.

To correct for a bias in intercepts, we could add bonus points to the scores for the minority group to correct for the amount of the systematic error, and to result in the same regression line. But if the minority group is over-predicted (as has often been the case where intercept differences have been observed), we would not want to use score adjustment to lower the minority group's scores.

15.2.1.1.3 Different intercepts and slopes

Predictive bias in terms of different intercepts and slopes exists when there are differences in the intercept and slope of the regression line between minority and majority groups. In cases of different intercepts and slopes, there is both differential validity (because the regression lines have different slopes), as well as varying under- and overestimation of groups' performance at particular scores. Different intercepts and slopes predictive bias is depicted in Figure 15.7.

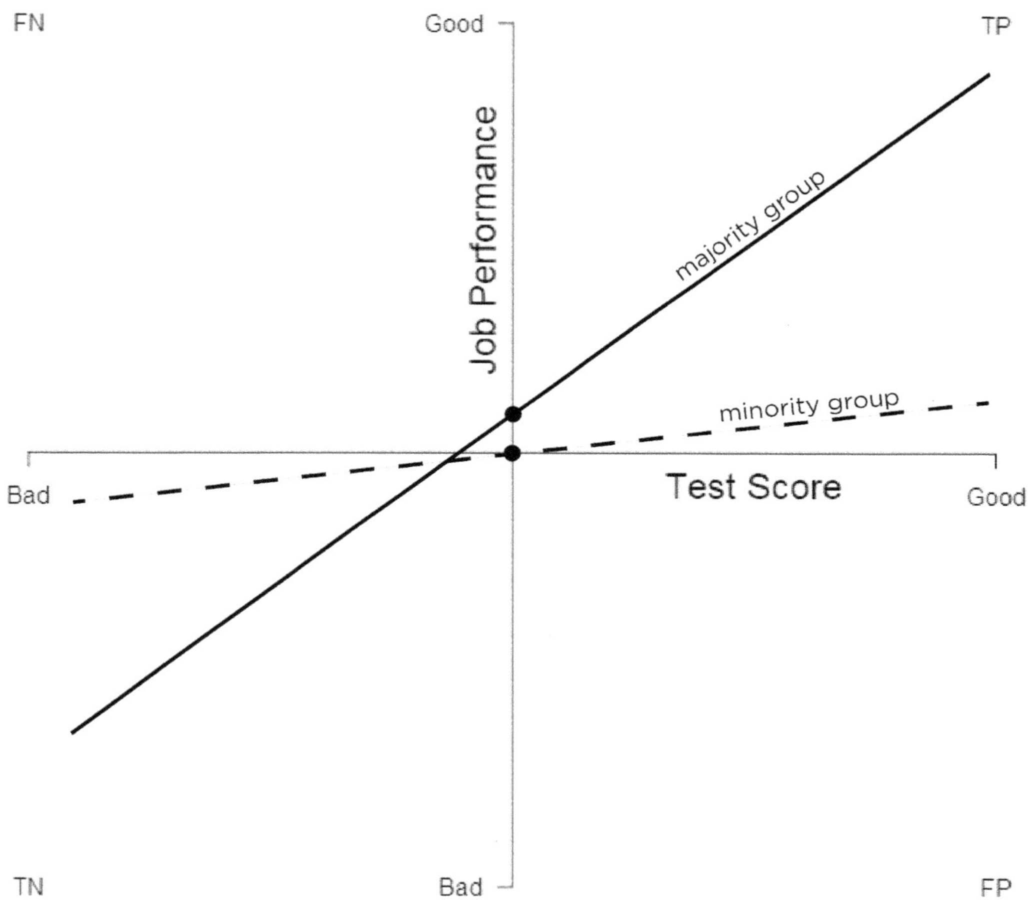

FIGURE 15.7 Test Bias: Different Intercepts and Slopes. TP = true positive; TN = true negative; FP = false positive; FN = false negative.

In instances of different intercepts and slopes predictive bias, a measure can simultaneously overestimate and underestimate a person's ability at different test scores. For instance, a measure can underestimate a person's ability at higher test scores and can overestimate a person's ability at lower test scores.

Different intercepts and slopes across groups is possibly more realistic than just different intercepts or just different slopes. However, different intercepts and slopes predictive bias is more complicated to study, represent, and resolve. It is difficult to examine because of complexity, and it is not easy to fix. Currently, we have nothing to address different intercepts and slopes predictive bias. We would need to use a different measure or measures for each group.

15.2.2 Test Structure Bias

In addition to predictive bias, another type of test bias is test structure bias. Test structure bias involves differences in internal test characteristics across groups. Examining test structure bias is different from examining the total score, as is used when examining predictive bias. Test structure bias can be identified empirically or based on theory/judgment.

Empirically, test structure bias can be examined in multiple ways.

15.2.2.1 Empirical Approaches to Identification

15.2.2.1.1 Item × group tests (ANOVA)

Item × Group tests in analysis of variance (ANOVA) examine whether the difference between groups on the overall score match comparisons among smaller items sets between groups. Item × Group tests are used to rule out that items are operating in different ways in different groups. If the items operate in different ways in different groups, they do not have the same meaning across groups. For example, if we are going to use a measure for multiple groups, we would expect its items to operate similarly across groups. So, if women show higher scores on a depression measure compared to men, we would also expect them to show similar elevations on each item (e.g., sleep loss).

15.2.2.1.2 Item response theory

Using item response theory, we can examine differential item functioning (DIF). Evidence of DIF, indicates that there are differences between group in terms of discrimination and/or difficulty/severity of items. Differences between groups in terms of the item characteristic curve (which combines the item's discrimination and severity) would be evidence against construct validity invariance between the groups and would provide evidence of bias. DIF examines stretching and compression of different groups. As an example, consider the item "bites others" in relation to externalizing problems. The item would be expected to show a weaker discrimination and higher severity in adults compared to children. DIF is discussed in Section 15.9.

15.2.2.1.3 Confirmatory factor analysis

Confirmatory factor analysis allows tests of measurement invariance (also called factorial invariance). Measurement invariance examines whether the factor structure of the underlying latent variables in the test is consistent across groups. It also examines whether the manifestation of the construct differs between groups. Measurement invariance is discussed in Section 15.10.

Even if you find the same slope and intercepts across groups in a prediction model, the measure would still be assessing different constructs across groups if the measure has a different factor structure between the groups. A different factor structure across groups is depicted in Figure 15.8.

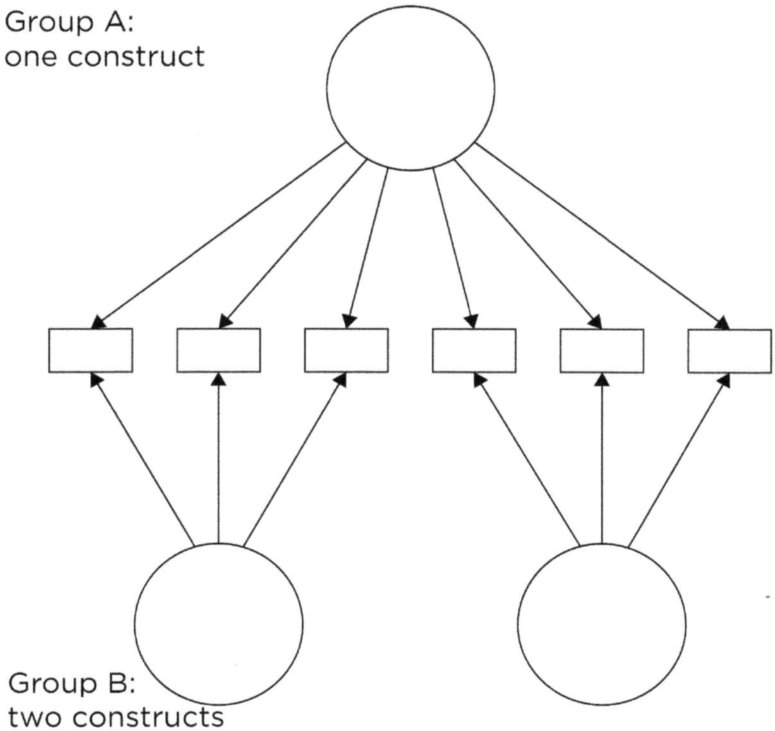

FIGURE 15.8 Different Factor Structure Across Groups.

An example of a different factor structure across groups is the differentiation of executive functions from two factors to three factors (inhibition, working memory, cognitive flexibility) across childhood (Lee et al., 2013).

There are different degrees of measurement invariance (for a review, see Putnick & Bornstein, 2016):

- Configural invariance: same number of factors in each group, and which indicators load on which factors are the same in each group (i.e., the same pattern of significant loadings in each group).
- Metric ("weak factorial") invariance: items have the same factor loadings (discrimination) in each group.
- Scalar ("strong factorial") invariance: items have the same intercepts (difficulty/severity) in each group.
- Residual ("strict factorial") invariance: items have the same residual/unique variances in each group.

15.2.2.1.4 Structural equation modeling

Structural equation modeling is a confirmatory factor analysis (CFA) model that incorporates prediction. Structural equation modeling allows examining differences in the underlying structure with differences in prediction in the same model.

15.2.2.1.5 Signal detection theory

Signal detection theory is a dynamic measure of bias. It allows examining the overall bias in selection systems, including both accuracy and errors at various cutoffs (sensitivity, specificity, positive predictive value, and negative predictive value), as well as accuracy across all possible cutoffs (the area under the receiver operating characteristic curve). While there may be similar predictive validity between groups, the type of errors we are making across groups might differ. It is important to decide which types of error to emphasize depending on the fairness goals and examining sensitivity/specificity to adjust cutoffs.

15.2.2.1.6 Empirical evidence of test structure bias

It is not uncommon to find items that show differences across groups in severity (intercepts) and/or discrimination (factor loadings). However, cross-group differences in item functioning tend to be small and not consistent across studies, suggesting that some of the differences may reflect Type I errors that result from sampling error and multiple testing. That said, some instances of cross-group differences in item parameters could reflect test structure bias that is real and important to address.

15.2.2.2 Theoretical/Judgmental Approaches to Identification

15.2.2.2.1 Facial validity bias

Facial validity bias considers the extent to which an average person thinks that an item is biased—i.e., the item has differing validity between minority and majority groups. If so, the item should be reconsidered. Does an item disfavor certain groups? Is the language specific to a particular group? Is it offensive to some people? This type of judgment moves into the realm of whether or not an item should be used.

15.2.2.2.2 Content validity bias

Content validity bias is determined by judgments of construct experts who look for items that do not do an adequate job assessing the construct between groups. A construct may include some content facets in one group, but it may include different content facets in another group, as depicted in Figure 15.9.

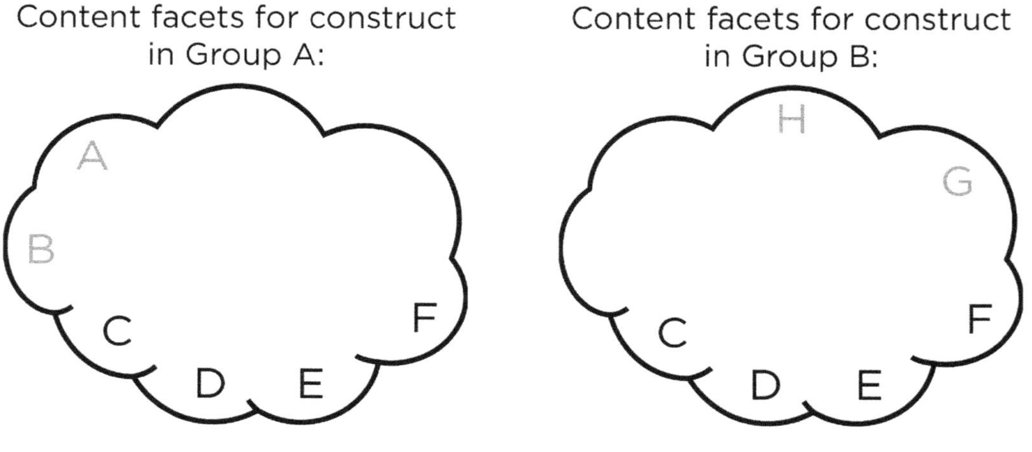

FIGURE 15.9 Different Content Facets in a Given Construct for Two Groups.

Examples include information questions and vocabulary questions on the Wechsler Adult Intelligence Scale. If an item is linguistically complicated, grammatically complex or convoluted, or a double negative, it may be less valid or predictive for rural populations and those with less education.

Also, stereotype threat may contribute to content validity bias. Stereotype threat occurs when people are or feel at risk of conforming themselves to stereotypes about their social group, thus leading them to show poorer performance in ways that are consistent with the stereotype. Stereotype threat may partially explain why some women may perform more poorly on some math items than some men.

Another example of content validity bias is when the same measure is used to assess a construct across ages even though the construct shows heterotypic continuity. Heterotypic continuity occurs when a construct changes in its behavioral manifestation with development (Petersen et al., 2020). That is, the same construct may look different at different points in development. An example of a construct that shows heterotypic continuity is externalizing problems. In early childhood, externalizing problems often manifest in overt forms, including physical aggression (e.g., biting) and temper tantrums. By contrast, in adolescence and adulthood, externalizing problems more often manifest in covert ways, including relational aggression and substance use. Content validity and facial validity bias judgments are often related, but not always.

15.3 Examples of Bias

As described in the overview in Section 15.1, there is not much empirical evidence of test bias (Brown et al., 1999; Hall et al., 1999; Jensen, 1980; Kuncel & Hezlett, 2010; Reynolds et al., 2021; Reynolds & Suzuki, 2012; Sackett et al., 2008; Sackett & Wilk, 1994). That said, some item-level bias is not uncommon. One instance of test bias is that, historically, women's grades in math and engineering classes tended to be underestimated by the Scholastic Aptitude Test [(SAT); M. J. Clark & Grandy (1984)]. Fernández & Abe (2018) review the evidence on other instances of test and item bias. For instance, test bias can occur if a subgroup is less familiar with the language, the stimulus material, or the response procedures, or if they have different response styles. In addition to test bias, there are known patterns of bias in clinical judgment, as described in Section 24.3.11.

15.4 Test Fairness

There is interest in examining more than just the accuracy of measures. It is also important to examine the *errors* being made and differentiate the weight or value of different kinds of errors (and correct decisions). Consider an example of an unbiased test, as depicted in Figure 15.10, adapted from L. S. Gottfredson (1994). Although the example is of a White group and a Black group, we could substitute any two groups into the example (e.g., males versus females).

The example is of an unbiased test between White and Black job applicants. There are no differences between the two groups in terms of slope. If we drew a regression line, the line

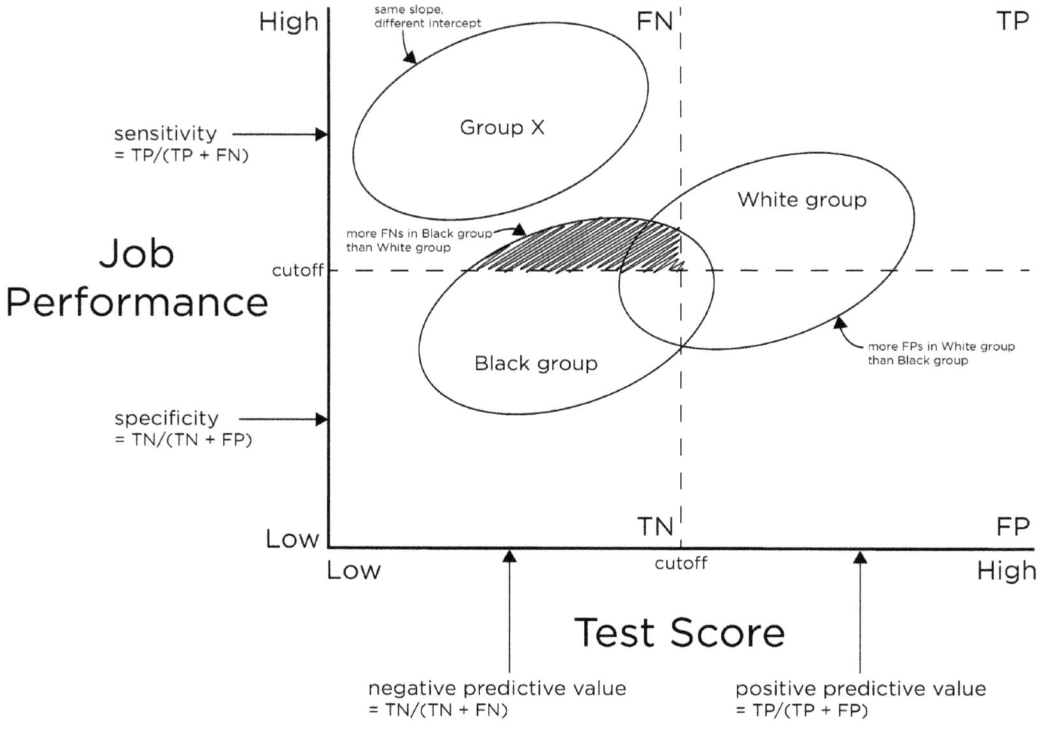

FIGURE 15.10 Potential Unfairness in Testing. The ovals represent the distributions of individuals' performance both on a test and a job performance criterion. TP = true positive; TN = true negative; FP = false positive; FN = false negative. (Adapted from L. S. Gottfredson (1994), figure 1, p. 958. Gottfredson, L. S. (1994). The science and politics of race-norming. *American Psychologist*, *49*(11), 955–963. https://doi.org/10.1037/0003-066X.49.11.955)

would go through the centroid of both ovals. Thus, the measure is equally predictive in both groups even though that the Black group failed the test at a higher rate than the White group. Moreover, there is no difference between the groups in terms of intercept. Thus, the performance of one group is not overestimated relative to the performance of the other group. To demonstrate what a different intercept would look like, Group X shows a different intercept. In sum, there is no predictive validity bias between the two groups. But just because the test predicts just as well in both groups does not mean that the selection procedures are *fair*.

Although the test is unbiased, there are differences in the *quality* of prediction: there are more false negatives in the Black group compared to the White group. This gives the White group an advantage and the Black group additional disadvantages. If the measure showed the same quality of prediction, we would say the test is fair. The point of the example is that just because a test is unbiased does not mean that the test is fair.

There are two kinds of errors: false negatives and false positives. Each error type has very different implications. False negatives would be when the test predicts that an applicant would perform poorly and we do not give them the job even though they would have performed well. False negatives have a negative effect on the applicant. And, in this example, there are more false negatives in the Black group. By contrast, false positives would be when we predict that an applicant would do well, and we give them the job but they perform poorly.

False positives are a benefit to the applicant but have a negative effect on the employer. In this example, there are more false positives in the White group, which is an undeserved benefit based on the selection ratio; therefore, the White group benefits.

In sum, equal accuracy of prediction (i.e., equal total number of errors) does not necessarily mean the test is fair; we must examine the types of errors. Merely ensuring accuracy does not ensure fairness!

15.4.1 Adverse Impact

Adverse impact is defined as rejecting members of one group at a higher rate than another group. Adverse impact is different from test validity. According to federal guidelines, adverse impact is present if the selection rate of one group is less than four-fifths (80%) the selection rate of the group with the highest selection rate.

There is much more evidence of adverse impact than test bias. Indeed, disparate impact of tests on personnel selection across groups is the norm rather than the exception, even when using valid tests that are unbiased, which in part reflect group-related differences in job-related skills (L. S. Gottfredson, 1994). Examples of adverse impact include:

- physical ability tests, which produce substantial adverse impact against women (despite overestimation of women's performance),
- cognitive ability tests, which produce substantial impact against some ethnic minority groups, especially Black and Hispanic people (despite overestimation of Black and Hispanic people's performance), even though cognitive ability tests tend to be among the strongest predictors of job performance (Sackett et al., 2008; Schmidt & Hunter, 1981), and
- personality tests, which produce higher estimates of dominance among men than women; it is unclear whether this has predictive bias.

15.4.2 Bias Versus Fairness

Whether a measure is accurate or shows test bias is a scientific question. By contrast, whether a test is fair and thus should be used for a given purpose is not just a scientific question; it is also an ethical question. It involves the consideration of the potential consequences of testing in terms of social values and consequential validity.

15.4.3 Operationalizing Fairness

There are many perspectives to what should be considered when evaluating test fairness (American Educational Research Association et al., 2014; Camilli, 2013; Committee on the General Aptitude Test Battery et al., 1989; Dorans, 2017; Fletcher et al., 2021; Gipps & Stobart, 2009; Helms, 2006; Jonson & Geisinger, 2022; Melikyan et al., 2019; Sackett et al., 2008; Thorndike, 1971; Zieky, 2006, 2013). As described in Fletcher et al. (2021), there are three primary ways of operationalizing fairness:

1. Equal outcomes: the selection rate is the same across groups.
2. Equal opportunity: the sensitivity (true positive rate; $1 -$ false negative rate) is the same across groups.
3. Equal odds: the sensitivity is the same across groups and the specificity (true negative rate; $1 -$ false positive rate) is the same across groups.

For example, the job selection procedure shows *equal outcomes* if the proportion of men selected is equal to the proportion of women selected. The job selection procedure shows *equal opportunity* if, among those who show strong job performance, the proportion of classification errors (false negatives) is the same for men and women. Receiver operating characteristic (ROC) curves are depicted for two groups in Figure 15.11. A cutoff that represents equal opportunity is depicted with a horizontal line (i.e., the same sensitivity) in Figure 15.11. The job selection procedure shows *equal odds* if (a), among those who show strong job performance, the proportion of classification errors (false negatives) is the same for men and women, and (b), among those who show poor job performance, the proportion of classification errors (false positives) is the same for men and women. A cutoff that represents equal odds is depicted where the ROC curve for Group A intersects with the ROC curve from Group B in Figure 15.11. The equal odds approach to fairness is consistent with a National Academy of Sciences committee on fairness (Committee on the General Aptitude Test Battery et al., 1989; L. S. Gottfredson, 1994). Approaches to operationalizing fairness in the context of prediction models are described by Paulus & Kent (2020).

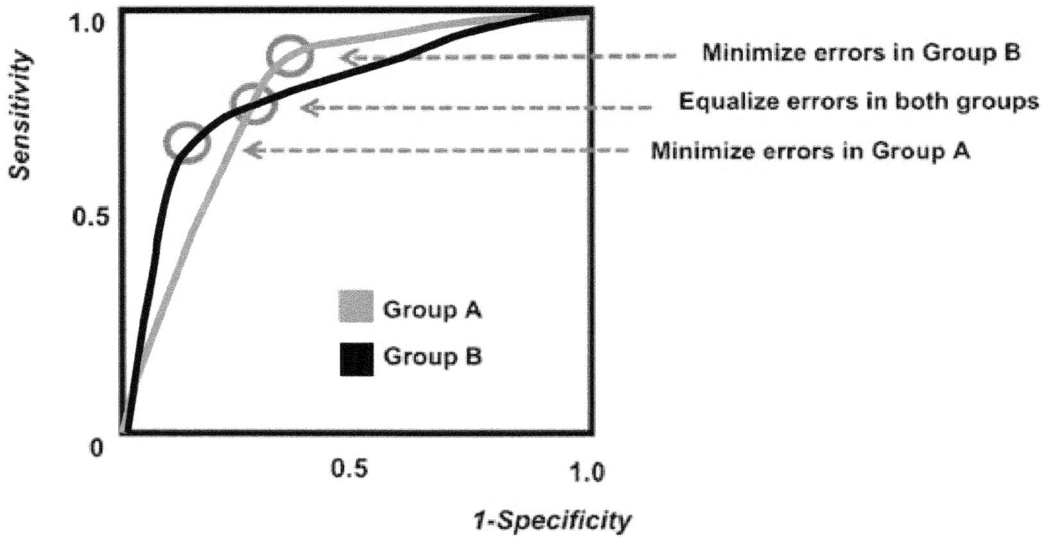

FIGURE 15.11 Receiver Operating Characteristic (ROC) Curves for Two Groups. (Figure reprinted from Fletcher et al. (2021), figure 2, p. 3. Fletcher, R. R., Nakeshimana, A., & Olubeko, O. (2021). Addressing fairness, bias, and appropriate use of artificial intelligence and machine learning in global health. *Frontiers in Artificial Intelligence*, *3*(116). https://doi.org/10.3389/frai.2020.561802)

It is not possible to meet all three types of fairness simultaneously (i.e., equal selection rates, sensitivity, and specificity across groups) unless the base rates are the same across groups or the selection is perfectly accurate (Fletcher et al., 2021). In the medical context, equal odds is the most common approach to fairness. However, using the cutoff associated with equal odds typically reduces overall classification accuracy. And, changing the cutoff for specific groups can lead to negative consequences. In the case that equal odds results in a classification accuracy that is too low, it may be worth considering using separate assessment procedures/tests for each group. In general, it is best to follow one of these approaches to fairness. It is difficult to get right, so try to minimize negative impact. Many fairness supporters argue for simpler rules. In the 1991 Civil Rights Act, score adjustments based on race, gender, and ethnicity (e.g., within-race norming or race-conscious score adjustments) were made illegal in personnel selection (L. S. Gottfredson, 1994).

Another perspective to fairness is that selection procedures should predict job performance and if they are correlated with any group membership (e.g., race, socioeconomic status, or gender), the test should not be used (Helms, 2006). That is, according to Helms, we should not use any test that assesses anything other than the construct of interest (job performance). Unfortunately, however, no measures like this exist. Every measure assesses multiple things, and factors such as poverty can have long-lasting impacts across many domains.

Another perspective to fairness is to make the selection procedures equal the number of successes within each group (Thorndike, 1971). According to this perspective, if you want to do selection, you should hire all people, then look at job performance. If among successful employees, 60% are White and 40% are Black, then set this selection rate for each group (i.e., hiring 80% White individuals and 20% Black individuals is not okay). According to this perspective, a selection system is only fair if the majority–minority differences on the selection device used are equal in magnitude to majority–minority differences in job performance. Selection criteria should be made based on prior distributions of success rates. However, you likely will not ever really know the true base rate in these situations. No one uses this approach because you would have a period where you have to accept everyone to find the percent that works. Also, this would only work in a narrow window of time because the selection pool changes over time.

There are lots of groups and subgroups. Ensuring fairness is very complex, and there is no way to accomplish the goal of being equally fair to all people. Therefore, do the best you can and try to minimize negative impact.

15.5 Correcting for Bias

15.5.1 What To Do When Detecting Bias

When examining item bias (using differential item functioning/DIF or measurement non-invariance) with many items (or measures) across many groups, there can be many tests, which will make it likely that DIF/non-invariance will be detected, especially with a large sample. Some detected DIF may be artificial or trivial, but other DIF may be real and important to address. It is important to consider how you will proceed when detecting DIF/non-invariance. Considerations of effect size and theory can be important for evaluating the DIF/non-invariance and whether it is negligible or important to address.

When detecting bias, there are several steps to take. First, consider what the bias indicates. Does the bias present adverse impact for a minority group? For what reasons might the bias exist? Second, examine the effect size of the bias. If the effects are small, if the bias does not present adverse impact for a minority group, and if there is no compelling theoretical reason for the bias, the bias might not be sufficient to scrap the instrument for the population. Some detected bias may be artificial, but other bias may be real. Gender and cultural differences have shown a number of statistically significant effects for a number of different assessment purposes, but many of the observed effects are quite small and likely trivial, and they do not present compelling reasons to change the assessment (Youngstrom & Van Meter, 2016).

However, if you find bias, correct for it! There are a number of score adjustment and non-score adjustment approaches to correct for bias, as described in Sections 15.5.2 and 15.5.3. If the bias occurs at the item level (e.g., test structure bias), it is generally recommended to remove or resolve items that show non-negligible bias. There are three primary options: (1) drop the item for both groups, (2) drop the item for one group but keep it for the other group, or (3) freely estimate the parameters for the item across groups. Addressing items that show larger bias can also reduce artificial bias in other items (Hagquist & Andrich, 2017). Thus, researchers are encouraged to handle item bias sequentially from high to low in magnitude. If the bias occurs at the test score level (e.g., predictive bias), score adjustments may be considered.

If you do not correct for bias, consider the impact of the test, procedure, and selection procedure when interpreting scores. Interpret scores with caution and provide necessary caveats in resulting papers or reports regarding the interpretations in question. In sum, it is important to examine the possibility of bias—it is important to consider how much "erroneous junk" you are introducing into your research.

15.5.2 Score Adjustment to Correct for Bias

Score adjustment involves adjusting scores for a particular group or groups.

15.5.2.1 Why Adjust Scores?

There may be several reasons to adjust scores for various groups in a given situation. First, there may be social goals to adjust scores. For example, we may want our selection device to yield personnel that better represent the nation or region, including diversity of genders, races, majors, social classes, etc. Score adjustments are typically discussed with respect to racial minority differences due to historical and systemic inequities. Our society aims to provide equal opportunity, including the opportunity to gain a fair share (i.e., proportional representation) of jobs. A diversity of perspectives in a job is a strength; a diversity of perspectives can lead to greater creativity and improved problem-solving. A second potential reason that we may want to apply score adjustment is to correct for bias. A third potential reason that we may want to apply score adjustment is to improve the fairness of a test.

15.5.2.2 Types of Score Adjustment

There are a number of potential techniques that have been used in attempts to correct for bias, i.e., to reduce negative impact of the test on an under-represented group. What is considered an under-represented group may depend on the context. For instance, men are under-represented compared to women as nurses, preschool teachers, and college students. However, men may not face the same systemic challenges compared to women, so even though men may show under-representation in some domains, it is arguable whether scores should be adjusted to increase their representation. Techniques for score adjustment include:

- Bonus points
- Within-group norming
- Separate cutoffs
- Top-down selection from different lists
- Banding
- Banding with bonus points
- Sliding band
- Separate tests
- Item elimination based on group differences

15.5.2.2.1 *Bonus points*

Providing bonus points involves adding a constant number of points to the scores of all individuals who are members of a particular group with the goal of eliminating or reducing group differences. Bonus points is used to correct for predictive bias differences in intercepts between groups. An example of bonus points is military veterans in placement for civil service jobs—points are added to the initial score for all veterans (e.g., add 5 points to test scores of all veterans). An example of using bonus points as a score adjustment is depicted in Figure 15.12.

Person	Group	Raw Score	Original Rank	Score Adjustment	Adjusted Score	Adjusted Rank
1	Majority	130	1		130	2
2	Majority	128	2		128	5
3	Majority	127	3		127	6
4	Minority	125	4.5	+5	130	1
5	Majority	125	4.5		125	7
6	Minority	124	6	+5	129	3
7	Minority	123	7	+5	128	4
8	Majority	120	8		120	9
9	Majority	119	9		119	10
10	Minority	118	10	+5	123	8

FIGURE 15.12 Using Bonus Points as a Scoring Adjustment.

There are several pros of bonus points. If the distribution of each group is the same, this will effectively reduce group differences. Moreover, it is a simple way of impacting test selection and procedure without changing the test, which is therefore a great advantage. There are several cons of bonus points. If there are differences in group standard deviations, adding bonus points may not actually correct for bias. The use of bonus points also obscures what is actually being done to scores, so other methods like using separate cutoffs may be more explicit. In addition, the simplicity of bonus points is also a great disadvantage because it is easily understood and often not viewed as "fair" because some people are getting extra points that others do not.

15.5.2.2.2 *Within-group norming*

A norm is the standard of performance that a person's performance can be compared to. Within-group norming treats the person's group in the sample as the norm. Within-group norming converts an individual's score to standardized scores (e.g., T scores) or percentiles within one's own group. Then, the people are selected based on the highest standard scores across groups. Within-group norming is used to correct for predictive bias differences in slopes between groups. An example of using within-group norming as a score adjustment is depicted in Figure 15.13.

There are several pros of within-group norming. First, it accounts for differences in group standard deviations and means, so it does not have the same problem as bonus points and is generally more effective at eliminating adverse impact compared to bonus points. Second, some general (non-group-specific) norms are clearly irrelevant for characterizing a person's functioning. Group-specific norms aim to describe a person's performance relative to people with a similar background, thus potentially reducing cultural bias. Third, group-specific norms may better reflect cultural, educational, socioeconomic, and other factors that may

Person	Group	Raw Score	Original Rank	Within-Group Percentile	Adjusted Rank
1	Majority	130	1	100	2
2	Majority	128	2	80	3
3	Majority	127	3	60	5
4	Minority	125	4.5	100	1
5	Majority	125	4.5	40	6
6	Minority	124	6	66.6	4
7	Minority	123	7	33.3	7
8	Majority	120	8	20	8
9	Majority	119	9	0	10
10	Minority	118	10	0	9

FIGURE 15.13 Using Within-Group Norming as a Scoring Adjustment.

influence a person's score (Burlew et al., 2019). Fourth, group-specific norms may increase specificity, and reduce over-pathologizing by preventing giving a diagnosis to people who might not show a condition (Manly & Echemendia, 2007).

There are several cons of within-group norming. First, group differences could be maintained if one decides to norm based on a reference sample or, when scores are skewed, a local sample, especially when using standardized scores. However, percentile scores will consistently eliminate adverse impact. Second, using group-specific norms may obscure background variables that explain underlying reasons for group-related differences in test performance (Manly, 2005; Manly & Echemendia, 2007). Third, group-specific norms do not address the problem if the measure shows test bias (Burlew et al., 2019). Fourth, group-specific norms may reduce sensitivity to detect conditions (Manly & Echemendia, 2007). For instance, they may prevent people from getting treatment who would benefit. It is worth noting that within-group norming on the basis of sex, gender, and ethnicity is illegal for the basis of personnel selection according to the 1991 Civil Rights Act.

As an example of within-group norming, the National Football League used to use race-norming for identification of concussions. The effect of race-norming, however, was that it lowered Black players' concussion risk scores, which prevented many Black players from being identified as having sustained a concussion and from receiving needed treatment. Race-norming compared the Black football players cognitive test scores to group-specific norms: the cognitive test scores of Black people in the general population (not to common norms). Using Black-specific norms assumed that Black football players showed lower cognitive ability than other groups, so a low cognitive ability score for a Black player was less likely to be flagged as concerning. Thus, the race-specific norms led to lower identified rates of concussions among Black football players compared to White football players. Due to the adverse impact, Black players sued the National Football League, and the league stopped the controversial practice of race-norming for identification of concussion (https://www.washingtonpost.com/sports/2021/06/03/nfl-concussion-settlement-race-norming/; archived at https://perma.cc/KN3L-5Z7R).

A common question is whether to use group-specific norms or common norms. Group-specific norms are a controversial practice, and the answer depends. If you are interested in a person's absolute functioning (e.g., for determining whether someone is concussed or whether they are suitable to drive), recommendations are to use common norms, not group-specific norms (Barrash et al., 2010; Silverberg & Millis, 2009). If, by contrast, you are interested in a person's *relative* functioning compared to a specific group, within-group norming could make sense if there is an appropriate reference group. The question about which norms to use are complex, and psychologists should evaluate the cost and benefit of each norm, and use the norm with the greatest benefit and the least cost for the client (Manly & Echemendia, 2007).

15.5.2.2.3 Separate cutoffs

Using separate cutoffs involves using a separate cutoff score per group and selecting the top number from each group. That is, using separate cutoffs involves using different criteria for each group. Using separate cutoffs functions the same as adding bonus points, but it has greater transparency—i.e., you are lowering the standard for one group compared to another group. An example of using separate cutoffs as a score adjustment is depicted in Figure 15.14.

Person	Group	Raw Score	Original Rank	Cutoff For Selection	Select?
1	Majority	130	1	128	Yes
2	Majority	128	2	123	Yes
3	Majority	127	3	128	No
4	Minority	125	4.5	123	Yes
5	Majority	125	4.5	128	No
6	Minority	124	6	123	Yes
7	Minority	123	7	123	Yes
8	Majority	120	8	128	No
9	Majority	119	9	128	No
10	Minority	118	10	123	No

FIGURE 15.14 Using Separate Cutoffs as a Scoring Adjustment. In this example, the cutoff for the majority group is 128; the cutoff for the minority group is 123.

15.5.2.2.4 Top-down selection from different lists

Top-down selection from different lists involves taking the best from two different lists according to a preset rule as to how many to select from each group. Top-down selection from different lists functions the same as within-group norming. An example of using top-down selection from different lists as a score adjustment is depicted in Figure 15.15.

15.5.2.2.5 Banding

Banding uses a tier system that is based on the assumption that individuals within a specific score range are regarded as having equivalent scores. So that we do not overestimate small score differences, scores within the same band are seen as equivalent—and the order of selection within the band can be modified depending on selection goals. The standard error of measurement (SEM) is used to estimate the precision (reliability) of the test scores, and it is used as the width of the band.

Person	Group	Raw Score	Original Rank	Selected? (Top 3 From Each Group)
1	Majority	130	1	Yes
2	Majority	128	2	Yes
3	Majority	127	3	Yes
4	Minority	125	4.5	Yes
5	Majority	125	4.5	No
6	Minority	124	6	Yes
7	Minority	123	7	Yes
8	Majority	120	8	No
9	Majority	119	9	No
10	Minority	118	10	No

FIGURE 15.15 Using Top-Down Selection From Different Lists as a Scoring Adjustment. In this example, the top three candidates are selected from each group.

Consider an example: if a person received a score with confidence interval of 18–22, then scores between 18 to 22 are not necessarily different due to random fluctuation (measurement error). Therefore, scores in that range are considered the same, and we take a band of scores. However, banding by itself may not result in increased selection of lower-scoring groups. The band provides a subsample of applicants so that we can use other criteria (other than the test) to select a candidate. Giving "minority preference" involves selecting members of minority group in a given band before selecting members of the majority group. An example of using banding as a score adjustment is depicted in Figure 15.16.

Person	Group	Raw Score	Original Rank	Band 1: [125, 130]	Band 2: [119, 124]	Band 3: [113, 118]	Adjusted Rank
1	Majority	130	1				2
2	Majority	128	2				3
3	Majority	127	3				4
4	Minority	125	4.5				1
5	Majority	125	4.5				5
6	Minority	124	6				6
7	Minority	123	7				7
8	Majority	120	8				8
9	Majority	119	9				9
10	Minority	118	10				10

FIGURE 15.16 Using Banding as a Scoring Adjustment.

The problem with banding is that bands are set by the standard error of measurement: you can select the first group from the first band, but then whom do you select after the first band? There is no rationale where to "stop" the band because there are indistinguishable scores on the edges of each band to the next band. That is, 17 is indistinguishable from 18 (in terms of its confidence interval), 16 is indistinguishable from 17, and so on. Therefore, banding works okay for the top scores, but if you are going to hire a lot of candidates, it is a problem. A solution to this problem with banding is to use a sliding band, as described later.

15.5.2.2.6 Banding with bonus points

Banding is often used with bonus points to reduce the negative impact for minority groups. An example of using banding with bonus points as a score adjustment is depicted in Figure 15.17.

Person	Group	Raw Score	Original Rank	Score Adjustment	Adjusted Score	Band 1: [126, 130]	Band 2: [121, 125]	Band 3: [116, 120]	Adjusted Rank
1	Majority	130	1		130				4
2	Majority	128	2		128				5
3	Majority	127	3		127				6
4	Minority	125	4.5	+5	130				1
5	Majority	125	4.5		125				7
6	Minority	124	6	+5	129				2
7	Minority	123	7	+5	128				3
8	Majority	120	8		120				9
9	Majority	119	9		119				10
10	Minority	118	10	+5	123				8

FIGURE 15.17 Using Banding with Bonus Points as a Scoring Adjustment.

15.5.2.2.7 Sliding band

Using a sliding band is a solution to the problem of which bands to use when using banding. Using a sliding band can help increase the number of minorities selected. Using the top band, you select all members of a minority group in the top band, then select members of the majority group with the top score of the band, then slide the band down (based on SEM), and repeat. You work your way down with bands though groups that are indistinguishable based on SEM, until getting a cell needed to select a relevant candidate.

For instance, if the top score is 22 and the SEM is 4 points, the first band would be: [18, 22]. Here is how you would proceed:

1. Select the minority group members who have a score between 18 to 22.
2. Select the majority group members who have a score of 22.
3. Slide the band down based on the SEM to the next highest score: [17, 21].
4. Select the minority group members who have a score between 17 to 21.
5. Select the majority group members who have a score of 21.
6. Slide the band down based on the SEM to the next highest score: [16, 20].
7. ...
8. And so on.

An example of using a sliding band as a score adjustment is depicted in Figure 15.18.

Person	Group	Raw Score	Original Rank	Band 1: [125, 130]	Band 2: [123, 128]	Band 3: [122, 127]	Band 4: [120, 125]	Band 5: [115, 120]	Band 6: [114, 119]	Adjusted Rank
1	Majority	130	1							2
2	Majority	128	2							5
3	Majority	127	3							6
4	Minority	125	4.5							1
5	Majority	125	4.5							7
6	Minority	124	6							3
7	Minority	123	7							4
8	Majority	120	8							9
9	Majority	119	9							10
10	Minority	118	10							8

FIGURE 15.18 Using a Sliding Band as a Scoring Adjustment.

In sum, using a sliding band, scores that are not significantly lower than the highest remaining score should not be treated as different. Using a sliding band has the same effects on decisions as bonus points that are the width of the band. For example, if the SEM is 3, it has the same decisions as bonus points of 3; therefore, any scores within 3 of the highest score are now considered equal.

A sliding band is popular because of its scientific and statistical rationale. Also, it is more confusing and, therefore, preferred by some because it may be less likely to be sued. However, a sliding band may not always eliminate adverse impact.

15.5.2.2.8 Separate tests

Using separate tests for each group is another option to reduce bias. For instance, you might use one test for the majority group and a different test for the minority group, making sure that each test is valid for the relevant group. Using separate tests is an extreme version of top-down selection and within-group norming. Using separate tests would be an option if a measure shows different slopes predictive bias.

One way of developing separate tests is to use empirical keying by group: different items for each group are selected based on each item's association with the criterion in each group. Empirical keying is an example of dustbowl empiricism (i.e., relying on empiricism rather than theory). However, theory can also inform the item selection.

15.5.2.2.9 Item elimination based on group differences

Items that show large group differences in scores can be eliminated from the test. If you remove enough items showing differences between groups, you can get similar scores between groups and can get equal group selection. A problem of item elimination based on group differences is that if you get rid of predictive items, then two goals, equal selection and predictive power, are not met. If you use this method, you often have to be willing for the measure to show decreases in predictive power.

15.5.2.3 Use of Score Adjustment

Score adjustment can be used in a number of different domains, including tests of aptitude and intelligence. Score adjustment also comes up in other areas. For example, the number of drinks it takes to be considered binge drinking differs between men (five) and women (four). Although the list of score adjustment options is long, they all really reduce to two ways:

1. Bonus points
2. Within-group norming

Bonus points and within-group norming are the techniques that are most often used in the real world. These techniques differ in their degree of obscurity—i.e., confusion that is caused not for scientific reasons, but for social, political, and dissemination and implementation reasons. Often procedures that are hard to understand are preferred because it is hard to argue against, critique, or game the system. Basically, you have two options for score adjustment. One option is to adjust scores by raising scores in one group or lowering the criterion in one group. The second primary option is to renorm or change the scores. In sum, you can change the scores, or you can change the decisions you make based on the scores.

15.5.3 Other Ways to Correct for Bias

Because score adjustment is controversial, it is also important to consider other potential ways to correct for bias that do not involve score adjustment. Strategies other than score adjustment to correct for bias are described by Sackett et al. (2001).

15.5.3.1 Use Multiple Predictors

In general, high-stakes decisions should not be made based on the results from one test. So, for instance, do not make hiring decisions based just on aptitude assessments. For example, college admissions decisions are not made just based on SAT scores, but also one's grades, personal statement, extracurricular activities, letters of recommendation, etc. Using multiple predictors works best when the predictors are not correlated with the assessment that has adverse impact, which is difficult to achieve.

There are larger majority–minority subgroup differences in verbal and cognitive ability tests than in noncognitive skills (e.g., motivation, personality, and interpersonal skills). So, it is important to include assessment of relevant noncognitive skills. Include as many relevant aspects of the construct as possible for content validity. For a job, consider as many factors as possible that are relevant for success, e.g., cognitive and noncognitive abilities.

15.5.3.2 Change the Criterion

Another option is to change the criterion so that the predictive validity of tests is less skewed. It may be that the selection instrument is not biased, but the way in which we are thinking about selection procedures is biased. For example, for judging the quality of universities, there are many different criteria we could use. It could be valuable to examine the various criteria, and you might find what is driving adverse effects.

15.5.3.3 Remove Biased Items

Using item response theory or confirmatory factor analysis, you can identify items that function differently across groups (i.e., differential item functioning/DIF or measurement non-invariance). For instance, you can identify items that show different discrimination/factor loadings or difficulty/intercepts by group. You do not just want to remove items that show mean-level differences in scores (or different rates of endorsement) for one group than another, because there may be true group differences in their level on particular items. If an item is clearly invalid in one group but valid in another group, another option is to keep the item in one group, and to remove it in another group.

Be careful when removing items because removing items can lead to poorer content validity—i.e., items may no longer be a representative set of the content of the construct. Removing items also reduces a measure's reliability and ability to detect individual differences (Hagquist, 2019; Hagquist & Andrich, 2017). DIF effects tend to be small and inconsistent; removing items showing DIF may not have a big impact.

15.5.3.4 Resolve Biased Items

Another option, for items identified that show differential item functioning using IRT or measurement non-invariance using CFA, is to resolve instead of remove items. Resolving items involves allowing an item to have a different discrimination/factor loading and/or difficulty/intercept parameter for each group. Allowing item parameters to differ across groups has a very small effect on reliability and person separation, so it can be preferable to removing items (Hagquist, 2019; Hagquist & Andrich, 2017).

15.5.3.5 Use Alternative Modes of Testing

Another option is to use alternative modes of testing. For example, you could use audio or video to present test items, rather than requiring a person to read the items, or write answers. Typical testing and computerized exams are oriented toward the upper-middle class, which is therefore a procedure problem! McClelland's (1973) argument is that we need more real-life testing. Real-life testing could help address stereotype threats and the effects of learning disabilities. However, testing in different modalities could change the construct(s) being assessed.

15.5.3.6 Use Work Records

Using work records is based on McClelland's (1973) argument to use more realistic and authentic assessments of job-relevant abilities. Evidence on the value of work records for personnel selection is mixed. In some cases, use of work records can actually increase adverse impact on under-represented groups because the primary group typically already has an idea of how to get into the relevant job or is already in the relevant job; therefore, they have a leg up. It would be acceptable to use work records if you trained people first and then tested, but no one spends the time to do this.

15.5.3.7 Increase Time Limit

Another option is to allot people more testing time, as long as doing so does not change the construct. Time limits often lead to greater measurement error because scores conflate pace and quality of work. Increasing time limits requires convincing stakeholders that job performance is typically not "how fast you do things" but "how well you do them"—i.e., that time does not correlate with outcome of interest. The utility of increasing time limits depends on the domain. In some domains, efficiency is crucial (e.g., medicine, pilot). Increasing time limits is not that effective in reducing group differences, and it may actually increase group differences.

15.5.3.8 Use Motivation Sets

Using motivation sets involves finding ways to increase testing motivation for minority groups. It is probably an error to think that a test assesses just aptitude; therefore, we should also consider an individual's motivation to test. Thus, part of the score has to do with ability and some of the score has to do with motivation. You should try to maximize each examinee's motivation, so that the person's score on the measure better captures their true ability score. Motivation sets could include, for example, using more realistic test stimuli that are clearly applicable to the school or job requirements (i.e., that have face validity) to motivate all test takers.

15.5.3.9 Use Instructional Sets

Using instructional sets involves coaching and training. For instance, you could inform examinees about the test content, provide study materials, and recommend test-taking strategies. This could narrow the gap between groups because there is an implicit assumption that the primary group already has "light" training. Using instructional sets aims to reduce error variance due to test anxiety, unfamiliar test format, and poor test-taking skills.

Giving minority groups better access to test preparation is based on the assumption that group differences emerge because of different access to test preparation materials. This could theoretically help to systematically reduce test score differences across groups. Standardized tests like the SAT/GRE/LSAT/GMAT/MCAT, etc. embrace coaching/training. For instance, the organization ETS gives training materials for free. After training, scores on standardized tests show some but minimal improvement. In general, training yields some improvement on quantitative subscales but minimal change on verbal subscales. However, the improvements tend to apply across groups, and they do not seem to lessen group differences in scores.

15.6 Getting Started

15.6.1 Load Libraries

```
library("petersenlab")
library("lavaan")
library("semTools")
library("semPlot")
library("mirt")
library("dmacs")
library("strucchange")
library("MOTE")
library("here")
library("tidyverse")
library("tinytex")
library("knitr")
library("kableExtra")
library("rmarkdown")
library("bookdown")
```

15.6.2 Prepare Data

15.6.2.1 Load Data

cnlsy is a subset of a data set from the Children of the National Longitudinal Survey of Youth Survey (CNLSY). The CNLSY is a publicly available longitudinal data set provided by the Bureau of Labor Statistics (https://perma.cc/EH38-HDRN). The CNLSY data file for these examples is located on the book's page of the Open Science Framework (https://osf.io/3pwza).

```
cnlsy <- read_csv(here("Data", "cnlsy.csv"))
```

15.6.2.2 Simulate Data

```
sampleSize <- 4000

set.seed(52242)

mydataBias <- data.frame(
  ID = 1:sampleSize,
```

```
  group = factor(c("male","female"),
                 levels = c("male","female")),
  unbiasedPredictor1 = NA,
  unbiasedPredictor2 = NA,
  unbiasedPredictor3 = NA,
  unbiasedCriterion1 = NA,
  unbiasedCriterion2 = NA,
  unbiasedCriterion3 = NA,
  predictor = rnorm(sampleSize, mean = 100, sd = 15),
  criterion1 = NA,
  criterion2 = NA,
  criterion3 = NA,
  criterion4 = NA,
  criterion5 = NA)

mydataBias$unbiasedPredictor1 <- rnorm(sampleSize, mean = 100, sd = 15)
mydataBias$unbiasedPredictor2[which(mydataBias$group == "male")] <-
  rnorm(length(which(mydataBias$group == "male")), mean = 70, sd = 15)
mydataBias$unbiasedPredictor2[which(mydataBias$group == "female")] <-
  rnorm(length(which(mydataBias$group == "female")),
        mean = 130, sd = 15)
mydataBias$unbiasedPredictor3[which(mydataBias$group == "male")] <-
  rnorm(length(which(mydataBias$group == "male")), mean = 130, sd = 15)
mydataBias$unbiasedPredictor3[which(mydataBias$group == "female")] <-
  rnorm(length(which(mydataBias$group == "female")), mean = 70, sd = 15)

mydataBias$unbiasedCriterion1 <- 1 * mydataBias$unbiasedPredictor1 +
  rnorm(sampleSize, mean = 0, sd = 15)
mydataBias$unbiasedCriterion2 <- 1 * mydataBias$unbiasedPredictor2 +
  rnorm(sampleSize, mean = 0, sd = 15)
mydataBias$unbiasedCriterion3 <- 1 * mydataBias$unbiasedPredictor3 +
  rnorm(sampleSize, mean = 0, sd = 15)

mydataBias$criterion1[which(mydataBias$group == "male")] <-
  .7 * mydataBias$predictor[which(mydataBias$group == "male")] +
  rnorm(length(which(mydataBias$group == "male")), mean = 0, sd = 5)
mydataBias$criterion1[which(mydataBias$group == "female")] <-
  .7 * mydataBias$predictor[which(mydataBias$group == "female")] +
  rnorm(length(which(mydataBias$group == "female")), mean = 0, sd = 5)
mydataBias$criterion2[which(mydataBias$group == "male")] <-
  .7 * mydataBias$predictor[which(mydataBias$group == "male")] +
  rnorm(length(which(mydataBias$group == "male")), mean = 10, sd = 5)
mydataBias$criterion2[which(mydataBias$group == "female")] <-
  .7 * mydataBias$predictor[which(mydataBias$group == "female")] +
  rnorm(length(which(mydataBias$group == "female")), mean = 0, sd = 5)
mydataBias$criterion3[which(mydataBias$group == "male")] <-
  .7 * mydataBias$predictor[which(mydataBias$group == "male")] +
  rnorm(length(which(mydataBias$group == "male")), mean = 0, sd = 5)
mydataBias$criterion3[which(mydataBias$group == "female")] <-
```

```
  .3 * mydataBias$predictor[which(mydataBias$group == "female")] +
  rnorm(length(which(mydataBias$group == "female")), mean = 0, sd = 5)
mydataBias$criterion4[which(mydataBias$group == "male")] <-
  .7 * mydataBias$predictor[which(mydataBias$group == "male")] +
  rnorm(length(which(mydataBias$group == "male")), mean = 0, sd = 5)
mydataBias$criterion4[which(mydataBias$group == "female")] <-
  .3 * mydataBias$predictor[which(mydataBias$group == "female")] +
  rnorm(length(which(mydataBias$group == "female")), mean = 30, sd = 5)
mydataBias$criterion5[which(mydataBias$group == "male")] <-
  .7 * mydataBias$predictor[which(mydataBias$group == "male")] +
  rnorm(length(which(mydataBias$group == "male")), mean = 0, sd = 30)
mydataBias$criterion5[which(mydataBias$group == "female")] <-
  .7 * mydataBias$predictor[which(mydataBias$group == "female")] +
  rnorm(length(which(mydataBias$group == "female")), mean = 0, sd = 5)
```

15.6.2.3 Add Missing Data

Adding missing data to dataframes helps make examples more realistic to real-life data and helps you get in the habit of programming to account for missing data.

`HolzingerSwineford1939` is a data set from the `lavaan` package (Rosseel et al., 2022) that contains mental ability test scores (`x1`–`x9`) for seventh- and eighth-grade children.

```
varNames <- names(mydataBias)
dimensionsDf <- dim(mydataBias[,-c(1,2)])
unlistedDf <- unlist(mydataBias[,-c(1,2)])
unlistedDf[sample(
  1:length(unlistedDf),
  size = .01 * length(unlistedDf))] <- NA
mydataBias <- cbind(
  mydataBias[,c("ID","group")],
  as.data.frame(
    matrix(
      unlistedDf,
      ncol = dimensionsDf[2])))
names(mydataBias) <- varNames

varNames <- names(HolzingerSwineford1939)
dimensionsDf <- dim(HolzingerSwineford1939[,paste("x", 1:9, sep = "")])
unlistedDf <- unlist(HolzingerSwineford1939[,paste("x", 1:9, sep = "")])
unlistedDf[sample(
  1:length(unlistedDf),
  size = .01 * length(unlistedDf))] <- NA
HolzingerSwineford1939 <- cbind(
  HolzingerSwineford1939[,1:6],
  as.data.frame(matrix(
    unlistedDf,
    ncol = dimensionsDf[2])))
names(HolzingerSwineford1939) <- varNames
```

15.7 Examples of Unbiased Tests (in Terms of Predictive Bias)

15.7.1 Unbiased Test Where Males and Females Have Equal Means on Predictor and Criterion

Figure 15.19 depicts an example of an unbiased test where males and females have equal means on the predictor and criterion. The test is unbiased because there are no significant differences in the regression lines (of `predictor` predicting `criterion`) between males and females.

```
summary(lm(
  unbiasedCriterion1 ~ unbiasedPredictor1 + group +
    unbiasedPredictor1:group,
  data = mydataBias))
```

```
Call:
lm(formula = unbiasedCriterion1 ~ unbiasedPredictor1 + group +
    unbiasedPredictor1:group, data = mydataBias)

Residuals:
   Min     1Q Median     3Q    Max
-54.62 -10.05  -0.03  10.37  66.81

Coefficients:
                               Estimate Std. Error t value Pr(>|t|)
(Intercept)                      0.9307     2.2951    0.41     0.69
unbiasedPredictor1               0.9970     0.0226   44.07   <2e-16 ***
groupfemale                     -1.1652     3.2505   -0.36     0.72
unbiasedPredictor1:groupfemale  -0.0044     0.0321   -0.14     0.89
---
Signif. codes:  0 '***' 0.001 '**' 0.01 '*' 0.05 '.' 0.1 ' ' 1

Residual standard error: 15.1 on 3913 degrees of freedom
  (83 observations deleted due to missingness)
Multiple R-squared:  0.496, Adjusted R-squared:  0.496
F-statistic: 1.29e+03 on 3 and 3913 DF,  p-value: <2e-16
```

15.7.2 Unbiased Test Where Females Have Higher Means Than Males on Predictor and Criterion

Figure 15.20 depicts an example of an unbiased test where females have higher means than males on the predictor and criterion. The test is unbiased because there are no differences in the regression lines (of `predictor` predicting `criterion`) between males and females.

```
summary(lm(
  unbiasedCriterion2 ~ unbiasedPredictor2 + group +
```

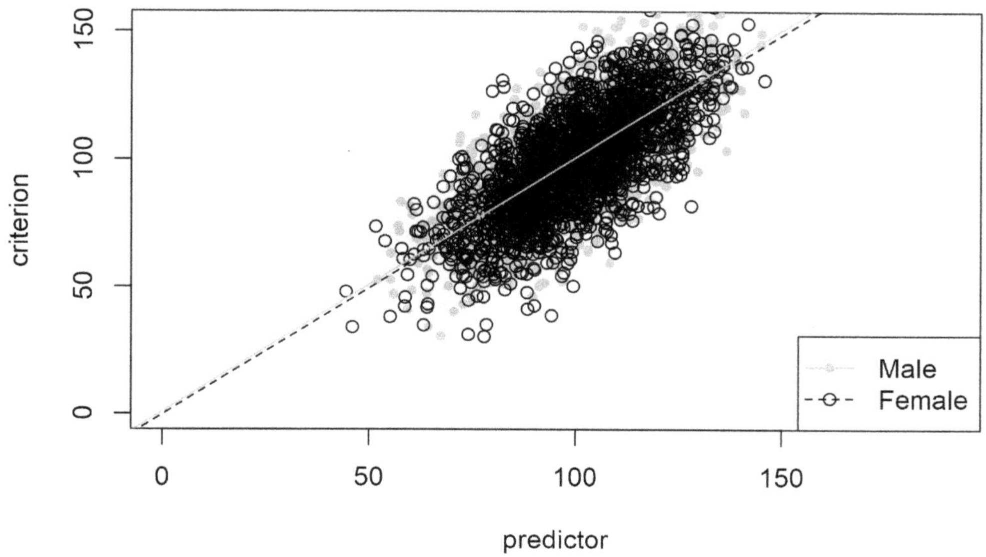

FIGURE 15.19 Unbiased Test Where Males and Females Have Equal Means on Predictor and Criterion.

```
    unbiasedPredictor2:group,
  data = mydataBias))


Call:
lm(formula = unbiasedCriterion2 ~ unbiasedPredictor2 + group +
    unbiasedPredictor2:group, data = mydataBias)

Residuals:
   Min     1Q Median     3Q    Max
-47.30  -9.99   0.01   9.86  53.79

Coefficients:
                               Estimate Std. Error t value Pr(>|t|)
(Intercept)                     -1.2933     1.5777   -0.82     0.41
unbiasedPredictor2               1.0201     0.0222   46.00   <2e-16 ***
groupfemale                      1.2129     3.2832    0.37     0.71
unbiasedPredictor2:groupfemale  -0.0150     0.0312   -0.48     0.63
---
Signif. codes:  0 '***' 0.001 '**' 0.01 '*' 0.05 '.' 0.1 ' ' 1

Residual standard error: 14.8 on 3919 degrees of freedom
```

```
  (77 observations deleted due to missingness)
Multiple R-squared:  0.841, Adjusted R-squared:  0.841
F-statistic: 6.92e+03 on 3 and 3919 DF,  p-value: <2e-16
```

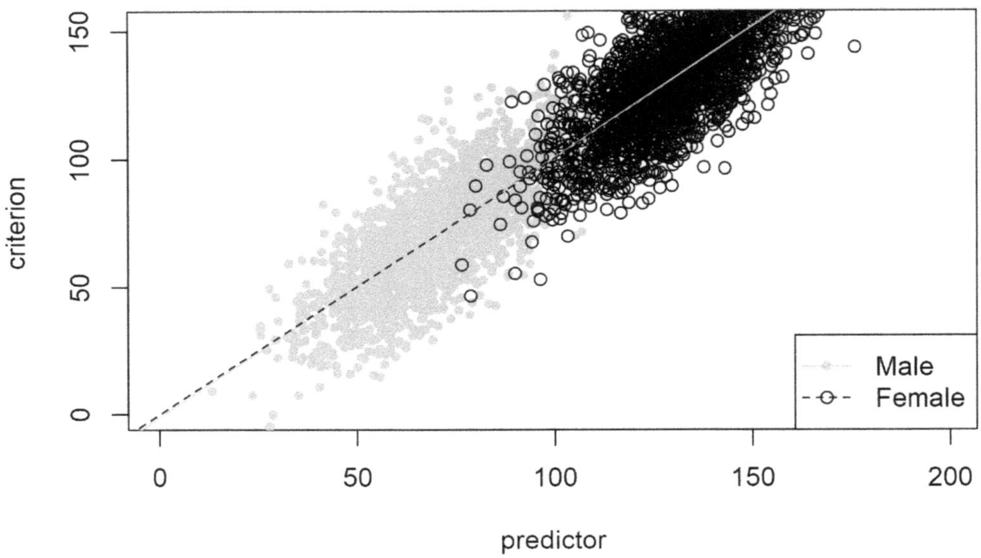

FIGURE 15.20 Unbiased Test Where Females Have Higher Means Than Males on Predictor and Criterion.

15.7.3 Unbiased Test Where Males Have Higher Means than Females on Predictor and Criterion

Figure 15.21 depicts an example of an unbiased test where males have higher means than females on the predictor and criterion. The test is unbiased because there are no differences in the regression lines (of `predictor` predicting `criterion`) between males and females.

```
summary(lm(
  unbiasedCriterion3 ~ unbiasedPredictor3 + group +
    unbiasedPredictor3:group,
  data = mydataBias))
```

```
Call:
lm(formula = unbiasedCriterion3 ~ unbiasedPredictor3 + group +
    unbiasedPredictor3:group, data = mydataBias)

Residuals:
    Min      1Q  Median      3Q     Max
```

```
-48.61 -10.12  -0.07   9.60  57.13

Coefficients:
                              Estimate Std. Error t value Pr(>|t|)
(Intercept)                    -1.6835     2.8499   -0.59     0.55
unbiasedPredictor3              1.0107     0.0218   46.37   <2e-16 ***
groupfemale                     1.4284     3.2623    0.44     0.66
unbiasedPredictor3:groupfemale -0.0119     0.0311   -0.38     0.70
---
Signif. codes:  0 '***' 0.001 '**' 0.01 '*' 0.05 '.' 0.1 ' ' 1

Residual standard error: 14.8 on 3916 degrees of freedom
  (80 observations deleted due to missingness)
Multiple R-squared:  0.838, Adjusted R-squared:  0.837
F-statistic: 6.73e+03 on 3 and 3916 DF,  p-value: <2e-16
```

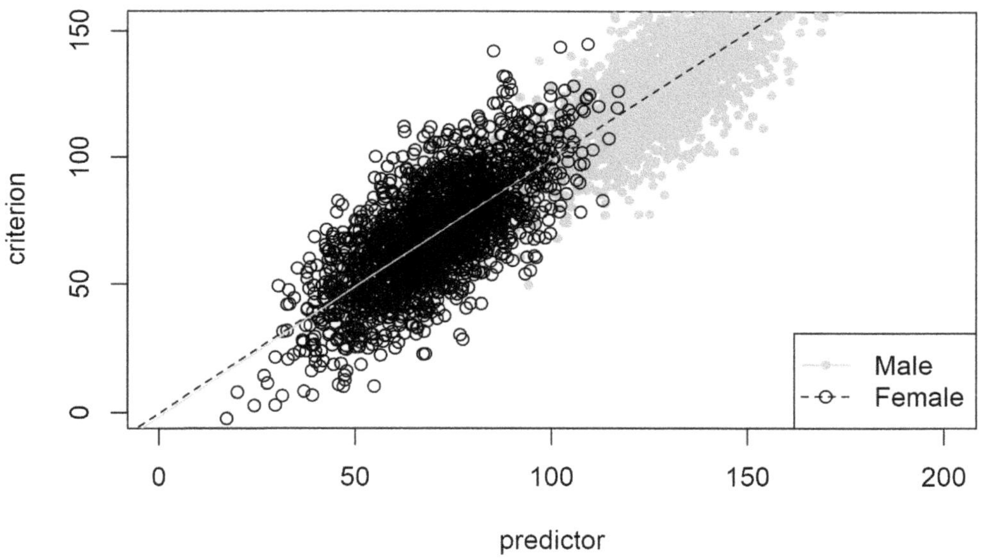

FIGURE 15.21 Unbiased Test Where Males Have Higher Means Than Females on Predictor and Criterion.

15.8 Predictive Bias: Different Regression Lines

15.8.1 Example of Unbiased Prediction (No Differences in Intercepts or Slopes)

Figure 15.22 depicts an example of an unbiased test where males and females have equal means on the predictor and criterion. The test is unbiased because there are no differences in the regression lines (of `predictor` predicting `criterion1`) between males and females.

```
summary(lm(
  criterion1 ~ predictor + group + predictor:group,
  data = mydataBias))
```

```
Call:
lm(formula = criterion1 ~ predictor + group + predictor:group,
    data = mydataBias)

Residuals:
    Min      1Q  Median      3Q     Max 
-18.831  -3.338   0.004   3.330  19.335 

Coefficients:
                      Estimate Std. Error t value Pr(>|t|)    
(Intercept)           -0.26436    0.74727   -0.35     0.72    
predictor              0.70173    0.00737   95.21   <2e-16 ***
groupfemale           -0.51586    1.05927   -0.49     0.63    
predictor:groupfemale  0.00600    0.01048    0.57     0.57    
---
Signif. codes:  0 '***' 0.001 '**' 0.01 '*' 0.05 '.' 0.1 ' ' 1

Residual standard error: 4.95 on 3908 degrees of freedom
  (88 observations deleted due to missingness)
Multiple R-squared:  0.822, Adjusted R-squared:  0.822 
F-statistic: 6.04e+03 on 3 and 3908 DF,  p-value: <2e-16
```

15.8.2 Example of Intercept Bias

Figure 15.23 depicts an example of a biased test due to intercept bias. There are differences in the intercepts of the regression lines (of `predictor` predicting `criterion2`) between males and females: males have a higher intercept than females. That is, the same score on the predictor results in higher predictions for males than females.

```
summary(lm(
  criterion2 ~ predictor + group + predictor:group,
  data = mydataBias))
```

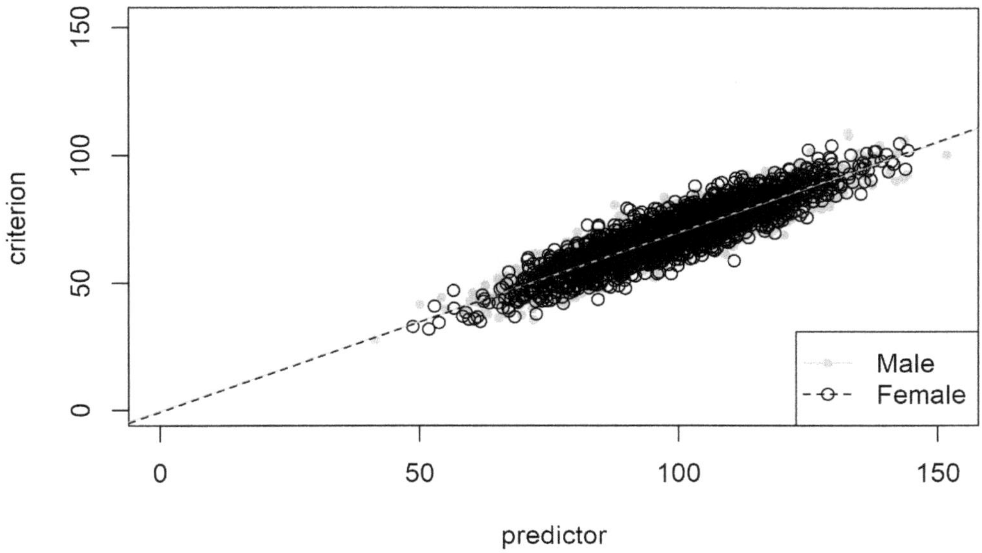

FIGURE 15.22 Example of Unbiased Prediction (No Differences in Intercepts or Slopes Between Males and Females).

```
Call:
lm(formula = criterion2 ~ predictor + group + predictor:group,
    data = mydataBias)

Residuals:
    Min      1Q  Median      3Q     Max
-18.685  -3.415  -0.038   3.398  18.086

Coefficients:
                       Estimate Std. Error t value Pr(>|t|)
(Intercept)            10.05405    0.76008   13.23   <2e-16 ***
predictor               0.69799    0.00750   93.07   <2e-16 ***
groupfemale           -10.28889    1.07417   -9.58   <2e-16 ***
predictor:groupfemale   0.00475    0.01062    0.45     0.65
---
Signif. codes:  0 '***' 0.001 '**' 0.01 '*' 0.05 '.' 0.1 ' ' 1

Residual standard error: 5.04 on 3913 degrees of freedom
  (83 observations deleted due to missingness)
Multiple R-squared:  0.845, Adjusted R-squared:  0.845
F-statistic: 7.12e+03 on 3 and 3913 DF,  p-value: <2e-16
```

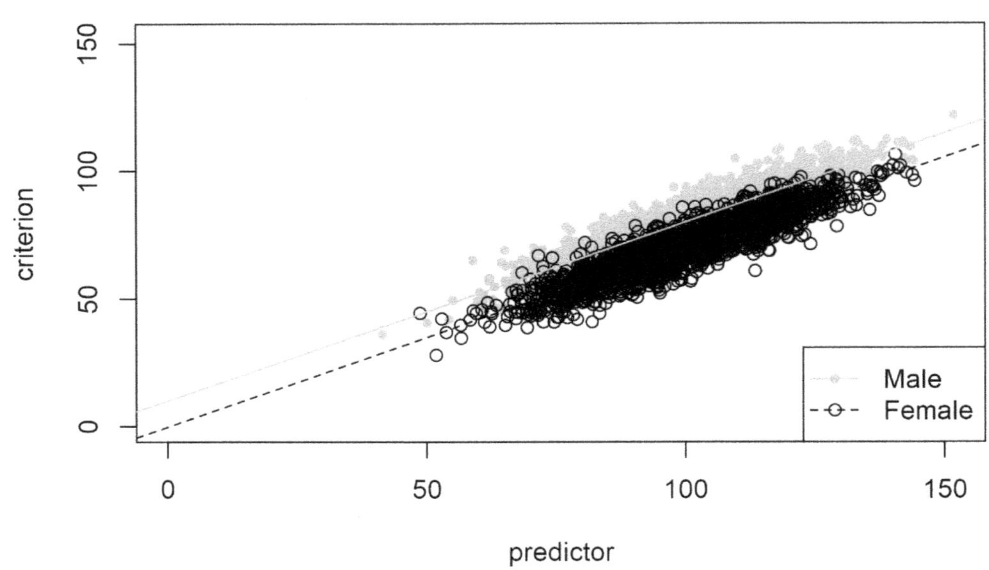

FIGURE 15.23 Example of Intercept Bias in Prediction (Different Intercepts Between Males and Females).

15.8.3 Example of Slope Bias

Figure 15.24 depicts an example of a biased test due to slope bias. There are differences in the slopes of the regression lines (of `predictor` predicting `criterion3`) between males and females: males have a higher slope than females. That is, scores have stronger predictive validity for males than females.

```
summary(lm(
  criterion3 ~ predictor + group + predictor:group,
  data = mydataBias))
```

```
Call:
lm(formula = criterion3 ~ predictor + group + predictor:group,
    data = mydataBias)

Residuals:
    Min      1Q  Median      3Q     Max
-18.318  -3.372   0.026   3.384  19.348

Coefficients:
                      Estimate Std. Error t value Pr(>|t|)
(Intercept)           -1.04194    0.75791   -1.37     0.17
predictor              0.70867    0.00748   94.80   <2e-16 ***
```

```
groupfemale              1.47853    1.07406    1.38     0.17
predictor:groupfemale -0.41323    0.01062  -38.91   <2e-16 ***
---
Signif. codes:  0 '***' 0.001 '**' 0.01 '*' 0.05 '.' 0.1 ' ' 1

Residual standard error: 5.03 on 3927 degrees of freedom
  (69 observations deleted due to missingness)
Multiple R-squared:  0.949, Adjusted R-squared:  0.949
F-statistic: 2.43e+04 on 3 and 3927 DF,  p-value: <2e-16
```

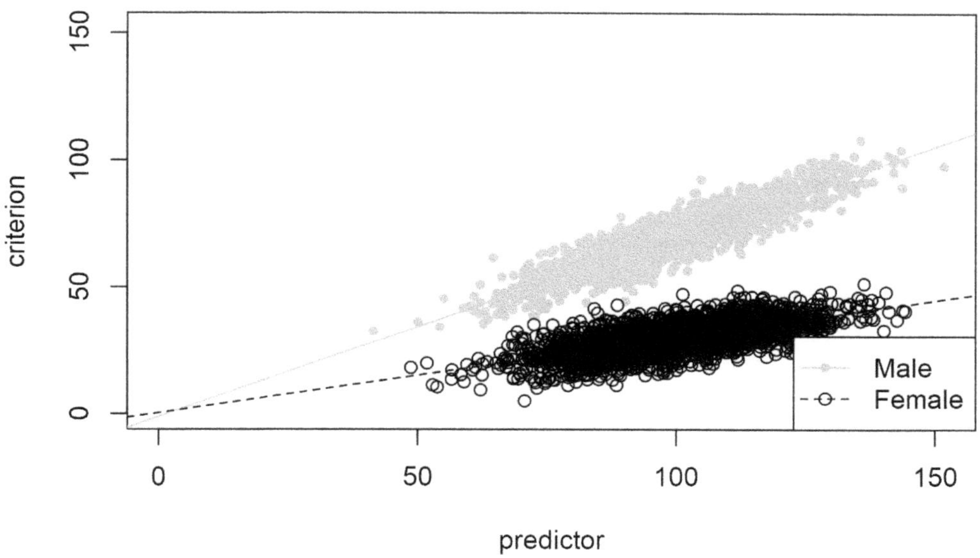

FIGURE 15.24 Example of Slope Bias in Prediction (Different Slopes Between Males and Females).

15.8.4 Example of Intercept and Slope Bias

Figure 15.25 depicts an example of a biased test due to intercept and slope bias. There are differences in the intercepts and slopes of the regression lines (of `predictor` predicting `criterion4`) between males and females: males have a higher slope than females. That is, scores have stronger predictive validity for males than females. Females have a higher intercept than males. That is, at lower scores, the same score on the predictor results in higher predictions for females than males; at higher scores on the predictor, the same score results in higher predictions for males than females.

```
summary(lm(
  criterion4 ~ predictor + group + predictor:group,
  data = mydataBias))
```

```
Call:
lm(formula = criterion4 ~ predictor + group + predictor:group,
    data = mydataBias)

Residuals:
    Min      1Q  Median      3Q     Max
-18.281  -3.440   0.027   3.320  17.882

Coefficients:
                      Estimate Std. Error t value Pr(>|t|)
(Intercept)           -0.27623    0.76708   -0.36     0.72
predictor              0.70218    0.00757   92.81   <2e-16 ***
groupfemale           29.15617    1.08625   26.84   <2e-16 ***
predictor:groupfemale -0.39202    0.01074  -36.49   <2e-16 ***
---
Signif. codes:  0 '***' 0.001 '**' 0.01 '*' 0.05 '.' 0.1 ' ' 1

Residual standard error: 5.1 on 3930 degrees of freedom
  (66 observations deleted due to missingness)
Multiple R-squared:  0.784, Adjusted R-squared:  0.784
F-statistic: 4.76e+03 on 3 and 3930 DF,  p-value: <2e-16
```

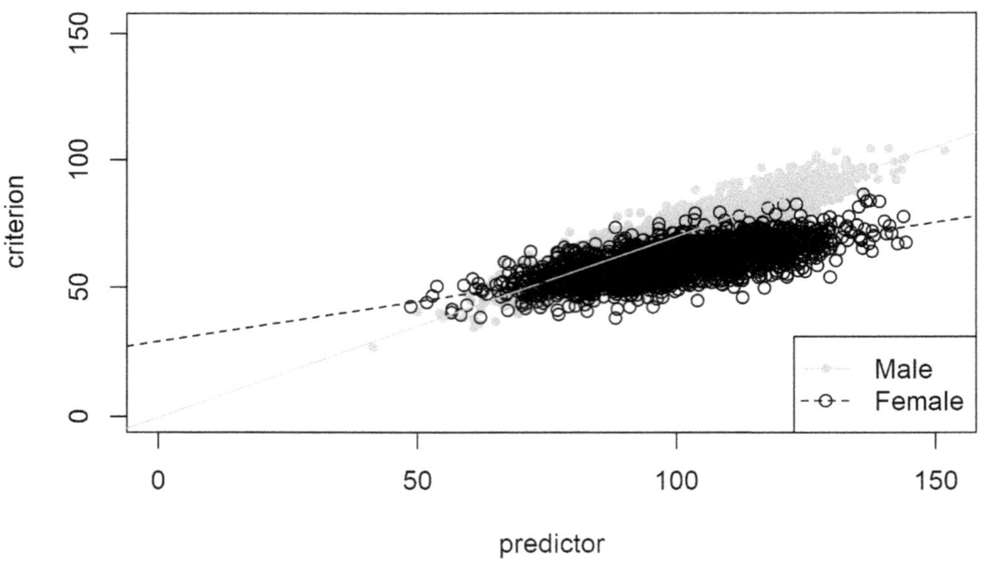

FIGURE 15.25 Example of Intercept and Slope Bias in Prediction (Different Intercepts and Slopes Between Males and Females).

15.8.5 Example of Different Measurement Reliability/Error Across Groups

In the example depicted in Figure 15.26, there are differences in the measurement reliability/error on the criterion between males and females: males' scores have a lower reliability (higher measurement error) on the criterion than females' scores. That is, we are more confident about a female's level on the criterion given a particular score on the predictor than we are about a male's level on the criterion given a particular score on the predictor.

```
summary(lm(
  criterion5 ~ predictor + group + predictor:group,
  data = mydataBias))
```

```
Call:
lm(formula = criterion5 ~ predictor + group + predictor:group,
    data = mydataBias)

Residuals:
    Min      1Q  Median      3Q     Max
-109.29   -7.06    0.08    6.84  108.43

Coefficients:
                      Estimate Std. Error t value Pr(>|t|)
(Intercept)            -9.2839     3.3262   -2.79   0.0053 **
predictor               0.7917     0.0328   24.14   <2e-16 ***
groupfemale             9.1245     4.7047    1.94   0.0525 .
predictor:groupfemale  -0.0908     0.0465   -1.95   0.0510 .
---
Signif. codes:  0 '***' 0.001 '**' 0.01 '*' 0.05 '.' 0.1 ' ' 1

Residual standard error: 22 on 3920 degrees of freedom
  (76 observations deleted due to missingness)
Multiple R-squared:  0.209, Adjusted R-squared:  0.208
F-statistic:  345 on 3 and 3920 DF,  p-value: <2e-16
```

15.9 Differential Item Functioning

Differential item functioning (DIF) indicates that one or more items functions differently across groups. That is, one or more of the item parameters for an item differs across groups. For instance, the severity or discrimination of an item could be higher in one group compared to another group. If an item functions differently across groups, it can lead to biased scores for particular groups. Thus, when observing group differences in level on the measure or group differences in the measure's association with other measures, it is unclear whether the observed group differences reflect true group differences or differences in the functioning of the measure across groups.

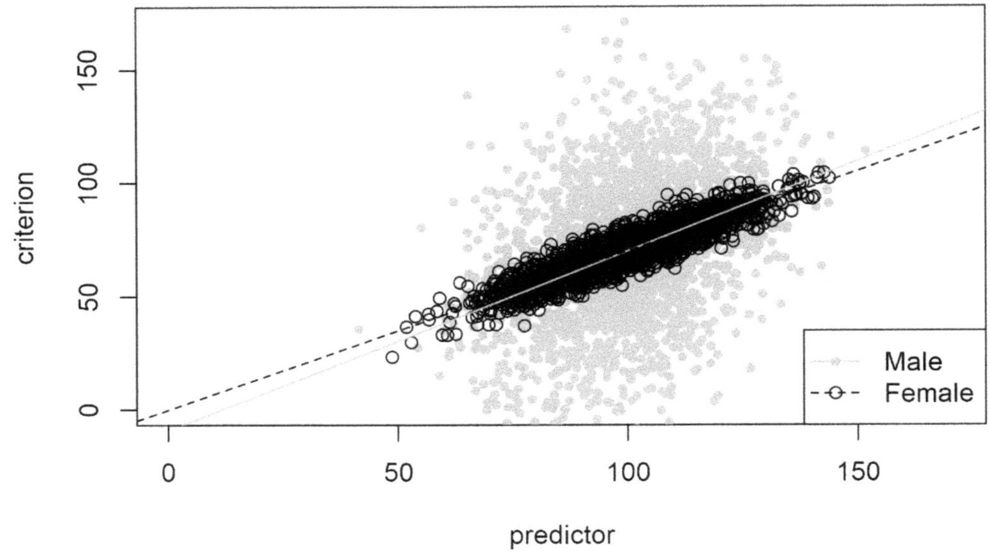

FIGURE 15.26 Example of Different Measurement Reliability/Error Across Groups.

For instance, consider an item such as "disobedience to authority", which is thought to reflect externalizing behavior in childhood. However, in adulthood, disobedience to authority could reflect prosocial functions, such as protesting against societally unjust actions, and may show weaker construct validity with respect to externalizing problems, as operationalized by a weaker discrimination coefficient in adulthood than in childhood. Tests of differential item functioning are equivalent to tests of measurement invariance.

Approaches to addressing DIF are described in Section 15.5.1. If we identify that an item shows non-negligible DIF, we have three primary options (described above): (1) drop the item for both groups, (2) drop the item for one group but keep it for the other group, or (3) freely estimate the parameters (discrimination and difficulty) for the item across groups.

Tests of DIF were conducted using the `mirt` package (Chalmers, 2020).

15.9.1 Unconstrained Model

15.9.1.1 Fit Model

```
unconstrainedModel <- multipleGroup(
  data = cnlsy[,c(
    "bpi_antisocialT1_1","bpi_antisocialT1_2","bpi_antisocialT1_3",
    "bpi_antisocialT1_4","bpi_antisocialT1_5","bpi_antisocialT1_6",
    "bpi_antisocialT1_7")],
  model = 1,
```

```
  group = cnlsy$sex,
  SE = TRUE)
```

15.9.1.2 Model Summary

Items that appear to differ:

- items 5 and 6 are more discriminating (a parameter) among females than males
- item 4 has higher difficulty/severity (b_1 and b_2 parameters) among males than females

```
coef(unconstrainedModel,
     simplify = TRUE,
     IRTpars = TRUE)
```

```
$female
$items
                       a     b1    b2
bpi_antisocialT1_1 1.657  0.029 2.451
bpi_antisocialT1_2 1.697  0.953 2.763
bpi_antisocialT1_3 1.069  0.650 2.585
bpi_antisocialT1_4 1.590  1.895 3.465
bpi_antisocialT1_5 2.008  1.281 2.936
bpi_antisocialT1_6 2.614  1.625 2.770
bpi_antisocialT1_7 0.807 -1.184 2.583

$means
F1
 0

$cov
   F1
F1  1


$male
$items
                       a     b1    b2
bpi_antisocialT1_1 1.507 -0.238 2.505
bpi_antisocialT1_2 1.853  0.582 2.455
bpi_antisocialT1_3 1.067  0.384 2.480
bpi_antisocialT1_4 1.729  1.165 2.765
bpi_antisocialT1_5 1.625  0.635 2.757
bpi_antisocialT1_6 1.677  1.494 2.873
bpi_antisocialT1_7 1.002 -0.986 2.143

$means
F1
 0

$cov
```

```
   F1
F1  1
```

15.9.2 Constrained Model

Constrain item parameters to be equal across groups (to use as baseline model for identifying DIF).

15.9.2.1 Fit Model

```
constrainedModel <- multipleGroup(
  data = cnlsy[,c(
    "bpi_antisocialT1_1","bpi_antisocialT1_2","bpi_antisocialT1_3",
    "bpi_antisocialT1_4","bpi_antisocialT1_5","bpi_antisocialT1_6",
    "bpi_antisocialT1_7")],
  model = 1,
  group = cnlsy$sex,
  invariance = c(c(
    "bpi_antisocialT1_1","bpi_antisocialT1_2","bpi_antisocialT1_3",
    "bpi_antisocialT1_4","bpi_antisocialT1_5","bpi_antisocialT1_6",
    "bpi_antisocialT1_7"),
    "free_means", "free_var"),
  SE = TRUE)
```

15.9.2.2 Model Summary

```
coef(
  constrainedModel,
  simplify = TRUE,
  IRTpars = TRUE)
```

```
$female
$items
                       a     b1    b2
bpi_antisocialT1_1 1.492  0.089 2.791
bpi_antisocialT1_2 1.713  0.978 2.883
bpi_antisocialT1_3 1.020  0.733 2.836
bpi_antisocialT1_4 1.686  1.687 3.265
bpi_antisocialT1_5 1.854  1.138 3.014
bpi_antisocialT1_6 2.040  1.779 3.034
bpi_antisocialT1_7 0.837 -0.952 2.697

$means
F1
 0

$cov
   F1
F1  1
```

```
$male
$items
                        a     b1    b2
bpi_antisocialT1_1 1.492  0.089 2.791
bpi_antisocialT1_2 1.713  0.978 2.883
bpi_antisocialT1_3 1.020  0.733 2.836
bpi_antisocialT1_4 1.686  1.687 3.265
bpi_antisocialT1_5 1.854  1.138 3.014
bpi_antisocialT1_6 2.040  1.779 3.034
bpi_antisocialT1_7 0.837 -0.952 2.697

$means
  F1
0.39

$cov
      F1
F1 1.054
```

15.9.3 Compare Model Fit of Constrained Model to Unconstrained Model

The constrained model and the unconstrained model are considered "nested" models. The constrained model is nested within the unconstrained model because the unconstrained model includes all of the terms of the constrained model along with additional terms. Model fit of nested models can be compared with a chi-square difference test.

```
anova(constrainedModel, unconstrainedModel)
```

```
                     AIC SABIC    HQ   BIC logLik      X2 df p
constrainedModel   34332 34403 34383 34476 -17143
unconstrainedModel 34247 34377 34341 34511 -17082 122.672 19 0
```

The constrained model fits significantly worse than the unconstrained model, which suggests that item parameters differ between males and females.

15.9.4 Identify DIF by Iteratively Removing Constraints from Fully Constrained Model

One way to identify DIF is to iteratively remove constraints from a model in which all parameters are constrained to be the same across groups. Removing constraints allows individual items to have different item parameters across groups, to identify which items yield a significant improvement in model fit when allowing their discrimination and/or severity to differ across groups. Items 1, 3, 4, 5, 6, and 7 showed DIF in discrimination and/or severity, based on a significant chi-square difference test.

TABLE 15.1 Differential Item Functioning in Terms of Discrimination and/or Severity.

Item	Groups	Converged	AIC	SABIC	HQ	BIC	χ^2	*df*	*p*
bpi_antisocialT1_1	female,male	TRUE	−11.90	−2.61	−5.22	6.92	17.90	3	0.000
bpi_antisocialT1_2	female,male	TRUE	1.89	11.18	8.57	20.71	4.11	3	0.250
bpi_antisocialT1_3	female,male	TRUE	−1.77	7.51	4.90	17.04	7.77	3	0.051
bpi_antisocialT1_4	female,male	TRUE	−14.22	−4.94	−7.54	4.60	20.22	3	0.000
bpi_antisocialT1_5	female,male	TRUE	−40.26	−30.98	−33.59	−21.45	46.26	3	0.000
bpi_antisocialT1_6	female,male	TRUE	−4.36	4.93	2.32	14.46	10.36	3	0.016
bpi_antisocialT1_7	female,male	TRUE	−24.69	−15.41	−18.02	−5.87	30.69	3	0.000

TABLE 15.2 Differential Item Functioning in Terms of Discrimination.

Item	Groups	Converged	AIC	SABIC	HQ	BIC	χ^2	*df*	*p*
bpi_antisocialT1_1	female,male	TRUE	−13.10	−10.00	−10.87	−6.82	15.10	1	0.000
bpi_antisocialT1_2	female,male	TRUE	−1.40	1.69	0.82	4.87	3.40	1	0.065
bpi_antisocialT1_3	female,male	TRUE	−3.54	−0.45	−1.32	2.73	5.54	1	0.019
bpi_antisocialT1_4	female,male	TRUE	−12.04	−8.95	−9.82	−5.77	14.04	1	0.000
bpi_antisocialT1_5	female,male	TRUE	−14.25	−11.15	−12.02	−7.98	16.25	1	0.000
bpi_antisocialT1_6	female,male	TRUE	0.83	3.92	3.05	7.10	1.17	1	0.279
bpi_antisocialT1_7	female,male	TRUE	1.97	5.06	4.19	8.24	0.03	1	0.858

15.9.4.1 Items That Differ in Discrimination and/or Severity

```
DIF(
  constrainedModel,
  c("a1","d1","d2"),
  scheme = "drop",
  simplify = TRUE)
```

15.9.4.2 Items That Differ in Discrimination

Items 1, 3, 4, and 5 showed DIF in discrimination, based on a significant chi-square difference test.

```
DIF(
  constrainedModel,
  c("a1"),
  scheme = "drop",
  simplify = TRUE)
```

15.9.4.3 Items That Differ in Severity

Items 1, 3, 4, 5, and 7 showed DIF in difficulty/severity, based on a significant chi-square difference test.

```
DIF(
  constrainedModel,
  c("d1","d2"),
```

TABLE 15.3 Differential Item Functioning in Terms of Severity.

Item	Groups	Converged	AIC	SABIC	HQ	BIC	χ^2	*df*	*p*
bpi_antisocialT1_1	female,male	TRUE	−10.05	−3.86	−5.60	2.49	14.05	2	0.001
bpi_antisocialT1_2	female,male	TRUE	0.11	6.30	4.56	12.65	3.89	2	0.143
bpi_antisocialT1_3	female,male	TRUE	−3.04	3.15	1.41	9.51	7.04	2	0.030
bpi_antisocialT1_4	female,male	TRUE	−16.10	−9.91	−11.65	−3.56	20.10	2	0.000
bpi_antisocialT1_5	female,male	TRUE	−40.90	−34.71	−36.44	−28.35	44.90	2	0.000
bpi_antisocialT1_6	female,male	TRUE	3.63	9.82	8.08	16.17	0.37	2	0.831
bpi_antisocialT1_7	female,male	TRUE	−23.57	−17.38	−19.12	−11.03	27.57	2	0.000

```
  scheme = "drop",
  simplify = TRUE)
```

15.9.5 Identify DIF by Iteratively Adding Constraints to Unconstrained Model

15.9.5.1 Items That Differ in Discrimination and/or Severity

Another way to identify DIF is to iteratively add constraints to a model in which all parameters are allowed to differ across groups. Adding constraints forces individual items to have the same item parameters across groups, to identify which items yield a significant worsening in model fit when constraining their discrimination and/or severity to be the same across groups. Items 1, 2, 3, 4, 5, and 6 showed DIF in discrimination and/or severity, based on a significant chi-square difference test.

```
difAddItems <- DIF(
  unconstrainedModel,
  c("a1","d1","d2"),
  scheme = "add",
  simplify = TRUE,
  plotdif = TRUE)
```

15.9.6 Compute Effect Size of DIF

Effect size measures of DIF were computed based on expected scores (Meade, 2010) using the `mirt` package (Chalmers, 2020). Some researchers recommend using a simulation-based procedure to examine the impact of DIF on screening accuracy (Gonzalez & Pelham, 2021).

15.9.6.1 Test-Level DIF

In addition to consideration of differential test functioning, we can also consider whether the test as a whole (i.e., the collection of items) differs in its functioning by group—called differential test functioning. Differential test functioning is depicted in Figure 15.27. Estimates of differential test functioning are in Table 15.4.

TABLE 15.4 Test-Level Differential Item Functioning.

Effect Size	Value
STDS	0.6052
UTDS	0.6414
UETSDS	0.6052
ETSSD	0.3652
Starks.DTFR	0.6085
UDTFR	0.6488
UETSDN	0.6103
theta.of.max.test.D	1.2157
Test.Dmax	1.1264

TABLE 15.5 Item-Level Differential Item Functioning.

	SIDS	UIDS	SIDN	UIDN	ESSD	theta.of.max.D	max.D	mean.ES.foc	mean.ES.ref
bpi_antisocialT1_1	0.08	0.08	0.08	0.08	0.27	−0.34	0.11	0.61	0.52
bpi_antisocialT1_2	0.09	0.09	0.09	0.09	0.32	1.05	0.18	0.35	0.26
bpi_antisocialT1_3	0.07	0.07	0.06	0.06	0.25	0.76	0.08	0.50	0.43
bpi_antisocialT1_4	0.11	0.11	0.12	0.12	0.57	2.55	0.40	0.21	0.10
bpi_antisocialT1_5	0.18	0.18	0.18	0.18	0.73	0.88	0.32	0.34	0.16
bpi_antisocialT1_6	0.07	0.08	0.07	0.08	0.40	1.10	0.17	0.15	0.08
bpi_antisocialT1_7	0.00	0.03	0.00	0.04	0.00	3.22	0.13	0.83	0.83

```
empirical_ES(
  unconstrainedModel,
  DIF = FALSE)
```

In general, the measure showed greater difficulty for females than for males. That is, at a given construct level, males were more likely than females to endorse the items. Otherwise said, it takes a higher construct level for females to obtain the same score on the measure as males.

```
empirical_ES(
  unconstrainedModel,
  DIF = FALSE,
  plot = TRUE)
```

15.9.6.2 Item-Level DIF

```
empirical_ES(
  unconstrainedModel,
  DIF = TRUE) %>%
  round(., 2)
```

Differential item functioning is depicted in Figure 15.28. Estimates of differential item functioning are given in Table 15.5.

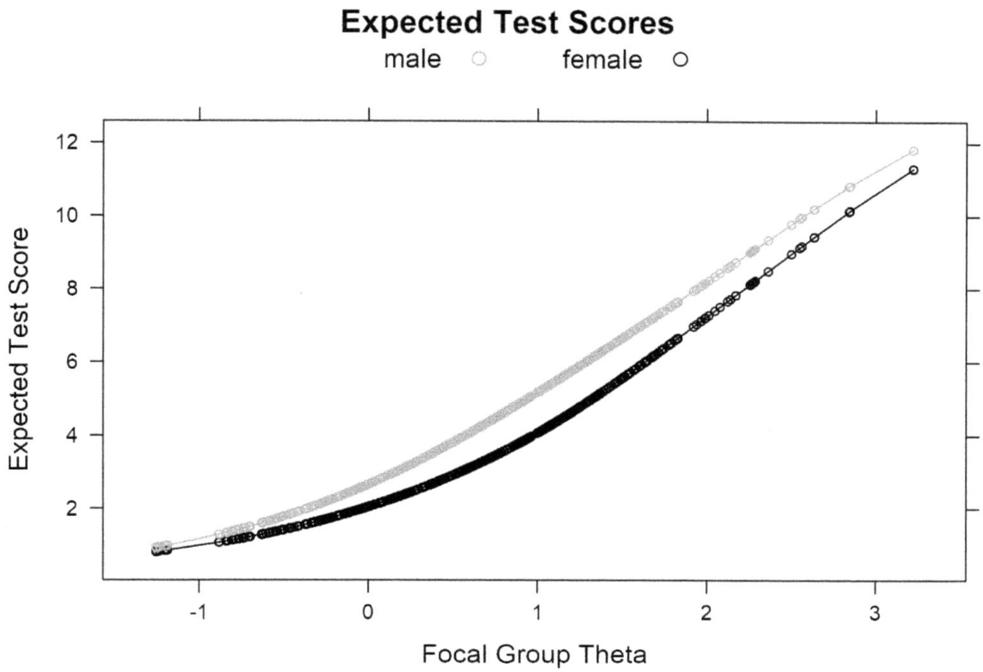

FIGURE 15.27 Differential Test Functioning by Sex.

The measure-level differences in functioning appear to be largely driven by greater difficulty of items 4 and 5 for females than males. That is, at a given construct level, males were more likely than females to endorse items 4 and 5, in particular. Otherwise said, it takes a higher construct level for females than males to endorse items 4 and 5.

```
empirical_ES(
  unconstrainedModel,
  DIF = TRUE,
  plot = TRUE)
```

15.9.7 Item Plots

Item response category characteristic curves by sex for item 4 are shown in Figure 15.29.

```
itemplot(
  unconstrainedModel,
  "bpi_antisocialT1_4",
  type = "trace")
```

Plots of item information functions by sex for item 6 are shown in Figure 15.30. Items 1, 5, and 6 showed greater information for females than for males. Items 2, 4, and 7 showed greater information for females than for males.

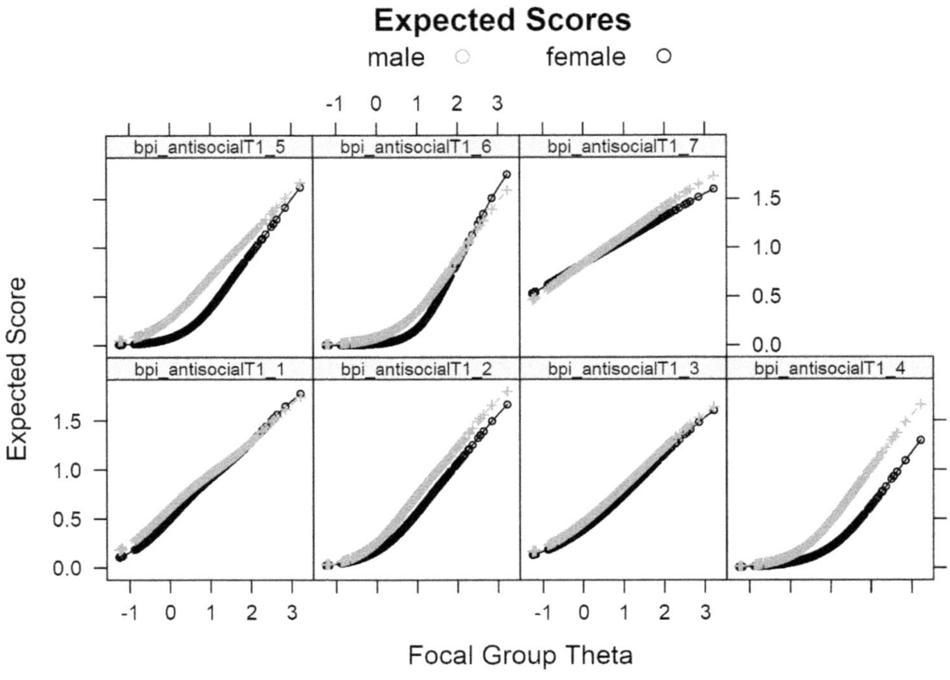

FIGURE 15.28 Differential Item Functioning by Sex.

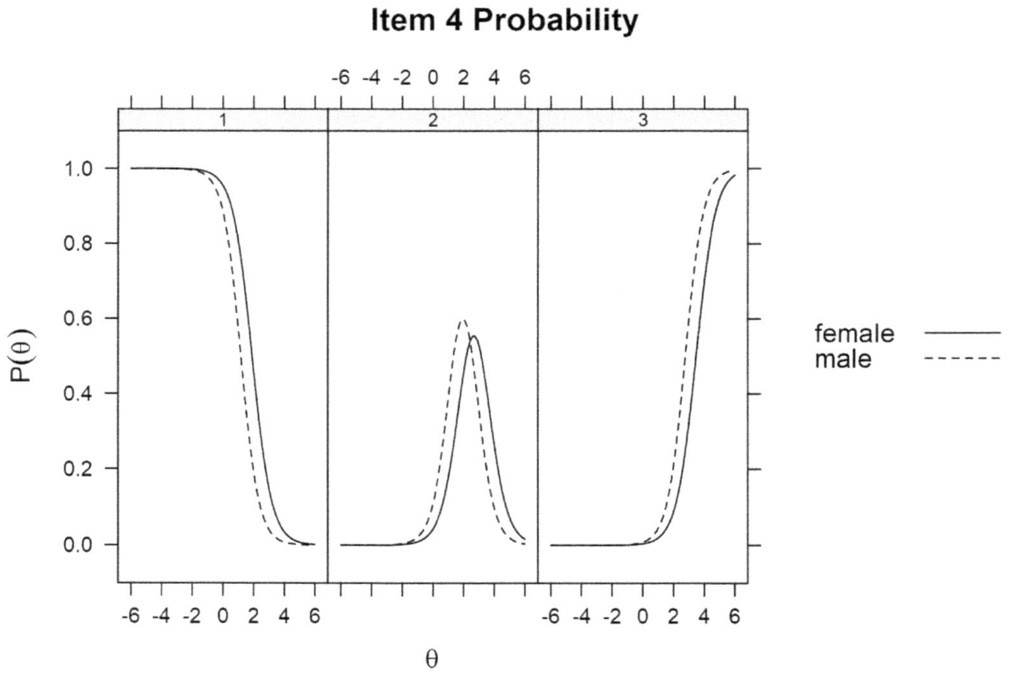

FIGURE 15.29 Item Response Category Characteristic Curves by Sex: Item 4.

```
itemplot(
  unconstrainedModel,
  "bpi_antisocialT1_6",
  type = "info")
```

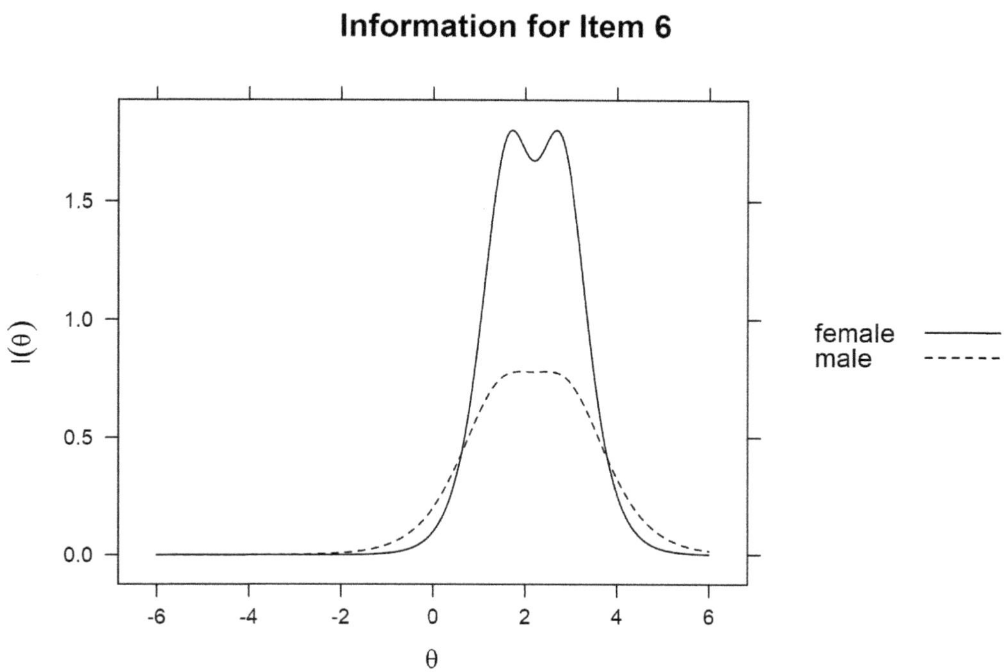

FIGURE 15.30 Item Information Curves by Sex: Item 6.

Plots of expected item scores by sex for items 4 and 6 are shown in Figures 15.31 and 15.32, respectively.

```
itemplot(
  unconstrainedModel,
  "bpi_antisocialT1_4",
  type = "score")
```

```
itemplot(
  unconstrainedModel,
  "bpi_antisocialT1_6",
  type = "score")
```

15.9.8 Addressing DIF

Based on the analyses above, item 5 shows the largest magnitude of DIF. Specifically, item 5 has a stronger discrimination parameter for women than men. So, we should handle item

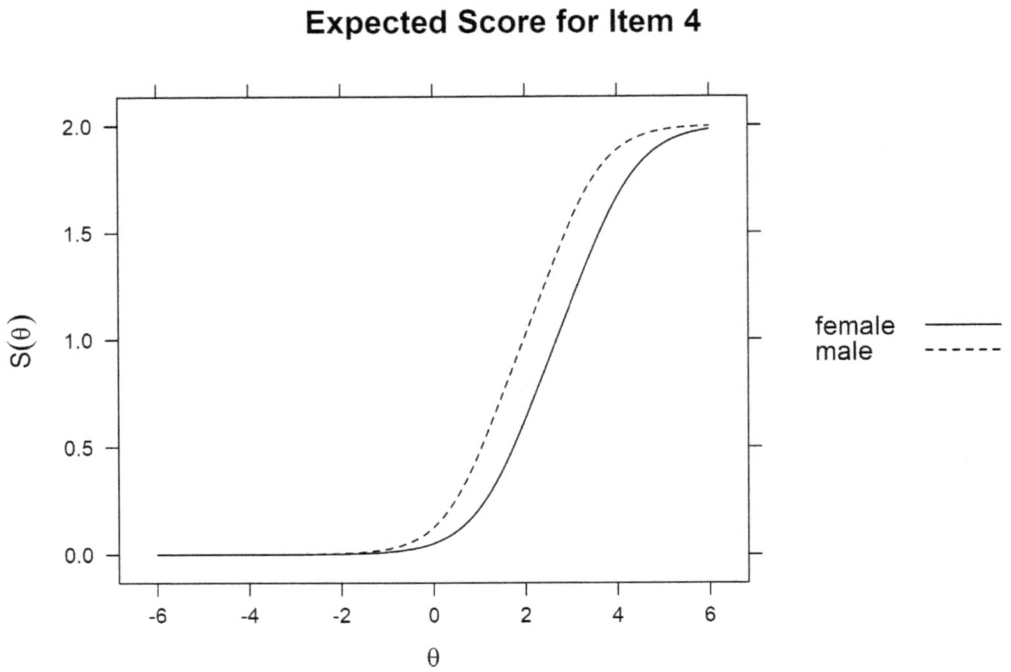

FIGURE 15.31 Expected Item Score by Sex: Item 4.

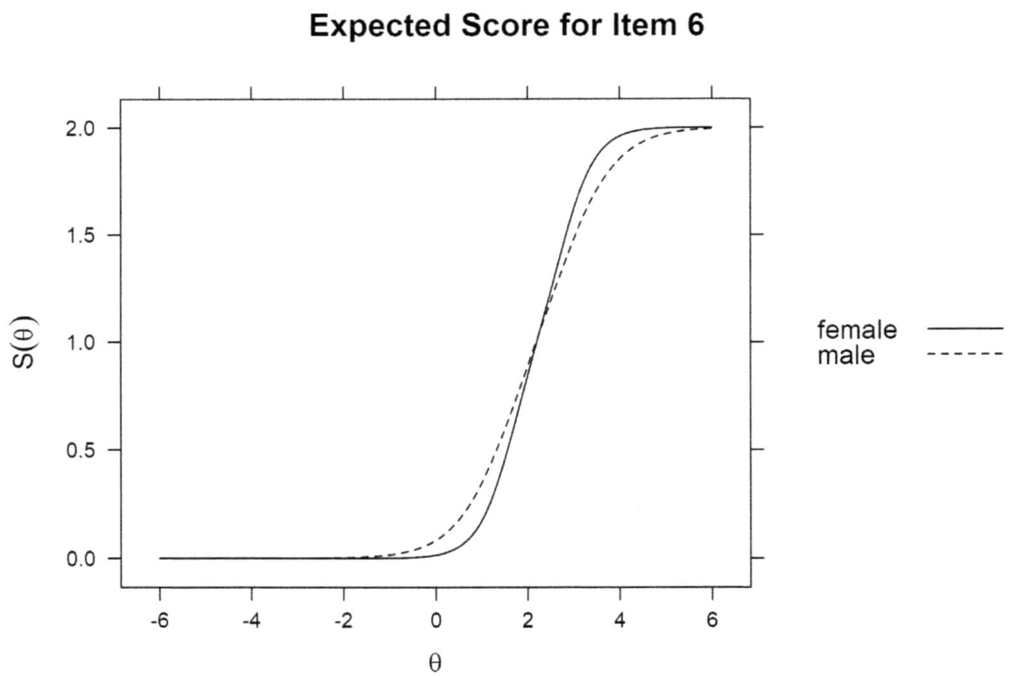

FIGURE 15.32 Expected Item Score by Sex: Item 6.

5 first. If we deem the DIF for item 5 to be non-negligible, we have three primary options: (1) drop item 5 for both men and women, (2) drop item 5 for men but keep it for women, or (3) freely estimate the parameters (discrimination and difficulty) for item 5 across groups.

15.9.8.1 Drop Item for Both Groups

The first option is to drop item 5 for both men and women groups. You might do this if you want to use a measure that has only those items that function equivalently across groups. However, this can lead to lower reliability and weaker ability to detect individual differences.

```
constrainedModelDropItem5 <- multipleGroup(
  data = cnlsy[,c(
    "bpi_antisocialT1_1","bpi_antisocialT1_2","bpi_antisocialT1_3",
    "bpi_antisocialT1_4","bpi_antisocialT1_6","bpi_antisocialT1_7")],
  model = 1,
  group = cnlsy$sex,
  invariance = c(c(
    "bpi_antisocialT1_1","bpi_antisocialT1_2","bpi_antisocialT1_3",
    "bpi_antisocialT1_4","bpi_antisocialT1_6","bpi_antisocialT1_7"),
    "free_means", "free_var"),
  SE = TRUE)

coef(constrainedModelDropItem5, simplify = TRUE)
```

15.9.8.2 Drop Item for One Group But Not Another Group

A second option is to drop item 5 for men but to keep it for women. You might do this if the item is invalid for men, but still valid for women. The coefficients show an item parameter for item 5 for men, but it was constrained to be equal to the parameter for women, and data were removed from the estimation of item 5 for men.

```
dropItem5ForMen <- cnlsy
dropItem5ForMen[which(
  dropItem5ForMen$sex == "male"),
  "bpi_antisocialT1_5"] <- NA

constrainedModelDropItem5ForMen <- multipleGroup(
  data = dropItem5ForMen[,c(
    "bpi_antisocialT1_1","bpi_antisocialT1_2","bpi_antisocialT1_3",
    "bpi_antisocialT1_4","bpi_antisocialT1_5","bpi_antisocialT1_6",
    "bpi_antisocialT1_7")],
  model = 1,
  group = dropItem5ForMen$sex,
  invariance = c(c(
    "bpi_antisocialT1_1","bpi_antisocialT1_2","bpi_antisocialT1_3",
    "bpi_antisocialT1_4","bpi_antisocialT1_5","bpi_antisocialT1_6",
    "bpi_antisocialT1_7"),
    "free_means", "free_var"),
  SE = TRUE)
```

```
coef(constrainedModelDropItem5ForMen, simplify = TRUE)
```

15.9.8.3 Freely Estimate Item To Have Different Parameters Across Groups

Alternatively, we can resolve DIF by allowing the item to have different parameters (discrimination and difficulty) across both groups. You might do this if the item is valid for both men and women, and it has importantly different item parameters nonetheless.

```
constrainedModelResolveItem5 <- multipleGroup(
  data = cnlsy[,c(
    "bpi_antisocialT1_1","bpi_antisocialT1_2","bpi_antisocialT1_3",
    "bpi_antisocialT1_4","bpi_antisocialT1_5","bpi_antisocialT1_6",
    "bpi_antisocialT1_7")],
  model = 1,
  group = cnlsy$sex,
  invariance = c(c(
    "bpi_antisocialT1_1","bpi_antisocialT1_2","bpi_antisocialT1_3",
    "bpi_antisocialT1_4","bpi_antisocialT1_6","bpi_antisocialT1_7"),
    "free_means", "free_var"),
  SE = TRUE)

coef(constrainedModelResolveItem5, simplify = TRUE)
```

15.9.8.4 Compare Model Fit

We can compare the model fit against the fully constrained model. In this case, all three of these approaches for handling DIF resulted in improvement in model fit based on AIC and, for the two nested models, the chi-square difference test.

```
anova(constrainedModel, constrainedModelDropItem5)
```

```
                              AIC SABIC    HQ   BIC logLik       X2   df
constrainedModel            34332 34403 34383 34476 -17143
constrainedModelDropItem5 30778 30840 30822 30903 -15369 3547.921 2913
                            p
constrainedModel
constrainedModelDropItem5 0
```

```
anova(constrainedModel, constrainedModelDropItem5ForMen)
```

```
                                    AIC SABIC    HQ   BIC logLik       X2
constrainedModel                  34332 34403 34383 34476 -17143
constrainedModelDropItem5ForMen 32179 32250 32230 32323 -16067 2152.722
                                  df   p
constrainedModel
constrainedModelDropItem5ForMen  0 NaN
```

TABLE 15.6 Differential Item Functioning After Resolving DIF in Item 5.

Item	Groups	Converged	AIC	SABIC	HQ	BIC	χ^2	*df*	*p*
bpi_antisocialT1_1	female,male	TRUE	−5.37	3.91	1.30	13.44	11.37	3	0.010
bpi_antisocialT1_2	female,male	TRUE	3.91	13.19	10.58	22.72	2.09	3	0.553
bpi_antisocialT1_3	female,male	TRUE	1.50	10.79	8.18	20.32	4.50	3	0.213
bpi_antisocialT1_4	female,male	TRUE	−26.45	−17.17	−19.77	−7.63	32.45	3	0.000
bpi_antisocialT1_5	female,male	TRUE	0.00	0.00	0.00	0.00	0.00	0	NaN
bpi_antisocialT1_6	female,male	TRUE	−9.91	−0.63	−3.23	8.91	15.91	3	0.001
bpi_antisocialT1_7	female,male	TRUE	−16.55	−7.27	−9.87	2.27	22.55	3	0.000

```
anova(constrainedModel, constrainedModelResolveItem5)
```

```
                                AIC SABIC    HQ   BIC logLik     X2 df p
constrainedModel              34332 34403 34383 34476 -17143
constrainedModelResolveItem5 34292 34372 34349 34455 -17120 46.274  3 0
```

15.9.8.5 Next Steps

Whichever of these approaches we select, we would then identify and handle the remaining non-negligent DIF sequentially by magnitude. For instance, if we chose to resolve DIF in item 5 by allowing the item to have different parameters across both groups, we would then iteratively drop constraints to see which items continue to show non-negligible DIF.

```
difDropItemsNew <- DIF(
  constrainedModelResolveItem5,
  c("a1","d1","d2"),
  scheme = "drop",
  simplify = TRUE)
```

Estimates of DIF after resolving item 5 are given in Table 15.6. Of the remaining DIF, item 4 appears to have the largest DIF. If we deem item 4 to show non-negligible DIF, we would address it using one of the three approaches above and then see which items continue to show the largest DIF, address it if necessary, then identify the remaining DIF, etc.

15.10 Measurement/Factorial Invariance

Before making comparisons across groups in terms of associations between constructs or their level on the construct, it is important to establish *measurement invariance* (also called *factorial invariance*) across the groups (Millsap, 2011). Tests of measurement invariance are equivalent to tests of differential item functioning. Measurement invariance can help provide greater confidence that the measure functions equivalently across groups, that is, the items have the same strength of association with the latent factor, and the latent factor is on the same metric (i.e., the items have the same level when accounting for the latent factor). For instance, If you observe differences between groups in level of depression without establishing measurement invariance across the groups, you do not know whether the differences observed reflect true group-related differences in depression or differences in the functioning of the measure across the groups.

Measurement invariance can be tested using many methods, including confirmatory factor analysis and IRT. CFA approaches to testing measurement invariance include multi-group CFA (MGCFA), multiple-indicator, multiple-causes (MIMIC) models, moderated nonlinear factor analysis (MNLFA), score-based tests (T. Wang et al., 2014), and the alignment method (Lai, 2021). The IRT approach to testing measurement (non-)invariance is to examine whether items show differential item functioning.

The tests of measurement invariance in confirmatory factor analysis (CFA) models were fit in the `lavaan` package (Rosseel et al., 2022). The examples were adapted from `lavaan` documentation: http://lavaan.ugent.be/tutorial/groups.html (archived at https://perma.cc/2FBK-RSAH). Procedures for testing measurement invariance are outlined in Putnick & Bornstein (2016). In addition to nested chi-square difference tests (χ^2_{diff}), we also demonstrate permutation procedures for testing measurement invariance, as described by Jorgensen et al. (2018). Also, you are encouraged to read about MIMIC models (Cheng et al., 2016; W.-C. Wang et al., 2009), score-based tests (T. Wang et al., 2014), and MNLFA that allows for testing measurement invariance across continuous moderators (Bauer et al., 2020; Curran et al., 2014; N. C. Gottfredson et al., 2019). MNLFA is implemented in the `mnlfa` package (Robitzsch, 2019). You can also generate syntax for conducting MNLFA in Mplus software (Muthén & Muthén, 2019) using the `aMNLFA` package (V. Cole et al., 2018). The alignment method allows many groups to be compared (Han et al., 2019).

Model fit of nested models can be compared with a chi-square difference test, as a way of testing measurement invariance. In this approach to testing measurement invariance, first model fit is evaluated in a configural invariance model, in which the same number of factors is specified in each group, and which indicators load on which factors are the same in each group. Then, successive constraints are made across groups, including constraining factor loadings, intercepts, and residuals across groups. The metric ("weak factorial") invariance model is similar to the configural invariance model, but it constrains the factor loadings to be the same across groups. The scalar ("strong factorial") invariance model keeps the constraints of the metric invariance model, but it also constrains the intercepts to be the same across groups. The residual ("strict factorial") invariance model keeps the constraints of the scalar invariance model, but it also constrains the residuals to be the same across groups. The fit of each constrained model is compared to the previous model without such constraints. That is, the fit of the metric invariance model is compared to the fit of the configural invariance model, the fit of the scalar invariance model is compared to the fit of the metric invariance model, and the fit of the residual invariance model is compared to the fit of the scalar invariance model.

The chi-square difference test is sensitive to sample size, and trivial differences in fit can be detected with large samples (Cheung & Rensvold, 2002). As a result, researchers also recommend examining change in additional criteria, including CFI, RMSEA, and SRMR (F. F. Chen, 2007). Cheung & Rensvold (2002) recommend a cutoff of $\Delta\text{CFI} \geq -.01$ for identifying measurement non-invariance. F. F. Chen (2007) recommends the following cutoffs for identifying measurement non-invariance:

- with a small sample size (total $N \leq 300$):
  - testing invariance of factor loadings:
    - $\Delta\text{CFI} \geq -.005$
    - supplemented by $\Delta\text{RMSEA} \geq .010$ or $\Delta\text{SRMR} \geq .025$
  - testing invariance of intercepts or residuals:

        * ΔCFI $\geq -.005$
        * supplemented by ΔRMSEA $\geq .010$ or ΔSRMR $\geq .005$
- with an adequate sample size (total $N > 300$):
    - testing invariance of factor loadings:
        * ΔCFI $\geq -.010$
        * supplemented by ΔRMSEA $\geq .015$ or ΔSRMR $\geq .030$
    - testing invariance of intercepts or residuals:
        * ΔCFI $\geq -.005$
        * supplemented by ΔRMSEA $\geq .015$ or ΔSRMR $\geq .010$

Little et al. (2007) suggested that researchers establish at least partial invariance of factor loadings (metric invariance) to compare covariances across groups, and at least partial invariance of intercepts (scalar invariance) to compare mean levels across groups. Partial invariance refers to invariance with some but not all indicators. So, to examine associations with other variables, invariance of at least some factor loadings would be preferable. To examine differences in level or growth, invariance of at least some factor loadings and intercepts would be preferable. Residual invariance is considered overly restrictive, and it is not generally expected that one establish residual invariance (Little, 2013).

Although measurement invariance is important to test, it is also worth noting that tests of measurement invariance and DIF rest on various fundamentally untestable assumptions related to scale setting (Raykov et al., 2020). For instance, to give the latent factor units, oftentimes researchers set one item's factor loading to be equal across time (i.e., the marker variable). Results of factorial invariance tests can depend highly on which item is used as the anchor item for setting the scale of the latent factor (Belzak & Bauer, 2020). And subsequent tests of measurement invariance then rest on the fundamentally untestable assumption that changes in the level of the latent factor precipitates the same amount of change in the item across groups. If this scaling is not proper, however, it could lead to improper conclusions. Researchers are, therefore, not conclusively able to establish measurement invariance.

Several possible approaches may help address this. First, it can be helpful to place greater focus on *degree* of measurement invariance and confidence (rather than presence versus absence of measurement invariance). To the extent that non-invariance is trivial in effect size, it provides the researcher with greater confidence that they can use the measure to assess a construct in a comparable way over time. A number of studies describe how to test the effect size of measurement invariance (Gunn et al., 2020; e.g., Liu et al., 2017) or differential item functioning (Gonzalez & Pelham, 2021; e.g., Meade, 2010). Second, there may be important robustness checks. I describe each in greater detail below. One important sensitivity analysis could be to see if measurement invariance holds when using different marker variables. This would provide greater evidence that their apparent measurement invariance was not specific to one marker variable (i.e., one particular set of assumptions). A second robustness check would be to use effects coding, in which the average of items' factor loadings is equal to 1, so the metric of the latent variable is on the metric of all of the items rather than just one item (Little et al., 2006). A third robustness check would be to use regularization, which is an alternative method to select the anchor items and to identify differential item functioning based on a machine learning technique that applies penalization to remove parameters that have little impact on model fit (Bauer et al., 2020; Belzak & Bauer, 2020).

Another issue with measurement invariance is that the null hypothesis that adding constraints across groups will not worsen fit is likely always false, because there are often at least slight differences across groups in factor loadings, intercepts, or residuals that reflect sampling variability. However, we are not interested in trivial differences across groups that reflect sampling variability. Instead, we are interested in the extent to which there are substantive, meaningful differences across the groups of large enough magnitude to be practically meaningful. Thus, it can also be helpful to consider whether the measures show *approximate measurement invariance* (Van De Schoot et al., 2015). For details on how to test approximate measurement invariance, see Van De Schoot et al. (2013).

When detecting measurement non-invariance in a given parameter (e.g., factor loadings, intercepts, or residuals), one can identify the specific items that show measurement non-invariance in one of two primary ways: (1) starting with a model that allows the given parameter to differ across groups, a researcher can iteratively add constraints to identify the item(s) for which measurement invariance fails, or (2) starting with a model that constrains the given parameter to be the same across groups, a researcher can iteratively remove constraints to identify the item(s) for which measurement invariance becomes established (and by process of elimination, the items for which measurement invariance does not become established).

Approaches to addressing measurement non-invariance are described in Section 15.5.1. If we identify that an item shows non-negligible non-invariance, we have three primary options (described above): (1) drop the item for both groups, (2) drop the item for one group but keep it for the other group, or (3) freely estimate the parameters (factor loadings and/or intercepts) for the item across groups.

Using the traditional chi-square difference test, tests of measurement invariance compare the model fit to a model with perfect fit. As the sample size grows larger, smaller differences in model fit will be detected as significant, thus rejecting measurement invariance even if the model fits well. So, it can also be useful to compare the model fit to a null hypothesis that the fit is poor, instead of the null hypothesis that the model is a perfect fit. *Chi-square equivalence tests* use the poor model fit as the null hypothesis. Thus, a significant chi-square equivalence test suggests that the equality constraints are plausible, providing support for the alternative hypothesis that the model fit is acceptable (Counsell et al., 2020).

15.10.1 Specify Models

15.10.1.1 CFA Model

```
cfaModel <- '
 visual  =~ x1 + x2 + x3
 textual =~ x4 + x5 + x6
 speed   =~ x7 + x8 + x9
'
```

15.10.2 Specify the Fit Indices of Interest

```
myAFIs <- c("chisq", "chisq.scaled",
            "rmsea", "cfi", "tli", "srmr",
            "rmsea.robust", "cfi.robust", "tli.robust")
moreAFIs <- NULL # c("gammaHat","gammaHat.scaled")
```

15.10.3 Configural Invariance

Specify the same number of factors in each group, and which indicators load on which factors are the same in each group.

15.10.3.1 Model Syntax

```
configuralInvarianceModel <- measEq.syntax(
  configural.model = cfaModel,
  data = HolzingerSwineford1939,
  ID.fac = "std.lv",
  group = "school")

configuralInvarianceSyntax <- as.character(configuralInvarianceModel)
```

15.10.3.2 Fit the Model

```
configuralInvarianceModel_fit <- cfa(
  configuralInvarianceSyntax,
  data = HolzingerSwineford1939,
  group = "school",
  missing = "ML",
  estimator = "MLR")
```

15.10.3.3 Model Fit

```
configuralInvarianceModelFitIndices <- fitMeasures(
  configuralInvarianceModel_fit)[c(
    "cfi.robust", "rmsea.robust", "srmr")]

configuralInvarianceModel_chisquare <- fitMeasures(
  configuralInvarianceModel_fit)[c("chisq.scaled")]

configuralInvarianceModel_chisquareScaling <- fitMeasures(
  configuralInvarianceModel_fit)[c("chisq.scaling.factor")]

configuralInvarianceModel_df <- fitMeasures(
  configuralInvarianceModel_fit)[c("df.scaled")]

configuralInvarianceModel_N <- lavInspect(
  configuralInvarianceModel_fit,
  what = "ntotal")
```

15.10.3.4 Effect Size of Non-Invariance

15.10.3.4.1 dMACS

The effect size of measurement non-invariance, as described by Nye et al. (2019), was calculated using the `dmacs` package (Dueber, 2019).

```
lavaan_dmacs(configuralInvarianceModel_fit)
```

```
$DMACS
   visual textual  speed
x1 0.2251      NA     NA
x2 0.1732      NA     NA
x3 0.3523      NA     NA
x4     NA  0.4265     NA
x5     NA  0.5748     NA
x6     NA  0.4770     NA
x7     NA      NA 0.3927
x8     NA      NA 0.2762
x9     NA      NA 0.1038

$ItemDeltaMean
     visual textual    speed
x1 -0.09092      NA       NA
x2  0.18253      NA       NA
x3 -0.38512      NA       NA
x4       NA  0.4869       NA
x5       NA  0.6445       NA
x6       NA  0.4690       NA
x7       NA      NA -0.35907
x8       NA      NA  0.10636
x9       NA      NA -0.02947

$MeanDiff
 visual textual   speed
-0.2935  1.6004 -0.2822
```

15.10.3.5 Equivalence Test

The `petersenlab` package (Petersen, 2024) contains the `equiv_chi()` function from Counsell et al. (2020) that performs an equivalence test: https://osf.io/cqu8v. An equivalence test evaluates the null hypothesis that a model is equivalent to another model. In this case, the equivalence test evaluates the null hypothesis that a model is equivalent to another model in terms of (poor) fit. Here, we operationalize a mediocre-fitting model as a model whose RMSEA is .08 or greater. So, the equivalence test evaluates whether our invariance model fits significantly better than a mediocre-fitting model. Thus, a statistically significant p-value indicates that our invariance model fits significantly better than the mediocre-fitting model (i.e., that invariance is established), whereas a non-significant p-value indicates that our invariance model does not fit significantly better than the mediocre-fitting model (i.e., that invariance is failed).

The chi-square equivalence test is non-significant, suggesting that the model fit of the configural invariance model is not acceptable (i.e., it is not better than the mediocre-fitting model). In other words, configural invariance failed.

```
equiv_chi(
  alpha = .05,
  chi = configuralInvarianceModel_chisquare,
  df = configuralInvarianceModel_df,
  m = 2,
  N_sample = configuralInvarianceModel_N,
  popRMSEA = .08)
```

```
              chi    Fml  popep popdelt  pval
chisq.scaled 70.9 0.2759 0.1536   39.48 0.147
```

15.10.3.6 Permutation Test

Permutation procedures for testing measurement invariance are described in Jorgensen et al. (2018). The permutation test evaluates the null hypothesis that the model fit is not worse than the best-possible fitting model. A significant p-value indicates that the model fits significanlty worse than the best-possible fitting model. A non-significant p-value indicates that the model does not fit significantly worse than the best-possible fitting model.

```
numPermutations <- 100
```

```
set.seed(52242)
configuralInvarianceTest <- permuteMeasEq(
  nPermute = numPermutations,
  modelType = "mgcfa",
  con = configuralInvarianceModel_fit,
  uncon = NULL,
  AFIs = myAFIs,
  moreAFIs = moreAFIs,
  parallelType = "multicore", #only 'snow' works on Windows
  iseed = 52242)
```

```
RNGkind("default", "default", "default")
set.seed(52242)

configuralInvarianceTest
```

```
Omnibus p value based on parametric chi-squared difference test:

Chisq diff    Df diff Pr(>Chisq)
    70.904     48.000      0.017


Omnibus p values based on nonparametric permutation method:
```

```
              AFI.Difference p.value
chisq                 71.443    0.59
chisq.scaled          70.904    0.57
rmsea                  0.061    0.59
cfi                    0.956    0.58
tli                    0.934    0.58
srmr                   0.067    0.53
rmsea.robust           0.072    0.56
cfi.robust             0.955    0.56
tli.robust             0.933    0.56
```

The *p*-values are non-significant, indicating that the model does not fit significantly worse than the best-possible fitting model. In other words, configural invariance held.

15.10.3.7 Path Diagram

A path diagram of the model is in Figures 15.33 (group 1) and 15.34 (group 2).

```
semPaths(
  configuralInvarianceModel_fit,
  what = "est",
  layout = "tree2",
  ask = FALSE,
  edge.label.cex = 1.2)
```

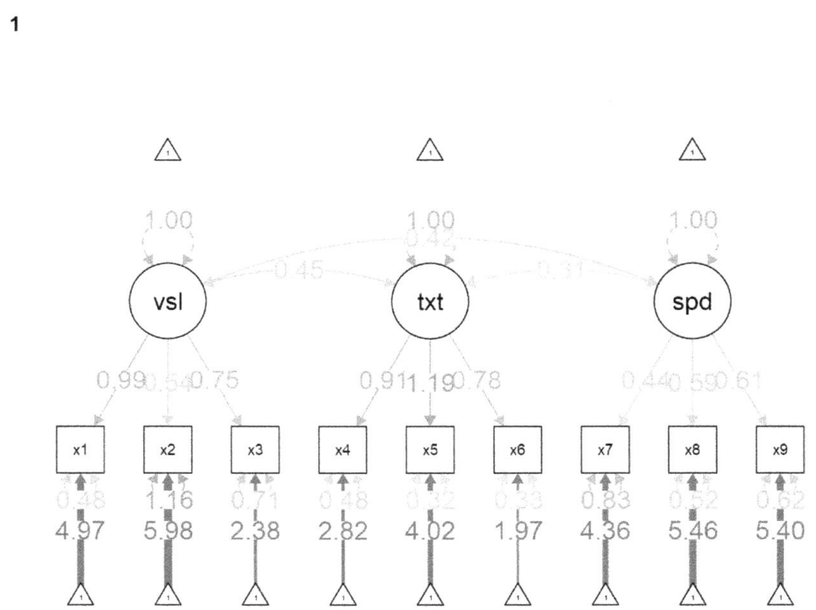

FIGURE 15.33 Configural Invariance Model in Confirmatory Factor Analysis (1 = Group 1; 2 = Group 2).

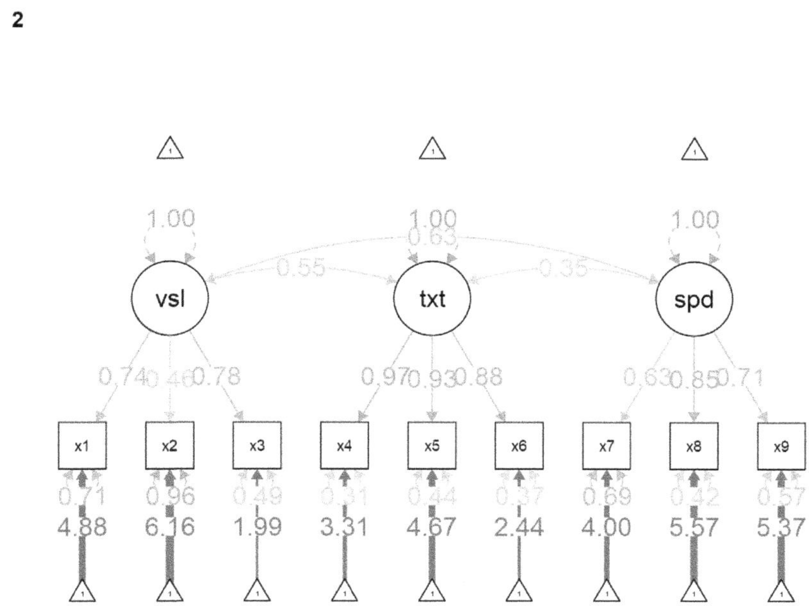

FIGURE 15.34 Configural Invariance Model in Confirmatory Factor Analysis (1 = Group 1; 2 = Group 2).

15.10.4 Metric ("Weak Factorial") Invariance Model

Specify invariance of factor loadings across groups.

15.10.4.1 Model Syntax

```
metricInvarianceModel <- measEq.syntax(
  configural.model = cfaModel,
  data = HolzingerSwineford1939,
  ID.fac = "std.lv",
  group = "school",
  group.equal = "loadings")

metricInvarianceSyntax <- as.character(metricInvarianceModel)
```

15.10.4.2 Fit the Model

```
metricInvarianceModel_fit <- cfa(
  metricInvarianceSyntax,
  data = HolzingerSwineford1939,
  group = "school",
```

```
  missing = "ML",
  estimator = "MLR")
```

15.10.4.3 Model Fit

```
metricInvarianceModelFitIndices <- fitMeasures(
  metricInvarianceModel_fit)[c(
    "cfi.robust", "rmsea.robust", "srmr")]

metricInvarianceModel_chisquare <- fitMeasures(
  metricInvarianceModel_fit)[c("chisq.scaled")]

metricInvarianceModel_chisquareScaling <- fitMeasures(
  metricInvarianceModel_fit)[c("chisq.scaling.factor")]

metricInvarianceModel_df <- fitMeasures(
  metricInvarianceModel_fit)[c("df.scaled")]

metricInvarianceModel_N <- lavInspect(
  metricInvarianceModel_fit, what = "ntotal")
```

15.10.4.4 Compare Model Fit

15.10.4.4.1 Nested model (χ^2) difference test

The configural invariance model and the metric ("weak factorial") invariance model are considered "nested" models. The metric invariance model is nested within the configural invariance model because the configural invariance model includes all of the terms of the metric invariance model along with additional terms. Model fit of nested models can be compared with a chi-square difference test, also known as a likelihood ratio test or deviance test. A significant chi-square difference test would indicate that the simplified model with additional constraints (the metric invariance model) is significantly worse fitting than the more complex model that has fewer constraints (the configural invariance model).

```
anova(configuralInvarianceModel_fit, metricInvarianceModel_fit)
```

```

Scaled Chi-Squared Difference Test (method = "satorra.bentler.2001")

lavaan NOTE:
    The "Chisq" column contains standard test statistics, not the
    robust test that should be reported per model. A robust difference
    test is a function of two standard (not robust) statistics.

                              Df  AIC  BIC Chisq Chisq diff Df diff
configuralInvarianceModel_fit 48 5492 5706  71.4
metricInvarianceModel_fit     54 5487 5679  78.0       5.15       6
                              Pr(>Chisq)
configuralInvarianceModel_fit
metricInvarianceModel_fit           0.53
```

The metric invariance model did not fit significantly worse than the configural invariance model, so metric invariance held. This provides evidence of measurement invariance of factor loadings across groups. Measurement invariance of factor loadings across groups provides support for examining whether the groups show different associations of the factor with other constructs (Little et al., 2007).

The `petersenlab` package (Petersen, 2024) contains a function to perform a Satorra-Bentler scaled chi-square difference test, where $c0$ and $c1$ are the scaling correction factor for the nested model and comparison model, respectively; $d0$ and $d1$ are the degrees of freedom of the nested model and comparison model, respectively; and $T0$ and $T1$ are the chi-square values of the nested model and comparison model, respectively.

```
metricInvarianceModel_chisquareDiff <-
  satorraBentlerScaledChiSquareDifferenceTestStatistic(
    T0 = metricInvarianceModel_chisquare,
    c0 = metricInvarianceModel_chisquareScaling,
    d0 = metricInvarianceModel_df,
    T1 = configuralInvarianceModel_chisquare,
    c1 = configuralInvarianceModel_chisquareScaling,
    d1 = configuralInvarianceModel_df)

metricInvarianceModel_chisquareDiff
```

```
chisq.scaled
       5.146
```

15.10.4.4.2 Compare other fit criteria

```
round(
  metricInvarianceModelFitIndices - configuralInvarianceModelFitIndices,
  digits = 3)
```

```
  cfi.robust rmsea.robust         srmr
      -0.009        0.003        0.007
```

15.10.4.4.3 Score-based test

Score-based tests of measurement invariance are implemented using the `strucchange` package and are described by T. Wang et al. (2014).

```
coef(metricInvarianceModel_fit)[1:9]

sctest(
  metricInvarianceModel_fit,
  order.by = HolzingerSwineford1939$school,
  parm = 1:9,
  functional = "LMuo")
```

15.10.4.4.4 Equivalence test

The chi-square equivalence test is non-significant, suggesting that the model fit is not acceptable.

```
equiv_chi(
  alpha = .05,
  chi = metricInvarianceModel_chisquare,
  df = metricInvarianceModel_df,
  m = 2,
  N_sample = metricInvarianceModel_N,
  popRMSEA = .08)
```

```
                chi    Fml  popep popdelt    pval
chisq.scaled 75.2 0.2926 0.1728   44.41 0.07603
```

Moreover, the equivalence test of the chi-square difference test is non-significant, suggesting that the degree of worsening of model fit is not acceptable. In other words, metric invariance failed.

```
metricInvarianceModel_dfDiff <-
  metricInvarianceModel_df - configuralInvarianceModel_df

equiv_chi(
  alpha = .05,
  chi = metricInvarianceModel_chisquareDiff,
  df = metricInvarianceModel_dfDiff,
  m = 2,
  N_sample = metricInvarianceModel_N,
  popRMSEA = .08)
```

```
               chi     Fml  popep popdelt   pval
chisq.scaled 5.146 0.02002 0.0192   4.934 0.1375
```

15.10.4.4.5 Permutation test

```
set.seed(52242)
metricInvarianceTest <- permuteMeasEq(
  nPermute = numPermutations,
  modelType = "mgcfa",
  con = metricInvarianceModel_fit,
  uncon = configuralInvarianceModel_fit,
  AFIs = myAFIs,
  moreAFIs = moreAFIs,
  parallelType = "multicore", #only 'snow' works on Windows
  iseed = 52242)
```

```
RNGkind("default", "default", "default")
set.seed(52242)
```

```
metricInvarianceTest
```

```
Omnibus p value based on parametric chi-squared difference test:

Chisq diff    Df diff Pr(>Chisq)
     5.146      6.000      0.525


Omnibus p values based on nonparametric permutation method:

             AFI.Difference p.value
chisq                 6.568    0.51
chisq.scaled          4.291    0.64
rmsea                -0.003    0.54
cfi                  -0.001    0.51
tli                   0.006    0.55
srmr                  0.007    0.47
rmsea.robust          0.003    0.12
cfi.robust           -0.009    0.13
tli.robust           -0.005    0.12
```

The *p*-values are non-significant, indicating that the model does not fit significantly worse than the configural invariance model. In other words, metric invariance held.

15.10.5 Scalar ("Strong Factorial") Invariance Model

Specify invariance of factor loadings and intercepts across groups.

15.10.5.1 Model Syntax

```
scalarInvarianceModel <- measEq.syntax(
  configural.model = cfaModel,
  data = HolzingerSwineford1939,
  ID.fac = "std.lv",
  group = "school",
  group.equal = c("loadings","intercepts"))

scalarInvarianceSyntax <- as.character(scalarInvarianceModel)
```

15.10.5.2 Fit the Model

```
scalarInvarianceModel_fit <- cfa(
  scalarInvarianceSyntax,
  data = HolzingerSwineford1939,
  group = "school",
  missing = "ML",
  estimator = "MLR")
```

15.10.5.3 Model Fit

```
scalarInvarianceModelFitIndices <- fitMeasures(
  scalarInvarianceModel_fit)[c(
    "cfi.robust", "rmsea.robust", "srmr")]

scalarInvarianceModel_chisquare <- fitMeasures(
  scalarInvarianceModel_fit)[c("chisq.scaled")]

scalarInvarianceModel_chisquareScaling <- fitMeasures(
  scalarInvarianceModel_fit)[c("chisq.scaling.factor")]

scalarInvarianceModel_df <- fitMeasures(
  scalarInvarianceModel_fit)[c("df.scaled")]

scalarInvarianceModel_N <- lavInspect(
  scalarInvarianceModel_fit, what = "ntotal")
```

15.10.5.4 Compare Model Fit

15.10.5.4.1 Nested model (χ^2) difference test

The metric invariance model and the scalar ("strong factorial") invariance model are considered "nested" models. The scalar invariance model is nested within the metric invariance model because the metric invariance model includes all of the terms of the metric invariance model along with additional terms. Model fit of nested models can be compared with a chi-square difference test, also known as a likelihood ratio test or deviance test. A significant chi-square difference test would indicate that the simplified model with additional constraints (the scalar invariance model) is significantly worse fitting than the more complex model that has fewer constraints (the metric invariance model).

```
anova(metricInvarianceModel_fit, scalarInvarianceModel_fit)
```

```

Scaled Chi-Squared Difference Test (method = "satorra.bentler.2001")

lavaan NOTE:
    The "Chisq" column contains standard test statistics, not the
    robust test that should be reported per model. A robust difference
    test is a function of two standard (not robust) statistics.

                          Df  AIC  BIC Chisq Chisq diff Df diff
metricInvarianceModel_fit 54 5487 5679  78.0
scalarInvarianceModel_fit 60 5495 5666  97.8       19.3       6
                          Pr(>Chisq)
metricInvarianceModel_fit
scalarInvarianceModel_fit     0.0037 **
---
Signif. codes:  0 '***' 0.001 '**' 0.01 '*' 0.05 '.' 0.1 ' ' 1
```

The scalar invariance model fit significantly worse than the configural invariance model, so scalar invariance did not hold. This provides evidence of measurement non-invariance of indicator intercepts across groups. Measurement non-invariance of indicator intercepts poses challenges to being able to meaningfully compare levels on the latent factor across groups (Little et al., 2007).

```
scalarInvarianceModel_chisquareDiff <-
  satorraBentlerScaledChiSquareDifferenceTestStatistic(
    T0 = scalarInvarianceModel_chisquare,
    c0 = scalarInvarianceModel_chisquareScaling,
    d0 = scalarInvarianceModel_df,
    T1 = metricInvarianceModel_chisquare,
    c1 = metricInvarianceModel_chisquareScaling,
    d1 = metricInvarianceModel_df)

scalarInvarianceModel_chisquareDiff
```

```
chisq.scaled
       19.29
```

15.10.5.4.2 Compare other fit criteria

```
round(
  scalarInvarianceModelFitIndices - metricInvarianceModelFitIndices,
  digits = 3)
```

```
  cfi.robust rmsea.robust         srmr
      -0.018        0.007        0.006
```

15.10.5.4.3 Score-based test

Score-based tests of measurement invariance are implemented using the `strucchange` package and are described by T. Wang et al. (2014).

```
coef(scalarInvarianceModel_fit)[10:18]

sctest(
  scalarInvarianceModel_fit,
  order.by = HolzingerSwineford1939$school,
  parm = 10:18,
  functional = "LMuo")
```

15.10.5.4.4 Equivalence test

The chi-square equivalence test is non-significant, suggesting that the model fit is not acceptable.

```
equiv_chi(
  alpha = .05,
```

```
  chi = scalarInvarianceModel_chisquare,
  df = scalarInvarianceModel_df,
  m = 2,
  N_sample = scalarInvarianceModel_N,
  popRMSEA = .08)
```

```
               chi    Fml popep popdelt   pval
chisq.scaled 94.37 0.3672 0.192   49.34 0.2039
```

Moreover, the equivalence test of the chi-square difference test is non-significant, suggesting that the degree of worsening of model fit is not acceptable. In other words, scalar invariance failed.

```
scalarInvarianceModel_dfDiff <-
  scalarInvarianceModel_df - metricInvarianceModel_df

equiv_chi(
  alpha = .05,
  chi = scalarInvarianceModel_chisquareDiff,
  df = scalarInvarianceModel_dfDiff,
  m = 2,
  N_sample = scalarInvarianceModel_N,
  popRMSEA = .08)
```

```
               chi     Fml  popep popdelt   pval
chisq.scaled 19.29 0.07505 0.0192   4.934 0.9162
```

15.10.5.4.5 Permutation test

```
set.seed(52242)
scalarInvarianceTest <- permuteMeasEq(
  nPermute = numPermutations,
  modelType = "mgcfa",
  con = scalarInvarianceModel_fit,
  uncon = metricInvarianceModel_fit,
  AFIs = myAFIs,
  moreAFIs = moreAFIs,
  parallelType = "multicore", #only 'snow' works on Windows
  iseed = 52242)


RNGkind("default", "default", "default")
set.seed(52242)

scalarInvarianceTest
```

```
Omnibus p value based on parametric chi-squared difference test:

Chisq diff    Df diff Pr(>Chisq)
```

```
    19.288      6.000      0.004


Omnibus p values based on nonparametric permutation method:

             AFI.Difference p.value
chisq                19.773    0.00
chisq.scaled         19.171    0.00
rmsea                 0.011    0.00
cfi                  -0.026    0.00
tli                  -0.025    0.00
srmr                  0.006    0.03
rmsea.robust          0.007    0.02
cfi.robust           -0.018    0.00
tli.robust           -0.015    0.01
```

The *p*-values are significant, indicating that the model fit significantly worse than the metric invariance model. In other words, scalar invariance failed.

15.10.6 Residual ("Strict Factorial") Invariance Model

Specify invariance of factor loadings, intercepts, and residuals across groups.

15.10.6.1 Model Syntax

```
residualInvarianceModel <- measEq.syntax(
  configural.model = cfaModel,
  data = HolzingerSwineford1939,
  ID.fac = "std.lv",
  group = "school",
  group.equal = c("loadings","intercepts","residuals"))

residualInvarianceSyntax <- as.character(residualInvarianceModel)
```

15.10.6.2 Fit the Model

```
residualInvarianceModel_fit <- cfa(
  residualInvarianceSyntax,
  data = HolzingerSwineford1939,
  group = "school",
  missing = "ML",
  estimator = "MLR")
```

15.10.6.3 Model Fit

```
residualInvarianceModelFitIndices <- fitMeasures(
  residualInvarianceModel_fit)[c(
```

```
  "cfi.robust", "rmsea.robust", "srmr")]

residualInvarianceModel_chisquare <- fitMeasures(
  residualInvarianceModel_fit)[c("chisq.scaled")]

residualInvarianceModel_chisquareScaling <- fitMeasures(
  residualInvarianceModel_fit)[c("chisq.scaling.factor")]

residualInvarianceModel_df <- fitMeasures(
  residualInvarianceModel_fit)[c("df.scaled")]

residualInvarianceModel_N <- lavInspect(
  residualInvarianceModel_fit,
  what = "ntotal")
```

15.10.6.4 Compare Model Fit

15.10.6.4.1 Nested model (χ^2) difference test

The scalar invariance model and the residual invariance model are considered "nested" models. The residual invariance model is nested within the scalar invariance model because the scalar invariance model includes all of the terms of the residual invariance model along with additional terms. Model fit of nested models can be compared with a chi-square difference test, also known as a likelihood ratio test or deviance test. A significant chi-square difference test would indicate that the simplified model with additional constraints (the residual invariance model) is significantly worse fitting than the more complex model that has fewer constraints (the scalar invariance model).

```
anova(scalarInvarianceModel_fit, residualInvarianceModel_fit)
```

```

Scaled Chi-Squared Difference Test (method = "satorra.bentler.2001")

lavaan NOTE:
    The "Chisq" column contains standard test statistics, not the
    robust test that should be reported per model. A robust difference
    test is a function of two standard (not robust) statistics.

                            Df  AIC  BIC Chisq Chisq diff Df diff
scalarInvarianceModel_fit   60 5495 5666  97.8
residualInvarianceModel_fit 69 5482 5620 102.6       4.15       9
                            Pr(>Chisq)
scalarInvarianceModel_fit
residualInvarianceModel_fit        0.9
```

In this instance, you do not need to examine whether residual invariance held because the preceding level of measurement invariance (scalar invariance) did not hold.

```
residualInvarianceModel_chisquareDiff <-
  satorraBentlerScaledChiSquareDifferenceTestStatistic(
```

```
    T0 = residualInvarianceModel_chisquare,
    c0 = residualInvarianceModel_chisquareScaling,
    d0 = residualInvarianceModel_df,
    T1 = scalarInvarianceModel_chisquare,
    c1 = scalarInvarianceModel_chisquareScaling,
    d1 = scalarInvarianceModel_df)

residualInvarianceModel_chisquareDiff
```

```
chisq.scaled
       4.149
```

15.10.6.4.2 Compare other fit criteria

```
round(residualInvarianceModelFitIndices - scalarInvarianceModelFitIndices,
      digits = 3)
```

```
  cfi.robust rmsea.robust         srmr
       0.012       -0.012        0.003
```

15.10.6.4.3 Score-based test

Score-based tests of measurement invariance are implemented using the `strucchange` package and are described by T. Wang et al. (2014).

```
coef(residualInvarianceModel_fit)[19:27]

sctest(
  residualInvarianceModel_fit,
  order.by = HolzingerSwineford1939$school,
  parm = 19:27,
  functional = "LMuo")
```

15.10.6.4.4 Equivalence test

The chi-square equivalence test is non-significant, suggesting that the model fit is not acceptable. The equivalence test of the chi-square difference test is non-significant, suggesting that the degree of worsening of model fit is not acceptable.

```
equiv_chi(
  alpha = .05,
  chi = residualInvarianceModel_chisquare,
  df = residualInvarianceModel_df,
  m = 2,
  N_sample = residualInvarianceModel_N,
  popRMSEA = .08)
```

```
               chi    Fml  popep popdelt    pval
chisq.scaled 97.52 0.3795 0.2208   56.75 0.06127
```

Moreover, the equivalence test of the chi-square difference test is non-significant, suggesting that the degree of worsening of model fit is not acceptable. In other words, residual invariance failed.

```
residualInvarianceModel_dfDiff <-
  residualInvarianceModel_df - scalarInvarianceModel_df

equiv_chi(
  alpha = .05,
  chi = residualInvarianceModel_chisquareDiff,
  df = residualInvarianceModel_dfDiff,
  m = 2,
  N_sample = residualInvarianceModel_N,
  popRMSEA = .08)
```

```
               chi     Fml  popep popdelt     pval
chisq.scaled 4.149 0.01614 0.0288   7.402 0.008112
```

15.10.6.4.5 Permutation test

```
set.seed(52242)
residualInvarianceTest <- permuteMeasEq(
  nPermute = numPermutations,
  modelType = "mgcfa",
  con = residualInvarianceModel_fit,
  uncon = scalarInvarianceModel_fit,
  AFIs = myAFIs,
  moreAFIs = moreAFIs,
  parallelType = "multicore", #only 'snow' works on Windows
  iseed = 52242)
```

```
RNGkind("default", "default", "default")
set.seed(52242)

residualInvarianceTest
```

```
Omnibus p value based on parametric chi-squared difference test:

Chisq diff    Df diff Pr(>Chisq)
     4.149      9.000      0.901


Omnibus p values based on nonparametric permutation method:

             AFI.Difference p.value
chisq                 4.797    0.94
chisq.scaled          3.156    0.95
rmsea                -0.008    0.93
cfi                   0.008    0.94
```

```
tli                0.019    0.96
srmr               0.003    0.79
rmsea.robust      -0.012    0.97
cfi.robust         0.012    0.97
tli.robust         0.024    1.00
```

The *p*-values are non-significant, indicating that the model did not fit significantly worse than the scalar invariance model.

15.10.7 Addressing Measurement Non-Invariance

In the example above, we detected measurement non-invariance of intercepts, but not factor loadings. Thus, we would want to identify which items show non-invariant intercepts across groups. When detecting measurement non-invariance in a given parameter (e.g., factor loadings, intercepts, or residuals), one can identify the specific items that show measurement non-invariance in one of two primary ways: (1) starting with a model that allows the given parameter to differ across groups, a researcher can iteratively add constraints to identify the item(s) for which measurement invariance fails, or (2) starting with a model that constrains the given parameter to be the same across groups, a researcher can iteratively remove constraints to identify the item(s) for which measurement invariance becomes established (and by process of elimination, the items for which measurement invariance does not become established).

15.10.7.1 Iteratively Add Constraints To Identify Measurement Non-Invariance

In the example above, we detected measurement non-invariance of intercepts. One approach to identify measurement non-invariance is to iteratively add constraints to a model that allows the given parameter (intercepts) to differ across groups. So, we can use the metric invariance model as the baseline model (in which item intercepts are allowed to differ across groups), and iteratively add constraints to identify which items show non-invariant intercepts across groups.

15.10.7.2 Iteratively Drop Constraints To Identify Measurement Non-Invariance

Another approach to identify measurement non-invariance is to iteratively drop constraints to a model that constrains the given parameter (intercepts) to be the same across groups. So, we can use the scalar invariance model as the baseline model (in which item intercepts are constrained to be the same across groups), and we can iteratively drop constraints to identify the items for which measurement invariance becomes established (relative to the metric invariance model which allows item intercepts to differ across groups), and therefore, identifies which items show non-invariant intercepts across groups.

15.10.7.3 Next Steps

After identifying which items show measurement non-invariance, we would evaluate the measurement non-invariance according to theory and effect sizes. We might start with the item with the largest measurement non-invariance. If we deem the measurement non-invariance for this item is non-negligible, we have three primary options: (1) drop the item for both groups, (2) drop the item for one group but keep it for the other group, or (3) freely estimate parameters for the item across groups. We would do this iteratively for the remaining items, by magnitude, that show non-negligible measurement non-invariance. Thus, our model might show partial scalar invariance—some items might have intercepts that are constrained to be the same across groups, whereas other items might have intercepts that are allowed to differ across groups. Then, we would test subsequent measurement invariance models (e.g., residual invariance) while keeping the partially freed constaints from the partial scalar invariance model. Once we establish the best fitting model that makes as many constraints that are theoretically and empirically justified for the purposes of the study, we would use that model in subsequent tests. As a reminder, full or partial metric invariance is helpful for comparing associations across groups, whereas full or partial scalar invariance is helpful for comparing mean levels across groups.

15.11 Conclusion

Bias is a systematic error. Test bias refers to a systematic error (in measurement, prediction, etc.) as a function of group membership. The two broad categories of test bias include predictive bias and test structure bias. Predictive bias refers to differences between groups in the relation between the test and criterion—i.e., different intercepts and/or slopes of the regression line between the test and the criterion. Test structure bias refers to differences in the internal test characteristics across groups, and can be evaluated with approaches such as measurement invariance and differential item function. When detecting test bias, it is important to address it, and there are a number of ways of correcting for bias, including score adjustment and other approaches that do not involve score adjustment. However, even if a test does not show bias, it does not mean that the test is fair. Fairness is not a scientific question but rather a moral, societal, and ethical question; there are many different ways of operationalizing fairness. Fairness is a complex question, so do the best you can and try to minimize any negative impact of the assessment procedures.

15.12 Suggested Readings

Putnick & Bornstein (2016); N. S. Cole (1981); Fernández & Abe (2018); Reynolds & Suzuki (2012); Sackett & Wilk (1994); Jonson & Geisinger (2022)

16

The Interview and the DSM

16.1 Overview

Clinical interviews are a form of conversation with a client, in which the conversation has explicit clinical goals including information gathering on the client. Sharp et al. (2013) provide an overview of the clinical interview. Interviews are the most widely used assessment technique in clinical psychology, yet there is very little done to explore their validity or ways to improve their validity. There is very little data on the validity of interviews. It is likely that there has been little research on the validity of interviews because the field has been riding the coattails of biological psychiatry, in which the tradition has been that the clinical interview is just assumed to be the "gold standard". However, this is based on theory, not data.

The problem is that we do not have a "gold standard" (Lilienfeld et al., 2015). We do not have any robust measure to compare interviews against to verify their accuracy—i.e., we do not have true knowledge about the pathophysiology as a strong indicator of disease status. Diagnoses are not directly observable concepts. Comparisons from one interviewer to another interviewer establishes inter-rater reliability (i.e., diagnostic agreement), but it does not establish diagnostic validity—i.e., the correspondence to truth about illness status.

To estimate diagnostic accuracy in the absence of a gold standard, one can use latent class models (Faraone & Tsuang, 1994), where you identify latent (unmeasured) class membership among participants using multiple observed variables. For example, you can identify a latent class membership based on multiple symptoms, raters or observers, and/or at multiple time points. High scores across symptoms, raters, and time points are more likely to reflect true illness. This is consistent with making diagnostic decisions using the LEAD standard: LEAD is an acronym for: **L**ongitudinal, **E**xpert, **A**ll **D**ata. So, the best approach may be to use LEAD data to evaluate diagnostic validity.

The latent class would be the illness status—i.e., whether the client "has" the disorder or not. Illness status is not directly observable, so we use observables to infer latent classes. Each person is assigned to a latent class with different probabilities to account for uncertainty. For example, Person A may be assigned a 75% probability of "having" depression, whereas the probability may be 13% for Person B. Then, we could treat the latent class estimate of illness status as the latent gold standard. Diagnoses based on LEAD data are not 100% valid; thus, they are a LEAD standard, not a gold standard. However, LEAD approaches are expensive and time-consuming, and they are not widely used.

16.2 Two Traditions: Unstructured and Structured Interviews

There are two primary traditions to the clinical interview: the unstructured interview and the structured interview.

16.2.1 Unstructured Interview

The unstructured interview is the oldest tradition of the clinical interview. It was the most widely used interview method until the late 1970s. The unstructured clinical interview came from a psychoanalytic theoretical orientation. In an unstructured interview, the clinician keeps the framework "in the head" of the information they want to extract from the client, including presenting problems, past treatments obtained, comorbid symptoms, etc.

An *unstructured interview* is an open-ended, free-flowing conversation between the clinician and client. According to psychoanalysis, the nondirective interview was believed to serve as a catalyst for the client's expression of their unconscious, for example by means of transference and free associations. *Transference* is when the client treats the therapist as if the therapist was an important figure in the client's past—for example, if the client treats the therapist as if the therapist were the client's parent. Notes were frowned upon because they were viewed as disrespectful to the client and a disruption of the flow of session.

A problem of the unstructured interview is that taking a different "conversation path" (i.e., asking different questions) or having a different clinician led to different information extracted from the client and to low inter-rater and test–retest reliability. The unstructured interview is susceptible to multiple forms of bias, such as halo effects when dealing with a polite client. Another important form of (cognitive) bias is confirmation bias, in which clinicians look for evidence that confirms their hypothesis about the client, which leads to the tendency to stop the interview once the first diagnosis is identified, and to fewer diagnoses. This is known as *diagnostic overshadowing*. The unstructured interview is also susceptible to race, gender, class bias, etc.

In general, unstructured interviews show low reliability. The low reliability of unstructured interviews is a result of several factors. One factor is information variance: different information is extracted from the client in each interview. Another factor that contributes to the low reliability of unstructured interviews is criterion variance, where different criteria are used to determine the presence or absence of a condition. Criterion variance was inadequate once criterion-based diagnosis came along. A third factor that contributes to the low reliability of unstructured interviews is varying levels of skill and knowledge of interviewers.

A potential advantage of the unstructured interview is that it can be good for non-specific aspects of interview. For instance, an unstructured interview can potentially be helpful for building rapport because the client feels the clinician's first goal is to understand them and their situation in order to provide help. Classic examples of an unstructured interview are provided in *The Psychiatric Interview* (1970) by Harry Stack Sullivan, who is a psychodynamically oriented clinician. Sullivan (1970)'s book provides a guide to understanding the unstructured interview. He described processes such as "reciprocal emotion," which he described as how the interviewer and interviewee influence each other and responses of the other through one's emotional tone.

16.2.2 Structured Interview

An important movement in the development of interviews was behavioral interviews that began in the 1960s. Behavioral interviews came from a cognitive-behavioral theoretical orientation. They started out as unstructured. However, behavioral interviews had a different set of goals from traditional unstructured interviews. Behavioral interviews sought to quantify aspects of behavior—for example, how often the symptoms occur. Behavioral interviews applied the A-B-C (antecedent-behavior-consequence) model. The A-B-C model tries to identify patterns of sequences that include the problem behavior. Specifically, the A-B-C model identifies things that came before the behavior (antecedents), and things that came after the behavior (consequences). This helps to identify precipitating and maintaining factors for the problem behavior, as well as strengths to bolster in treatment. It provides helpful ways to generate information and helps with case conceptualization. The behavior interviews eventually led to more structured versions, called structured interviews.

An example of a structured clinical interview is the Structured Clinical Interview for DSM (SCID). Structured interviews were developed to solve the problem of reliability. In a *structured interview*, a pre-determined domain of questions is asked in a pre-defined way. A fully structured interview provides a script to use to ask each question (to standardize wording), and in a particular order, with a decision tree and branching logic to choose subsequent questions based on the responses given.

For a structured diagnostic interview, the diagnostic criteria for a disorder are codified, and the exact language is provided to ask about each symptom. Then, the responses are scored and integrated in a systematic way, and the diagnosis is determined in a systematic way.

Structured interviews show higher reliability compared to unstructured interviews due to: less information variance because the clinician extracts similar information from a given client, and less criterion variance because the clinician makes diagnostic decisions using the same criteria. Interviews differ in their continuum or degree of structure, from semi-structured to structured. In general, convergent validity improves as the degree of structure for an interview increases (Widiger, 2002).

When very structured, even a layperson could perform the interview. Taken to the extreme, a human interviewer becomes unnecessary; the entire interview can be recorded and done by a computer. In these cases, inter-rater reliability approaches perfection. However, this removes the role of clinical judgment, which can lead to errors if the client misinterprets the computer-administered question or describes a behavior that is not actually clinically concerning. Therefore, structured interviews reduce the amount of training necessary for a clinician to administer, but they lose the potential positive qualities of unstructured interview: e.g., the capacity for better rapport; clients may not feel understood, cared about, or that they are working with an expert. Therefore, semi-structured interviews were developed.

16.2.2.1 Semi-Structured Interview

Semi-structured interviews provide some leeway in how the clinician asks questions and the pace of the questions, so the clinician can ask questions in their own words and ask follow-up questions or restate questions using the client's own words. Semi-structured interviews are still structured in that they are still asking about the same range of problems as a structured interview, to avoid confirmation bias, and they provide a structured way to score diagnostic criteria and assign diagnoses, to ensure consistency across therapists. A well-designed semi-structured interview balances improvements in validity—due to greater clinical judgment and probing—with the tradeoff in lower inter-rater reliability due to idiosyncratic decisions.

A semi-structured interview also allows clarifying the meaning of questions and response choices.

Conducting semi-structured interviews requires more training and there is frequent discussion, in the literature, of their problems, and it takes a long time to become really skilled. This can become an issue with highly trained individuals because they sometimes "screw around" with the interview (i.e., do things differently because they believe their approach is superior) and bypass the structure, leading to an unstructured interview.

In addition to degree of structure, interviews also differ in their degree of specialization. Some interviews are general/broad, including the SCID. Other interviews are specific to particular domains, such as the Semi-Structured Assessment for the Genetics of Alcoholism (SSAGA), which assesses alcohol use disorder. As you get further away from the construct, you lose valued information and the interview becomes less and less helpful. Specialized interviews provide the maximum amount of information in the area of interest, and they take less time, which is why they are popular in research.

A review of structured and semi-structured diagnostic interviews is provided by Summerfeldt et al. (2010).

16.2.3 Structured Versus Unstructured Interviews

Structured interviews show higher reliability than unstructured interviews, in terms of both inter-rater and test–retest reliability. Inter-rater reliability of a clinical interview is typically estimated based on the degree of agreement between an interviewer and an observer of the interview. That is, most often inter-rater reliability of interviews is estimated based on two raters of the same interview content. However, this does not necessarily capture different styles of different interviewers. Therefore, the typical estimates of inter-rater reliability of interviews do not capture all parts of the reliability of the measure.

Test–retest reliability of a clinical interview, is usually evaluated by conducting interviews of the same client separated (typically) by 2 weeks, often by a different interviewer. However, different ratings might be made at each time point if the diagnosis (e.g., depression) fluctuates over time or especially if the disorder is influenced by variation of the context. Therefore, changes in symptoms can contribute to differences in reliability over time—or, alternatively, differences could be due to differences in interviewers. Because of conflating differences in raters and time, test–retest reliability tends to be lower than inter-rater reliability in evaluating the reliability of interviews.

Fully structured diagnostic interviews typically deliver inter-rater reliability Cohen's kappa (κ) estimates of .80 or higher. By contrast, estimates of inter-rater agreement between clinicians conducting unstructured interviews usually are near zero, which indicates that their agreement is no better than chance. Cohen's kappa ranges from -1 (perfect disagreement) to $+1$ (perfect agreement). A kappa greater than .75 would be considered good inter-rater reliability.

Despite the increased reliability of using structured and semi-structured interviews compared to unstructured interviews, many clinicians are reluctant to use structured and semi-structured interviews. Clinicians often feel that structured interviews impinge upon their professional autonomy and believe that structured interviews will damage rapport, even though semi-structured interviews have been shown to increase rapport. Clients prefer structured approaches, feeling that the clinician has a more comprehensive understanding of the client's needs. Clinicians prefer to use their expertise, insight, and judgment. However, their judgment is what results in lower reliability and validity. Unstructured interviews are much more widely used in practice despite the advantages of structured interviews in terms of reliability and validity, because clinicians tend to prefer them.

Clinicians using unstructured approaches tend to diagnose fewer conditions than structured interviews detect. This likely reflects confirmation bias and diagnostic overshadowing.

16.3 Other Findings Regarding Interviews

There are other notable patterns regarding clinical interviews. Inter-rater reliability of Diagnostic and Statistical Manual of Mental Disorders (DSM) diagnoses is better for some conditions than others, but in general it is not very good. This provides further evidence that DSM-defined diagnostic categories are not "real" in a phenomenological sense. Moreover, there is considerable evidence that these diagnostic categories are better conceptualized as dimensional than categorical (Markon et al., 2011). Therefore, a better understanding of the structure of psychopathology may lead to a more valid diagnostic system.

Low inter-rater reliability of interviews could be a result of either low sensitivity or low specificity. Even if one is high but the other is low, you will get low inter-rater reliability.

It is worth noting that the clinical interview is not merely a tool for assessment. A clinical interview can be used as a form of intervention (i.e., therapeutic interview). For instance, motivational interviewing is a therapeutic interview that is often used as a treatment for substance use.

16.4 Best Practice for Diagnostic Assessment

There are several best practice approaches for conducting diagnostic assessment. As discussed earlier, when possible, it is best to follow the LEAD standard: **l**ongitudinal, **e**xpert, **a**ll **d**ata. Have the assessment conducted by an expert or multiple experts in the domain(s) of interest. Have multiple people who are experts on the client (e.g., parent, teacher, friend, sibling, self) report on the person's behavior. Use rating scales to generate the contending hypotheses, and then pick structured or semi-structured interview modules to use for follow-up to examine and rule out hypotheses. Incorporate multiple forms of information, e.g., interviews, rating scales, observations, objective/direct/performance-based measures, and school/work/legal records. If possible, include an observational measure and an objective/direct/performance-based measure of diagnostic-relevant behavior. Examples of observational measures include parent–child play in the clinic paired with a cleanup command to see how parents give commands, how children respond to the parent's commands, and how parents respond to their child's noncompliance. Examples of more objective measures could include biological assessments, such as polysomnography, or performance-based assessments, such as intelligence tests and academic achievement tests.

There are many important skills when conducting a clinical interview, including:

- Taking a nonjudgmental stance
- Active listening
- Empathy

- Authenticity
- Effective use of silence
- Paraphrasing
- Summarizing
- Providing a sense of hope

16.5 DSM and ICD

The Diagnostic and Statistical Manual of Mental Disorders (DSM) provides the list of mental disorders and the diagnostic criteria for mental health treatment providers. It is published by the American Psychiatric Association and is used in the United States. The equivalent list of mental disorders and diagnostic criteria for mental health providers outside of the United States is the International Classification of Diseases (ICD). However, the ICD also includes diseases that are not considered mental disorders. Collectively, the DSM and ICD represent the diagnostic system for mental disorders. A goal of DSM and ICD is to define different "mental disorders" to make sure people get the services they need.

16.5.1 Strengths

There are several strengths of the DSM and ICD. First, they can facilitate communication about disorders with other mental health providers; they provide a common language to describe complex behavioral presentations. Second, ideally, the DSM and ICD also guide treatment selection, especially if people are homogeneous within a disorder in terms of their symptoms, course, etiology, and treatment response. Third, diagnosis is used to justify payment for services from third-party payers (e.g., insurance companies, government). Fourth, diagnosis can be normalizing and empowering to some clients. It may help people learn that other people are experiencing similar challenges, and it may give them hope that there is something that can be done to address it. Fifth, the DSM/ICD promotes research in psychopathology, in terms of epidemiology (the disorder distribution in the population), etiology (causes of the disorder), course (how the disorder plays out over time), and treatment (including development and evaluation of interventions).

16.5.2 Concerns

However, there are also key concerns with the DSM and ICD. One potential concern with the DSM and ICD is stigmatization. The goal of the DSM/ICD is not to label people. Labeling people can be an unfortunate consequence, however, and it can be stigmatizing because mental disorders often carry a stigma. A second concern is that we may be pathologizing normality. Mental disorders are not infrequent. Estimates of lifetime prevalence of mental disorders are around 75% (Schaefer et al., 2017). That is, three out of four people will experience a mental disorder at some point in their life. Thus, abnormality as defined by the DSM and ICD are *normal*. Another concern with the DSM and ICD is that they medicalize and pathologize problems in living as mental illnesses, and they obscure the role of environmental factors such as poverty (Gambrill, 2014). Moreover, diagnoses specified in the DSM and ICD ignore causes and etiology—they do not provide explanations for behavior (Fried, 2022).

Ideally, a diagnostic system should have validity and utility. For instance, the diagnoses in a diagnostic system should have construct validity. That is, the diagnostic categories should reflect truth, reality, or the existence of the construct (i.e., diagnostic validity). Diagnostic validity is the extent to which the diagnostic category accurately captures the abnormal phenomenon of interest. Typical indicators of diagnostic validity are homogeneity (similarity) across people receiving a given diagnosis in terms of etiology, course, treatment response, etc. Utility means that the diagnostic system should help clinical decision-making, in terms of ease of use (e.g., saving time), facilitating communication with others, and in treatment planning. However, diagnostic systems (DSM and ICD) have serious concerns with both validity and utility. The diagnostic system has serious concerns with validity, in terms of whether the diagnostic categories defined by the DSM/ICD are actually real. There is great heterogeneity (variability) between people with the same diagnosis, in terms of symptom profiles, etiologies, course, and treatment outcomes (Fried, 2022). For instance, there are over 600,000 ways in terms of differing symptom profiles that a person can meet criteria for post-traumatic stress disorder (Galatzer-Levy & Bryant, 2013). As another example, two people diagnosed with conduct disorder can share zero symptoms. Subtypes can attempt to address this problem, but there is little support for the validity of these subtypes. Many disorder subtypes and features are not based on empirical data—instead, they are based on expert judgment, consensus, and politics. Moreover, which diagnoses a person experiences at a given time do not portend the types of diagnoses they will experience in the future—people show considerable diagnosis switching from one disorder to another (and even across diagnostic families—e.g., from an externalizing disorder to an internalizing or thought disorder) across development (Caspi et al., 2020).

There is also strong comorbidity (co-occurence) across disorders. A person who meets criteria for one disorder is likely to also meet criteria for other disorders (Caspi et al., 2020). Many disorders often co-occur within an individual, including major depressive disorder and generalized anxiety disorder, which suggests that they may share an underlying liability and do not reflect distinct categories. This complicates treatment and challenges the validity of the diagnostic system.

Another challenge is regarding the coverage of the diagnostic system, including the number of categories and which are represented. How many disorders/categories should there be? Do we have too many categories? There are hundreds of possible diagnoses, including 541 disorders in the DSM-5 (Blashfield et al., 2014). Do we have too few diagnoses? Clinicians often use "Not Otherwise Specified" or "Unspecified" for diagnoses, which suggests that the current diagnostic categories do not cover the variability of clients' presentations. How thinly should we "split" the categories? Some people are "splitters" and tend to split categories into as many categories as possible. Other people are "lumpers" and tend to lump categories together so there are fewer categories.

The diagnostic system also has serious concerns with utility, in terms of lengthy criterion sets that are time-consuming and difficult to assess in practice (Mullins-Sweatt & Widiger, 2009). One possible way to address the time-consuming nature of using lengthy criterion sets is to use prototypal matching instead of criterion sets. Prototypal matching involves having the clinician rate the similarity of the client to a narrative description of a prototypical person with the disorder. However, prototypal matching could result in lower inter-rater reliability (compared to using criterion sets) because of idiosyncratic judgments. There is a tradeoff between assessment time and validity. The clinician's time can be saved by using computerized interviews or computerized tests. Another way to save the clinician's time is to use self-report inventories as a screening device followed by an interview that is specific to the most relevant conditions identified by the screen.

The diagnostic system includes arbitrary thresholds that do not facilitate social and clinical decision-making. Current diagnostic categories do not provide much utility in terms of determining the appropriate treatment.

No single biological substrate has been identified for any psychological disorder that has high enough sensitivity and specificity to be useful for diagnosis or for predicting response to treatment (Tiego et al., 2023). This is because the DSM/ICD-based psychological disorders are fictive categories. The DSM/ICD-defined categories do not exist in nature. This does not dismiss the importance of what people are experiencing, which is very real. A person's experience of depression is real, but the construct of major depressive disorder—as defined by the DSM/ICD—is not real. Mental disorders are not a concrete thing. Psychological disorders are social constructs. Mental disorders are not something that people "have"; rather, they are something that people "do" or "experience". The mental disorders in the DSM/ICD are merely a description of behaviors. They are fuzzy concepts with vague boundaries. They are subjective, often without a clear "yes" or "no" as to whether someone meets criteria for a particular disorder. Mental disorders are defined in relation to cultural, social, and familial norms and values. That is, they are socially defined not biologically. The boundaries between normality and abnormality vary across cultures. Thus, the diagnostic categories in the DSM/ICD may not involve "biological pathology"—they do not carve nature at its joints.

Researchers have examined biology-related differences in people with versus without mental disorders, and they have found some differences, but these biology-related differences are not able to classify perfectly because the categories are defined socially in terms of behaviors, and not in terms of biology.

Another concern with the DSM and ICD is their conceptualization of psychopathology as binary. The DSM and ICD treat most disorders as categorical phenomena that are binary in nature: either you have a disorder or you do not. There is no gray in this conceptualization of psychopathology. However, research has shown that the difference between "normal" and "abnormal" behavior frequently is one of degree rather than kind (Markon et al., 2011). Thus, a dimensional approach to classification may provide more valid portrayal of many clinical phenomena than the categorical approach used by the DSM and ICD.

There is also potential for bias in the diagnostic system or its application, especially against people with particular disorders. For instance, some therapists will not treat people with particular disorders, especially certain types of personality disorders (e.g., borderline personality disorder, antisocial personality disorder), because of perceived challenges. The diagnostic system also might overestimate abnormality in women (e.g., premenstrual dysphoric disorder) or racial/ethnic minorities.

In general, reliability of diagnoses is low. The inter-rater reliability of diagnoses tends to be low (Lobbestael et al., 2011). Moreover, test–retest reliability is also relatively low. A client might cycle back and forth between diagnosis and no diagnosis based on one or a few symptoms. For instance, major depressive disorder is given a diagnosis with 5 or more symptoms, but no diagnosis is given with 4 or fewer symptoms. The fluctuation of symptoms and disorder status across time suggests that a binary approach to diagnosis is inaccurate.

It will thus be important to improve our diagnostic system. For instance, it will be important for the diagnostic system to account for the dimensional nature of constructs so that the diagnostic system better carves nature at its joints (better validity) and is flexible to allow different optimal thresholds for different social and clinical decisions (better utility). One argument against dimensional diagnostic systems is that treatment decisions are often binary (e.g., whether or not to provide treatment). However, decisions in practice can be dimensional too, and can reflect different levels of treatment, including, for example, the dosage of medication, the frequency and intensity of therapy, and the degree of hospitalization.

16.5.3 Alternative Structures of Psychopathology

Emerging evidence suggests that alternative models of psychopathology may provide a better fit to its structure. Models that have captured the greatest attention include hierarchical (higher-order) models of psychopathology, including the *p*-factor (Caspi et al., 2014; Smith et al., 2020) and the hierarchical taxonomy of psychopathology [HiTOP; Kotov et al. (2017); Kotov et al. (2021)]. The *p*-factor is the general factor of psychopathology, akin to the general factor of intelligence (g), and it attempts to account for the fact that many forms of psychopathology show strong covariation and co-occurrence. The *p*-factor (Caspi et al., 2014; Smith et al., 2020) is a hierarchical model of psychopathology in which the *p*-factor subsumes three lower-order dimensions of psychopathology: internalizing problems (e.g., depression, anxiety, obsessive-compulsive disorder), externalizing problems (e.g., conduct disorder, ADHD), and thought-disordered problems (e.g., autism, schizophrenia).

In the HiTOP model (Kotov et al., 2017, 2021), a *p*-factor influences super spectra, including emotional dysfunction, psychosis, and externalizing problems. Emotional dysfunction subsumes somatoform and internalizing problems (e.g., sexual problems, eating pathology, fear, distress, and mania). Psychosis subsumes thought disorder and detachment. Externalizing problems are subdivided into disinhibited externalizing and antagonistic externalizing. Both disinhibited and antagonistic externalizing subsume antisocial behavior, whereas disinhibited externalizing subsumes heavy substance use.

A third alternative conceptualization of psychopathology is the National Institute of Mental Health (NIMH) Research Domain Criteria (RDoC). RDoC is described in Chapter 19.

Another emerging technique is network approaches that model the covariation among symptoms (McNally, 2021).

16.6 Conclusion

Interviews can be administered (a) in a free-flowing way as unstructured interviews, (b) in a way that asks questions in a pre-defined way with a pre-defined order and pre-defined scoring criteria as structured interviews, or (c) as semi-structured interviews that blend structured interviews with freedom to ask follow-up questions. In general, reliability and validity improves as the degree of structure for an interview increases.

The Diagnostic and Statistical Manual of Mental Disorders (DSM) and the International Classification of Diseases (ICD) provide the list of mental disorders and the diagnostic criteria for mental health treatment providers. The DSM and ICD have potential strengths, including (ideally) facilitating communication, guiding treatment selection, providing justification for payment for services, providing a normalizing and empowering effect for some clients, and promoting research in psychopathology. However, there are key concerns of the DSM and ICD, including concerns with stigmatization, pathologizing normality, poor coverage, binary classification, obscuring environmental factors, no biological criteria, potential bias, and low reliability, validity, and utility. There are alternatives to the DSM and ICD for conceptualizing psychopathology. Alternative structures of psychopathology include hierarchical structures such as the *p*-factor and the hierarchical taxonomy of psychopathology (HiTOP).

16.7 Suggested Readings

Sommers-Flanagan & Sommers-Flanagan (2016)

17

Objective Personality Testing

17.1 Overview

There are two main types of personality tests: objective personality tests and projective personality tests. Of course, no measure is truly "objective" but some measures are more or less so. In a so-called *objective personality test* (or structured personality test), a stimulus is presented to a respondent, who makes a closed-ended (constrained) response, such as True/False or Likert ratings. Examples of objective personality or symptomatology tests include the Minnesota Multiphasic Personality Inventory (MMPI) and the Beck Depression Inventory (BDI). In a *projective personality test*, an ambiguous stimulus is presented to a respondent, who is asked to make an open-ended response. Examples of projective personality tests include the Rorschach Inkblot Test and the Thematic Apperception Test (TAT). Projective tests have largely fallen by the wayside now, but it is still helpful to think about their potential advantages. Projective tests are described in further detail in Chapter 18.

17.1.1 Projective Personality Tests

In a projective personality test, the client's response is not limited. Projective personality tests were designed from a psychodynamic perspective, and they are supposed to have limitless variability and therefore a freer access to the client's internal world. However, Card V of the Rorschach Inkblot Test looks like a moth or a bat, and around 90% of respondents likely give that response (Wiggins, 1973), so projective tests are not completely limitless. Projective personality tests are designed to have ambiguous content. This is, in part, to make them hard to figure out what is being assessed. That is, they tend to have low face validity. However, even so-called objective personality tests can have items that are ambiguous and that function similarly to a projective test. For instance, one of the items on the original MMPI asks respondents whether they like mechanics magazines. But in modern times, many people have never looked at a mechanics magazine. So, it becomes like a Rorschach question because the client starts to think about other factors.

Scoring of projective tests does not rely on the client's insight, so projective tests might get past social desirability of clients' responses and potential defensiveness. Therefore, projective tests are potentially difficult to fake. *Faking good* means to present oneself as better (or in a more positive light) than one actually is, whereas *faking bad* means to present oneself as worse (or in a more negative light) than one actually is. Faking or feigning responses often happens for incentives due to external reasons. For instance, a client may want to fake good on a test if it allows them to get a job or to win custody of a child. By contrast, a client may want to fake bad to receive disability insurance or to be pronounced not guilty by reason of insanity.

As of 1995, the TAT and Rorschach were the #5 and #6 most widely used assessments, respectively, by clinical psychologists (Watkins et al., 1995). However, they and other projective techniques have lost considerable ground since then.

17.1.2 Objective Personality Tests

In contrast to projective personality tests, objective personality tests, the client's responses are substantially constrained to the possible answers. Moreover, objective personality tests tend to be cheap and fast to administer, and they can be scored by computers now. In addition, objective tests have more reliable scoring than projective tests. It takes a very long time to score the Rorschach Inkblot Test, and it still has very low reliability. With an objective test, by contrast, scoring reliability approaches perfection. The earliest examples of objective personality tests were the MMPI and the Strong Vocational Interest Blank. The MMPI assesses personality, whereas the Strong Vocational Interest Blank assessed preferences for different jobs or professions. An overview of objective personality tests is provided by Wiggins (1973).

17.2 Example of an Objective Personality Test: MMPI

The MMPI is an example of a so-called "objective" personality test. But the MMPI and other objective personality tests are not truly objective. Consider an example of a True/False item from the MMPI: "I hardly ever notice my heart pounding and I am seldom short of breath". The item is intended to assess somatic symptom disorder, with a response of "false" being more indicative of disorder. But there are other factors that could influence a person's response to the question besides whether the person has somatic symptom disorder. Figure 17.1 depicts how a person's response to the question could be influenced by several factors. A comorbidity of somatic symptom disorder could make it more likely that a person answers with a response of "false", in line with somatic symptom disorder. In addition, a person's insight ability may influence whether they answer with a response of "false." Also, people who exercise more may experience a pounding heart and shortness of breath more frequently (i.e., while exercising), and therefore answer with a response of "false". In sum, the item and the test as a whole is clearly not "objective" because constructs in the questions are not clearly defined. What does a "pounding heart" mean? How much is "hardly ever"? People may define "seldom" differently.

There are multiple forms of measurement error for a given item. For instance, there are situational sources of measurement error. Consider the item, "I hardly ever notice my heart pounding, and I am seldom short of breath". For example, how many stairs the participant climbed to get to the lab could influence their response to the question. Other situational factors could include whether they are dehydrated, whether they have a cold or are sick, and what they did over the past week. Another form of measurement error could result from the purpose of test taking. It is important to consider the purpose of the assessment. For example, if the assessment is for disability payments or to get a physical job, such as a firefighter, it may change a person's answers. Response biases, such as social desirability, could also influence a person's answers. In addition, memory limitations of the person could influence their responses.

There have been multiple versions of the MMPI. J. R. Graham et al. (2022) provide an overview of how the MMPI was developed. The original MMPI was developed using the

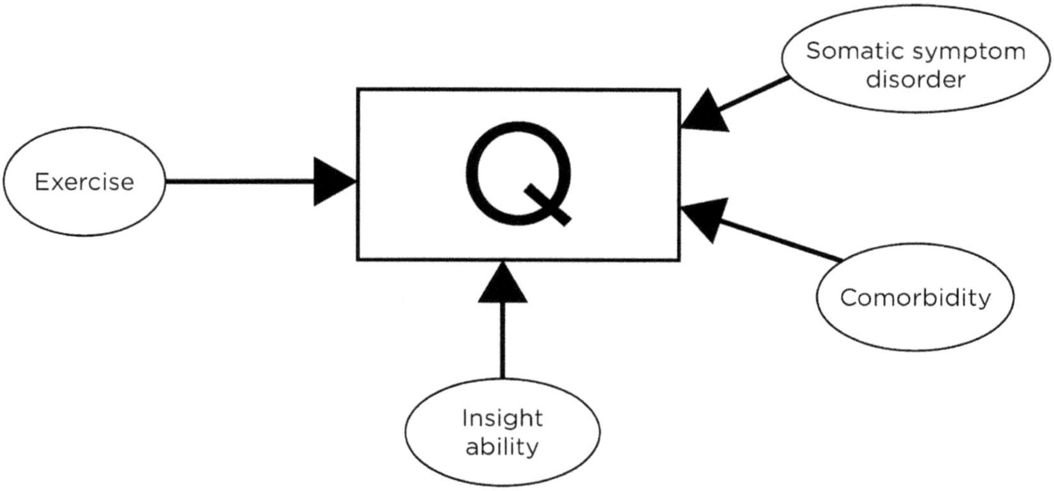

FIGURE 17.1 Various Factors That Could Influence a Respondent's Answer to the True/False Question: "I hardly ever notice my heart pounding, and I am seldom short of breath".

external approach to scale construction. The second version of the MMPI (MMPI-2) placed greater emphasis on content validity of the items, on removing items with outdated or offensive language, and on updating the norms to be more representative. Later, restructured versions of the MMPI-2 were created, which became known as the MMPI-2-Restructured Forms (MMPI-2-RF). Evidence on the MMPI-2-RF is reviewed by Sellbom (2019). The latest version of the MMPI is the MMPI-3.

17.3 Problems with Objective True/False Measures

There are a number of problems with objective True/False measures. However, the problems are not necessarily unique to objective personality measures or to True/False measures.

One problem is related to the response biases of acquiescence and disacquiescence. *Acquiescence* occurs when the person agrees in response to items regardless of item content. Acquiescence occurs oftentimes when the participant is just going along because they think the experimenter may want them to have certain characteristics, therefore they often just say "TRUE" a lot. That is, they may want to please the investigators. *Disacquiescence*, by contrast, is when the person disagrees in response to the items regardless of item content. Disacquiescence is also called opposition bias. Disacquiescence may occur if the person does not think they have the disorder or problem of the characteristics being explored.

True/False measures, just like other questionnaire formats, are influenced by multiple sources of variation. In an objective personality test, there is a high demand on respondents. For instance, on the MMPI, respondents must be aware of recall over an unspecified period of time, which can cause confusion. The high demand on respondents can lead to inaccuracy of individuals' reading of the items. Additional sources of information could influence the respondents' answers to the item, "I hardly ever notice my heart pounding, and I am seldom short of breath". Some respondents may be intoxicated while answering questions, which could influence physiological experiences. Some respondents may have comorbordities that influence their responses. Psychological and medical comorbidities could cause difficulty in interpreting the questions. For example, the respondent may wonder whether the investigator is inquiring about heart beating that reflects anxiety versus heart beating that reflects high blood pressure.

In addition, there are effort differences that influence people's responding. There has been a recent resurgence in how to assess respondents' effort. There are often limits to predicting phenomena due to individuals not putting effort into answering questions. Other potential sources of variation in an item could include psychopathology, stress, physical fitness, age, and gender. For instance, older people are more likely to notice shortness of breath because their lung capacity is less than what it used to be. Moreover, women are more likely to say "FALSE" to this item than men, but the item has less social desirability bias than some other items, so women could be putting in more effort and giving different responses than men.

In sum, lots of factors beyond the construct of interest can influence a response on an item. It is valuable to scan through your measures and consider what goes into a person's answers. It is important to keep the content in mind of all things contributing to scores, and you should consider these potential factors when interpreting results!

Another problem with some questions is compound questions, also called double-barreled questions. Double-barreled questions following the structure: T/F: X + Y. An example of a compound question is, "True or False: Cars should be faster and safer". It is unclear which components of a compound question people are responding to. In conclusion, every objective test is partly projective—that is, the stimuli are interpreted in different ways by different people.

17.4 Approaches to Developing Personality Measures

There are three primary approaches to developing personality measures and other scales:

1. An external approach to scale construction, also called an empirical approach or criterion-keyed approach
2. A deductive approach to scale construction, also called a rational, theoretical, or intuitive approach
3. An inductive approach to scale construction, also called an internal or item-metric approach

However, these approaches are not mutually exclusive and can be combined.

17.4.1 External Approach to Scale Contruction

The external approach to developing a personality measure is also called the empirical approach or the criterion-keyed approach. The external approach relies on an external criterion. In general, a criterion-keyed approach examines scores on items in relation to the criterion, and selects items that are associated with the criterion, regardless of the item content. The MMPI is an example of a scale that was developed using the external approach. For the MMPI, the criterion was a group (i.e., a criterion group approach), or more accurately, multiple groups: patients with different disorders and controls. The original

MMPI was not developed based on theory (e.g., theoretical understanding of the construct of depression); instead, it was developed based on items' empirical associations with a criterion group. Because an external approach relies on an external criterion, if people lose interest in the scale criterion, the scale loses interest.

Consider the development of the MMPI as an example of a measure that was developed using the external approach to scale construction. The developers grouped people together based on their criterion status, for example one group of people with schizophrenia and a control group that does not have mental disorders. How did they develop the test? The idea of the external approach is to let nature decide what goes into the test. So, the MMPI developers sampled thousands of questions very broadly from pre-existing questionnaires of personality, symptoms, etc. Then, they had the criterion groups (e.g., schizophrenia) and control groups answer the questions. They examined the item responses to determine which items discriminate between groups (i.e., which items are associated with criterion group status). And if an item(s) is good at discriminating between the criterion and control groups, the items are selected for the measure. It was purely empirical business—i.e., dustbowl empiricism. In sum, using an external approach, item selection depends on the discriminatory power of each item to inform about an external criterion of interest. Such an approach does not require having any theoretical assumptions about item functioning.

17.4.1.1 Pros

There are several pros of using the external approach to develop measures:

- You do not need to know anything—it requires no theory or theoretical knowledge about disorders and their etiology
- There is likely to be some generalizability of the utility of the measure in the future because there is some carryover of criterion-related validity
- The measure has some practical utility given its relation to criteria of interest
- "Subtle items" with poor face validity can be selected solely based on their discriminatory power. Subtle items are items that neither you nor the respondent predicted would show differences between groups. Subtle items provide an advantage that the data are moving beyond our ignorance. It is also an advantage that clients cannot fake subtle items as well as they can more obvious items.

17.4.1.2 Cons

There are also cons of using the external approach to develop measures:

- Measures developed using the external approach have lower content validity and/or face validity because they include subtle items. For example, the original version of the MMPI had low content validity and face validity. Using the external approach, it is possible to construct a scale that makes no sense due to lack of consideration of face validity.
- The success of the external approach depends highly on the quality of the criterion and control groups—if a criterion falls out of favor as an indicator of the construct (or interest fades), then the utility of the test decreases because it is no longer applicable.
- Items will not always generalize because the generalizability depends on the representativeness of the sample and the quality of the groups—if you select poor groups, it is not a representative sample, which results in a biased measure. The validity of the scale depends on the representativeness of your groups in regard to the criterion of interest. It is possible that your findings might not be generalizable if your sample is not—this is especially problematic when you rely only on data and not on theory.

  - An example of the importance of the representativeness of the sample comes from the original MMPI. The norms of the original MMPI were based on largely White participants from Scandinavian, German, and Irish descent in the Midwestern U.S., with an average of an 8th-grade education. The norms became known as "Minnesota farmers". Therefore, "Minnesota normals" (i.e., the control group) were pretty "dull" normals. In addition, to be included in the norms, the respondents for the MMPI had to be waiting in the hospital (not everyone does that for family in the hospital) and had to be kind enough to take a 4–5 hour measure for psychologists (not all would do this). For all of these reasons, there were issues with poor generalizability of the original MMPI norms in the broader population. A scale is most likely to be valid when it is used with similar populations and in similar conditions.
- Shrinkage often occurs when using a measure developed using an external approach. As described in Section 10.4, *shrinkage* is when variables with stronger predictive power in the original data set tend to show somewhat smaller predictive power (smaller validity coefficients) when applied to new groups. When variables are selected empirically, they tend to show less predictive power (smaller validity coefficients) when applied to new groups during cross-validation. Shrinkage reflects a model over-fitting, because it is somewhat capitalizing on chance in selecting items. Many subtle items may be instances of Type I error (false positives). Shrinkage is especially likely when the original sample is small and/or unrepresentative and the number of variables considered for inclusion is large.
- Externally developed measures also have a problem of communicability (Burisch, 1984). For something to have meaning to others, it should have connection to constructs, which may not be true for many measures developed using the external approach.
- It can take a long time to develop measures using the external approach, and they tend to be longer to administer because of having more items. For instance, there are 567 items in the MMPI-2.

17.4.1.3 MMPI Examples

Paul Meehl wrote his dissertation to develop the K scale of the MMPI to attempt to detect faking good. In the context of the MMPI, faking good would involve under-reporting of symptoms. He developed the K scale based on all positive qualities that around half of people typically endorse. So, it is not obvious that the items reflect faking good, and if someone is trying to respond in a socially desirable way, they endorse more of these positive qualities. There is also a "faking bad" version of the scale, too. The "faking bad" (F) scale was developed as an attempt to detect malingering (over-reporting of symptoms).

However, the MMPI could pathologize normality in some cases. Some psychotic patients may have been identified as "faking bad" because they actually have had a lot of odd experiences. And very healthy people may have gotten higher score on "faking good", but they just may be very positive and well-adjusted. As examples from the original MMPI from 1940, male teenagers tended to have elevated scores on the psychopathy and mania scales. Graduate students, including female graduate students, tended to have higher "masculine" scores on the Masculinity/Femininity (Mf) scale. This shows that non-clinical samples can still have "clinical" scores. In the 1930s–1940s, there was an emphasis on developing empirically based measures, where the researchers rely on data, not theory as had previously been emphasized.

17.4.2 Deductive Approach to Scale Construction

The deductive approach to developing a personality measure is also called a rational, theoretical, or intuitive approach. Using a *deductive approach*, the choice and definition of constructs precede and govern the formulation of items. Item pools are generated using theoretical considerations, and item selection depends on possessing a rich theoretical knowledge about the construct and selecting which items assess the construct the best. In a deductive approach, the measure developer deduces the content; they do not rely on criterion data to select the content. Deducing the content involves thinking and talking about the construct, and having experts write items that they think would do well in eliciting information about the construct. The measure developer deduces from the construct which items to use. Therefore, the deductive approach completely depends on our ability to understand a given construct and translate this understanding to the generation of item content that will be understood by the examinees in such a way that it elicits accurate ratings for the construct of interest. Most assessments are developed using the deductive approach.

17.4.2.1 Pros

There are several pros of using the deductive approach to develop measures:

- Using the deductive approach is fast, easy, and short. Generating such scales requires few people, and is often fast and accurate. It does not typically take as much time to develop a measure using the deductive approach. Moreover, it allows the possibility of short scales that are quick to administer. By contrast to short scales developed by the deductive approach, the MMPI (developed using the external approach) is very long.
- Measures developed (well) using the deductive approach are always content valid because of the reliance on theory—items tend to be prototypical of the construct.
- Measures developed using the deductive approach are usually face valid, more likely than external approach. Face validity is often an advantage, but not always. Face validity can help with disseminability, because others may be more likely to adopt it if it appears to assess what it claims to assess. However, face validity is not desirable when trying to prevent faking good or faking bad.
- Measures developed using the deductive approach tend to have better communicability—i.e., how comprehensible the information communicated is to the examiner based on the responses.

17.4.2.2 Cons

There are also cons of using the deductive approach to develop measures:

- If your theory or understanding is wrong, your scale will be wrong!
- Additionally, if the construct itself is vague, and there is overlap between constructs, scales may be difficult to differentiate between them, making it difficult to establish discriminant validity. Many theories and constructs overlap. Therefore, measures often overlap—even measures with very different names! For example, consider the Rosenberg Self-Esteem Scale and the Spielberger State–Trait Anxiety Inventory below.

Items on the Rosenberg Self-Esteem Scale include:

- "At times I think I am no good at all"
- "I certainly feel useless at times"
- "On the whole, I am satisfied with myself"

Items on the Spielberger State–Trait Anxiety Inventory (STAI):

- "I lack self-confidence"
- "I feel inadequate"
- "I feel satisfied with myself"

17.4.3 Inductive Approach to Scale Construct

The inductive approach to developing a personality measure is also called an internal or item-metric approach. The inductive approach is an empirical, data-driven approach for scale construction, in which scales are derived from the pre-existing internal associations between items. A large pool of items is selected, and scales are generated from the item pools based on the structure of the internal association between items. The inductive approach assumes that universal laws exist for personality structure, that is, that there is a natural structure. The hope is that personality has simple structure: that each item loads onto (i.e., reflects) one and only one factor. It is the hope of the inductive approach that there is simple structure because it makes the natural structure easier to detect using available methods.

The inductive approach is empirical because the answers come from within the data. But the inductive approach differs from the external approach. In the inductive approach, the data come from the internal structure of the measure's items. The empirical approach is also based on empirical data. Science involves prediction and both the inductive and empirical approach use prediction. The empirical approach examines how items predict some external criterion. By contrast, the inductive approach examines how items predict or relate to each other. The goal of the inductive approach is to "describe nature at its joints".

According to the inductive approach, once you understand constructs, you can understand how they are connected to each other. The external approach does not really care about the items themselves. In the inductive approach, you need to use theoretical knowledge to interpret findings. The deductive approach uses theory up front to make the scale. The inductive approach concerns itself with the items and what inferences can be made. The method helps group the large set of items into subscales based on clusters of items that covary most strongly with each other using factor analysis, and it drops items with a low item–total correlation, factor loading, or discrimination parameter.

Factor analysis is used for the inductive approach to developing measures. It is used to evaluate the internal structure of a measure, and ideally, the structure of a construct. Factor analysis is considered to be a "pure" data-driven method for structuring data, but as noted in Section 6.1.4, the "truth" that we get depends heavily on the decisions we make regarding the parameters of our factor analysis. In sum, factor analysis is not purely inductive because the result is influenced by many decisions by the investigator. Even though the inductive approach (factor analysis) is empirical, theory and interpretability should also inform decisions.

17.4.3.1 Pros

There are several pros of using the inductive approach to develop measures:

- The inductive approach yields estimates of associations between items and can arrive at estimates of a simple, homogeneous construct.
- You do not need to know much to use the inductive approach (relative to the deductive approach): just use the items you have and use a data reduction approach.
- The inductive approach can derive short, homogeneous scales. Then, you can see how constructs relate to other constructs.
- The inductive approach is a "purer" method of scale construction because it relies on the natural structure of the data, and no theoretical knowledge or validation to a criterion is required on the front end of scale development.
- The data are allowed to "speak for themselves".

17.4.3.2 Cons

There are also cons of using the inductive approach to develop measures:

- The inductivists (i.e., users of the inductive approach) hope that a simple structure exists within a set of items and that this structure can meaningfully differentiate between constructs. If there is no simple structure, interpretations of scales that emerge can be difficult.
- In addition, this approach is not "pure" because the structure we get depends on the analysis decisions we make. The answers you get depend on the decisions you make, and there really is no basis on which to make decisions. This is called indeterminacy. There are a number of decisions in factor analysis, including decisions such as the number of factors and the nature of factors—i.e., how to interpret them.
- Factor analysis is not straightforward, and depends on decisions made along the way. Therefore, some argue because so much is in the hands of the investigator that factor analysis is really a semi-empirical approach.
- SPSS likely contributes to the problem because it makes so many decisions for you, and many have no idea what they are doing! SPSS is for ease of use, but it is limiting. In SPSS, you can use principal component analysis (PCA) for item extraction. Investigators often determine how many components/factors to keep based on the criterion of keeping components with eigenvalues greater than 1, often use orthogonal rotation of data, etc. Factor analysis and PCA are described in Chapter 6.

17.4.4 Hybrid Approach

The preceding discussion described the three primary approaches to developing objective personality measures. However, the approaches can be mixed. For instance, one could write a large set of items based on theory (i.e., the deductive approach) and then pick items to keep based on their criterion-related validity (i.e., the external approach), and group them into scales based on their internal structure (i.e., the inductive approach). There is not strong evidence for the superiority of any of the approaches compared to the others.

17.5 Measure Development and Item Selection

Despite not having strong evidence for the superiority of any of the approaches to scale construction, best practices to measure development include:

- Start with theory to define the construct and create item pools, using a deductive approach.
  - Be inclusive at this stage. Create more items than you will actually use—even if items are only tangentially related—so you have a broad pool of items.
  - Include items of other constructs to establish the boundaries of the construct, i.e., discriminant validity.
- Then, test these item pools, and consider their empirical relations to revise and/or drop items. Ideally, you would test the items in large and heterogeneous samples that are representative of the population.
  - Examine the items in relation to external criteria, using an empirical approach.
  - Examine items in relation to each other, using an inductive approach. This likely involves factor analysis and/or item response theory.

    * We want items, collectively, to span the full range of difficulty/severity of the construct in the target range of interest. It is important for the items to have accuracy (i.e., strong discrimination and information) in the target range of interest on the construct (e.g., low, medium, and/or high). The target range of interest depends on the purpose of the assessment, as described in Section 8.1.7.1. For example, items used for diagnosis should focus on higher levels of the construct, whereas items used for screening should identify those with elevated risk but might not need to discriminate at higher levels. For assessing individual differences, you would want items that discriminate across the full range, including at the lower end.
    * Items should show some internal consistency, as evidenced by an inter-item or item–total correlation, but items should not be too highly inter-correlated. If items are too highly correlated, then they are redundant and do not provide unique information. Inter-item correlations should only be moderate, e.g., should range from approximately .15 to .50. But items should be highly correlated with the latent factor representing the target construct. That is, the items should have a high discrimination or a strong factor loading.
- Then, interpret the results and label the factors based on theory.
- Evaluate multiple aspects of reliability and validity of the scale.

Other ideas in scale development are discussed by Burisch (1984), L. A. Clark & Watson (1995), L. A. Clark & Watson (2019), and Loevinger (1957).

17.5.1 Response Scale

Evidence suggests that there may not be benefits of having more than six response options for Likert-scale items that assess personality (Simms et al., 2019).

17.6 Emerging Techniques

One emerging technique for developing personalized models of personality is the group iterative multiple model estimation (GIMME) model (Wright et al., 2019), as described in Section 22.5.5.

17.7 Flawed Nature of Self-Assessments

It is a common finding that people tend to overestimate their skill and abilities—most people tend to describe themselves as "above average", which is statistically impossible. People are over-confident, and they overestimate the likelihood of achieving desirable outcomes and underestimate how long it will take to complete future projects. Self-report is only weakly associated with people's actual behavior.

There are there prominent ways in which self-assessment has been shown to be flawed:

- response bias
- ambiguity of items
- lack of insight by people to rate themselves

17.7.1 Response Bias

One way that self-assessment has been shown to be flawed is in terms of response bias. Bias involves a systematic measurement error. For instance, it is not uncommon for participants to fake good or fake bad on assessments due to situational reasons or due to how questions are worded. When answering questions, many people desire to seem better than they are. This phenomenon is called social desirability bias, which is a form of method bias in which people systematically adjust their responses to reflect more socially desirable attributes. The degree of a person's faking has been shown to be related to social desirability bias (Bensch et al., 2019). If you want to want to know the true prevalence of a given behavior, you can deal with social desirability bias using a randomized response model, as described in Section 3.10.3.1. There are indicators of response bias that are worth considering (Burchett & Ben-Porath, 2019).

17.7.2 Ambiguity of Items

Another way that self-assessment has been shown to be flawed is in the ambiguity of items. People tend to have a difficult time providing an accurate characterization of their skills on tasks that are poorly defined or ambiguous. For example, what does it mean to be a "warm" parent? Beyond this, even the language on self-assessments can be highly ambiguous. For example, how often is "rarely"? Such questions can systematically skew answers to self-assessments.

17.7.3 Lack of Insight by People To Rate Themselves

A third way that self-assessment has been shown to be flawed is due to respondents' lack of insight into the required information to make good self-assessments. People often make poor judgments because they lack the required skills and information necessary to have insight into their actual performance, or they neglect it when it is available. The lack of insight into poor judgments can also be caused by errors of omission—in which they do not know that they have made a mistake because they do not know what the best alternative would have been. Also, people infrequently get feedback from others on the constructs we are attempting to assess—as a result, their self-views are not informed by objective feedback.

17.7.4 Ways to Improve Self-Assessment

Ways to improve self-assessment are described by Dunning et al. (2004):

- Use clear items that are behaviorally specific
- Provide frequent, timely, objective, and individualized feedback
- Use self-testing, following some delay of time after studying the material
- Review one's past performance
- Use peer assessment
- Target the motivational basis of the over-confidence
- Benchmark—compare one's performance against others' performance
- Introduce "desirable difficulties" to instruction, such as spreading training over several sessions and varying the circumstances of the training. These challenges can harm the speed that students learn but leaves them better able to retain what they learned and to transfer it to new situations in the future.
- To account for over-confidence, add in safety factors and buffer time. For instance, add 30%–50% extra time to all time-completion estimates for projects.

17.7.5 Satisficing (Versus Optimizing)

There have been new developments in gaining insight into the cognitive processes by which respondents generate answers to survey questions (Krosnick, 1999).

17.7.5.1 Optimizing

Optimizing involves a respondent responding optimally to a question—i.e., responding in an unbiased and thorough manner. There are four cognitive steps or stages that respondents must complete to answer a question optimally:

1. They interpret the question
2. They search their memory for relevant information
3. They integrate all relevant information into a single judgment
4. They use that judgment to select a response

The complexity of the cognitive processes one must engage in when giving an optimal answer requires a lot of cognitive effort. Giving such effort can happen for a variety of reasons: desire of self-expression, being altruistic, desire for gratification, etc. The extent to which such motivations inspire a person to engage in the cognitive requirements to respond to questions in an unbiased and thorough manner is referred to as optimization. Optimizing deals with how hard the person worked and how much they care about giving their best response.

17.7.5.2 Satisficing

If, for some reason, a person is not motivated to expend the cognitive effort required to make an optimal response, and instead settle for a satisfactory response, they are said to be *satisficing*. That is, they are expending less effort that prevents obtaining the optimal answer. There are two types of satisficing: weak satisficing and strong satisficing. In *weak satisficing*, respondents execute all four cognitive steps, they are just less diligent about doing so, and they settle on selecting a satisfactory answer rather than the optimal answer. Weak satisficing may lead to selecting earlier response options without careful evaluation of later response options, which is susceptible to confirmation bias. In *strong satisficing*, a respondent skips the retrieval and judgment steps, interprets the question superficially and selects an answer based on what they think will be a reasonable (or "satisfactory") response. Their answer is not reflective of a person's actual feelings about the construct of interest. Answers could also be selected arbitrarily.

There are several conditions when satisficing is most likely to occur:

- The greater the task difficulty
- The lower the respondent's ability
- The lower the respondent's motivation
- When "No opinion" responses are an option

In sum, to reduce the likelihood of satisficing, match the task to the participant's ability, make sure they have motivation to respond correctly, and do not provide a "no opinion" response option.

17.8 Observational Assessments

Given the challenges with self- and informant-report of personality, it can also be worth considering observational assessments. For example, one observational approach to assessing personality involves a "thin-slice" approach, in which observers briefly assess people's personality via observations across a range of situations or contexts (Tackett, Lang, et al., 2019). Observational ratings of personality can then be combined with self- and informant-rated personality in a multitrait-multimethod matrix (Tackett, Lang, et al., 2019).

17.9 Structure of Personality

The most well-supported structure of personality is the five-factor model of personality. The highest-order dimensions of the five-factor model are defined by the Big Five. The Big Five are known by the acronym OCEAN: **O**penness to experience (versus closed-mindedness), **C**ontientiousness (versus disorganization), **E**xtraversion (versus intraversion), **A**greeableness (versus disagreeableness), and **N**euroticism (versus emotional stability).

17.10 Personality Across the Lifespan

As described by Costa Jr. et al. (2019), individual differences (i.e., rank order) in personality are relatively stable from middle childhood to old age. On average, neuroticism tends to decline, and agreeableness and contientiousness tend to increase with age (Costa Jr. et al., 2019). It is unclear how extraversion and openness to new experiences change across the life span.

17.11 Conclusion

In an *objective personality test*, a stimulus is presented to a respondent, who makes a closed-ended response, such as True/False or Likert ratings. An example of an objective personality test is the Minnesota Multiphasic Personality Inventory (MMPI). There are three primary approaches to developing personality measures and other scales. One is the external approach, in which items are selected based on their association with an external criterion. A second approach is the deductive approach, in which items are deduced based on theory. A third approach is the inductive approach, in which items are selected based on the internal association between items that are intended to assess the same construct. Guidelines for measurement development are provided. Nevertheless, relying on self-report and self-assessment is prone to key weaknesses including response bias, ambiguity of items, lack of insight, and satisficing. There are ways to improve self-assessment, but it can also be helpful to supplement self-assessments with informants' ratings and with observational assessments.

17.12 Suggested Readings

Burisch (1984); Dunning et al. (2004); Krosnick (1999)

18

Projective Personality Testing

18.1 Overview

Surveys consistently show projective measures to be among the most commonly used assessment devices in clinical psychology, school psychology, and neuropsychology (see Youngstrom & Van Meter, 2016). There has been some decline in their usage, in part due to managed care and in part due to criticisms, but they are still widely used.

Frank (1939) presents a problem to solve—how best to assess personality—and his proposed solution. He sought to develop a predictive model of people's personality and behavior based on how people process information. The approach of predictive modeling has worked in other areas of psychology. According to their conceptual framework, people exist in multiple spheres:

1. in the common public world of nature (i.e., as humans)
2. as members of their social and cultural groups
3. as individuals in their private worlds of highly idiosyncratic meanings, significances, and feelings (i.e., personality)

When psychologists try to assess people's private worlds (personalities), they are not seeking to assess the cultural and social norms—instead they seek to assess the peculiarities of the individual. Psychodynamic theorists viewed standardized tests as a measure of how much a person conforms to the expectations of a cultural group, not as a measure of the person as an individual. Psychodynamic theorists viewed personality as a dynamic process of how a person organizes their experience according to the unique individual's private world. They viewed projective measures as an "x-ray of the soul" that reveals its components and organization, including the state, condition, and maturation of the organism.

Projective measures are an indirect method used to assess the internal organization and composition of an individual organism. According to the conceptual framework, projective measures allowed examiners to get a glimpse into this dynamic process and their private world by observing the examinee's response to various "fields." *Fields* are ambiguous stimuli consisting of objects, materials, and experiences with relatively little structure and cultural patterning. Psychodynamic theorists hypothesized that an individual's personality projects onto the field their way of seeing life, their meanings, significances, patterns, and feelings.

Projection, according to Freud (1911), is a defense mechanism by which people unconsciously attribute their negative personality traits and impulses to others. According to a psychodynamic framework, psychopathology is hypothesized to be caused by unconscious motives, conflicts, and memories. In this framework, defense mechanisms keep us unaware of the painful contents of the unconscious. However, attributing negative characteristics to others does not appear to be effective in reducing anxiety or keeping one unaware of one's own negative characteristics.

Projective measures were thought to be a way to access a person's unconscious. When presented with a field (an ambiguous stimulus), the person has to organize the field, interpret the material, and react affectively to it. Therefore, according to the framework, projective measures elicit a projection of the individual person's private world, that is how they organize their life space. Psychoanalysts seek to assess "what one cannot or will not say" because the person does not know themselves well enough, and is unaware of what they are revealing about themselves through their projections. According to this perspective, the person rarely has an understanding of themselves or awareness of what their activities signify.

18.1.1 Categorization of Responses

The psychoanalysis separates projections (i.e., responses to the ambiguous stimuli) into categories, such as:

- Constitution: forming a holistic entity or "Gestalt"
- Interpretive: describing what a stimulus-situation means to them
- Cathartic: discharging affect or feeling upon the stimulus-situation for emotional release
- Constructive: building with the materials in a way that reflects something meaningful about their life

18.1.2 Projective Hypothesis

Psychodynamic theorists are less concerned with psychometrics (reliability and validity) from statistical correlations across many people. Instead, they seek to assess one person in many ways to see how they structure their life space. They would argue that the projective measures are valid if the examinee provides similar response configurations across stimuli and situations.

Projective measures are based on the projective hypothesis. According to the *projective hypothesis*, whatever a person does when exposed to an ambiguous stimulus will reveal important aspects of the person's personality. An ancillary hypothesis to the projective hypothesis is that indirect responses are more valid than direct responses. Indirect responses are responses to ambiguous stimuli, whereas direct responses are responses to interviews or questionnaires.

18.1.3 Projective Measures

Projective measures are measures in which an ambiguous stimulus is presented to the respondent, who is asked to make an open-ended response. There is theoretical strength behind projective measures in that they have good goals, but they are based on poor implementation. The goal of projective measures is to discover things that do not depend on self-knowledge and the person's ability or willingness to share it. Projective measures aim to bypass defense mechanisms so that they assess characteristics the person has and which the person is not consciously aware of. For example, projective measures aim to assess characteristics the person does not recognize or wants to hide.

Examples of projective measures include the Rorschach Inkblot Test, the Thematic Apperception Test (TAT), Draw-A-Person Test, and drawing a family (Kinetic Family Drawing).

Most projective techniques do **not** have:

- standardized stimuli and testing instructions,
- systematic algorithms for scoring responses to stimuli, or
- well-calibrated norms for comparing responses with those of other people

There are various types of projective measures, including measures that use:

- association techniques, often with an ambiguous form—e.g., inkblot, clouds, or word association tests
- construction techniques, often with artistic media—e.g., human figure drawing or story creation methods like the Thematic Apperception Test (TAT). Thematic perception involves writing or telling stories about a series of pictures.
- completion techniques—e.g., sentence completion tests
- arrangement or selection techniques
- expression techniques, often with movement or play—e.g., projective doll play, puppetry, or hand-writing analysis. Play is often used by psychoanalysts as a projective measure with children because it is thought that children have fewer defenses to hide behind (compared to adults) and are less aware of how much they are revealing through their play. For instance, psychoanalysts believe that children who have been abused will reveal that in their play configurations with dolls.

The Rorschach Inkblot Test is a classic example of a projective measure. It was designed by Swiss psychiatrist Hermann Rorschach in 1921. It was initially designed as an instrument for studying perception, but it became to be conceived of as a test of personality pathology. It was conceived by psychoanalysts as an "x-ray of the soul." The Rorschach Inkblot Test has low face validity, and is therefore potentially difficult to fake. For instance, a person may fake good (present as if they are better than they are) in the context of a custody evaluation or job interview, whereas a person may fake bad (present as if they are worse than they are) in the context of an evaluation for disability claims or of the person's sanity to stand trial.

In 1968, a projectively oriented, classic textbook was published, titled *The Interpretation of Psychological Tests.* The textbook provides case examples of a patient. Examiners were trying to decide if the patient was psychotic, and they interpret her crystallized intelligence from the Wechsler Adult Instelligence Scale based on Rorschach scores ("insufficiency of ego strength"). The examiners attributed her lack of consistency across items not to the inconsistency in the test (and its stimuli), but to her own inconsistencies.

18.1.4 Why Not Use Projective Measures?

Projective measures can be considered examples of performance-based assessments. It can be helpful to include performance-based assessments as part of a broader assessment battery to avoid exclusive reliance on self-report. From this perspective, one might think that it could be beneficial to use projective measures. However, there are many reasons not to use projective measures. First, projective measures can be very time consuming: both for the client and the psychologist, in terms of administration, scoring, and interpretation. Second, unlike other observational and performance-based measures, projective measures provide very little information. You could just ask clients questions on a questionnaire or in an interview. Consider the example of assessing a client for depression. Instead of relying on the client to report relatively color-less items in the Rorschach, why not ask them (and others) how their mood is and observe their energy and affect? Thus, projective measures have an incremental validity problem. The scientific status of projective measures is described in further detail later in the chapter in Section 18.4.

18.2 Examples of Projective Measures

In this chapter, two projective measures are described in detail. The first is the Rorschach Inkblot Test and the second is the Thematic Apperception Test (TAT).

18.2.1 Rorschach Inkblot Test

The Rorschach Inkblot Test was designed by Hermann Rorschach in 1921 and has ten inkblots, five of which are black and white, and five of which contain color. The measure is composed of three phases, depending on whether one is using the Comprehensive System (CS) (Exner, 1974; Exner & Erdberg, 2005) or the Rorschach Performance Assessment System (R-PAS) (Meyer et al., 2011). The phases include: (1) the Free Association (CS) or Response (R-PAS) Phase, (2) the Inquiry (CS) or Clarification (R-PAS) Phase, and (3) the Follow-Up Phase.

In the "Free Association" or "Response" phase, the examinee is handed one inkblot card at a time and is asked what they see. The stimuli were designed with an aim to provide the least amount of intrinsic information; the test developers did not want to impose intrinsic information from concrete stimuli. The inkblots start completely black and white, then they move to grayscale, which was considered to be "easier emotionally" for clients, and then color inkblots are shown, which was considered more challenging emotionally. The clinician intends not to guide the examinee to particular responses, but they also want to hear more than one response. The idea is that eventually, with additional responses, the examinee will get to be less censored.

After finishing the response phase, the clinician moves to the "Inquiry" or "Clarification" phase, in which the examiner reminds the examinee of the examinee's responses and asks where on the card the examinee saw their responses and what about the inkblot made it look like that. The clinician inquires what part of the card includes the image the examinee had described. The examinee then identifies the location in the card, i.e., whether it is the whole card or particular parts of the card, or excluded parts (negative space) of the card. It involves asking the examinee what exactly they saw, and what (determinants) made them see that. It also involves examining whether they use integration to complete the whole picture. Or if they are more defensive, it is hypothesized that the examinee will pick out a little part of the picture when describing what they see. Then, they are asked to flip the card around. The inquiry phase can last a long time, sometimes 1 hour or more.

In the open-ended "Follow-Up" phase, the examiner tries to learn what the examinee was thinking and the process that may have led to the response obtained (Choca & Rossini, 2018). The examiner may use a technique called "testing the limits". This may involve additional questions or observations. For instance, questions might ask why a respondent may not see what many others see. Did the person see two insects or two people? Were they males or females? Observations might include noting that the examinee provided many responses.

18.2.1.1 Variables

There are a number of variables that are often scored in a Rorschach administration. Here are some of the ones that can be scored:

- Latency to respond
  - Let the examinee stew for a while because the first response is the least interesting because it is the most obvious.
- How are they holding the card? How do they turn the card? How many times do they turn the card?
- What content do they see and describe in the inkblot?
  - Do they see sexual content? Violent content?
- Location: did the examinee see the whole blot as a picture or just one particular area of the blot, or excluded parts (negative space) of the card?
- Determinants: the characteristics of what the image looked like to the respondent
  - Form: form or shape features
  - Movement: hypothesized to reflect intelligence
  - Color: lack of color is hypothesized to reflect depression
  - Shading: e.g., texture
  - Form dimension: e.g., three-dimensionality
  - Pairs and reflections: identical objects

18.2.1.2 Scoring

The clinician then can spend several hours scoring, and there are many different potential indices. Whether the content described by the examinee is considered good or bad is based on textbook judgments. This could represent an example of an illusory correlation. An *illusory correlation* is the tendency to perceive associations between signs and psychopathology even when they do not exist.

John Exner (1974) developed standardized rules for administration and scoring, which improved the reliability of scores. The Exner system, also known as the "Comprehensive System" (CS) (Exner, 1974; Exner & Erdberg, 2005) is the most widely used scoring system for the Rorschach. But there are still major problems with the system. A more recent scoring system has been developed, known as the Rorschach Performance Assessment System (R-PAS) (Meyer et al., 2011). R-PAS has limited research on its use by those outside of its developers, but it likely has similar problems with validity and utility.

18.2.2 Thematic Apperception Test

The Thematic Apperception Test (TAT) is described by Lindzey (1952). The TAT was developed by Christiana Morgan and Henry Murray in 1935 (Morgan & Murray, 1935). The TAT is more about storytelling, and having the examinee tell a story. So, unlike the Rorschach, storytelling is allowed in the TAT. It was developed by scientists, and there has been a lot of research on the TAT.

The TAT aims to get a better understanding of underlying motivations (e.g., achievement motivation), and it is thought by psychoanalysts to assess implicit motives, unlike self-attributed motives assessed by self-report instruments. Most stimuli in the TAT involve humans, but the situations are ambiguous.

Examinees' responses on the TAT are strongly predictive of various motivations, but they are no more predictive than just asking people their motivations. Motivations that are intended to be assessed by the TAT include: achievement motivation, need for power, need for affiliation, and object relations. Object relations are people's mental representations of other people.

The administrator picks cards to administer that "pull" at issues of interest related to the respondent's presenting difficulties. As a result, the TAT is non-standardized. The examiner asks the examinee what is going on in the picture, what the characters are thinking and feeling, what led up to it, and how it ended.

The examiner might examine the respondent's response latency, and writes down all words of the response. They would examine who the examinee is relating to and identifying with. The examiner seeks to identify patterns and commonalities across stories in response to different TAT cards.

Towards the end of the story, there is very little information from the card, so the respondent has to fill in the story. Thus, psychoanalysts believe that responses at the end of the story are the most "pure", and come from the inside (as opposed to external factors).

The examiner pays attention for themes that are consistent across cards. However, fantasy behavior is not the same as actual behavior. For instance, telling violent stories is not the same as being violent. The horror author Stephen King is an apt example of how describing violence does not mean that the person is violent.

18.3 Most Widely Used Assessments for Children

Projective assessments are widely used. As of 2002, the top 30 most widely used assessments for children (Cashel, 2002) include:

- Wechsler Intelligence Scale for Children
- Child Behavior Checklist
- And then many projective techniques, including:
  - Sentence completion
  - Draw-A-Person test (with psychodynamic oriented scoring)
  - House–Tree–Person Technique
  - Kinetic Family Drawing
  - Rorschach Inkblot Test
  - Thematic Apperception Test (TAT)
  - Children's Apperception Test (Children's TAT)

In sum, seven of the most widely used assessments for children are projective tests.

18.4 Evaluating the Scientific Status of Projective Measures

Given that projective assessments are so widely used, it would be expected that they have a strong scientific status. Lilienfeld et al. (2000) evaluated the scientific status of projective techniques. To evaluate the scientific status of the Rorschach Inkblot Test (or any other projective measure), we would assess across several domains of evidence, as described below. Evaluation of the Rorschach Inkblot Test is provided by Wood and colleagues (1996a, 1996b; 2001).

18.4.1 Utility of Norms

One consideration to evaluate is the utility of the norms. This includes assessing if the normative information on which scoring of the test is based sets the cut-off accurately for those with and without maladaptive behavior, across cultural and minority groups. Of note, the Rorschach does not correctly distinguish between those with and without maladaptive behavior, and it does not lead to unbiased estimates for ethnic minorities. In addition, we cannot evaluate the norms because they are not published.

In terms of the Exner norms, they showed somewhat higher reliability than the original Rorschach norms, but they did not show strong evidence for validity. The Exner norms are not well-calibrated. The Exner norms result in over-diagnosis and over-pathologizing of normality. And they are not representative and generalizable: there are ethnic and cultural biases.

18.4.2 Reliability of Scores

Another important consideration of projective measures is the reliability of scores. This would include evaluating both inter-rater reliability and test–retest reliability. For the Rorschach, the inter-rater reliability depends on the subscale of diagnosis, and has to be much lower than that of objective techniques, especially in field settings. Field reliability refers to reliability in actual practice rather than ideal reliability in optimal conditions of a controlled lab study. The reliability and standardization of administration of the Rorschach is also questionable. The test–retest reliability is also low—but high enough to be passable for research settings—but it should be used with caution in clinical diagnostic settings.

18.4.3 Influence of Measurement Error on Scores

Another important consideration is the influence of measurement error on scores: one aspect of the Rorschach in particular that can lead to measurement error is the effect of response frequency on test validity. If people provide more answers, which is correlated with intelligence, these people are more likely to express a deviant answer indicative of maladjustment.

18.4.4 Validity

A crucial consideration of the scientific status is their validity. Validity is not a yes/no thing. It is important to ask what the validity is for what purpose? Rorschach responses can be moderately valid indicators of creativity. Projective drawings have moderate validity for drawing ability. But are projective tests valid for their typical purposes in clinical psychology? For instance, do they have diagnostic accuracy? Their accuracy for their typical purposes in clinical psychology is discussed below.

18.4.4.1 Criterion-Related Validity

Criterion-related validity would consider whether the diagnosis given on the basis of the Rorschach aligns with an external criterion of an actual diagnosis. For the Rorschach, the answer is: not really. Scores have some relation to psychosis and thought disorders, but they are not strongly related to other aspects of psychopathology. Research designs comparing diagnostic versus control groups often overestimate predictive validity of the Rorschach compared to what it would be in practice because clinicians are typically interested in low base rate phenomena for which predictive accuracy will be lower.

18.4.4.2 Convergent Validity

Convergent validity would consider whether Rorschach findings correspond to the findings of more reliable objective tests such as the Minnesota Multiphasic Personality Inventory? The answer is also no.

18.4.4.3 Incremental Validity

In terms of incremental validity, a frequent argument by proponents of projective tests is that, "I don't use the Rorschach/TAT in isolation but in combination with other measures". But does the inclusion of the Rorschach lead to improvements in the validity of diagnoses of clinicians? No. In many cases, it has *decremental* validity—it decreases predictive or diagnostic accuracy (Garb et al., 2005).

18.4.4.4 Treatment Utility

Treatment utility considers whether it is worth the vast amount of time spent administering, scoring, and interpreting the measure (2–3 hours)? The answer is also no. You can assess psychopathology more accurately with more reliable and less time-consuming measures, including interviews, questionnaires, and demographic data. Projective measures present actual costs in addition to opportunity costs. Actual costs of projective measures include that they are expensive and time-consuming for training, and are time-consuming to administer, score, and interpret. Opportunity costs of projective measures include that they take time away from other, more useful procedures.

18.4.5 Summary

Hence, we would not say the scientific status of the Rorschach is very positive. The evidence does not provide the evidence necessary to call projective measures "tests". No known projective measures have enough power to justify their lengthy use. Considering the important role that assessments can play in clinical decision-making that influences people's lives, it seems unethical to use projective techniques, as they are currently designed and used.

18.5 Conclusion

Projective measures are measures in which an ambiguous stimulus is presented to the respondent, who is asked to make an open-ended response. Projective measures were developed based on psychodynamic theory and the projective hypothesis that whatever a person does when exposed to an ambiguous stimulus will reveal important aspects of the person's personality. The goal of projective measures is to discover things that do not depend on self-knowledge and the person's ability or willingness to share it. Projective measures aim to bypass defense mechanisms so that they assess characteristics the person has and which the person is not consciously aware of. Examples of projective measures include the Rorschach Inkblot Test, the Thematic Apperception Test (TAT), Draw-A-Person Test, and drawing a family (Kinetic Family Drawing). However, there are many problems with projective measures: most projective techniques do **not** have standardized stimuli and testing instructions, systematic algorithms for scoring responses to stimuli, or well-calibrated norms for comparing responses with those of other people. Their scientific status is not strong in terms of utility of norms, reliability, influence of measurement error, or validity. In addition, they can be very time-consuming, and they provide very little information. Thus, there are many reasons not to use projective measures.

18.6 Suggested Readings

Lilienfeld et al. (2000)

19

Psychophysiological and Ambulatory Assessment

There are a number of alternative conceptualizations of psychopathology compared to the conceptualization of psychopathology provided in the Diagnostic and Statistical Manual of Mental Disorders (DSM). One alternative conceptualization of psychopathology is the p-factor (Caspi et al., 2014; Smith et al., 2020). The p-factor is a hierarchical view of psychopathology that accounts for covariation among various kinds of psychopathology. The p-factor is a general psychopathology factor, similar to the general intelligence factor (g), and has three sub-factors: internalizing problems, externalizing problems, and thought-disordered problems. Hierarchical conceptualizations tend to be advanced by lumpers, who group similar forms of psychopathology together, as opposed to splitters, who tend to split forms of psychopathology into separate categories.

Another hierarchical view of psychopathology is HiTOP, the Hierarchical Taxonomy of Psychopathology (Kotov et al., 2017, 2021).

A third conceptualization of psychopathology is presented by the Research Domain Criteria, also called (RDoC), from the National Institute of Mental Health (NIMH). Recommendations for conducting assessment in a transdiagnostic way that is consistent with HiTOP and RDoC are provided by Stanton et al. (2020).

19.1 NIMH Research Domain Criteria

The National Institute of Mental Health (NIMH) has funded research to understand the etiology of mental illnesses and how best to intervene. Historically, NIMH funded considerable work on traditional DSM-based diagnostic categories. However, work studying DSM-defined diagnostic categories has not had as much impact as NIMH would have liked. So, the NIMH led an initiative known as the Research Domain Criteria, also called RDoC, to provide a template for research on psychopathology.

An overview of RDoC is provided by Kozak & Cuthbert (2016). There are several ways in which RDoC is different from the DSM. Compared to the DSM, RDoC is dimensional, not categorical. RDoC views psychopathology as existing on continua, not as discrete categories. Another difference is that RDoC works from the ground up, starting with brain–behavior relations, and linking those to clinical symptoms. By contrast, the DSM is top-down, starting with diagnostic categories and determining what fits in those categories based on behavioral symptoms. However, as discussed in Section 16.5.2, diagnoses are fictive categories that have poor diagnostic validity. The DSM-defined categories are based on behavioral presentations; that is, disorders are not things that people "have"; they are things that people "do".

The same behavior can occur for different underlying reasons, a principle known as equifinality. Different neurodevelopmental trajectories may underlie the same behavior for two different people. Behavioral presentations in the same disorder are heterogeneous. The pathophysiology in a given DSM category is not unitary. DSM categories also share symptoms and show lots of co-occurrence, so they are not entirely distinct. The DSM has resulted in the reification of these fictive diagnostic categories.

RDoC is a template for psychopathology research that consists of dimensional constructs integrating elements of psychology and biology. It incorporates a wider range of data, and multiple levels of analysis, including genetics, brain structure and function, and physiology. By contrast, the DSM only incorporates symptoms. In RDoC, there is a focus on narrower dimensions, such as cognition, emotion, reward seeking, fear, learning, memory, motivation, and perception, rather than disorders. The focus on narrow dimensions is based on the idea that there is greater potential to relate biological processes to simpler, lower-order, narrower dimensions of psychological constructs compared to disorders. These narrower dimensions of psychological constructs can be related to important clinical dimensions. Psychopathology is thought to represent extremes on the psychobiological distribution, e.g., high fearfulness in phobia versus low fearfulness in psychopathy. Thus, psychophysiological processes are a key emphasis in RDoC (G. A. Miller et al., 2016).

19.1.1 RDoC Matrix

The RDoC matrix is a matrix of two dimensions: six domains by eight units of analysis. In the RDoC matrix, domains are constructs that include elements, processes, mechanisms, and responses. The domains include: negative valence systems (i.e., negative affect: fear, anxiety, etc.), positive valence systems (i.e., positive affect: reward processing), cognitive systems (attention, perception, language, cognitive control, working memory), social processes (attachment, social communication, empathy), arousal and regulatory systems (sleep, circadian rhythms), sensorimotor systems (e.g., motor actions).

In the RDoC matrix, units of analysis are classes of measurement that are similar to levels of analysis. Units of analysis include: genes, molecules, cells, circuits, physiology, behaviors, self-reports, and paradigms.

The RDoC matrix is presented in Figure 19.1.

In the RDoC framework, there is theoretical neutrality of the units of analysis. No unit of analysis is thought to be more important than any other; they are each thought to be important in their own right. That is why they are referred to as *units* of analysis rather than *levels* of analysis. "Levels" connotes order from basic to higher-order, and the developers of RDoC wanted to avoid suggesting that one level underlies another.

RDoC dimensional constructs are meant to be integrative rather than reductionistic. It involves moving away from the subjectivist tradition and moving toward a heterophenomenological approach. The subjectivist tradition is one in which subjective experience is deemed the primary measure of a phenomenon (e.g., fear). The heterophenomenological approach combines multiple units of analysis to identify phenomena.

The domains and constructs will need to be added and refined with further research. The RDoC matrix is just a tentative and incomplete starting template. The goal is to understand the bridge (i.e., mechanisms) that links the different units of analysis for the same construct, for example, how the biological and psychological bases of fear influence each other. Examples of mechanisms include endophenotypes, that are heritable, "unobservable", intermediary traits that signify disease liability, and that mediate the association between genotype and phenotypic expressions of psychopathology. An example of an endophenotype is depicted in Figure 19.2.

Domain	Construct	Subconstruct	Genes	Molecules	Cells	Circuits	Physiology	Behavior	Self-Report	Paradigms
Negative Valence Systems	Acute Threat ("Fear")									
	Potential Threat ("Anxiety")									
	Sustained Threat									
	Loss									
	Frustrative Nonreward									
Positive Valence Systems	Reward Responsiveness	Reward Anticipation Initial Response to Reward Reward Satiation								
	Reward Learning	Probabilistic and Reinforcement Learning Reward Prediction Error Habit								
	Reward Valuation	Reward (Probability) Delay Effort								
Cognitive Systems	Attention									
	Perception	Visual Perception Auditory Perception Olfactory/Somatosensory/ Multimodal/Perception								
	Declarative Memory									
	Language									
	Cognitive Control	Goal Selection Updating, Representation, and Maintenance Response Selection Inhibition/Suppression Performance Monitoring								
	Working Memory	Active Maintenance Flexible Updating Limited Capacity Interference Control								
Social Processes	Affiliation and Attachment									
	Social Communication	Reception of Facial Communication Production of Facial Communication Reception of Non-Facial Communication Production of Non-Facial Communication								
	Perception and Understanding of Self	Agency Self-Knowledge								
	Perception and Understanding of Others	Animacy Perception Action Perception Understanding Mental States								
Arousal and Regulatory Systems	Arousal									
	Circadian Rhythms									
	Sleep-Wakefulness									
Sensorimotor Systems	Motor Actions	Action Planning and Selection Sensorimotor Dynamics Initiation Execution Inhibition and Termination								
	Agency and Ownership									
	Habit - Sensorimotor									
	Innate Motor Patterns									

FIGURE 19.1 National Institute of Mental Health (NIMH) Research Domain Criteria (RDoC) Matrix.

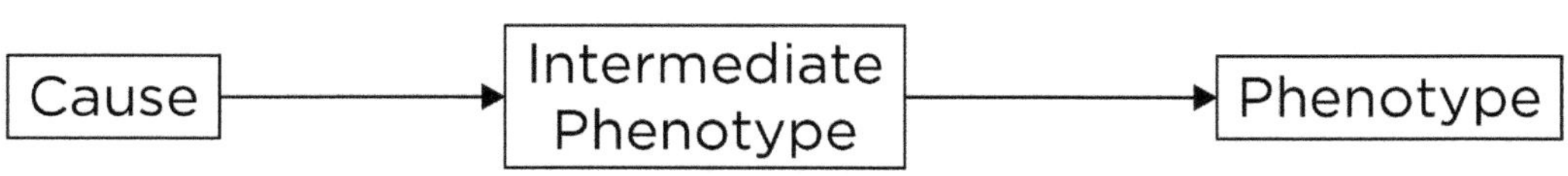

FIGURE 19.2 Example of an Endophenotype.

The idea is that genes influence endophenotypes and that endophenotypes lead to the phenotype. An endophenotype is similar to "intermediate phenotype", but an intermediate phenotype does not have the requirement of a genetic cause. An example of an intermediate phenotype is depicted in Figure 19.3. Endophenotypes and intermediate phenotypes are different from biomarkers, which are biological indicators (i.e., correlates) that are not necessarily causal. All endophenotypes are biomarkers, but not all biomarkers are endophenotypes.

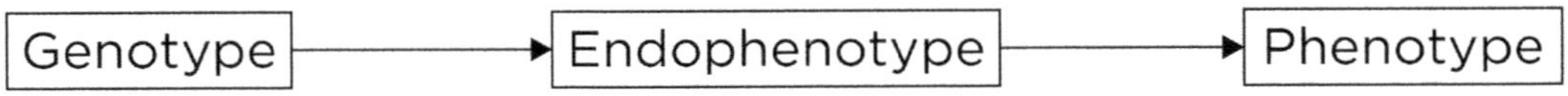

FIGURE 19.3 Example of an Intermediate Phenotype.

One dimension that the RDoC does not include is development. It has been a challenge incorporating development into the RDoC matrix (Conradt et al., 2021; Durbin et al., 2022).

When considering the RDoC matrix, it is important to consider the RDoC dimensions—domains of functioning and units of analysis—within the context of environmental and developmental influences (Lupien et al., 2017; Woody & Gibb, 2015), as depicted in Figure 19.4.

19.2 Psychophysiological Measures

Examples of psychophysiological measures include electroencephalography (EEG), event-related potential (ERP), (functional) magnetic resonance imaging (f)MRI, computerized axial tomography (CAT), magnetoencephalography (MEG), functional near infrared spectroscopy (fNIRS), electrocardiography (ECG or EKG), electromyography (EMG), electrooculography (EOG), eyetracking, and actigraphy. G. A. Miller et al. (2007) provide an overview of neuroimaging techniques for clinical assessment.

EEG caps can include 256 electrode sensors from millisecond to millisecond, with strong temporal resolution, yielding lots of data. Having more sensors allows better estimates of spatial localization. Psychophysiological measures are relevant because lots of behavior problems have important physiological facets. But it is not always clear whether biological processes cause psychopathology or the reverse, or whether there are third variable confounds that influence both psychophysiology and behavior problems (that explain why they are associated, even though they are non-causally related).

Psychophysiological measures are not invulnerable to basic measurement issues, including reliability and validity. Psychophysiological measures tend to be more expensive than questionnaire measures, so people traditionally were reluctant to consider issues of reliability and validity.

Galton and Cattell, nearly 200 years ago, were more interested in direct measures, like grip strength, than self-report. Hans Berger made the first EEG recording in 1924: EEG has been around a long time.

19.2.1 Reliability

Reliability matters, especially when you are examining individual differences (Dubois & Adolphs, 2016). From a generalizability theory point of view, we could examine the consistency

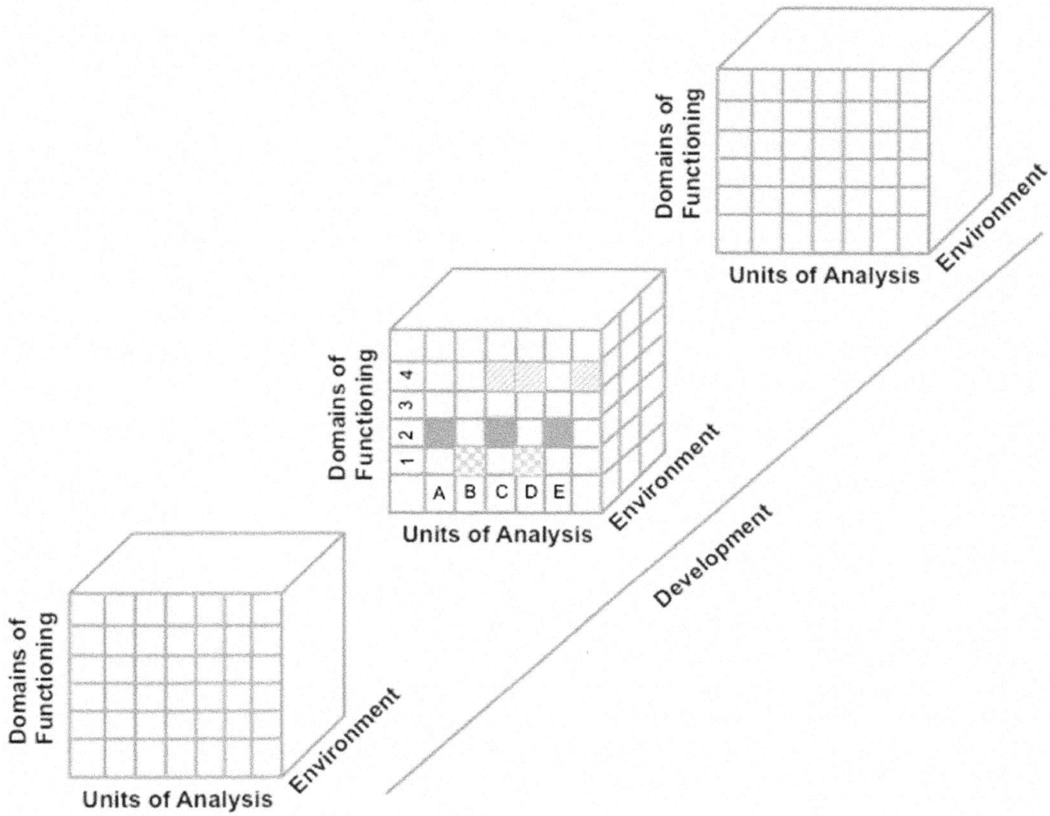

FIGURE 19.4 Schematization Representation (from an Original idea from Woody & Gibb (2015)) of the Four-Dimensional Matrix of the RDoC Framework. Each row represents a sub-domain of functioning that could be studied in different studies or in a single study. Each column represents a unit of analysis. The different matrices are represented as a function of the environmental and developmental dimensions. For example, the domain of functioning in figure could represent the 'Negative Valence System' where '1' represents acute threat or fear, '2' represents potential threat of anxiety, '3' represents sustained threat, and '4' represents loss. The units of analysis could be represented by 'A' Genes; 'B' Stress Hormones; 'C' EEG; 'D' Brain imaging, and 'E': Metabolic markers. Each row of this schematized RDoC matrix represents a particular study (e.g., the gray boxes in Row #1 could represent a study measuring acute threat of fear as a function of stress hormones and brain imaging in an adult population) and the results of various studies are represented by the different filled boxes represented in rows and columns. Environmental and developmental factors could be added to all of these studies. (Figure reprinted from Lupien et al. (2017), figure 1, p. 9. Lupien, S. J., Sasseville, M., François, N., Giguère, C. E., Boissonneault, J., Plusquellec, P., Godbout, R., Xiong, L., Potvin, S., Kouassi, E., & Lesage, A. (2017). The DSM5/RDoC debate on the future of mental health research: implication for studies on human stress and presentation of the signature bank. *Stress*, *20*(1), 2-18. https://doi.org/10.1080/10253890.2017.1286324)

or inconsistency of scores across facets and factors to determine which ones matter and which ones do not matter. Important considerations for evaluating reliability are discussed by Calamia (2019).

Internal consistency involves examining the consistency of scores across trials to demonstrate that the measure assesses the same thing across trials. An example of internal consistency that could be applied to psychophysiological data is split-half reliability.

Another important form of reliability is test–retest reliability, which involves examining the consistency of scores across time. You could examine the consistency of individual differences across time, i.e., stability, and the consistency of scores within a person across time, i.e., repeatability. An example of repeatability would be examining a Bland-Altman plot.

Another important form of reliability is inter-rater reliability, which involves examining the consistency of scores across raters or processing methods. The goal is to generalize across instruments (machines, operators, etc.) to identify the reliability of the general method and not just the reliability of a particular operator or machine.

Parallel-forms reliability would involve examining the consistency of scores across slightly different stimuli thought to reflect the same cognitive processes. For instance, one could examine the reliability of scores across trials, time, raters, and stimuli. And if the reliability is low, it would be important to follow up to determine why the reliability is low.

It can be beneficial to conduct sensitivity analyses. Sensitivity analyses evaluate the robustness of findings by examining the extent to which findings differ based on changes in methods. For instance, you could examine whether findings differ when using different processing methods. If findings are consistent when using different processing methods, this provides further confidence in your findings because they do not appear to be due to the processing method chosen. However, if the findings differ across processing methods, it tells you that the processing method has an important consequence in relation to your outcome of interest. Sensitivity analysis can help you learn more about the phenomenon of interest.

19.2.2 Lots of Data

Psychophysiological measures yield lots of data. Some of the variance in the data reflects garbage (noise), some of the variance in the data reflects signal. So, when collecting lots of information, there's a possibility of finding an effect merely by chance. There are many researcher degrees of freedom. There are many brain voxels. There are often multiple conditions. And there are many ways to analyze the data. The researcher degrees of freedom can lead to *p*-hacking.

An example of the potential problem with researcher degrees of freedom is the "dead salmon study" (Bennett et al., 2009, 2010). In the study, activation was detected in voxels of a dead salmon during fMRI scanning. The false positive activation detected was due to a failure to account for many multiple comparisons. The point of the dead salmon study was not to invalidate fMRI—it was to show the importance of how rich data should be analyzed to adjust for multiple testing to lower the rate of Type I errors.

When dealing with lots of data, over-fitting is a common issue. As described in Section 4.3.1.3.3.3, over-fitting involves explaining noise variance, a finding which would not generalize to a new sample. To avoid over-fitting when examining individual differences, such as with a correlation, it can be helpful to cross-validate the findings in an independent sample or in a hold-out sample. A hold-out sample is when you sub-divide a sample into a training and test data set. You develop the model on the training data set and see how the findings cross-validate on the hold-out (test) data set. Cross-validation requires larger sample (typically $N > 100$), which is difficult with psychophysiological measures. Most samples with psychophysiological data are relatively small, and as a result, have low power (Button et al., 2013b, 2013a). With lots of data, researcher degrees of freedom, a small sample, and a statistical significance filter, reported findings have inflated estimates of effect sizes and poor replicability (Loken & Gelman, 2017).

One way to deal with the large data is to reduce the massive data down, and to use scoring and algorithms. For instance, you can examine the reliability of the scoring system, versus the reliability of the person conducting the scoring system. For data reduction, principal component analysis (PCA) is a useful technique.

Historically, psychophysiological data were averaged across subjects (group averaging) to improve the signal-to-noise ratio. For example, data were averaged for a clinical group versus controls. However, we think of psychopathology as dimensional and involving individual differences. There have been recent attempts to examine data at the individual differences level.

Issues such as reliability and validity are even more crucial when trying to make inferences about individual differences. It is important to remove as much noise as possible without sacrificing signal. Movement artifacts in psychophysiological measurements can lead to poor data quality. It is important to correct for artifacts because they do not occur at random. For example, patients with attention-deficit hyperactivity disorder (ADHD) and schizophrenia will likely show more movement artifacts than controls. One approach is to regress out the artifact (e.g., heart rate), if you have an independent measure of the artifact. If you do not have an independent measure of the artifact, you can use independent component analysis (ICA) to separate independent components of data and to remove artifacts.

19.2.3 Validity

Consideration of aspects of validity are crucial for any measure, including psychophysiological measures.

Consideration of construct validity, whether the measure actually assesses what it intends to assess, is crucial. For instance, performance on a measure of counting back by 7 is associated with many domains, including psychosis, anxiety, impulsivity, intelligence, etc. It is a measure of many constructs. It is important for our measures to have convergent validity in that they are associated with what they should be associated with, but also discriminant validity, in that they should not be associated with things that we do not expect them to be associated with.

If the research identifies activation in a specific part of the brain in association with the task, it is important to consider whether it is the same region across participants. For instance, the researcher should consider whether they are using a single atlas/head model for the whole sample or whether they are using a personalized atlas for each participant. Often, a given brain region is involved in lots of different cognitive processes and behaviors. This raises construct validity questions.

Ask yourself, "What is the evidence to support my interpretation of these effects?" Evidence is strengthened by showing evidence of convergent and discriminant validity. For example, differential deficits can provide stronger evidence of an effect. For instance, people with schizophrenia show deficits, abnormalities, or differences in many different brain processes—but an important question is whether they show relatively greater abnormalities in a given neural process than another neural process. This helps inform the specificity of the process (as opposed to other processes) for explaining differences in the condition of interest.

Another important question is: what is considered baseline? For heart rate reactivity and many psychophysiological measures, a comparison is made to a "baseline", which yields a contrast or difference score. But what should be considered "baseline"? There are many different possibilities for what could be considered "baseline," and each could yield different results. And, time during a participant's visit to the lab might not provide a good baseline because people may be anxious about being in a psychology lab. In addition, participants' brains are not resting during "resting-state".

Another important consideration is the ecological validity of the measures. Measures are often assessed in contexts and with stimuli that are not naturalistic. Psychophysiological measures may not reflect a participant's typical functioning. A goal would be to use more naturalistic contexts and task paradigms. Another challenge that biological measures have is in relating the biological criteria to actual behavior in the real world. It is not sufficient to show group differences on a biological measure; the researcher needs to show that the biological measure is associated with particular behaviors, that is, an independent measure in the same subjects.

When reliability and validity of psychophysiological measures are improved, a goal is to have norms for their use, so you know where a person stands compared to the population on the measure of interest.

19.2.4 Examples

19.2.4.1 Ambulatory Assessment

An ambulatory assessment is a measurement strategy designed to acquire minimally disruptive measures of a person engaging in normal activities in their natural environment. Ambulatory biosensors are assessment tools that measure physiological or motor activity (Haynes & Yoshioka, 2007). Ecological momentary assessment (EMA) is an example of an ambulatory assessment. Ambulatory assessment allows rich measurement including, for example, audio, pictures, video, geolocation (global positioning system [GPS]), and physical activity (accelerometer). Ambulatory assessment may provide more precise measurement of phenotypes because they can assess contextual and environmental influences.

Ambulatory assessments can collect many measurements passively, without the respondent needing to do anything. Ambulatory assessment minimizes retrospective reporting biases because they can assess people in the moment. They also allow alerts and notifications for compliance reminders so that the participant completes the measurement. And they allow context-based triggers based on GPS. Queries can be random, event-based, time-based, or location-based. Some research suggests that event-based reporting may be preferable compared to signal-based reporting because participants may report that the target behavior occurs more frequently when using event-based reporting compared to signal-based reporting (Himmelstein et al., 2019).

Ambulatory assessments can also connect to external sensors via Bluetooth to record, for instance, blood pressure. They can provide data with high temporal resolution; for example, they can provide measurement samples from second to second or even millisecond to millisecond. When dealing with rich data, one important question is the level of granularity you want to analyze the data: seconds, days, weeks, etc. The optimal granularity depends on the research question.

Ambulatory assessment might provide opportunities for developing idiographic (personalized) models of the inter-relations among thoughts, feelings, behavior, physiology, and context (Wright & Zimmermann, 2019).

In addition, ambulatory assessment might have utility for intervention. For instance, it could help provide a just-in-time intervention when an event or context occurs. Ambulatory assessment can also be used for self-monitoring. And alerts can be used to increase homework compliance.

The three most popular versions of ambulatory biosensors are those that monitor cardiovascular activity (e.g., heart rate and blood pressure), physical activity (e.g., actigraph and pedometer), and cortisol levels. However, other ambulatory biosensors assess EEG, respiration, muscle tension, blood glucose, skin conductance, and other processes.

An applied example of an ambulatory biosensor is actigraphy. Actigraphy is the tracking of physical movement. Actigraphy uses an actigraph device. An actigraphy is a watch-like device attached to the wrist or ankle that has an accelerometer. Smartphones can also serve as actigraphs because they have accelerometers. Actigraphy is a peripheral measure because it assesses gross motor movements. Actigraphy is also frequently used as a corresponding index of sleep because limb movements occur less frequently during sleep. Actigraphy is considered a better index of sleep than self-/informant-report, but not as good as polysomnography (PSG). However, actigraphy allows for greater ecological validity than a sleep study conducted in the lab, because a person can wear it while sleeping in their own bed at home.

In prior work, we took hundreds of sleep variables from actigraphy and using PCA to reduce the data down to key independent dimensions of sleep deficit: activity (sleep quality), (late) timing, (short) duration, and night-to-night variability (Staples et al., 2019).

19.2.4.1.1 Pros

Pros of ambulatory assessment include:

- Ambulatory biosensors do not rely on participants to report their experience; they provide information about constructs that is derived from a different method—and they are useful in a multimethod assessment strategy. Ambulatory biosensors lead to an increase in incremental validity and can improve specificity of decisions.
- Ambulatory biosensors are highly sensitive to change—they can track rapid changes in the variable of interest, with rapid timecourses (i.e., strong temporal resolution or precision).
- Ambulatory biosensors are portable, and have potential for greater ecological validity. Biosensor variables collected in naturalistic settings are often only weakly associated with biosensor variables collected in lab settings, possibly due to reactivity in a lab setting.
- Ambulatory biosensors allow concurrent evaluation of contexts that influence psychophysiological responses.

19.2.4.1.2 Cons

Cons of ambulatory assessment include:

- Ambulatory biosensors are expensive—they are potentially not cost-efficient depending on the use—i.e., they are potentially too expensive for clinical use.
- Some devices can be intrusive, cumbersome, and technical.
- There is limited psychometric evaluation conducted with many ambulatory methods. Ambulatory biosensors are potentially unreliable. In addition, ambulatory biosensors are potentially not accurate for certain trait levels. For example, heart rate devices may be

less accurate at high levels of physical activity. Ambulatory biosensors may not generalize well across time, devices, labs, and raters.
- The research investigator has less experimental control.
- There are practical challenges in conducting assessments outside of the research laboratory, as discussed by Holmlund et al. (2019) and Raugh et al. (2019).

19.2.4.2 Other Examples

Other examples of psychophysiological measures include eyetracking, which is used to assess attention, and wearables, which are smart "textiles" or clothing that has embedded biosensors.

19.2.5 Virtual Reality

Virtual reality (VR) is an emerging approach to assessment that allows structured assessment in simulated but life-like situations. It provides the investigator greater experimental control compared to ambulatory assessment approaches. Considerations in using virtual reality and other immersive technological approaches to assessment are described by Roberts et al. (2019).

19.2.6 Using Psychophysiological Measures

Ideally, we would be able to combine psychophysiological measures as objective measures with other measures, e.g., a performance-based assessment or self-/informant-report, in a multimethod measurement of constructs, as suggested by Patrick et al. (2019). Psychophysiological measures as part of a multimethod assessment approach helps to address the bias of participants and the bias in clinical judgment of clinicians. Ambulatory measures can provide incremental validity and increase the specificity of clinical judgment. Recommendations for using psychophysiological measures include using them in an ecologically valid way, including ambulatory approaches that allow ecological momentary assessment of contexts that influence psychophysiological responses, and conducting recordings over lengthy periods (Raugh et al., 2019). Recommendations for using ambulatory assessment in research on psychopathology are provided by Trull & Ebner-Priemer (2020).

Challenges exist in selecting the granularity of analysis—how fine-grained to assess at each level of analysis—and how to combine measures across multiple levels of analysis because each may operate at different timescales. One option is to use multimodal imaging, e.g., simultaneous recordings of EEG and fMRI or EEG and fNIRS, to cancel out weaknesses of each. For instance, EEG has stronger temporal resolution than fMRI—it provides a faster timecourse—but EEG has weaker spatial resolution than fMRI—it provides less accurate estimates of where in the brain the neural activity is occurring.

It is worth considering combining multiple measures in a latent variable framework using, for example, factor analysis or structural equation modeling.

Given the costs, challenges, and time-consuming nature of psychophysiological data collection, science may be best positioned to address reliability and validity issues by sharing and combining data sets through consortia and open science. Consortia and data-sharing can help ensure large enough sample sizes for adequate statistical power, especially for individual difference analyses. Larger samples would also allow cross-validation of analyses in independent samples using out-of-sample prediction.

19.3 Conclusion

The National Institute of Mental Health (NIMH) provided the Research Domain Criteria (RDoC) as an alternative structure of psychopathology. Compared to the DSM, RDoC is dimensional and it works from the ground up, starting with brain–behavior relations, and linking those to clinical symptoms. RDoC spans multiple domains—such as positive and negative valience systems—and units of analysis, including genes, molecules, cells, circuits, physiology, behaviors, self-reports, and paradigms.

Psychophysiological measures include electroencephalography (EEG), event-related potential (ERP), (functional) magnetic resonance imaging (f)MRI, computerized axial tomography (CAT), magnetoencephalography (MEG), functional near infrared spectroscopy (fNIRS), electrocardiography (ECG or EKG), electromyography (EMG), electrooculography (EOG), eyetracking, and actigraphy. Psychophysiological measures are not invulnerable to basic measurement issues, including reliability and validity. Another important consideration of psychophysiological measures is how to handle the rich data without increasing the likelihood of Type I errors.

Another class of measurement includes ambulatory assessment. Ambulatory assessment is designed to acquire minimally disruptive measures of a person engaging in normal activities in their natural environment. Ambulatory assessment allows rich measurement including, for example, audio, pictures, video, geolocation (global positioning system [GPS]), and physical activity (accelerometer). Ambulatory biosensors are assessment tools that measure physiological or motor activity, such as those that monitor cardiovascular activity (e.g., heart rate and blood pressure), physical activity (e.g., actigraph and pedometer), cortisol levels, EEG, respiration, muscle tension, blood glucose, skin conductance, and other processes. Virtual reality is an emerging approach that allows structured assessment in simulated but life-like situations.

19.4 Suggested Readings

G. A. Miller et al. (2007); Haynes & Yoshioka (2007)

20

Computers and Adaptive Testing

20.1 Computer-Administered/Online Assessment

Computer-administered and online assessments have the potential to be both desirable and dangerous (Buchanan, 2002). The potential is to have a mental health screening instrument online that a person fills out, is automatically scored, and automatic feedback is provided with suggestions to follow a particular course of action. This would save the clinician time and could lead to a more productive therapy session. As an example, our clients complete a brief measure of behavioral issues on a tablet when they arrive and are in the waiting room. This is an example of measurement-based care, in which the participant's treatment response is assessed throughout treatment to help determine whether treatment is working or not, and whether to try something different.

20.1.1 Advantages

There are many advantages of computer-administered or online assessment:

- Computer-administered and online assessment requires less time on the part of the clinician and administrators than traditional assessment methods. They do not need the clinician to administer and score the assessment, and scores can be entered directly into the client's chart.
- Computer-administered and online assessments tend to be less costly than traditional assessment methods.
- Computer-administered and online assessments can increase access to services because some people can complete the assessment who otherwise would not be able to complete it. For example, some people may be restricted by geographic or financial circumstances. You can provide the questionnaire in multiple languages and modalities, including written, spoken, and pictorial.
- People may disclose more information to a computer than to a person. The degree of one's perceived anonymity matters. Perceived anonymity may be especially important for information on sensitive yet important issues, such as suicidality, homicidality, abuse, neglect, criminal behavior, etc.
- Computerized and online assessment has the potential to be more structured and the potential to do a more comprehensive and accurate assessment than an in-person interview, which tends to be less structured and more biased by clinical judgment (Garb, 2007).
- Computerized and online assessment tends to provide more comprehensive information than is usually collected in practice. Structured approaches tend to ask more questions. Computers can increase the likelihood that the client answers all questions, because it can prevent clients from skipping questions. Computers can apply "branching logic" to adapt which questions are asked based on the participant's responses (i.e., adaptive testing) to more efficiently gain greater coverage. Clinicians tend not to ask questions about important

issues. Clinicians fail to examine disorders other than the hypothesized ones, which is known as diagnostic overshadowing due to the confirmation bias of looking for evidence-confirming information rather than disconfirming evidence. In general, computers give more diagnoses than clinicians. Clinicians often miss co-occurring disorders. Doing a more comprehensive assessment normalizes that people can and do experience the behavioral issues that they are asked about, and can increase self-disclosure. Greater structure leads to higher inter-rater reliability, less bias, and greater validity.
- Computerized and online assessment lends itself to continuous monitoring during treatment for measurement-based care. Measurement-based care has been shown to be related to better treatment outcomes. Computerized or online assessment may be important in risk assessment that might otherwise go unrecognized. Treatment utility of computerized assessment has been demonstrated for suicide and substance use.

20.1.2 Validity Challenges

There are a number of challenges to the validity of computer-administered and online assessment:

- The impersonality of computers; however, this does not seem to be a strong threat.
- Lack of control in the testing situation.
- The possibility that extraneous factors can influence responses.
- Language and cultural differences; it is difficult to ask follow-up questions to assess understanding unless a clinician is present.
- Inability to observe the client's body language or nonverbals.
- Computers are not a great medium to assess constructs that could be affected by computer-related anxiety.
- Some constructs show different ratings online versus in-person.
- Computer-administered and online assessment may require different norms and cutoffs than paper-and-pencil assessment. Different norms could be necessary, for example, due to increased self-disclosure and higher ratings of negative affect in computer-administered assessment compared to in-person assessment.
- Careless and fraudulent responding can be common when recruiting an online sample to complete a survey (Chandler et al., 2020). Additional steps may need to be taken to ensure high-quality responses such as CAPTCHA (or reCAPTCHA), internet protocol (IP) verification of location, and attention or validity checks.

In general, online assessments of personality seem generally comparable to their paper-and-pencil versions, but their psychometric properties are not identical. In general, computer-administered and online assessments yield the same factor structure as in-person assessments, but particular items may not function in the same way across computer versus in-person assessments.

20.1.3 Ethical Challenges

There are important ethical challenges of using computer-administered and online assessments:

- The internet and app stores provide a medium for the dissemination and proliferation of quackery. Businesses sell access to assessment information despite no evidence of the reliability or validity of the measure.
- When giving potentially distressing or threatening feedback, it is important to provide opportunities for follow-up sessions or counseling. When using online assessment in research,

you can state that release of test scores is not possible, and that participants should consult a professional if they are worried or would like a professional assessment.

- An additional ethical challenge of computer-administered and online assessment deals with test security. The validity of many tests is based on the assumption that the client is not knowledgeable about the test materials. Detailed information on many protected tests is available on the internet (Ruiz et al., 2002), and it could be used by malingerers to fake health or illness.
- Data security is another potential challenge of computer-administered and online assessments, including how to protect HIPAA compliance in the clinical context.

20.1.4 Best Practices

Below are best practices for computer-administered and online assessments:

- Only use measures with established reliability and validity, unless you are studying them, in which case you should evaluate their psychometrics.
- Have a trained clinician review the results of the assessment.
- Combine computer-administered assessment with clinical judgment. Clients can be expected to make errors completing the assessment, so ask necessary follow-up questions after getting results from computer-administered assessments. Asking follow-up questions can help avoid false positive errors in diagnosis. Check whether a client mistakenly reported something; or whether they under-/over-reported psychopathology.
- Provide opportunities for follow-up sessions or counseling if distressing or threatening feedback is provided.
- It may be important to correct for a person's level of experience with computers when using computerized tasks for clinical decision-making (Lee Meeuw Kjoe et al., 2021).

20.2 Adaptive Testing

Adaptive testing involves having the respondent complete only those items that are needed to answer an assessment question. It involves changing which items are administered based on responses to previous items, and administering only a subset of the possible items. Adaptive testing is commonly used in intelligence testing, achievement testing, and aptitude testing. Adaptive testing is not yet commonly used for personality or psychopathology assessment. Most approaches to assessment of personality and psychopathology rely on conventional testing approaches using classical test theory. But many structured clinical interviews, use decision rules to skip a diagnosis, module, or section if a decision rule is not met. Adaptive testing has also been used with observational assessments (e.g., Granziol et al., 2022).

A goal of adaptive testing is to get the most accurate estimate of a person's level on a construct with the fewest items possible. Ideally, you would get similar results between adaptive testing and conventional testing that uses all items, when adaptive testing is done well.

There are multiple approaches to adaptive testing. Broadly, one class of approaches uses manual administration, whereas another class of approaches uses computerized adaptive testing (CAT) based on item response theory (IRT).

20.2.1 Manual Administration of Adaptive Testing (Adaptive Testing without IRT)

Manual administration of adaptive testing involves moving people up and down in the item difficulty according to their responses. Approaches to manual administration of adaptive testing include using "skip rules", basal and ceiling criteria, and the countdown method.

20.2.1.1 Skip Rules

Many structured clinical interviews, such as the Structured Clinical Interview for DSM Disorders (SCID) and Mini-International Neuropsychiatric Interview (MINI), use decision rules to skip a diagnosis, module, or section if a decision rule is not met. The skip rules allow the interviews to be more efficient and therefore clinically practical.

20.2.1.2 Basal and Ceiling Approach

One approach to manual administration of adaptive testing involves establishing a respondent's basal and ceiling level. The basal level is the difficulty level at which the examinee answers almost all items correctly. The respondent's ceiling level is the difficulty level at which the examinee answers almost all items incorrectly. The basal and ceiling criteria set the rules for establishing the basal and ceiling level for each respondent and for when to terminate testing.

The goal of adaptive testing is to administer the fewest items necessary to get an accurate estimate of the person's ability, to save time and prevent the respondent from becoming bored from too-easy items or frustrated from too-difficult items. The basal and ceiling approach starts testing at the recommended starting point for a person's age or ability level. The examiner scores as items are administered. If the person gets too many items wrong in the beginning, the examiner moves to an earlier starting point, i.e., provides easier items, until the respondent gets most items correct, which establishes their basal level. Then, after establishing the respondent's basal level, the examiner proceeds forward to progressively more difficult items until they reach their ceiling level, i.e., they get too many wrong in some set, which establishes their ceiling level.

20.2.1.3 Countdown Approach

The countdown approach of adaptive testing is a variant of the variable termination criterion approach to adaptive testing. It classifies the respondent into one of two groups—elevated or not elevated—based on whether they exceed the cutoff criterion on a given scale. The cutoff criterion is usually the raw score on the scale that corresponds to a clinical elevation.

Two countdown approaches include (1) the classification method and (2) the full scores on elevated scales (FSES) method. The countdown approach to adaptive testing is described by Forbey & Ben-Porath (2007).

20.2.1.3.1 Classification method

Using the classification method to the countdown approach of adaptive testing, the examiner stops administering items once elevation is either ruled in or ruled out. The classification method only tells you *whether* a client produced an elevated score on the scale. It does not tell you their actual score on that scale.

20.2.1.3.2 Full scores on elevated scales method

Using the full scores on elevated scales method to the countdown approach of adaptive testing, the examiner stops administering items only if elevation is ruled out. The approach generates a score on that scale only for people who produced an elevated score.

20.2.1.4 Summary

When doing manual administration with clinical scales, you see the greatest item savings when ordering items from least to most frequently endorsed (i.e., from most to least difficulty) so you can rule people out faster. Ordering items in this way results in a 20–30% item savings on the Minnesota Multiphasic Personality Inventory (MMPI), and corresponding time savings. Comparative studies using the MMPI tend to show comparable results (i.e., similar validity) between the countdown adaptive method and the conventional testing method. That is, the reduction in items does not impair the validity of the adaptive scales. However, you can get even greater item savings when using an IRT approach to adaptive testing. Using IRT, you can order the administration of items differently for each participant to administer the next item that will provide the most information (i.e., precision) for a respondent's ability given their responses on all previous items.

20.2.2 CAT with IRT

Computerized adaptive testing (CAT) based on IRT is widely used in educational testing, including the Graduate Record Examination (GRE) and the Graduate Management Admission Test (GMAT), but it is not widespread in mental health measurement for two reasons: (1) it works best with large item banks; large item banks are generally unavailable for mental health constructs; and (2) mental health constructs are multidimensional and CAT using IRT has primarily been restricted to unidimensional constructs, such as math achievement. However, that is changing; there are now multidimensional IRT approaches that allow simultaneously estimating people's scores on multiple dimensions, as described in Section 8.6. For example, the higher-order construct of externalizing problems includes sub-dimensions including aggression and rule-breaking.

A CAT is designed to locate a person's level on the construct (theta) with as few items as possible. CAT has potential for greater item savings than the countdown approach, but it has more assumptions. IRT can be used to create CATs using information gleaned from the IRT model's item parameters, including discrimination and difficulty (or severity). The item's discrimination indicates how strongly the item is related to the construct. For a strong measure, you want highly discriminating items that are strongly related to the construct. In terms of item difficulty/severity, you want items that span the full distribution of difficulty/severity so they are non-redundant.

An IRT-based CAT starts with a highly discriminating item at the 50th percentile of the distribution (severity) (or at whatever level is the best estimate of the person's ability/severity before the CAT is administered). Then, based on the participant's response, it generates a provisional estimate of the person's level on the construct and administers the item that will provide the most information. For example, if the respondent gets the first item correct, the CAT administers a highly discriminating item that might be at the 75th percentile of the distribution (severity). And so on, based on the participants' responses.

As described in Section 8.1.6, item information is how much measurement precision for the construct is provided by a particular item. In other words, iitem information indicates how much the item reduces the standard error of measurement; i.e., how much the item reduces uncertainty of our estimate of the respondent's construct level. An IRT-based CAT continues to generate provisional estimates of the person's construct level and updates it based on new responses. The CAT tries to find the construct level where the respondent keeps getting items right and wrong (or endorsing versus not endorsing) 50% of the time. This process continues until the uncertainty in the person's estimated construct level is smaller than a pre-defined threshold—that is, when we are fairly confident (to some threshold) about a person's construct level.

CAT is a promising approach that saves time because it tailors which items are administered to which person and in which order based on their construct level to get the most reliable estimate in the shortest time possible. It administers items that are appropriate to the person's construct level, and it does not administer items that are way too easy or way too hard for the person, which saves time, boredom, and frustration. It shortens the assessment because not all items are administered, and it typically results in around 50% item savings or more. It also allows for increased measurement precision, because you are drilling down deeper (i.e., asking more items) near the person's construct level. You can control the measurement precision of the CAT because you can specify the threshold of measurement precision (i.e., standard error of measurement) at which testing is terminated. For example, you could have the CAT terminate when the standard error of measurement of a person's construct level becomes less than 0.2.

However, CATs assume that if you get a more difficult item correct, you would have gotten easier items correct, which might not be true in all contexts (especially for constructs that are not unidimensional). For example, just because a person does not endorse low-severity symptoms does not necessarily mean that they will not endorse higher-severity symptoms, especially when assessing a multidimensional construct.

Simpler CATs are built using unidimensional IRT. But many aspects of psychopathology are not unidimensional and would violate assumptions of unidimensional IRT. For example, the externalizing spectrum includes sub-dimensions including aggression, disinhibition, and substance use. You can use multidimensional IRT to build CATs, though this is more complicated. For instance, you could estimate a bifactor model in which each item (e.g., "hits others") loads onto the general latent factor (e.g., externalizing problems) and its specific sub-dimension (e.g., aggression versus rule-breaking). Computerized adaptive testing of mental health disorders is reviewed by Gibbons et al. (2016).

Well-designed CATs show equivalent reliability and validity to their full-scale counterparts. By contrast, many short forms are not as accurate as their full-scale counterparts. Part of the reason that CATs tend to do better than short forms is that the CATs are adaptive; they determine which items to administer based on the participant's responses to prior items, unlike short forms. For guidelines on developing and evaluating short forms, see Smith et al. (2000).

20.3 Getting Started

20.3.1 Load Libraries

```
library("petersenlab")
library("mirtCAT")
```

```
library("MOTE")
library("here")
library("tidyverse")
library("tinytex")
library("knitr")
library("kableExtra")
library("rmarkdown")
library("bookdown")
```

20.4 Example of Unidimensional CAT

The computerized adaptive test (CAT) was fit using the `mirtCAT` package (Chalmers, 2021). The example of a CAT with unidimensional data is adapted from `mirtCAT` documentation: http://philchalmers.github.io/mirtCAT/html/unidim-exampleGUI.html (archived at https://perma.cc/3ZW4-DAUR)

20.4.1 Define Population IRT Parameters

```
set.seed(52242)
nitems <- 100
itemnames <- paste("Item.", 1:nitems, sep = "")
a <- matrix(rlnorm(nitems, meanlog = .2, sdlog = .3))
d <- matrix(rnorm(nitems, mean = 0, sd = 1))
pars <- data.frame(a1 = a, d = d, g = 0.2)
```

20.4.2 Fit IRT Model

```
mod <- generate.mirt_object(pars, "3PL")
```

20.4.3 Model Summary

```
modItemParameters <- coef(
  mod,
  simplify = TRUE,
  IRTpars = TRUE)$items
```

20.4.4 Model Plots

A test characteristic curve of the measure is shown in Figure 20.1.

```
plot(mod)
```

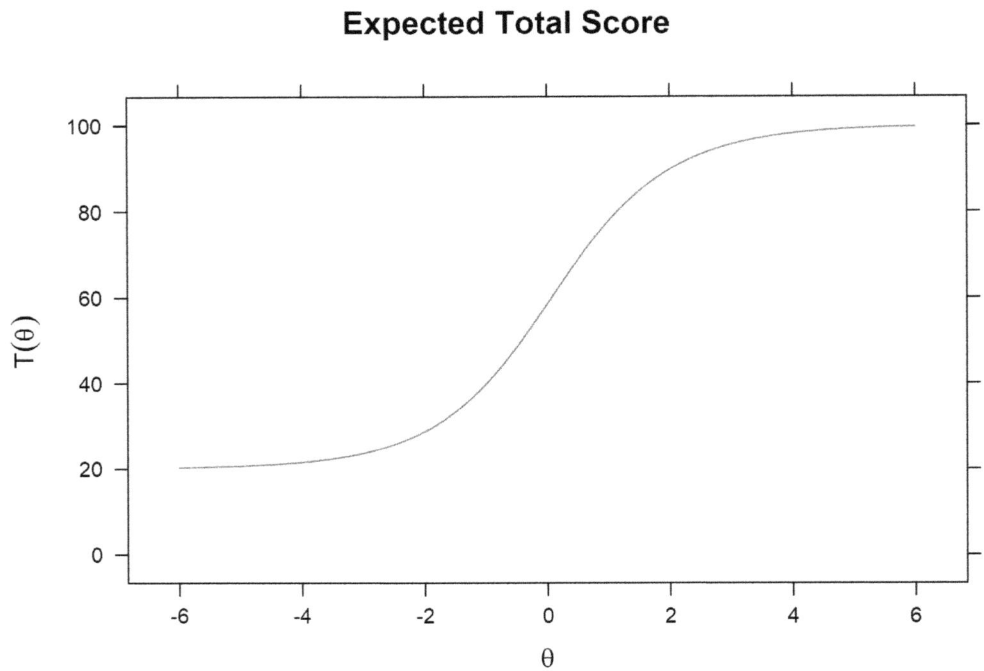

FIGURE 20.1 Test Characteristic Curve.

The test information and standard error of measurement as a function of the person's construct level (theta; θ) is in Figure 20.2. The test appears to measure theta (θ) with $SE < .4$ within a range of -1.5 to 2.

```
plot(
  mod,
  type = "infoSE",
  theta_lim = c(-3, 3))
```

20.4.5 Item Plots

You can examine item characteristic curves using the following syntax:

```
plot(mod, type = "trace", theta_lim = c(-3, 3))
```

You can examine item information curves using the following syntax:

```
plot(mod, type = "infotrace", theta_lim = c(-3, 3))
```

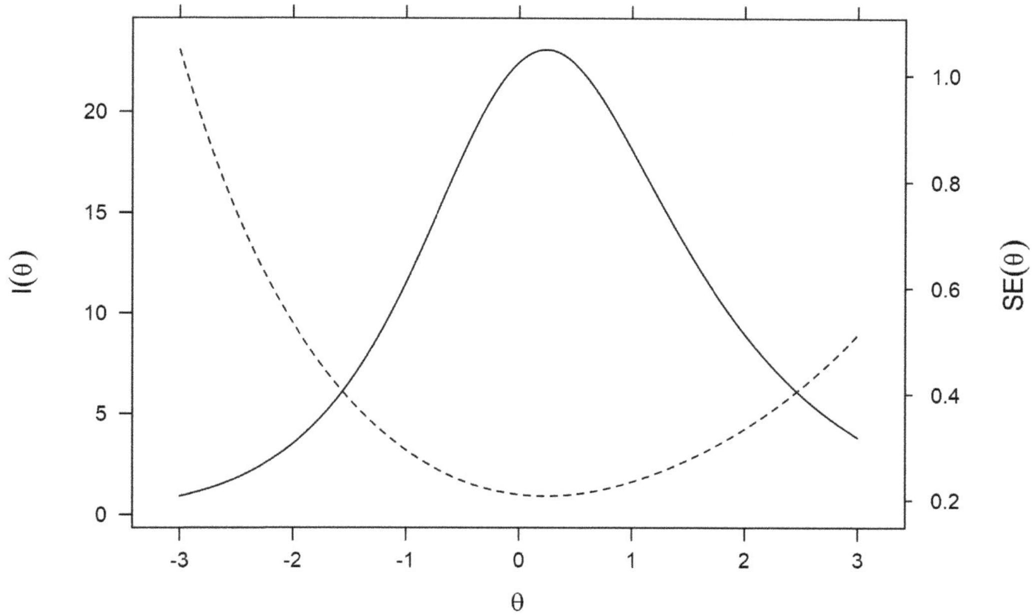

FIGURE 20.2 Test Information and Standard Error of Measurement.

- Item 30 would be a good starting item; it has a difficulty closest to the 50th percentile ($b = 0.019$) and a high discrimination ($a = 1.834$).
- Item 70 would be a good starting item; it has a difficulty closest to the 50th percentile ($b = -0.051$) and a high discrimination ($a = 2.141$).
- Item 86 is an easy item ($b = -2.303$).
- Item 16 is a difficult item ($b = 2.062$).
- Item 53 has a low discrimination ($a = 0.572$).

Item characteristic curves and information curves for Item 30 are shown in Figure 20.3.

```
itemplot(
  object = mod,
  item = "Item.30",
  "infotrace",
  main = "")
```

20.4.6 Create Math Items

```
questions <- answers <- character(nitems)
choices <- matrix("a", nitems, 5)
spacing <- floor(d - min(d)) + 1 #easier items have more variation
```

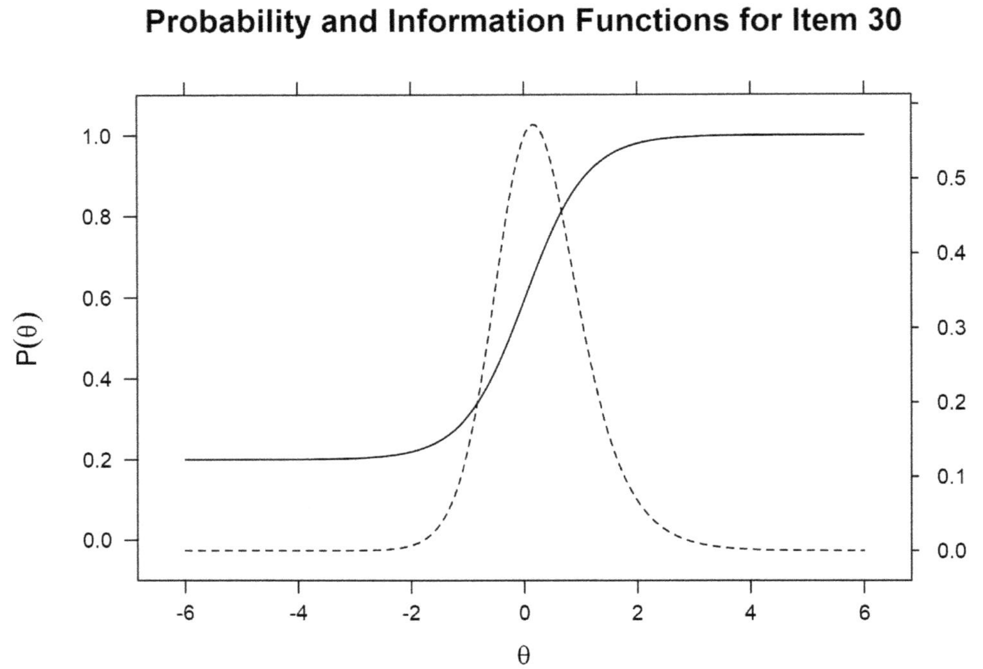

FIGURE 20.3 Item Characteristic Curves and Information Curves for Item 30.

```
for(i in 1:nitems){
  n1 <- sample(1:100, 1)
  n2 <- sample(101:200, 1)
  ans <- n1 + n2
  questions[i] <- paste(n1, " + ", n2, " = ?", sep = "")
  answers[i] <- as.character(ans)
  ch <- ans + sample(c(-5:-1, 1:5) * spacing[i,], 5)
  ch[sample(1:5, 1)] <- ans
  choices[i,] <- as.character(ch)
}

df <- data.frame(
  Questions = questions,
  Answer = answers,
  Option = choices,
  Type = "radio")
```

20.4.7 Run Computerized Adaptive Test

Set the minimum standard error of measurement for the latent trait (theta; θ) that must be reached before stopping the CAT. You can lengthen the CAT by lowering the minimum standard error of measurement, or you can shorten the CAT by raising the minimum standard error of measurement.

```
minimum_SEM <- .3
```

Run the CAT and stop once the standard error of measurement for the latent trait (theta; θ) becomes 0.3 or lower.

```
result <- mirtCAT(
  df,
  mod,
  start_item = "MI",
  method = "EAP",
  criteria = "MI",
  design = list(min_SEM = minimum_SEM))

RNGkind("default", "default", "default")
```

20.4.8 CAT Results

```
print(result)
```

```
 n.items.answered Theta_1 SE.Theta_1
               27  0.2389     0.2975
```

```
summary(result)
```

```
$final_estimates
          Theta_1
Estimates  0.2389
SEs        0.2975

$raw_responses
 [1] "230" "170" "167" "177" "175" "216" "177" "218" "184" "191" "184"
[12] "202" "294" "204" "200" "204" "264" "242" "177" "189" "267" "200"
[23] "235" "149" "248" "180" "239"

$scored_responses
 [1] 1 1 1 1 0 1 0 1 1 1 0 1 0 1 0 1 0 1 0 1 1 0 1 0 1 1 1

$items_answered
 [1] 70 54 92 19 43 23 97 30  1 41 40 31 89  5 66 96 48 79  7 88 75 59
[23] 13 26 71 81 29

$thetas_history
      Theta_1
 [1,]  0.0000
 [2,]  0.4057
 [3,]  0.7815
 [4,]  0.9751
```

```
 [5,]  1.1562
 [6,]  0.7421
 [7,]  0.8464
 [8,]  0.5304
 [9,]  0.6257
[10,]  0.7129
[11,]  0.7810
[12,]  0.6338
[13,]  0.6792
[14,]  0.5229
[15,]  0.5590
[16,]  0.3680
[17,]  0.4110
[18,]  0.3113
[19,]  0.3506
[20,]  0.1783
[21,]  0.2191
[22,]  0.2576
[23,]  0.1699
[24,]  0.2023
[25,]  0.1356
[26,]  0.1602
[27,]  0.1960
[28,]  0.2389

$thetas_SE_history
      Theta_1
 [1,]  1.0000
 [2,]  0.9069
 [3,]  0.8093
 [4,]  0.7266
 [5,]  0.6879
 [6,]  0.6098
 [7,]  0.5592
 [8,]  0.5193
 [9,]  0.4821
[10,]  0.4631
[11,]  0.4487
[12,]  0.4224
[13,]  0.4080
[14,]  0.3919
[15,]  0.3778
[16,]  0.3693
[17,]  0.3568
[18,]  0.3507
[19,]  0.3409
[20,]  0.3438
[21,]  0.3332
[22,]  0.3252
[23,]  0.3240
[24,]  0.3164
```

```
[25,]  0.3148
[26,]  0.3076
[27,]  0.3018
[28,]  0.2975

$terminated_sucessfully
[1] TRUE
```

20.4.8.1 CAT Standard Errors

Standard errors of measurement of a person's estimated construct level (theta; θ) as a function of the item (presented in the order that items were administered as part of the CAT) are shown in Figure 20.4.

Initially, the respondent got the first items correct, which raised the estimate of their construct level. However, as the respondent got more items incorrect, the CAT converged upon the estimate that the person has a construct level around $theta = 0.24$, which means that the person scored slightly above average (i.e., 0.24 standard deviations above the mean).

```
plot(result, SE = 1, main = "")
```

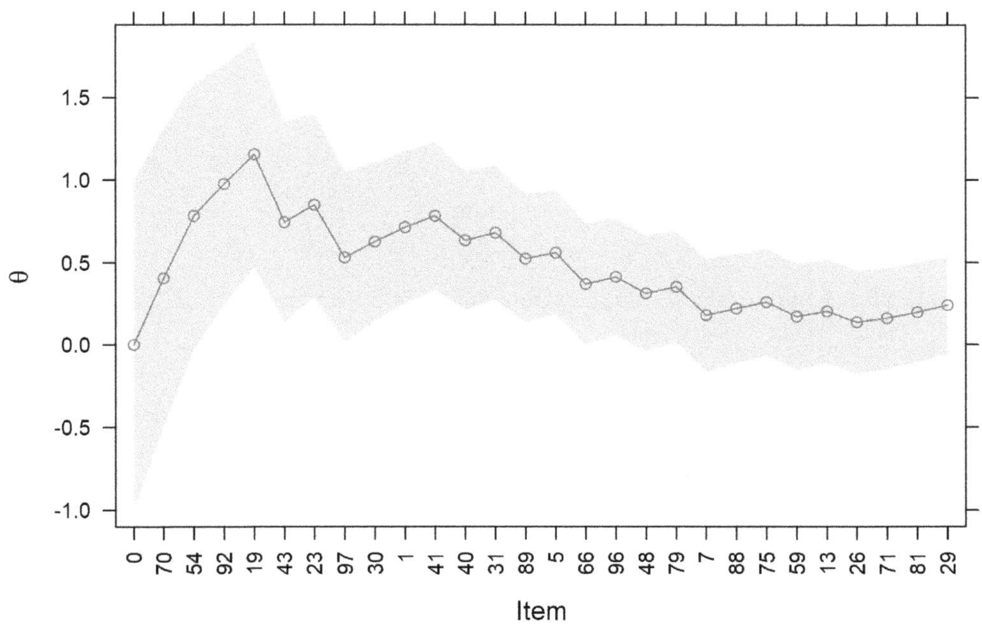

FIGURE 20.4 Standard Errors of Measurement Around Theta in a Computerized Adaptive Test.

20.4.8.2 CAT 95% Confidence Interval

Ninety-five percent confidence intervals of a person's estimated construct level (theta; θ) as a function of the item (presented in the order that items were administered as part of the CAT) are shown in Figure 20.5.

```
plot(result, SE = qnorm(.975), main = "")
```

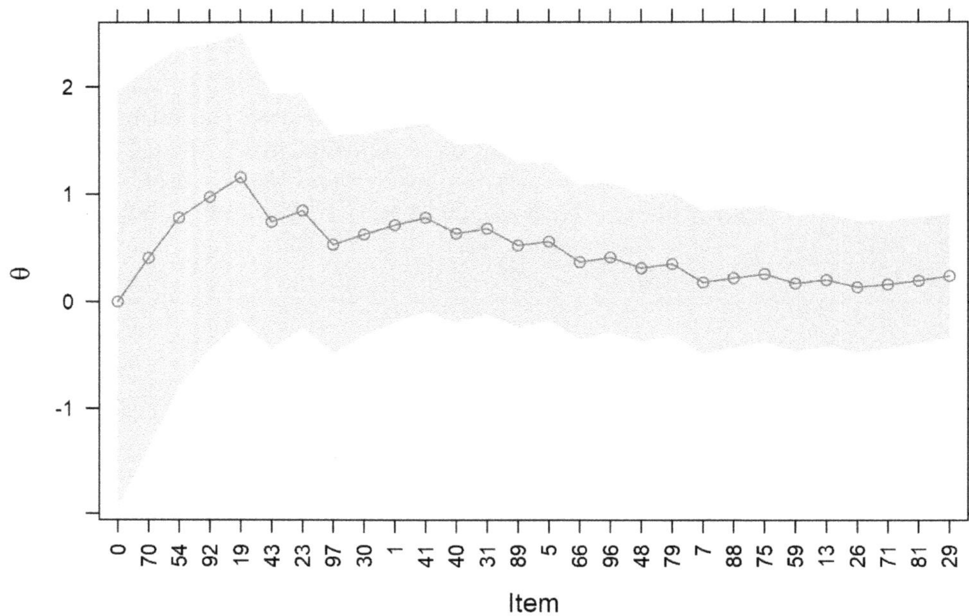

FIGURE 20.5 Computerized Adaptive Test 95% Confidence Interval of Theta.

20.5 Creating a Computerized Adaptive Test From an Item Response Theory Model

You can create a computerized adaptive test from any item response theory model.

20.5.1 Create Items

For instance, below we create a matrix with the questions and response options from the graded response model that we fit in Section 8.9 in Chapter 8 on item response theory.

```
numItemsGRM <- nrow(coef(
  gradedResponseModel,
  simplify = TRUE,
```

```
  IRTpars = TRUE)$items)

questionsGRM <- c(
  "Science and technology make our lives more comfortable.",
  "Science and new technology will make work more interesting.",
  "Science and technology will provide more opportunities for future generations.",
  "The benefits of science are greater than any harmful effect it may have."
)

responseOptionsGRM <- c(
  "strongly disagree",
  "disagree to some extent",
  "agree to some extent",
  "strongly agree"
)

numResponseOptionsGRM <- length(responseOptionsGRM)

choicesGRM <- matrix("a", numItemsGRM, numResponseOptionsGRM)

for(i in 1:numItemsGRM){
  choicesGRM[i,] <- responseOptionsGRM
}

dfGRM <- data.frame(
  Questions = questionsGRM,
  Option = choicesGRM,
  Type = "radio")
```

20.5.2 Run Computerized Adaptive Test

Then you can create and run the computerized adaptive model:

```
resultGRM <- mirtCAT(
  dfGRM,
  gradedResponseModel,
  start_item = "MI",
  method = "EAP",
  criteria = "MI",
  design = list(min_SEM = minimum_SEM))
```

20.6 Conclusion

Computer-administered and online assessments have the potential to be both desirable and dangerous. They have key advantages; at the same time, they have both validity and ethical challenges. Best practices for computer-administered and online assessments are provided. Adaptive testing involves having the respondent complete only those items that are needed to answer an assessment question, which can save immense time without sacrificing validity (if done well). There are many approaches to adaptive testing, including manual administration—such as skip rules, basal and ceiling criteria, and the countdown approach—and computerized adaptive testing (CAT) using item response theory. A CAT is designed to locate a person's level on the construct with as few items as possible. A CAT administers the items that will provide the most information based on participants' previous responses. CAT typically results in the greatest item savings—around 50% item savings or more.

20.7 Suggested Readings

Buchanan (2002); Gibbons et al. (2016)

21

Behavioral Assessment

21.1 Overview

In other chapters, we discuss using psychophysiological assessment, cognitive assessment, and other assessment techniques. Psychology is often concerned about understanding behavior. To assess behavior, one approach would be to observe people. Observing people allows seeing the dynamic of the behavior unfold in relation to other processes. Observations might also allow getting around examinees' response biases such as social desirability.

Behavioral observation provides a temporal stream of behavior to see which behaviors precede other behaviors. An overview of observational assessment is provided by Girard & Cohn (2016). When conducting observations, it is important to consider the context and the environment.

21.1.1 Approaches

Examples of behavioral assessment include naturalistic behavioral observation, analogue (structured) observation, self-monitoring/diary, behavior ratings (e.g., informant report), and self-report. Self-report is essentially retrospective self-monitoring.

Naturalistic behavioral observation involves observing a person in their natural context or habitat. For instance, it might involve a person in their home, at school, at work, or their everyday interpersonal interactions. The observer is like a "fly on the wall" in that they want to exert as little effect as possible on the person's behavior. The observation occurs within normal situational contexts and under naturally occurring reinforcements and consequences. Naturalistic observations were the origins of behavioral assessment.

Analogue observation, also called structured observation, is the observation of a person in a contrived environment (Haynes, 2001). The goal of analogue observation is for the contrived situation to be analogous to the situations that the client is likely to encounter in their natural environment. For instance, the examiner might set up similar conditions in a lab or therapy room. Analogue observations can differ in the degree to which the observation is structured, but they are typically more structured than naturalistic observation. Analogue observations might involve role-plays, family or marital interaction tasks, and compliance (do/don't) tasks. As an example, the observer might observe role-played scenarios in which the person engages in one or more simulated social interactions.

Behavioral observation has occurred for a long time. In the 1960s, research included work on Pavlov's classical conditioning and Skinner's operant conditioning. Their work involved ethology, the scientific examination of animal behavior. Their work involved observing rodents and other mammals. In her work, Jane Goodall observed primates.

21.2 Contexts for Observing

There are multiple contexts in which we can observe people. Here are just a few examples:

- Classrooms
- Homes
- In the community; for example, you could take a client out into the world to see how they interact with others
- Group homes
- Psychiatric hospitals

Token economies for people with schizophrenia were based on behavioral assessment in psychiatric hospitals. A token economy is a contingency management system based on operant conditioning. Operant conditioning occurs when the frequency of behavior is influenced by the outcomes of the behavior. In a token economy, a secondary reinforcer, such as a token or symbol, is given to the client for matching the target behavior, which can be exchanged for back-up reinforcers. For instance, a token may be given to the client for making their bed. The tokens could then be turned in for back-up reinforcers. Back-up reinforcers include material reinforcers such as food, money, and cigarettes; services, such as having your room cleaned; and privileges such as getting to make a phone call. Token economies have been shown to work and to influence people's behavior, especially the negative symptoms of schizophrenia. However, token economies are not widely used because of political issues.

21.3 Costs of Behavioral Observation

Behavioral observations are costly due to people and time. The cost limits the amount of observation time that is possible, which raises questions about how typical and representative the participant's behavior was during the observation period relative to their everyday life. The limited amount of observation time raises questions about reliability and external validity, that is the generalizability of the person's behavior in the situation to their typical functioning.

A gold standard for naturalistic observations would be to observe someone in their natural context across more than one day, time, situation, and context with more than one rater to get a more robust sampling of the person's behavior. But it is costly to do this, and is therefore uncommon in practice.

21.4 Dependent Variable

After (or during) the observation, we need to turn the observation into information that can be useful. To do that, we create a dependent variable using behavioral coding. Behavioral coding involves observing behavior and quantifying it, that is turning behavior into numbers that can be analyzed to make inferences. During observation, you can measure the frequency of the behavior (how many times a behavior occurs), which is a useful measure of individual differences. But you may want to know the stream of behavior, so you know when the behavior occurred. So, you might make a coding sample at regular intervals (e.g., every 6 seconds). Coding systems can differ in their granularity with which they treat time. In *event-based coding*, the coder codes whenever a discrete behavior occurs—i.e., the behavior has discrete start and stop points. For example, an event-based coding system may determine when a person is talking. Event-based coding allows assessing the number, duration, and sequence of behaviors with high temporal precision.

In *interval-based coding*, the coder codes during specified spans of time that are called intervals. Intervals can be of any length. Shorter intervals provide more temporal precision but are more burdensome to code. Longer intervals provide less temporal precision but are less burdensome to code. An example of interval-based coding would be coding the extent of positive affect that a person showed during each 10-second interval.

Coding can focus on the small units of behavior or what the behavior means. *Sign-based coding* involves focusing on small units of behavior, such as movements. *Message-based coding* involves focusing on the meaning of the behavior using theory. For example, message-based coding might attempt to code examinees' emotional states. Sign-based coding requires a lesser degree of inference, has less subjectivity, and has higher inter-rater reliability than message-based coding. On the other hand, message-based coding is potentially more theoretically interesting than sign-based coding.

21.5 Functional Behavioral Assessment/Analysis

One goal of behavioral assessment is to determine the function of the problem behavior. Every behavior has a function, reason, or purpose (or multiple ones). If you can determine the function(s) of the behavior, you may be able to help the client learn more adaptive ways of accomplishing their goals. To determine the function(s) of behavior, functional behavioral assessments (FBAs) are commonly conducted, especially in schools. FBA involves identifying the patterns of sequences that involve the problem behavior, noting the following:

- The time
- The context
- What led up to the problem behavior (antecedents)
- What problem behavior occurred
- What happened after the problem behavior (consequences)
- How the situation resolved

An FBA is based on the antecedent-behavior-consequence (A-B-C) model. The idea of the A-B-C model is that every behavior is a function of its antecedents and consequences. The goal of the A-B-C model is to identify common patterns of antecedents and consequences. Examples of antecedents include insufficient sleep, a change in routine, and an ineffective command. Examples of consequences include giving attention, and getting to play without having to pick up the toys. By identifying the patterns of antecedents and consequences, we can generate hypotheses for the function of the behavior. For example, a possible hypothesis for a function of given problem behavior might be to get attention, to get out of doing what they do not want to do (escape or avoidance), to get access to a preferable activity or object, or to engage in sensory stimulation (e.g., rocking).

You can design treatment to change the antecedents and consequences to show them more adaptive ways of behaving. One approach to case conceptualization or case formulation is the "5 Ps": protective factors, predisposing factors, precipitating factors, perpetuating factors, and prognosis. Treatment would focus on addressing the perpetuating (maintaining) factors, and helping the client identify the triggering (precipitating) factors and how to handle those, while building on their strengths (protective factors) and considering their vulnerabilities (predisposing factors), with the intensity of treatment matched to the prognosis.

21.6 Mental Status Exam

A mental status exam is a structured assessment of a client's cognition, affect, etc. A mental status exam is often used in psychiatric hospitals to quickly "size up" a patient. Mental status exams are also useful in outpatient settings. For training clinicians, it can be useful to get in the habit of performing mental status exams.

21.7 Reliability

It is important to consider the reliability of behavioral observations. From a generalizability perspective, we aim to generalize behavioral observations across, raters, contexts, and time points. Thus, inter-rater reliability and test–retest reliability are especially relevant. Averaging ratings across multiple raters can yield scores that are more reliable than the scores from the individual raters, assuming both raters have inter-rater reliability.

21.8 Validity

Validity is also an important consideration of behavioral observations. In general, little attention has been paid to validity of observational measures, particularly those used in clinical practice. This is a content validity problem. When coding, the examiner makes choices about what to code; they are not "writing down the real thing".

21.8.1 Reactivity

Another concern of observational measures is response biases, such as faking good, faking bad, and impression control. For instance, people may act differently because they are being observed, which is a form of *reactivity*. People could be behaving better or worse than they typically do, but observation tends to push people to the extremes.

21.8.2 Coding

Regarding coders and observers, it is ideal during training to provide them immediate corrective feedback. It is ideal for them to be blind to hypotheses, so they are not biased in favor of a particular outcome. It can be helpful to periodically compare coders' ratings to criterion ratings that are accepted as the gold-standard ratings to prevent coder drift. Coder drift occurs when there are changes in coders' ratings over time. You can evaluate intra-observer reliability by having them rate the same (video-recorded) behavior at two different time points. You can have two or more raters code at least a subset of the participants, to establish inter-rater reliability.

21.9 Forms of Measurement

There are several forms of measurement that behavioral assessments can take. One form of measurement from observation is notes, which involves qualitative data. For rating scales, the form of measurement is often Likert scales. Likert scales assess the observer's impression of the examineee's behavior, which is a simpler way of getting the same information as many approaches to video coding. Rating scales can be completed in the context of, for example, a home observation, parent report, teacher report, or school observation.

It can be helpful to examine correlations between these different methods and contexts. Having multiple forms of measurement is great for research but is difficult to do in clinical practice because it comes at a tremendous expense. There is also difficulty in observing what you want to observe. For example, aggression is a relatively low base rate phenomenon, so the client may not engage in aggressive behavior during the observation window. There are also questions of the incremental validity of naturalistic observational assessments because simpler measures (including analogue assessments) could get at the same thing.

21.10 Analogue (Structured) Observational Assessments

Analogue or structured assessments use tasks that evoke individual differences in the behavior of interest. For instance, in our lab we have forbidden toys on a shelf, and we see how the children and parents handle that situation when they are in the room together, then when the parent is occupied on the phone, and then when the parent leaves the room and the child is alone in the room. In the clinic, we have a parent tell their child to clean up the toys so we can observe how the parent gives the command and how the child responds. To study marital conflict, researchers may have the couple provide a list of topics they disagree about, and have them have a discussion about one of those topics to evoke an argument in the lab. To study stress and anxiety, or to perform exposure in the clinic, the clinician or researcher may have the client/participant give a public speech in a simulated session.

The goal of analogue assessments is that the tasks should have content validity. That is, the tasks should be relevant to the target construct, and they should be representative of the tasks the person is likely to face in their natural environment by sampling all facets that affect the behavior problem in the natural environment.

Analogue assessment can lead to greater frequency of target behavior through the use of contrived situations or stimuli, compared to naturalistic observation. For instance, non-compliance might occur more often when doing a compliance task in the lab than when observing a child in their natural environment. Therefore, the frequency or rate of behavior may not generalize to the natural context. But the functional relations of the behavior in relation to other behaviors, such as antecedents and consequences, may generalize. Thus, they can help identify potential intervention targets.

Analogue assessment is most useful for assessing behaviors that are difficult or rare to observe in the natural environment but that are frequent in the analogue environment. For example, analogue assessment is particularly useful for assessing socially sensitive behavior problems such as verbal aggression, panic, and oppositional behavior.

Analogue assessment can be sensitive to change, and therefore can be a clinically useful measure of treatment gains or failure. A client who cannot demonstrate a skill in the clinic may not be able to demonstrate a skill in the real world. But just because they show a skill in a session does not necessarily mean they will be able to use it in the real world.

In terms of reliability and validity, analogue/structured assessments tend to show greater reliability than naturalistic observations. Analogue assessments tend to show greater internal validity than naturalistic observations. That is, analogue assessments are more likely to reflect causal factors because they have more control of when and how the stimuli are presented. However, analogue assessments show weaker ecological validity than naturalistic observations and therefore tend to show weaker external validity. That is, analogue assessments yield lower generalizability than naturalistic observations because analogue assessments may not be as reflective of their functioning in the real world. Nevertheless, analogue assessments tend to show greater clinical utility, in terms of incremental validity and cost-effectiveness than naturalistic observations, when they are done well.

21.11 Self-Monitoring

Self-monitoring involves observing and recording one's own behaviors, thoughts, emotions, bodily sensations, events, etc. Given the expense of conducting behavioral observations, you can train people to be their own observers, which has better portability. Phone apps can now be used to track many different processes, such as mood, sleep, and nutrition. These are examples of electronic diaries. An overview of research on self-monitoring and electronic diaries is provided by Korotitsch & Nelson-Gray (1999) and Piasecki et al. (2007).

Self-monitoring provides a great deal of information at a low cost. There are several benefits of self-monitoring. Self-monitoring can help characterize the problem and the presumed causal or maintaining factors. Self-monitoring can also contribute to greater objective self-awareness. In addition, self-monitoring can be used to track treatment progress. Furthermore, self-monitoring can be helpful for assessing covert behaviors that are hidden to outside observers, such as obsessions, paranoid thoughts, and sexual problems.

Self-monitoring is a component of most empirically supported treatments. In addition, the extent to which clients complete self-monitoring is predictive of treatment effectiveness. As an example of self-monitoring in therapy, in parent management training, we have parents track (tally) the frequency of their child's compliance, noncompliance, and aggression each day during the week between sessions as homework. Self-monitoring provides a more objective way to track treatment progress than retrospective reports or satisfaction ratings because clients track the specific behavior the moment it occurs. We modify treatment in response to the information gained from tracking. We also become more aware of the situations and contexts in which the behavior occurs, so it is predictable and the client can better anticipate, prepare for, and control the problem.

Based on principles of measurement-based care, assessment does not just occur at the outset of treatment; it should continue throughout treatment. And self-monitoring helps parents become more aware of the actual frequency of the problem behavior. For instance, they might have over- (or under-)estimated how often a behavior occurs. Thus, self-monitoring can lead to a change in people's perceptions of the behavior. Also, some children will misbehave less at home or school due to reactivity because they know they are being observed, so this can be a way of kick-starting some behavioral improvement.

Reactivity is the change in a behavior for the mere reason that the behavior is being observed. There are often changes in a behavior in response to self-monitoring—typically, the client experiences behavioral improvement. Self-monitoring might increase awareness of how often a problem behavior is happening and their perceived predictability and control of the behavior. Self-monitoring is now considered an empirically supported treatment for a number of conditions, including academic/conduct problems, addictive behaviors, anxiety and depression, disordered eating, physical health problems, psychosis, and insomnia. That is, assessment is a form of intervention!

However, there are challenges to self-monitoring. One challenge is how to evaluate the reliability of self-monitoring. Another challenge is how to handle if the client fills out the whole tracking sheet retrospectively, all at once, right before session—this is called "backfilling". In addition, there is a possibility of inaccuracy and distortion with self-monitoring due to the respondent not having been trained on how to observe the phenomenon of interest. To counter this, in parent management training, we explicitly define what counts as an instance of compliance, noncompliance, and aggression. Another challenge with self-monitoring is that it involves respondent burden because it requires compliance by the client. To handle noncompliance with self-monitoring, it can be helpful to "get procedural" and to discuss with the client when they will track, where they will put the tracking sheet, etc. It can also be helpful to perform advance troubleshooting: help the client anticipate obstacles and how they will address them. For instance, if the client feels that they might forget to do the tracking, have them set a timer. Self-monitoring has lower reliability and validity than behavioral observation, but it is still useful and widely used because it is cheap and easy to obtain lots of information that can lead to behavioral improvement.

21.12 Behavior Rating Scales

Behavior rating scales include self- or informant ratings on a checklist of behaviors assessing particular construct(s). An example assessment system that uses behavior rating scales is the Achenbach System of Empirically Based Assessment (ASEBA) that includes the Child Behavior Checklist (CBCL), Teacher's Report Form (TRF), Adult Self-Report, etc. The ASEBA is an empirically based assessment of psychopathology, rather than a DSM-focused assessment.

Behavior rating scales are widely used in research and clinical settings. They are relatively cheap and easy to administer and score. Item response theory techniques reveal issues with different levels of Likert scale anchors of rating scales. For example, people assign different meanings to the levels "never", "sometimes", and "a lot". It is often better to have the rater describe or provide the numeric amount. For example: "How many times during the last week did your child physically hit someone else?"

Behavior rating scales are typically retrospective where the rater has to reflect back and estimate the frequency of behaviors and people's responses to the environment. Retrospective ratings can have challenges with validity due to inaccurate memory recall.

21.13 Assessment of Therapeutic Process

Other behavioral assessments include assessments of therapeutic process. Example assessments of therapeutic process include having a video recording of a session and then coding it in a naturalistic setting. For a therapist, the naturalistic setting is the therapeutic context.

An example of assessment of the therapeutic process could include assessing the clinician's adherence and competence. Assessing adherence would involve coding whether the therapist is following the treatment protocol and manual, that is, the degree to which the clinician shows treatment fidelity. Assessing the clinician's competence would involve coding how skilled the therapist is in providing the treatment. Coding clinician competence in most treatments, including cognitive behavioral therapy, would not be a moment-to-moment coding; instead, the coder would examine the sequence of interactions between client and therapist.

21.14 Conclusion

Examples of behavioral assessment include naturalistic behavioral observation, analogue (structured) observation, self-monitoring/diary, behavior ratings (e.g., informant report), and self-report. A gold standard for naturalistic observations is to observe people in their natural context across more than one day, time, situation, and context with more than one rater to get a more robust sampling of the person's behavior. Compared to naturalistic observation, analogue assessments tend to show greater reliability and internal validity but lower external validity. A useful approach to identify the function of a given behavior is to identify patterns of sequences according to the antecedent-behavior-consequence (A-B-C) model as part of a functional behavior assessment. Another useful approach is self-monitoring, which provides a lot of information at low cost and is therefore a component of most empirically supported treatments.

21.15 Suggested Readings

Girard & Cohn (2016)

22

Repeated Assessments Across Time

22.1 Overview

Repeated measurement enables examining within-person change in constructs. Relating within-person change in a construct to within-person change in another construct provides a stronger test of causality compared to simple bivariate correlations. Identifying that within-person change in construct X predicts later within-person change in construct Y does not necessarily indicate that X causes Y but it provides stronger evidence consistent with causality than a simple bivariate association between X and Y. As described in Section 4.3.1.3.3.1, there are three primary reasons a correlation between X and Y does not necessarily mean that X causes Y: First, the association could reflect the opposite direction of effect, where Y actually causes X. Second, the association could reflect the influence of a third variable that influences both X and Y (i.e., a confound). Third, the association might be spurious.

If you find that within-person changes in sleep predict later within-person changes in mood, that is a stronger test of causality because (a) it demonstrates temporal precedence; it attenuates the possibility that the association is due to the opposite direction of effect; and (b) it accounts for all time-invariant confounds that differ between people (e.g., birth order) because the association is examined *within* the individual. That is, the association examines whether the person's mood is better when they get more sleep compared to when that same person gets less sleep. The association could still be due to time-varying confounds, but you can control for specific time-varying confounds if you measure them.

Repeated measurement also enables examination of the developmental timing of effects and sensitive periods. Furthermore, repeated measures designs are important for tests of mediation, which are tests of hypothesized causal mechanisms.

Repeated measurement involves more complex statistical analysis than cross-sectional measurement because multiple observations come from the same person, which would violate assumptions of traditional analyses that the observations (i.e., the residuals) are independent and uncorrelated. Mixed-effects modeling (i.e., mixed modeling, multilevel modeling, hierarchical linear modeling) and other analyses, such as structural equation modeling, can handle the longitudinal dependency or nesting of repeated measures data.

Repeated measurement can encompass many different timescales, such as milliseconds, days, or years.

22.1.1 Comparison of Approaches

Research designs can be compared in terms of their internal validity—the extent to which we can be confident about causal inferences. A cross-sectional association is depicted in Figure 22.1:

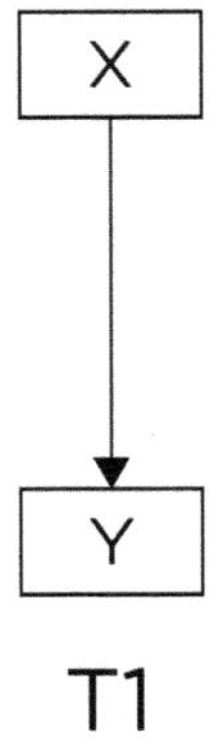

FIGURE 22.1 Cross-Sectional Association.

Among observational/correlational research designs, cross-sectional designs tend to have the weakest internal validity. That is, if we observe a cross-sectional association between X and Y, we have little confidence that X causes Y. Consider a lagged association, which is a slightly better approach:

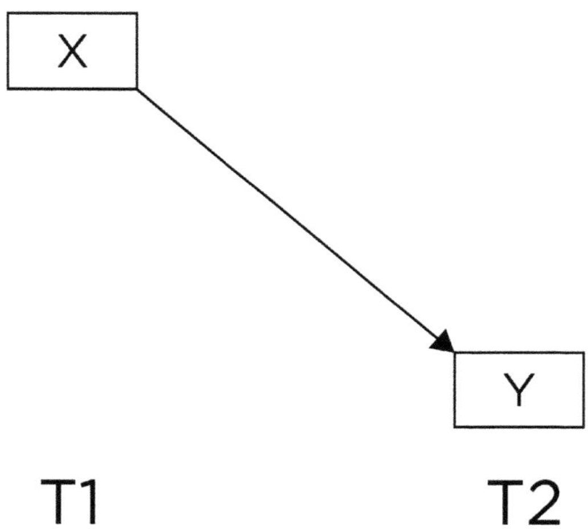

FIGURE 22.2 Lagged Association.

A lagged association has somewhat better internal validity than a cross-sectional association because we have greater evidence of temporal precedence—that the influence of the predictor *precedes* the outcome because the predictor was assessed before the outcome and it shows a predictive association. However, part of the association between the predictor with later levels of the outcome could be due to prior levels of the outcome that are stable across time. Thus, consider an even stronger alternative—a lagged association that controls for prior levels of the outcome:

A lagged association controlling for prior levels of the outcome has better internal validity than a lagged association that does not control for prior levels of the outcome. When we control for prior levels of the outcome in the prediction, we are essentially predicting (relative) change. Predicting change provides stronger evidence consistent with causality because it uses the individual as their own control and controls for many time-invariant confounds.

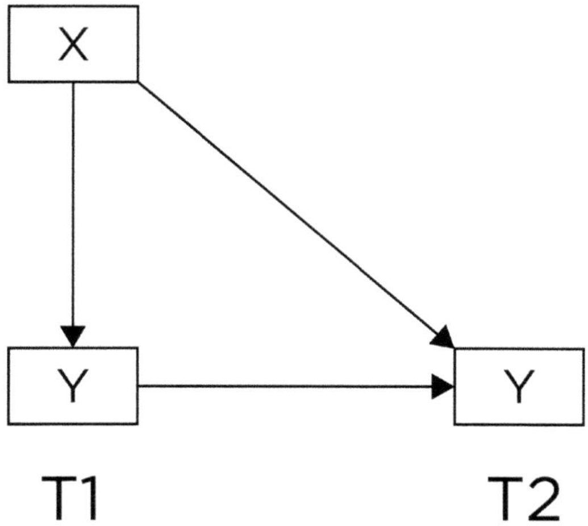

FIGURE 22.3 Lagged Association, Controlling for Prior Levels of the Outcome.

However, consider an even stronger alternative—lagged associations that control for prior levels of the outcome and that simultaneously test each direction of effect:

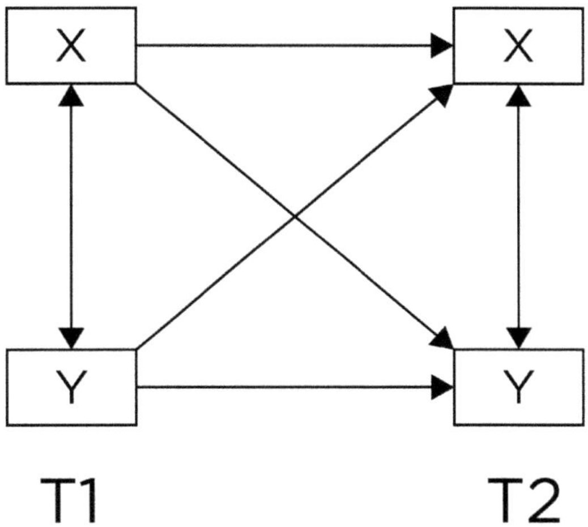

FIGURE 22.4 Lagged Association, Controlling for Prior Levels of the Outcome, Simultaneously Testing Both Directions of Effect.

Lagged associations that control for prior levels of the outcome and that simultaneously test each direction of effect provide the strongest internal validity among correlational/observational designs, especially when examining whether within-person changes in the predictor predict later within-person changes in the outcome (and vice versa). Such a design can help better clarify which among the variables is the chicken and the egg—which variable is more likely to be the cause and which is more likely to be the effect. Or, if there are bidirectional, transactional effects, what the magnitude of each direction of effect is. The cross-lagged panel model and dual latent change score model are examples of models that include lagged associations that control for prior levels of the outcome and that simultaneously test each direction of effect. However, consider an even stronger model—lagged associations that control for prior levels of the outcome and for random intercepts and that simultaneously test each direction of effect:

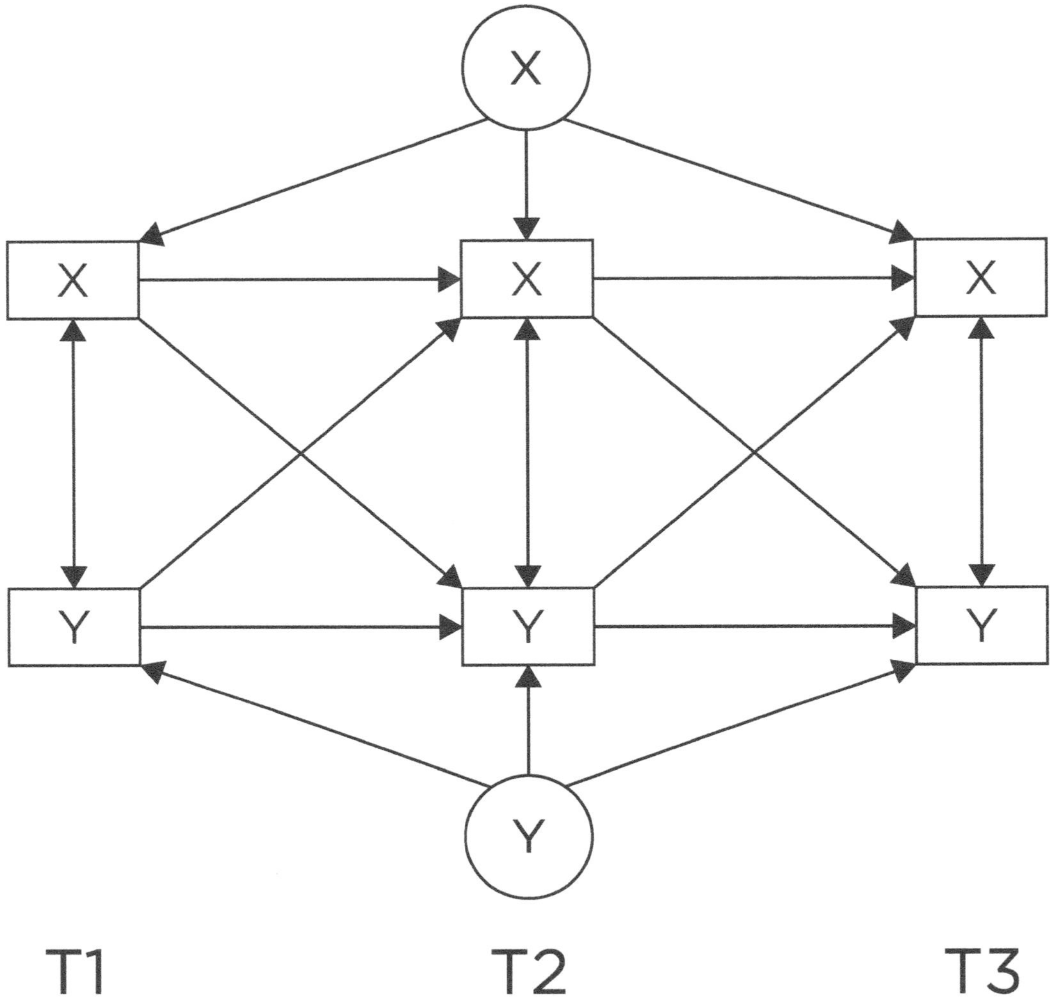

FIGURE 22.5 Lagged Association, Controlling for Prior Levels of the Outcome and Random Intercepts, Simultaneously Testing Both Directions of Effect.

Some researchers have called into question the cross-lagged panel model (Berry & Willoughby, 2017; Hamaker et al., 2015). A stronger alternative may be a cross-lagged model that controls for stable between-person differences (i.e., random intercepts) (Hamaker et al., 2015). This is known as a random intercepts cross-lagged panel model.

22.2 Examples of Repeated Measurement

Below are some examples of repeated measurement.

22.2.1 Alcohol Timeline Followback

A clinically relevant example of repeated measurement is the Alcohol Timeline Followback, published by Sobell & Sobell (2008). The Alcohol Timeline Followback is a method for retrospectively assessing the quantity of alcohol consumption on a daily basis. It provides retrospective estimates of people's drinking using a calendar of the number of drinks consumed each day. The time frame can vary from 30 days to 360 days. The participant is given detailed instructions to enhance the accuracy of recall and reporting of their behavior.

Moreover, a specific definition is provided of what counts as a drink. The measure is intended to provide a detailed record of patterns of alcohol use to guide treatment and assess treatment outcome. The measure provides many summary statistics and norms are available.

The measure has several clinical uses. First, it can provide personalized feedback to the client regarding their drinking behavior compared to the population as part of enhancing their motivation to change, in a motivational interviewing framework. Second, the measure can help identify high- and low-risk periods for a client to help them prevent relapse.

Because the measure provides detailed information with norms, it can be more useful than global estimates of drinking derived from less structured clinical interviews. The detailed instructions help respondents remember more accurately, so the clinician or researcher can examine how people's heavy substance use influences other processes like parenting.

22.2.2 Ambulatory Assessment

We discussed ambulatory assessment in Section 19.2.4.1. Ambulatory assessment includes an array of methods used to study people in their natural environment. There is a proliferation of smartphone apps for ambulatory assessment. And the ambulatory assessments often, because of their temporal resolution, provide repeated measurements.

For instance, Carpenter et al. (2016) depicted the examination, during a drinking episode, of self-reported drinking in relation to physiological indices including skin temperature, heart rate, breathing rate, physical activity, and in relation to self-reported sadness and mood dysregulation. The self-reported indices were assessed on various intervals (e.g., every 15 minutes) and upon various events (e.g., when they take a drink). However, the physiological indices were assessed continuously from moment to moment. These different timescales pose challenges for how to examine them in relation to each other.

Matthews et al. (2016) provided an example of how they developed an ambulatory assessment using a smartphone app to assess the dynamic process of bipolar disorder. Regularity of social rhythms is disrupted in bipolar disorder, so the authors developed an app to help assess social rhythms. The authors used a participatory design in which they involved the patients in the development of the app to ensure it worked well for them. The app tracked the occurrence and timing of daily events, such as getting out of bed, starting your day, having dinner, and going to bed. It also passively detected daily events ("social rhythms") with many sensors on the smartphone using information from the light, accelerometer, and microphone of the smartphone. And the app used a machine learning algorithm to estimate level of physical activity and social interaction.

22.3 Test Revisions

An important part of repeated measurements deals with test revisions. Tests are revised over time. Some test revisions are made to be consistent with improvements in the understanding of the construct. Other test revisions are made to make the norms more up-to-date. For instance, the Weschler Adult Intelligence Scale has multiple versions (WAIS-3, WAIS-IV, etc.). There are important considerations when dealing with test revisions.

When you assess people at different times, whether the same people at multiple time points (such as in a longitudinal study) or different people at different times, challenges may result in comparing scores across time. There can be benefits of keeping the same measure across ages or across time for comparability of scores. However, it is not necessarily good to use the same measure across ages or at different times merely for the sake of mathematical comparability of scores. If a measure was revised to improve its validity or if a measure is not valid at particular ages, it may make sense to use different measures across ages or across time. You would not want to use a measure at a given age if it is not valid at that age. Likewise, it does not make sense to use an invalid measure at a later time point if a more valid version becomes available, even if it was used at an earlier time point. That is, even if a measure's scores are *mathematically* comparable across ages or time, they may not be *conceptually* comparable across ages or time. If different measures are used across ages or across time, there may be ways to link scores from the different measures to be on the same scale, as described in Section 22.8.4.1.3.

One interesting phenomenon of time-related changes in scores is the Flynn effect, in which the population scores on intelligence tests rise around 3 points every decade. That is, intelligence, as measured by tests of cognitive abilities, increases from generation to generation. Test revisions can hide effects like the Flynn effect if we just keep using score transformations instead of raw scores.

To observe a person's (or group's) growth, it is recommended to use raw scores rather than standardized scores that are age-normed, such as T scores, z scores, standard scores, and percentile ranks (Moeller, 2015). Age-normed scores prevent observing growth at the person level and at the group level (e.g., changes in means or variances over time). T scores ($M = 50$, $SD = 10$), z scores ($M = 0$, $SD = 1$), and standard scores ($M = 100$, $SD = 15$) have a fixed mean and standard deviation. Percentile ranks have a fixed range (0–100).

22.4 Change and Stability

A key goal of developmental science is to assess change and stability of people and constructs. Stability is often referred to in a general way. For instance, you may read that intelligence and personality show "stability" over time. However, this is not a useful way of describing the stability of people and/or constructs because stability is not one thing. There are multiple types of stability, and it is important to refer to the types of stability considered.

Types of stability include, for instance, stability of level, rank order (individual differences), and structure. Stability of level refers to whether people show the same level on the construct over time. For example, stability of level considers whether people stay the same in their level of neuroticism across childhood to adulthood. Stability of people's level is evaluated with the coefficient of repeatability.

Mean-level stability refers to whether the mean level stays the same across time. For example, mean-level stability considers whether the population average stays the same in their level of neuroticism across childhood to adulthood. Mean-level stability is evaluated by examining mean-level age-related differences; for instance, with a t-test or ANOVA, or by examining whether the construct is associated with age.

Rank-order stability refers to whether individual differences stay the same across time. For instance, rank-order stability considers whether people who have higher neuroticism than their peers as children also tend to have higher neuroticism than their peers as adults. Rank-order stabiliy is evaluated by examining the association of people's level at T1 with people's level at T2 (e.g., correlation coefficient or regression coefficent).

Stability of structure considers whether the structure of the construct stays the same across ages. For instance, stability of structure considers whether personality is characterized by the same five factors across ages (i.e., openness, conscientiousness, extraversion, agreeableness, and neuroticism). Stability of structure is examined using longitudinal factorial invariance.

People and constructs can show stability in some types and not others. For instance, although intelligence and personality show *relative* stability in structure and rank-order, they do not show *absolute* stability in level. Even though *individual differences* in intelligence and personality show relative stability, people tend to change across time in their absolute level of intelligence and various personality factors across ages. For instance, neuroticism decreases in later adulthood. Examining age-normed scores would preclude identifying mean-level change because age-normed scores have a fixed mean. Moreover, examining a strong correlation of intelligence and personality scores across time merely indicates that individual differences show relative stability; it does not indicate whether individuals show absolute stability in level.

22.5 Assessing Change

There are many important considerations for assessing change, that is, changes in a person's level on a construct across time. There is a key challenge in assessing change between two time points. If a person's score differs between two time points, how do you know that the differences across time reflect a person's true change in their level on the construct rather than measurement error, such as regression to the mean? Regression to the mean occurs if an extreme observation on a measure at time 1 (T1) more closely approximates the person's mean at later time points, including time 2 (T2). For instance, clients with high levels of symptomatology tend to get better with the mere passage of time, which has been known as the self-righting reflex.

22.5.1 Inferring Change

The inference of change is strengthened to the extent that:

a. the magnitude of the difference between the scores at the two time points is large (i.e., a large effect size)
b. the measurement error (unreliability) at both time points is small

c. the measure has the same meaning and is on a comparable scale at each time point (i.e., the measure's scores show measurement invariance across time)
d. evidence suggests that the differences across time are not likely to be due to potential confounds of change such as practice effects, cohort effects, and time-of-measurement effects.

Measurement error can be reduced by combining multiple measures of a construct into a latent variable, such as in structural equation modeling (SEM) or item response theory (IRT).

To detect change, it is important to use measures that are sensitive to change. For instance, the measures should not show range restriction owing to ceiling effects or floor effects.

22.5.2 Potential Confounds of Change

Potential confounds of change include practice effects, cohort effects, and time-of-measurement effects.

22.5.2.1 Practice Effects

It is important to consider the potential for practice or retest effects (Hertzog & Nesselroade, 2003). Practice/retest effects occur to the extent that a person improves on a task assessed at multiple time points for reasons due to the repeated assessment rather than true changes in the construct. That is, a person is likely to improve on a task if they complete the same task at multiple time points, even if they are not changing in their level on the construct. Practice and retest effects are especially likely to be larger the closer in time the retest is to the prior testing. Improvement in scores across time might not reflect people's true change in the construct; thus, you might not be able to fairly compare people's scores who have completed the task different numbers of times.

In sum, the ages and frequency of assessment should depend on theory.

22.5.2.2 Cohort Effects

It is also important to consider the potential for cohort effects (Hertzog & Nesselroade, 2003). Cohorts often refer to birth cohorts—people who were born at the same time (e.g., the same year). Cohorts tend to have some similar experiences at similar ages, including major events (e.g., 9/11 terrorist attacks, assassination of John F. Kennedy, bombing of Pearl Harbor) and economic or socio-political climates (e.g., the Great Depression, coronavirus pandemic, Cold War, World War II). These collective differences in the different experiences between different cohorts may lead to apparent age-related differences between cohorts that are not actually due to age differences per se, but rather to differences in the experiences between the cohorts.

22.5.2.3 Time-of-Measurement Effects

It is also important to consider time-of-measurement effects. For instance, people's general anxiety may be higher, on average, during the coronavirus pandemic. Thus, some apparent age-related differences might be due to the time of measurement (i.e., a pandemic) rather than age.

22.5.3 When and How Frequently to Assess

Key questions arise in terms of when (at what ages or times) and how often to assess the construct. If the measurement intervals are too long, you might miss important change in between. If the measurement intervals are too frequent, differences might reflect only measurement error. The Nyquist theorem provides guidance in terms of how frequently to assess a construct. According to the Nyquist theorem, in order to accurately reproduce a signal, you should sample it at twice the highest frequency you wish to detect. For instance, to detect a 15 Hz wave, you should sample it at least at 30 Hz (Hertz means times per second). Thus, the frequency of assessment should be as frequent as, if not more frequent than, the highest frequency of change you seek to observe.

22.5.4 Difference Scores

As described in Section 3.5.8, difference scores (also called change scores) can have limitations because they can be less reliable than each of the individual measures that compose the difference score. The reliability of individual differences in change scores depends on the extent to which: (a) the measures used to calculate the change scores are reliable, and (b) the variability of true individual differences in change is large—that is, there are true individual differences in change.

22.5.4.1 Superior Approaches to Difference Scores

There are several options that are better than traditional difference scores or change scores. Instead of difference scores, use autoregressive cross-lagged models, latent change score models, or growth curve models.

22.5.4.1.1 Autoregressive cross-lagged models

Autoregressive cross-lagged models (aka cross-lagged panel models) can be fit in path analysis or SEM. Cross-lagged panel models examine relative change in a variable, that is, change in individual differences in the variable, but not changes in level on the variable. Such a model allows examining whether one variable predicts *relative* change in another variable. The cross-lagged panel model tests whether individuals with low levels of X *relative to others* experience subsequent *rank-order increases* in Y (Evans & Shaughnessy, in press; Orth et al., 2021). By contrast, the random-intercepts cross-lagged panel model tests whether, when individuals experience *lower-than-their-own usual levels* of X, they experience subsequent increases in Y *relative to their usual level* (Evans & Shaughnessy, in press; Orth et al., 2021). As an example of a cross-lagged panel model, we conducted a collaborative study that examined whether language ability predicts later behavior problems controlling for prior levels of behavior problems—that is, whether language ability predicts a person's change in behavior problems relative to the change among other people in the sample (Petersen et al., 2013; Petersen & LeBeau, 2021). Cross-lagged panel models predict relative (rank-order) change, not absolute change in level. For tests of absolute change, models such as change score models or growth curve models are necessary.

22.5.4.1.2 Latent change score models

Latent change score models can be fit in SEM. Unlike autoregressive cross-lagged models, latent change score models examine *absolute* change—that is, people's changes in level. With latent change score models, you can examine change in latent variables that reflect the common variance among multiple measures. Latent variables are theoretically error-free (at least of random error), so latent change scores can be perfectly reliable, unlike traditional difference scores, whose reliability is strongly influenced by the measurement unreliability of the specific measures that compose them. Latent change score models are described by R. A. Kievit et al. (2018).

22.5.4.1.3 Growth curve models

Growth curve models can be fit in mixed-effects modeling or SEM. Growth curve models require three or more time points to be able to account for measurement error in terms of the shape of a linear trajectory. Growth curve models examine absolute change, i.e., changes in level. Growth curve models include an intercept (starting point) and slope (amount of change), but you can model other nonlinear forms of change as well, such as quadratic, logistic, etc. with more time points. Growth curve models correct for measurement error in the shape of the person's trajectory. In addition, growth curve models can examine risk and protective factors as predictors of the intercepts and slopes. For instance, we examined risk and protective factors that predict the development of externalizing problems (Petersen et al., 2015).

22.5.5 Nomothetic Versus Idiographic

The approaches described above (autoregressive cross-lagged models, latent change score models, and growth curve models) tend to be nomothetic in nature. That is, they are interested in examining group-level phenomena and assume that all people come from the same population and can be described by the same parameters of change. That is, they assume a degree of homogeneity, even though they allow each person to differ in their intercept and slope. This nomothetic (population) approach differs from an idiographic (individual) approach. In clinical work, we are often interested in making inferences or predictions at the level of the individual person, consistent with an idiographic approach. But fully ignoring the population estimates is unwise because they tend to be more accurate than individual-level judgments. Further, individual-level predictions may not generalize to the population. Nomothetic modeling approaches can be adapted to examine change for different subgroups if there are theoretically different populations. Approaches that examine different subgroups include group-based trajectory models, latent class growth models, and growth mixture models (Fontaine & Petersen, 2017; van der Nest et al., 2020).

For instance, Moffit (1993, 2006b, 2006a) created the developmental taxonomy of antisocial behavior with the support of these approaches. Moffitt identified one subgroup that showed very low levels of antisocial behavior across the lifespan, which she labeled the "low" group. She identified one subgroup that showed antisocial behavior only in childhood, which she labeled the "childhood-limited" group. She hypothesized that the antisocial behavior among the childhood-limited group was influenced primarily by genetic factors and the early environment. She identified another subgroup that showed antisocial behavior only in adolescence, which she labeled the "adolescent-limited"group. She hypothesized that the antisocial behavior among the adolescent-limited group was largely socially mediated. She identified another subgroup that showed antisocial behavior across the lifespan, which she labeled the "life-course persistent" group. She hypothesized that the "life-course persistent" group reflected neuropsychological deficits.

Idiographic approaches for personalized modeling of psychopathology are described by Wright & Woods (2020). An example of an approach that combines an idiographic (person-centered) approach with a nomothetic (population) approach to understand change is the group iterative multiple model estimation (GIMME) model, as described by Beltz et al. (2016) and Wright et al. (2019). The GIMME model is a data-driven approach to identifying person-specific time-series models. The approach first identifies the associations among constructs that replicate across most participants. The group-level associations are then used as a starting point for identifying person-specific associations. Thus, the GIMME model provides an approach for developing personalized time-series models. The choices on which model to use depend on the research question and should be guided by theory.

22.5.6 Structural Equation Modeling

Structural equation modeling (SEM) allows multiple dependent variables. This provides a key advantage in longitudinal designs, such that two constructs can each be represented by a dependent variable that is predicted by the other. If examining changes in two constructs in the context of SEM, you could examine for instance whether one precedes the other in prediction, to better understand which might cause which and to help tease apart the chicken and the egg. For instance, in collaboration, I found that low language ability predicts later behavior problems stronger than behavior problems predict later language ability, suggesting that, if they are causally related, that language ability is more likely to have a causal effect on behavior problems than the reverse (Petersen et al., 2013).

22.5.7 Attrition and Systematic Missingness

Rates of attrition in longitudinal studies can be substantial and missingness is often not completely at random. There is often selective and systematic attrition. For example, attrition often differs as a function of socioeconomic status and other important factors. It is important to use approaches that examine and account for systematic missingness. It can be helpful to use full-information maximum likelihood (FIML) in SEM to make use of all available data. Multiple imputation is another approach that can be helpful for dealing with missingness. With multiple imputation, you can use predictors that might account for missingness, such as socioeconomic status and demographic factors. You can help account for practice effects with planned missingness designs in which participants are randomly assigned to receive or not receive a given measurement occasion.

22.5.8 Measurement Invariance

Just like measurement or factorial invariance can be tested and established across genders, races, ethnicities, cultures, etc. to ensure measurement equivalence, it can also be tested across ages or times. The goal is to establish longitudinal measurement invariance, i.e., measurement invariance across ages, so that you know that you are assessing the same construct over time in a comparable way so that you know that differences across time reflect true change. To examine longitudinal measurement invariance, you can use SEM or IRT. In SEM, you could examine whether measures have the same intercepts, factor loadings, and residuals across ages. In IRT, you could examine whether items show differential item functioning, versus whether they show the same difficulty and discrimination across ages.

But there are times when we would expect a construct would, theoretically, fail to show longitudinal factorial invariance, as in the case of heterotypic continuity, described in Section 22.8.

22.6 Types of Research Designs

Schaie (1965), Baltes (1968), and Schaie & Baltes (1975) proposed various types of research designs, in terms of the various combinations of age, period (i.e., time of measurement), and cohort. Age refers to a person's chronological age at the time of measurement. Period refers to the time of measurement (e.g., April 12, 2014 at 7:53 AM). Cohort refers to a person's time (e.g., year) of birth (e.g., 2003). If you know two of these (e.g., age and period), you can determine the third (e.g., cohort). Here are types of research designs based on combinations of age, period, and cohort:

- cross-sectional
- cross-sectional sequences
- time-lag
- longitudinal
- longitudinal sequences
  - time-sequential
  - cross-sequential
  - cohort-sequential

These research designs are depicted by age and cohort in Figure 22.6 and by time of measurement and cohort in Figure 22.7. Although the depictions of cohort-sequential and cross-sequential designs differ from the depictions by Schaie (2005) (i.e., they are reversed), they are consistent with contemporary definitions of these designs (Little, 2013; Masche & Dulmen, 2004; Whitbourne, 2019).

22.6.1 Cross-Sectional Design

A *cross-sectional* design involves multiple participants, often spanning different ages, assessed at one time of measurement. A cross-sectional design is a single factor design, where the researcher is interested in comparing effects of one factor: age. However, in a cross-sectional design, cohort (i.e., birth year) is confounded with age differences. Thus, observed age-related differences could reflect cohort differences rather than true age differences. Additionally, sampling differences at each age could yield non-comparable age groups.

Cross-sectional designs are thus limited in their ability to describe developmental processes including change and stability over time (Kraemer et al., 2000). Any age-related differences are confounded with cohort differences and are strongly influenced by between age-group sampling variability. Cross-sectional studies are useful for preliminary data on validity of measures for the age groups, and for examining whether the age differences are in the expected direction. Cross-sectional studies are less costly and time-consuming than longitudinal studies. Therefore, they are widely used and provide a useful starting point.

However, findings from cross-sectional studies can differ from findings examining the same people over time, which violates the convergence assumption. In cross-sectional studies, the convergence assumption is the assumption that cross-sectional age differences and longitudinal age changes converge onto a common trajectory. However, it has been shown, for example, that cross-sectional studies overestimate age-related cognitive declines compared to following the same people over time in a longitudinal study (Ackerman, 2013).

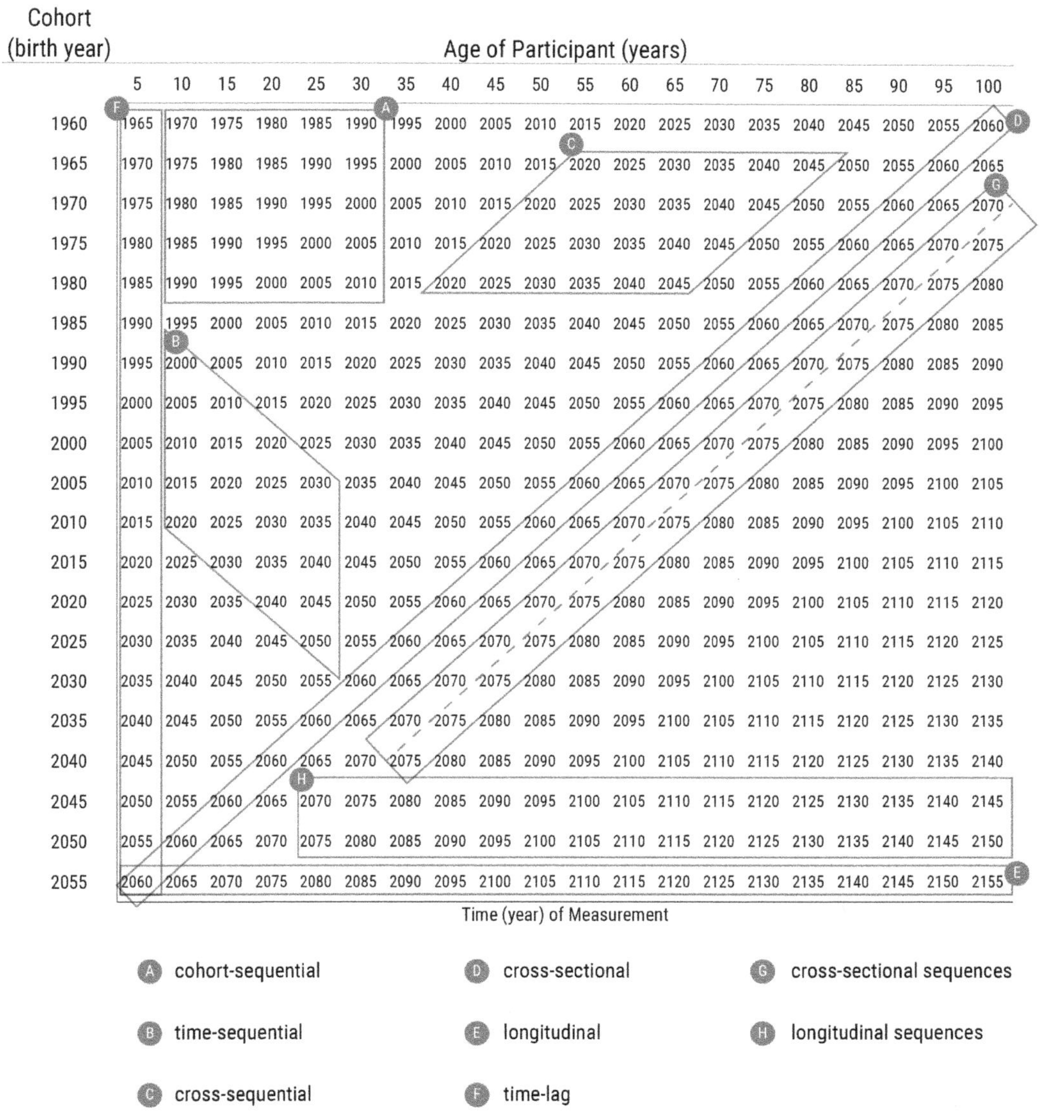

FIGURE 22.6 Research Designs by Age and Cohort. Values in the cells are the times (years) of measurement. Dashed line indicates different participants were assessed at each time of measurement.

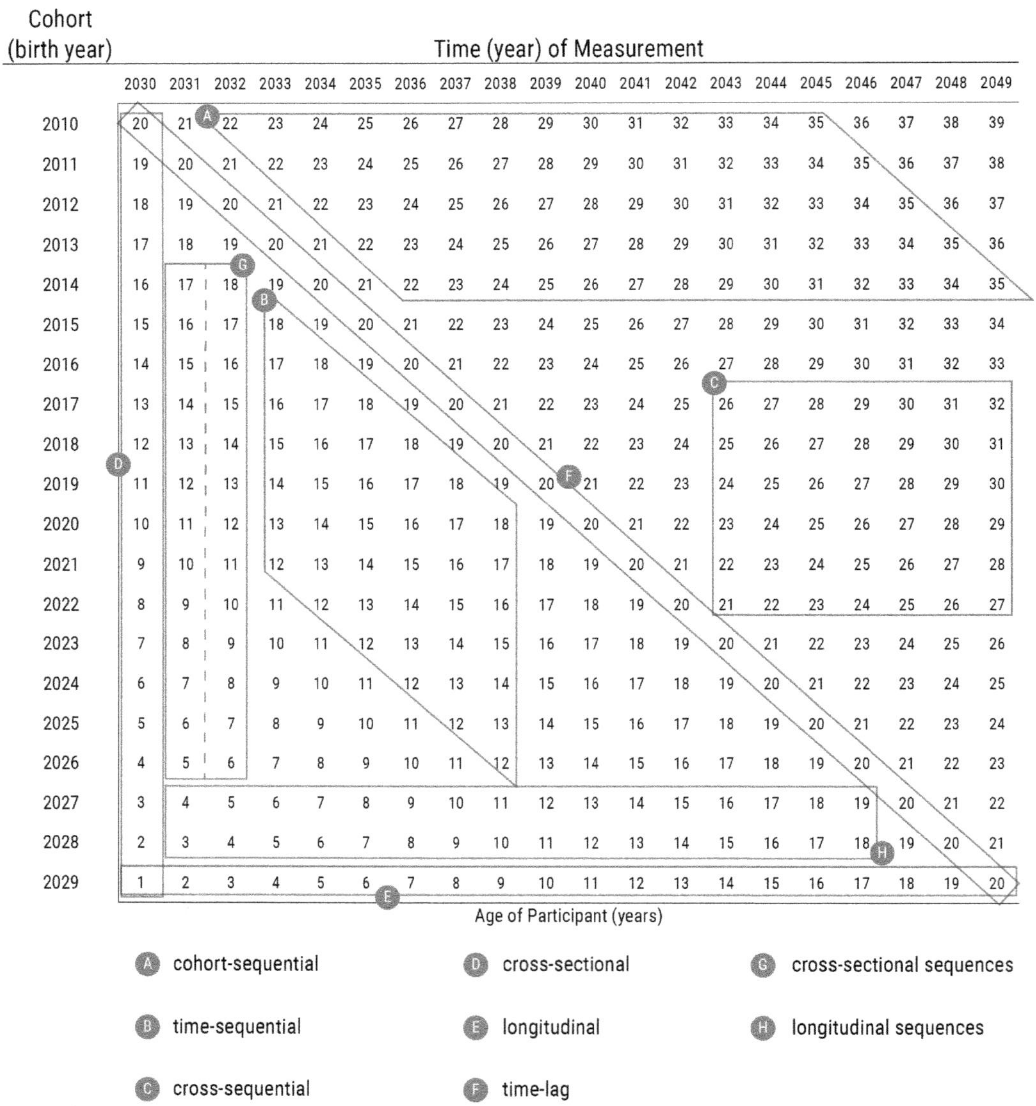

FIGURE 22.7 Research Designs by Time of Measurement and Cohort. Values in the cells are ages of the participants. Dashed line indicates different participants were assessed at each time of measurement.

22.6.2 Cross-Sectional Sequences Design

A *cross-sectional sequences* design involves successive cross-sectional studies of different participants at different times of measurement. In a cross-sectional sequences design, cohort and time-of-measurement are confounded with age differences. Thus, observed age-related differences could reflect cohort differences or time-of-measurement differences rather than true age differences. This poses challenges for using cross-sectional sequences to estimate age-related changes due to time-related effects such as the Flynn effect.

22.6.3 Time-Lag Design

A time-lag design involves participants from different cohorts assessed at the same age. The time-lag design is a single factor design: the researcher specifies one factor: cohort. However, time of measurement is confounded with cohort. Thus, any cohort differences could reflect different times of measurement.

22.6.4 Longitudinal Design

A *longitudinal* design involves following the same participants over time. The single-cohort longitudinal design is a single factor design: the researcher specifies one factor: age. However, in a single-cohort longitudinal design, cohort and time of measurement are confounded with age. Thus, any observed changes with age could be due to time-of-measurement effects or cohort effects (instead of people's true change).

22.6.5 Longitudinal Sequences Design

A *longitudinal sequences* design involves following multiple cohorts across time. There are three types of longitudinal sequence designs: time-sequential, cross-sequential, and cohort-sequential designs. The three types of longitudinal sequences are depicted in Figure 22.8 as a function of which two factors are specified by the researcher.

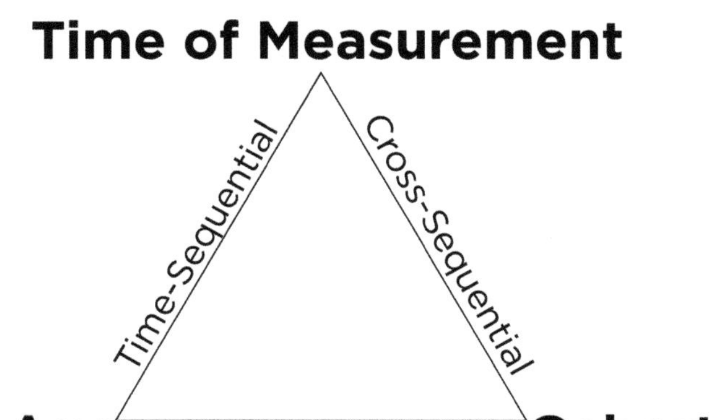

FIGURE 22.8 Types of Longitudinal Sequences as a Function of Which Two Factors are Specified by the Researcher.

22.6.5.1 Time-Sequential Design

A *time-sequential* design is depicted in Figure 22.9. In a time-sequential design, multiple age groups are assessed at multiple times (Whitbourne, 2019). It is a repeated cross-sectional design, with some participants followed longitudinally. Additional age groups are added to a time-lag design, with some of the participants assessed at more than time point. In other words, the age range is kept the same and is repeatedly assessed (with only some participants being repeatedly assessed). The two factors a researcher specifies in a time-sequential design are age and time of measurement. A time-sequential design can be helpful for identifying age differences while controlling for time-of-measurement differences, or for identifying time-of-measurement differences while controlling for age differences. However, cohort effects are confounded with the interaction of age and time of measurement (Whitbourne, 2019). Thus, observed differences as a function of age or time of measurement could reflect cohort effects.

Age of Participant	Time (year) of Measurement	
	2030	2040
10 years old	2020	2030
20 years old	2010	2020
	Cohort (birth year)	

FIGURE 22.9 Time-Sequential Research Design.

22.6.5.2 Cross-Sequential Design

A *cross-sequential* design is depicted in Figure 22.10. In a cross-sequential design, multiple cohorts are assessed at multiple times (Whitbourne, 2019). It is a cross of a cross-sectional and longitudinal design. It starts as a cross-sectional study with participants from multiple cohorts, and then all participants are followed longitudinally (typically across the same duration). It is also called an accelerated longitudinal design. The two factors a researcher specifies in a cross-sequential design are time of measurement and cohort. A cross-sequential design can be helpful for identifying cohort differences while controlling for time-of-measurement differences, or for identifying time-of-measurement differences while controlling for cohort differences. However, age differences are confounded with the interaction between cohort and time of measurement. Thus, observed differences as a function of cohort or time of measurement could reflect age effects.

22.6.5.3 Cohort-Sequential Design

A *cohort-sequential* design is depicted in Figure 22.11. In a cohort-sequential design, multiple cohorts are assessed at multiple ages (Whitbourne, 2019). It starts multiple cohorts at the same age and then follows them longitudinally (typically across the same duration). It is like starting a longitudinal study at the same age over and over again. The two factors a researcher specifies in a cohort-sequential design are age and cohort. A cohort-sequential design can be helpful for identifying age differences while controlling for cohort differences, or for identifying cohort differences while controlling for age differences. However, time-of-measurement effects are confounded with the interaction of age and cohort (Whitbourne, 2019). Thus, observed differences as a function of age or cohort could reflect time-of-measurement effects.

Time (year) of Measurement	Cohort (birth year)	
	2010	2020
2030	20 years old	10 years old
2040	30 years old	20 years old
	Age of Participant	

FIGURE 22.10 Cross-Sequential Research Design.

Age of Participant	Cohort (birth year)	
	2020	2030
5 years old	2025	2035
10 years old	2030	2040
	Time (year) of Measurement	

FIGURE 22.11 Cohort-Sequential Research Design.

22.7 Using Sequential Designs to Make Developmental Inferences

Which research design you select should depend on which change function you are most interested in: age, cohort, or time of measurement. However, age is not the only metric for development; time after an exposure (e.g., puberty onset, school entry) can also be an important time metric. There are many other potential metrics of time for studying development.

To have greater confidence that age-related differences reflect true change (development) rather than effects of cohort or time of measurement, we would conduct all three sequential designs. To the extent that the age-related effects in the time-sequential and cohort-sequential designs are stronger than the cohort- and time-of-measurement effects in the cross-sequential design, we have confidence that the observed age-related differences reflect development (Whitbourne, 2019). Moreover, there is an entire set of analytic approaches, known as age-period-cohort analysis (Yang & Land, 2013), whose goal is to disentangle the effects of age, period, and cohort.

22.8 Heterotypic Continuity

Heterotypic continuity is the persistence of an underlying construct with behavioral manifestations that change across development (Caspi & Shiner, 2006; Cicchetti & Rogosch, 2002; Petersen et al., 2020). Patterson (1993) described antisocial behavior like a chimera. A chimera is a mythical creature with a body of a goat that, with development, grows the head of a lion and then a tail of a snake. Patterson (1993) conceptualized antisocial behavior across development as having an underlying essence of oppositionality that is maintained while adding more mature features with age, including the ability to inflict serious damage with aggression and violence. Other analogies of heterotypic continuity include the change from water to ice or steam, and the metamorphosis of a caterpillar to a butterfly—the same construct shows different manifestations across development.

The various types of continuity, including homotypic continuity, heterotypic continuity, and phenotypic continuity, in addition to discontinuity are depicted in Figure 22.12.

22.8.1 How to Identify Heterotypic Continuity

Heterotypic continuity can be identified or quantified as changes in the factor structure (i.e., content) of a construct across time. The content of a measure includes the facets assessed by a given measure, such as individual behaviors, questionnaire items, or sub-dimensions of a broader construct. The content of the measure can be compared to content of a construct to evaluate the content validity of the measure.

Heterotypic continuity is present to the extent that the content of a construct shows cross-time changes in: people's rank-order stability, the content's level on the construct, and how strongly the content reflects the construct. Cross-time changes in people's rank-order stability indicate changes in the degree of stability of individual differences in the construct across time, and they are examined with correlation of the content across time.

The content's level on the construct is similar to the inverse of frequency, prevalence, or base rate of the content. The content's level on the construct is examined with item difficulty (severity) in IRT or with intercepts in SEM. For example, the item "sets fires" has a higher item severity than the item "argues" because setting fires is less frequent than arguing.

How strongly the content reflects the construct, conceptually is the degree of a content's construct validity, and it is examined with item discrimination in IRT or with factor loadings in SEM. For example, the item "hits others" has a higher item discrimination than "eats ice cream" for the construct of externalizing problems because hitting others is more strongly related to the construct (compared to eating ice cream).

Externalizing problems are an example of a construct that changes in behavioral manifestation with development (F. R. Chen & Jaffee, 2015; J. L. Miller et al., 2009; Moffitt, 1993; Patterson, 1993; Petersen et al., 2015; Petersen & LeBeau, 2022; Wakschlag et al., 2010). The content of externalizing problems show changes in the magnitude of rank-order stability, changes in the content's level on the construct, and changes in how strongly the construct reflect the construct. For example, inattention shows increases in the magnitude of rank-order stability with age (Arnett et al., 2012). Drinking alcohol becomes more frequent in adolescence compared to childhood, so its item severity decreases. Threatening other people is more strongly associated with externalizing problems in adolescence than in early childhood (Lubke et al., 2018). Moreover, externalizing content, including disobedience and

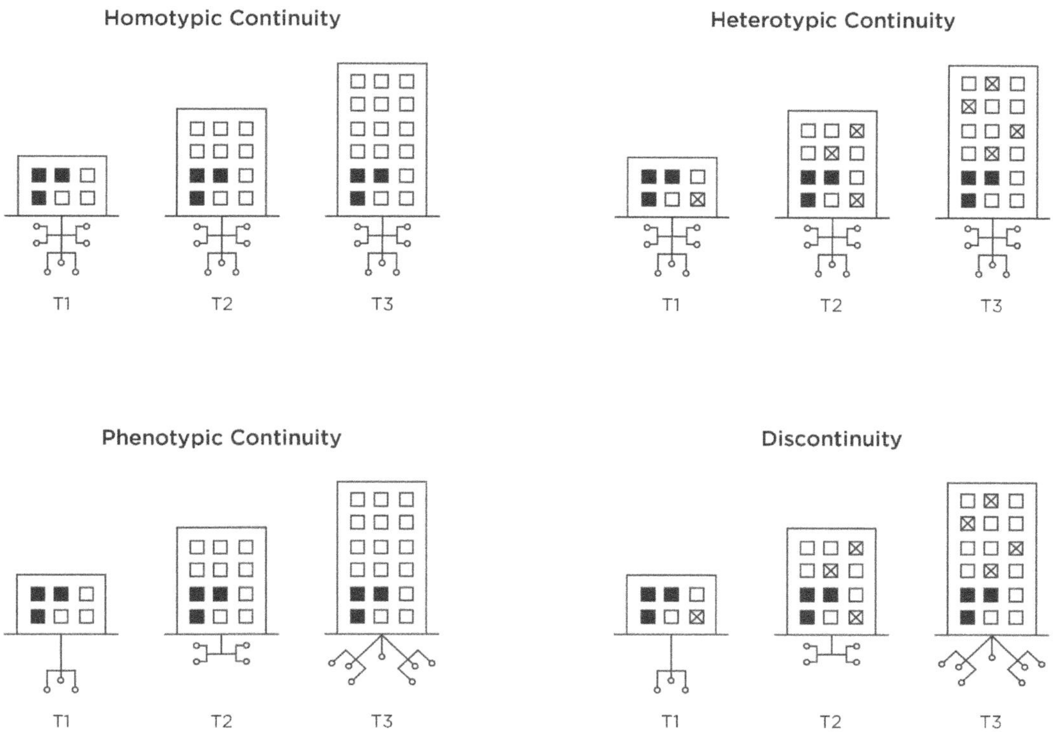

FIGURE 22.12 The Three Types of Continuity in Addition to Discontinuity in the Form of a 2 (Behavioral Manifestation, Underlying Processes) × 2 (Same Versus Different Across Time) Latin Square. 'T1,' 'T2,' and 'T3' reflect time points 1, 2, and 3, respectively. The illustrations above the lines are buildings, representing the surface structure (i.e., behavioral manifestation). The illustrations below the lines depict the underlying processes supporting the buildings at each time point. The squares on the buildings are windows. The black windows represent content facets that are active across all time points (i.e., age-common content). The windows that contain Xs represent content facets that are active at some but not all time points (i.e., age-unique content). The white windows represent content facets that are inactive, and therefore they are not part of the construct at that time point. The increasing size of the buildings at later time points reflects growth with development. The top row of the Latin square involves the same underlying processes across time, whereas the bottom row involves different underlying proccesses across time. The left column of the Latin square involves the same behavioral manifestation across time, whereas the right column involves a different behavioral manifestation across time. Homotypic continuity (top left) describes the same behavioral manifestation with the same underlying process (i.e., construct) across development. Heterotypic continuity (top right) describes the same underlying process with a different behavioral manifestation across development. Phenotypic continuity (or functional discontinuity) (bottom left) describes the same behavior with different underlying processes across development. Discontinuity (bottom right) describes different behavioral manifestations with different underlying processes across development. Thus, in both homotypic continuity and heterotypic continuity, the active content facets reflect the same construct or underlying process across time, whereas in phenotypic continuity and discontinuity, the active content facets do not reflect the same construct across time. (Figure reprinted from Petersen et al. (2020), figure 1, p. 2. Petersen, I. T., Choe, D. E., & LeBeau, B. (2020). Studying a moving target in development: The challenge and opportunity of heterotypic continuity. *Developmental Review*, *58*, 100935. https://doi.org/10.1016/j.dr.2020.100935 Copyright ©Elsevier. Used with permission.)

biting, likely change in meaning with developoment. In childhood, disobedience could be an indicator of externalizing problems. In adulthood, disobedience could serve prosocial functions, including protesting against societally unjust actions, and thus it shows weaker construct validity for externalizing problems. In general, in early childhood, externalizing problems often manifest in overt forms, such as physical aggression and temper tantrums. Later in development, externalizing problems tends to manifest in covert forms, such as indirect aggression, relational aggression, and substance use (J. L. Miller et al., 2009).

In addition to externalizing problems, other constructs also likely show heterotypic continuity across development. For instance, internalizing problems may show heterotypic continuity (Weems, 2008; Weiss & Garber, 2003) such that anxiety precedes depression (Garber & Weersing, 2010). In addition, somatic complaints such as headaches, stomachaches, and heart pounding are more strongly associated with and more common in those with internalizing problems in childhood than adulthood (Petersen et al., 2018). Other constructs that show heterotypic continuity include inhibitory control (Petersen et al., 2016; Petersen, Bates, et al., 2021), substance use (Schulenberg & Maslowsky, 2009), sleep states (Blumberg, 2013), and temperament (Putnam et al., 2008). In addition, constructs that are typically assessed with different measures across ages also likely show heterotypic continuity, including language ability (Petscher et al., 2018), nonverbal ability (McArdle & Grimm, 2011), working memory (McArdle et al., 2009), and academic skills (Tong & Kolen, 2007). In sum, many constructs show heterotypic continuity.

22.8.2 The Problem

Heterotypic continuity poses challenges for longitudinal assessment. According to the maxim, "what we know depends on how we know it". If a construct changes in manifestation across time, and the measures do not align with the changing manifestation, the scores will not validly assess individuals' growth. Failing to account for heterotypic continuity leads to misidentified trajectories of people's growth (F. R. Chen & Jaffee, 2015) and to trajectories that are less able to detect people's change (Petersen et al., 2018; Petersen, LeBeau, et al., 2021). Thus, it is important that our measurement and statistical schemes account for heterotypic continuity when a construct changes in manifestation across time. These measurement and statistical schemes are discussed below.

22.8.3 Ways to Assess a Construct Across Development

There are three ways of assessing a construct across development:

1. All possible content
2. Only the common content
3. Only the construct-valid content

Assume content A is construct-valid at T1, content B is content-valid at T1 and T2, and content C is content-valid at T2. All possible content would assess: ABC at T1, ABC at T2. Only the common content would assess: B at T1, B at T2. Only the construct-valid content would assess: AB at T1, BC at T2. A depiction of assessing only the construct-valid content is in Figure 22.13.

22.8.3.1 All Possible Content

There are advantages and disadvantages of each. Advantages of using all possible content include that it is comprehensive and allows examining change in each content facet. However,

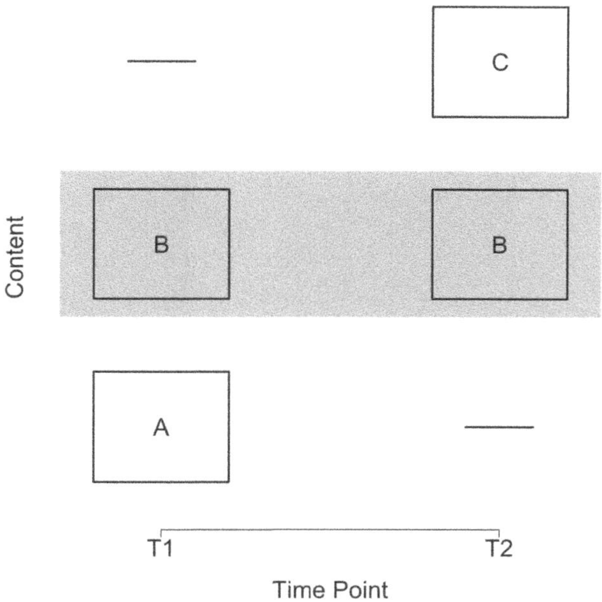

FIGURE 22.13 Using Only the Construct-Valid Content at Each Age. Content set A corresponds to content that is construct-valid at only T1. Content set B corresponds to content that is construct-valid at both T1 and T2. Content set C corresponds to content that is construct-valid at only T2. The *common content* (content set B) is highlighted in gray. The three approaches to assessing a construct over time are as follows: (1) using *all possible content* across all ages: ABC at T1 and T2, (2) using *only common content* across all ages: B at T1 and T2, or (3) using *only construct-valid content* at each age: AB at T1 and BC at T2. (Figure reprinted from Petersen, LeBeau, et al. (2021), figure 1, p. e3. Petersen, I. T., LeBeau, B., & Choe, D.E. (2021). Creating a developmental scale to account for heterotypic continuity in development: A simulation study. *Child Development*, *92*(1), e1–e19. https://doi.org/10.1111/cdev.13433 Copyright ©John Wiley & Sons. Used with permission.)

it also has key disadvantages. First, it is inefficient and assesses lots of items. Second, it could assess developmentally inappropriate content. And in the case of heterotypic continuity, it assesses content that lacks construct validity, i.e., there are item intrusions.

22.8.3.2 Only the Common Content

Advantages of using only the common content include that it is efficient and may exclude developmentally inappropriate content. Moreover, it permits examining consistent content across ages. However, it also has key disadvantages. First, it results in fewer items and a loss of information. In particular, it may involve a systematic loss of content that reflects very low or very high levels on the construct. Third, and due to the loss of information, it may be less sensitive to developmental change. And in the case of heterotypic continuity, it assesses content that lacks content validity because all important facets of the construct are not assessed—i.e., there are item gaps.

22.8.3.3 Only the Construct-Valid Content

There are disadvantages to using only the construct-valid content. First, it is more time-intensive than assessing only the common content. Second, it uses a different measure across time, which can pose challenges to ensuring scores across time are comparable. Nevertheless, the approach has important advantages. First, it is more efficient than using all possible content. Second, it retains content validity and construct validity. And in the case of heterotypic continuity, it is recommended. Developmental theory requires that we account for changes in the construct's expression!

Many measures are used outside the age range for which they were designed and validated to use. Many measures for children and adolescents are little more than downward extensions of those developed for use with adults (Hunsley & Mash, 2007). Use of the same measure across ages does not ensure measurement equivalence. The problem is that even if the same measure is used across ages, the measure may lack construct validity at some ages. Thus heterotypic continuity may require different measures at different ages to retain construct validity. But, then there is the challenge of how to assess change when using different measures across time.

22.8.4 Accounting for Heterotypic Continuity

To account for heterotypic continuity, it is recommended to use different measures across time. Specifically, it is recommended to use (only) the construct-valid content at each age when the content is valid for assessing the construct. To ensure scores are comparable across time, despite the differing measures, it is important to take steps to ensure statistical and theoretical equivalence of scores across time.

22.8.4.1 Ensuring Statistical Equivalence

Historically, there have been various attempts to handle different measures across time to ensure statistical equivalence of scores—i.e., that measures are on the same mathematical metric.

22.8.4.1.1 Age-norming

Age-norming includes standardized scores (e.g., T scores, z scores, standard scores) and percentile ranks. However, as discussed in Section 22.3, standardized scores prevent observing individuals' or groups' absolute change over time. Moreover, despite putting scores on the same mathematical metric, they do not ensure scores are on the same conceptual metric. Thus, age-norming is not recommended for putting different measures onto the same score to account for heterotypic continuity and examine individuals' growth.

22.8.4.1.2 Average or proportion scores

Average and proportion scores account for the different numbers of items in each measure. However, average and proportion scores assume that measures do not differ in difficulty or discrimination. Thus, average and proportion scores are not recommended to account for heterotypic continuity and examine individuals' growth.

22.8.4.1.3 Developmental scaling

A third approach to ensure statistical equivalence of measures is developmental scaling, which is also called vertical scaling (see Figure 22.14) and is a form of data harmonization. In developmental scaling, measures that differ in difficulty and discrimination are placed on the same scale using the common content. The common content sets the scale, but all content (including both age-common content and age-differing content) estimate each person's score on that scale. There are several approaches to developmental scaling, including Thurstone scaling, factor analysis, and IRT.

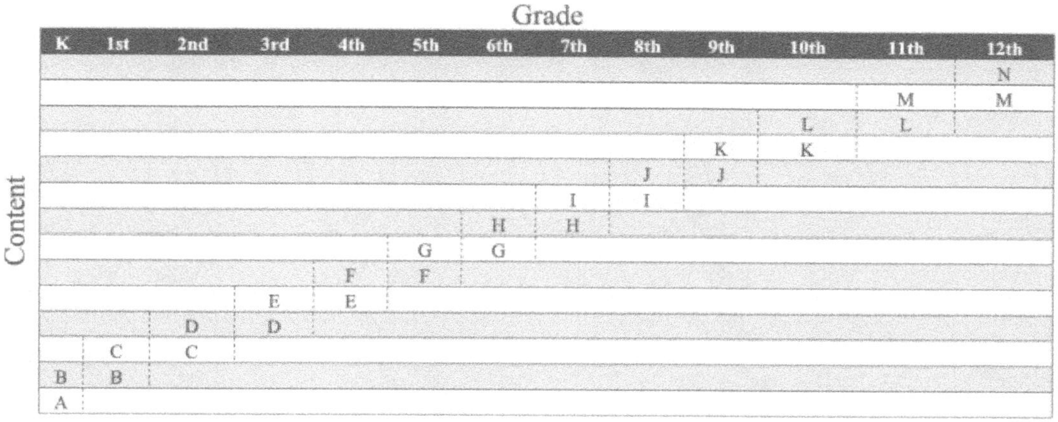

FIGURE 22.14 Illustrative Example of a Vertical Scaling Design That Uses Common Content to Link the Different Measures at Adjacent Ages to be on the Same Scale. For example, content set B is administered at both kindergarten and 1st grade, and is the common content used to link scores at 1st grade to the same scale as kindergarten scores. Content set A is the unique content at kindergarten; content set C is the unique content at 1st grade (but it is common content with content set C at 2nd grade). The unique content represents age-specific manifestations of the construct. The procedure of linking measures that differ in difficulty to be on the same scale is called vertical scaling (as opposed to horizontal scaling) because the measures, especially in educational settings, tend to increase in difficulty with age (relative to a given level of ability; as depicted above with the upward-trend). Thus, vertical scaling is particularly useful for linking different measures across ages to be on the same scale. Horizontal scaling, by contrast, links different measures that have the same difficulty (commonly at the same age). To better align with the breadth of constructs in developmental psychology, we use the term 'developmental scaling' instead of vertical scaling to refer to putting measures across development on the same scale. (Figure reprinted from Petersen et al. (2020), figure 3, p. 9. Petersen, I. T., Choe, D. E., & LeBeau, B. (2020). Studying a moving target in development: The challenge and opportunity of heterotypic continuity. *Developmental Review, 58*, 100935. https://doi.org/10.1016/j.dr.2020.100935 Copyright ©Elsevier. Used with permission.)

Thurstone scaling aligns the percentile scores of two measures based on z scores on the common content. It is an observed score approach. An example of Thurstone scaling is provided by Petersen et al. (2018).

Factor analysis allows estimation of a latent variable using different content over time. An example of a factor analysis approach to developmental scaling is provided by S. Wang et al. (2013). IRT finds scaling parameters that put people's scores from the different measures on the same metric, and it links the measures' scales based on the difficulty and discrimination of the common content. Examples of an IRT approach to developmental scaling are provided by Petersen et al. (2018), Petersen, LeBeau, et al. (2021), Petersen & LeBeau (2021), and Petersen & LeBeau (2022).

The IRT approach to developmental scaling is depicted in Figure 22.15.

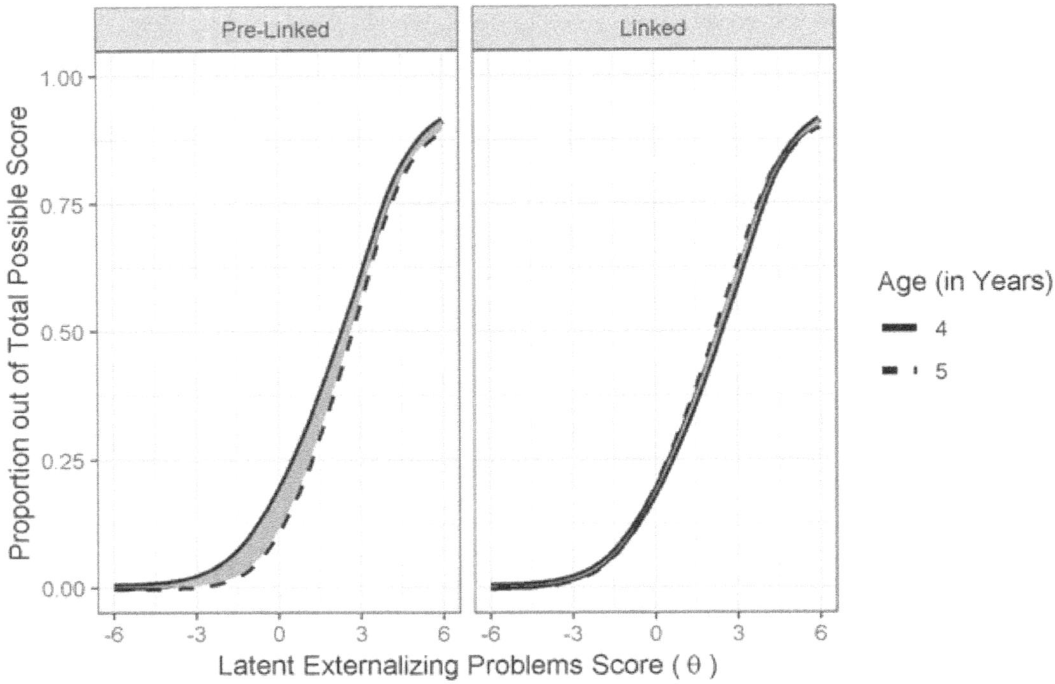

FIGURE 22.15 Effect of Linking the Latent Externalizing Problems Scores, θ, Across Ages, Using Mother-Reported Externalizing Problems at Ages 4 and 5 as an Example. The left panel illustrates the test characteristic curves representing the model-implied proportion out of total possible scores across the latent externalizing problems score at age 4 and 5, before the linking process. The right panel illustrates the test characteristic curves after the linking process. The shading between the ages 4 and age 5 test characteristic curves represents differences between the two test characteristic curves in terms of discrimination and/or severity, where larger differences reflect scores that are less comparable. Linking minimizes differences between the discrimination and severity of the common items. Discrimination is depicted by the steepness of the slope at the inflection point of the test characteristic curve. Severity is represented by the value on the x-axis at the inflection point of the test characteristic curve. The left panel indicates that the externalizing problem items showed higher severity at age 5 than at age 4. The right panel shows considerably smaller differences between the two test characteristic curves, which provides empirical evidence that the linking successfully placed the latent externalizing problem scores across age on a more comparable scale (i.e., more similar discrimination and severity of the common items). (Figure reprinted from Petersen & LeBeau (2021), figure 1, p. 7. Petersen, I. T., & LeBeau, B. (2021). Language ability in the development of externalizing behavior problems in childhood. *Journal of Educational Psychology*, *113*(1), 68–85. https://doi.org/10.1037/edu0000461 Copyright ©American Psychological Association. Used with permission.)

22.8.4.2 Ensuring Theoretical Equivalence

A number of pieces of evidence can provide support for the theoretical equivalence of measures. The goal is for the measures to have construct validity invariance—the measure should assess the same construct across time. The content that is assessed at each age should be based on theory. The assessed content should reflect the same construct at relevant ages—i.e., the content should show construct validity at each age it is assessed. Second, the content should adequately sample all aspects of construct—i.e., the content should show content validity. Second, assuming the construct is thought to be relatively stable, the measures should show test–retest reliability, at least in the short term. In addition, the measures should show convergent and discriminant validity. Furthermore, the measures assessed should show a similar factor structure across time, based on factor analysis. In addition, the measures should have high internal consistency reliability.

22.8.5 Are There Measures That Can Span the Lifespan?

There are measures that attempt to span the lifespan, including the NIH Toolbox (Weintraub et al., 2013) and the Minnesota Executive Function Scale (Carlson & Zelazo, 2014). However, we would argue that a single (non-adaptive) measure would not be able to validly assess the same construct across development if the construct shows heterotypic continuity. The content must change with changes in the construct's expression in order to remain valid for the construct given its changing behavioral manifestation.

Adaptive testing may help to achieve this goal. However, just because something is on the same mathematical metric does not mean it is on the same conceptual metric. The same challenge can be relevant for many different types of data, including questionnaire items, reaction time, event-related potentials (ERPs), electrocardiography (ECG/EKG), and functional magnetic resonance imaging (fMRI).

22.8.6 Why Not Just Study Development in a Piecewise Way?

If heterotypic continuity poses such challenges, why not just study development in a piecewise way? Although there can be benefits to examining development in a piecewise way, relying on a fixed set of content restricts our ability to see growth over a longer time and our ability to understand key developmental transitions. The pathways to outcomes can be just as important as the outcomes themselves. Consistent with the principle of *multifinality*, the same genetic and environmental influences can lead to different outcomes for different people. Conversely, consistent with the principle of *equifinality*, different genetic and environmental influences can lead to the same outcome for different people.

Longitudinal studies allow understanding antecedent-consequent effects, better estimation of change than difference scores derived from two time points, and separating age-related from cohort effects.

22.8.7 Why Not Just Study Individual Behaviors?

If higher-order constructs show heterotypic continuity, why not just study individual behaviors? Individual behaviors can also show changes in meaning. Moreover, there is utility in examining constructs rather than individual behaviors. Theoretical constructs have better psychometric properties, including better reliability than individual behaviors due to the principle of aggregation (Rushton et al., 1983). Moreover, constructs are theoretically and empirically derived. You can always reduce to a lower-level unit, and this reductionism can result in a loss of utility.

22.8.8 Summary

In summary, it is important to pay attention to whether constructs change in expression across development. Use different measures across time to align with changes in the manifestation of the construct. Use developmental scaling approaches to link different measures onto the same scale. Use theoretical considerations to ensure the measures reflect the same construct across development. In doing so, we will be better able to study development across the lifespan.

22.9 Conclusion

Repeated measurement is a design feature that can provide stronger tests of causality compared to concurrent associations. By repeatedly assessing multiple constructs, we can examine lagged associations that control for prior levels of the outcome and that simultaneously test each direction of effect. There are many important considerations for assessing change. The inference of change is strengthened to the extent that (a) the magnitude of the difference between the scores at the two time points is large, (b) the measurement error at both time points is small, (c) the measure has the same meaning and is on a comparable scale at each time point, (d) the differences across time are not likely to be due to potential confounds of change such as practice effects, cohort effects, and time-of-measurement effects. Difference scores, though widely used, can have limitations because they can be less reliable than each of the individual measures that compose the difference score. Instead of using traditional difference scores to represent change, consider other approaches such as autoregressive cross-lagged models, latent change score models, or growth curve models.

There are a variety of types of research designs based on combinations of age, period, and cohort: cross-sectional, cross-sectional sequences, time-lag, longitudinal, and longitudinal sequences, such as time-sequential, cross-sequential, and cohort-sequential designs. Which research design you select should depend on which change function you are most interested in: age, cohort, or time of measurement. However, any single research design has either age, cohort, or time of measurement confounded, so the strongest inferences come from inferences drawn from more than one research design.

When considering people's change, it is important to consider changes in the behavioral manifestation of constructs, known as heterotypic continuity. Heterotypic continuity can be identified as changes in the factor structure (i.e., content) of a construct across time. Use different measures across time to align with changes in the manifestation of the construct. Use developmental scaling to link different measures onto the same scale. Use theoretical considerations to ensure the measures reflect the same construct across development.

22.10 Suggested Readings

Petersen et al. (2020); Hertzog & Nesselroade (2003)

23

Assessment of Cognition

23.1 Overview

Cognitive-behavioral therapy (CBT) is the most effective treatment we have for many mental health conditions, especially depression and anxiety. The cognitive therapy component of CBT assumes that thoughts mediate the influences of the environment on emotions and behavioral responses. In general, cognitions and cognitive processes play a key role in many psychological theories. Therefore, cognitions and distorted cognitions are assumed to be a key construct to assess. However, there are many challenges to cognitive assessment. Some consider cognitions to be fictitious entities or epiphenomenal to people's experience—i.e., that is, they are not a causal process, but rather they are a by-product of neural and biological processes.

23.2 Aspects of Cognition Assessed

Multiple aspects of cognition can be assessed, including cognitive products, processes, and structures or organization. Cognitive products include a person's conscious thoughts or imaginal images. Cognitive processes include how a person transforms the environmental input and how they take meaning from it. Cognitive structures and organization include the hypothesized structures that a person has to guide information processing.

Consider an example of a person with an anxiety disorder. Cognitive products for the person may include having the thought, "I'm going to make a fool of myself, and everyone will think I'm stupid". The person's cognitive processes may involve the overestimation of personal risk. The person's cognitive structures may include "danger" schemas that, when activated, lead to attention bias toward threat stimuli. Though, this finding is under question because of challenges to the reliability of the dot-probe task, which has been frequently used to examine attentional bias.

23.3 Approaches to Assessing Cognition

The general approaches to assessing cognition include endorsement methods and production methods. Endorsement methods for assessing cognition contain a predetermined set of thoughts that participants identify or rate, such as a checklist. Using production methods, participants generate or recall their thoughts, i.e., the method involves free response. The psychometric status is currently stronger for endorsement methods; however, increasing attention is being given to production methods. Approaches to assessing cognition are reviewed by Dunkley et al. (2019).

23.3.1 Self-Reports of Cognition

Self-reports of cognition can either be in written or interview format and comprise most of the cognitive assessment techniques that are regularly used in clinical practice. Few of the other approaches to assessing cognition are used routinely in clinical practice. In a self-report of cognition, the participant must reflect on and report about their own cognitive style. Thus, self-report of cognition involves introspection.

Self-reports of cognition are still used in CBT, to learn about people's cognitive styles, their attributions to life events or a specific negative event, and their expectancies. Expectancies include, for instance, what the person anticipates happening.

23.3.1.1 Pros

Pros of self-reports of cognition include:

- They are cheap, easy to score and administer, and are able to be useful in clinical practice.
- They are sensitive to treatment effects. Cognitive therapy advocates would argue that changes in cognitions mediate treatment changes (i.e., they are thought to be a causal mechanism that explains how therapy works).
- They are standardized, normed, and have been psychometrically validated.

23.3.1.2 Cons

Despite the fact that these techniques are so popular, there are still some major drawbacks to these approaches. Cons of self-reports of cognition include:

- They require a participant to have insight into their cognitions that they can report on—such insight is not always typical. Nisbett & Wilson (1977) published a classic study titled, "Telling more than we can know: Verbal reports on mental processes". The study was based on the idea that people believe they were thinking particular things; however, they reported thoughts on things that would not have been possible for them to know. Findings such as these challenge the validity of self-reported cognition.
- They require a person to reflect upon their cognitions, retrospectively recalling what they were thinking in various situations.
- At least in the written format, which is often used as an endorsement method, participants are limited to responding to the experimenter-generated choice options—which can lead people into having certain thoughts and make people endorse thoughts that they did not actually have.

23.3.2 Think-Aloud Approaches (Thought Listing)

In think-aloud approaches, the participant is asked to verbalize their cognitions in the form of a continuous monologue while performing some task, and responses are recorded for later evaluation. In this way, thoughts are assessed concurrently with their occurrence. In some approaches, such as Articulated Thoughts in Simulated Situations (ATSS), thoughts are assessed in simulated situations that are geared towards eliciting certain emotions—the "situations" can be presented in video, audiotape, or virtual reality format. In a think-aloud approach, the participant lists their thoughts, so the approach is also called "thought listing".

The purpose of think-aloud approaches is to avoid retrospection, and to create a situation in the lab that resembles a real-world situation to see what thoughts or what stream of thoughts are generated. Think-aloud approaches are reviewed by Davison et al. (1997).

23.3.2.1 Examples

Examples of think-aloud assessments of cognition include video replay and private speech.

23.3.2.1.1 Video replay

Video replay is also called videotape thought reconstruction. In videotape thought reconstruction, the examiner video records the interaction, then replays the video for the examinee, and asks the examinee what they were thinking during that moment. It is more proximal than retrospective report. The act of re-watching a video of oneself can be strange, and there is commonly reactivity to that.

23.3.2.1.2 Private speech

Another example of think-aloud cognition is children's private speech. Young children sometimes talk out loud to themselves to guide their behavior, and the speech is not serving a communicative function. This is known as private or self-directed speech. Private speech is most common among 2- to 7-year-olds, and it provides insight into their cognition, often while performing a challenging task.

23.3.2.2 Pros

Pros of think-aloud approaches include:

- Participants are asked to report on cognitions at the same time or just after the thoughts are occurring, so they are less sensitive to retrospective recall bias.
- Responses are not limited to experimenter-selected choices—all cognitions can be assessed. The constraints are made in terms of how the thoughts are coded and analyzed by the experimenter, not in terms of the unstructured and open-ended thoughts that the participant can provide.
- Specific situations of interest to the research team can be explored. For example, the examiner can examine the respondent in situations that are thought to evoke particular cognitive processes, including situations that might be impractical due to low frequency or that are unethical to assess in their natural context. For example, an examiner could examine a person's self-reported thoughts in response to social criticism for someone with social anxiety.

23.3.2.3 Cons

Cons of think-aloud approaches include:

- Performance is susceptible to observer effects. Observer effects are changes in the person's response because they are being watched or recorded. That is, response biases may be present because the person's responses are not anonymous.
- Social desirability bias: people may censor negative or disturbing thoughts and may describe their thoughts in a way that portrays themselves in a more positive light.
- It can be difficult to generate the thoughts. There are individual differences in people's awareness of their cognitions.

- Think-aloud approaches can interrupt the thought flow—we think faster than we can speak, so verbalizing thoughts can alter the thoughts. That is, talking about thoughts interferes with the task itself.
- It can be difficult to get a whole narrative of thoughts from think-aloud approaches.
- It can be difficult to code the qualitative thoughts and reduce them down to meaningful data. And coders may attribute different meaning to a thought than was intended by the respondent.
- Think-aloud approaches tend to be lower in ecological validity because they typically occur in the lab rather than in a naturalistic context.

23.3.3 Random Thought Sampling

The purpose of thought sampling is to quantify characteristics or aspects of thinking in an ecologically valid context. By ecologically valid, we mean that the situation closely represents the specific situations under which the person usually exists. In a random thought sampling procedure, participants are given a beeper or some other device that beeps randomly. When the person hears the beep, they must record what they are doing and what they are thinking—either quantitatively or qualitatively. The person hears a beep, and jots down the thought they were having when the beep occurred, so it is retrospective back a second.

In the experience sampling method (ESM), the examiner can also ask participants to report the context in which the experience occurred. This can be helpful for those with schizophrenia who are hallucinating to help link the hallucinations to particular situations or contexts. Thought sampling and ESM are described by Hurlburt (1997).

23.3.3.1 Pros

Pros of random thought sampling include:

- The delay of recall is instantaneous—hence participants are not forced to recall what they were thinking.
- The situations are ecologically valid in that they are occurring in situations that the person actually experiences, rather than a lab.
- Random thought sampling gets at what people are actually thinking about rather than what they think they are thinking about.
- Random thought sampling is better able to detect fluctuations in thoughts than retrospective approaches, and it is better able to detect co-variation with other processes, such as mood.
- Random thought sampling involves less interference with the interaction. Presumably, the "flow" of a situation is not interrupted; although it very well might be.
- A client's reactivity could show therapeutic benefit.

23.3.3.2 Cons

Cons of random thought sampling include:

- It assesses narrow slices of time.
- Because it assesses narrow slices of time, it is hard to capture the whole sequence of events.
- It is odd to be interrupted by a beeper.
- Random thought sampling could elicit reactivity such that thinking about one's thoughts could change thoughts or create thoughts.

- Random thought sampling only accesses the contents of the consciousness, like the approaches discussed earlier. That is, the respondent has to be aware of the thoughts in order to write them down. There are likely many cognitive processes that nobody is aware of.
- The written-down thoughts have to be coded.
- Because random thought sampling typically occurs in an ecologically valid context, the experimenter has less experimental control of the situation, context, and stimuli. Consequently, the experimenter is less likely to discover relations between rare but theoretically important processes.

23.3.4 Cognitive Science Approaches

Cognitive science approaches to assessing cognition include a range of non-mutually exclusive approaches, including performance-based measures, cognitive modeling, and cognitive neuroscience approaches. These cognitive science approaches are different from the approaches described earlier in that they do not rely on respondents reporting their thoughts. Cognitive science approaches try to assess a person's cognitions based on behavior or neural functioning. For instance, using performance-based measures and cognitive modeling, the approaches are based on behavioral performance and then use a model to try to estimate what is happening cognitively—the participants just have to engage and process information.

23.3.4.1 Performance-Based Measures

Performance-based measures are used to assess many domains and constructs, including attention, executive functions, inhibitory control, memory, decision-making, categorization, etc. Examples of performance-based measures include the Stroop test, Iowa Gambling Task (IGT), and implicit cognition tasks such as the Implicit Association Test. In many performance-based tasks, respondents' accuracy and reaction times are evaluated when there are competing demands.

23.3.4.2 Cognitive Modeling

Cognitive modeling attempts to decompose behavioral performance into different indices that reflect different sub-processes, such as working memory and processing speed. Behavior is complex and is influenced by many different processes, such as cognitive, motivational, and response processes. If you observe that a person shows behavioral deficits, it can be helpful to know what specific process is responsible for the behavioral deficits.

It can be difficult to use multiple behavioral tasks to decompose basic processes because any task taps multiple cognitive processes, including likely overlapping processes, and each is affected by measurement error. Cognitive modeling seeks to identify the "hidden processes" that underlie behavioral performance in complex tasks. Cognitive modeling generally requires a lot of data—for example, many trials—but it can be used with small sample sizes.

Busemeyer & Stout (2002) provide an example of cognitive modeling of the IGT to identify the sub-processes that account for behavioral performance deficits in Huntington's Disease. The IGT attempts to simulate real-life decision-making based on learning from decisions that have different probabilities of rewards and punishments. In the IGT, participants are presented with four virtual decks on a computer screen. They pick a card each turn, and have to select from one of the four decks. Some decks reward the player more often and some decks penalize the player more often. The player has to figure out which decks to pick from based on statistical probabilities.

Busemeyer & Stout (2002) compared and tested competing models for the task based on different theoretical possibilities. With cognitive models, the aim is to achieve a combination of accuracy and parsimony (simplicity). Busemeyer & Stout (2002) selected a model with three parameters: a cognitive process, a motivational process, and a response mechanism. A cognitive process was examined with an updating rate parameter, which describes a person's memory for past sequences produced by each deck. A motivational process was examined with the attention weight parameter, which describes the amount of attention a person allocated to gains versus losses. A response mechanism, such as recklessness and/or impulsivity, was assessed with threshold parameter, which describes the sensitivity of the choice mechanisms to the expectancies.

Busemeyer & Stout (2002) found that people with Huntington's Disease showed deficits in the updating rate and threshold parameters but not in the attention weight parameter. In particular, the people with Huntington's Disease were more reactive to recent information and forgot old information more rapidly, and they became less sensitive with training and produced more random behavior. But people with Huntington's Disease did not show deficits in how much attention they allocated to losses.

Other examples of clinically relevant cognitive model include cognitive modeling approaches to better understand cognitive processes in sexual aggression and eating disorders (Treat et al., 2007).

23.3.4.3 Challenges

Despite the advantages of not relying on participants' recall of their thoughts, there are challenges to using cognitive science approaches to assess cognition.

23.3.4.3.1 Reliability of difference scores

One challenge related to the use of performance-based assessment of cognition is that many such tasks involve difference scores. A difference score involves the subtraction of one score from another score. In performance-based assessments of cognition, many tasks subtract scores, especially accuracy or reactive time, in one condition from scores in another condition. For example, the most-often used dependent variable in the Flanker task, Stroop task, stop-signal task, and dot-probe task is a difference score. For instance, in the Flanker task, the reaction time to incongruent (interference) stimuli is subtracted from the reaction time to congruent stimuli.

The problem is that difference scores tend to be lower in reliability than other scores because differences depend on the reliability of both indices in the subtraction, as described in Section 3.5.8. Difference scores tend to be lower in reliability than each of the indices that compose it, especially when the two indexes are correlated. Therefore, scores on these tasks tend to be less reliable than scores on other tasks that do not involve difference scores. To be reliable, difference scores require high reliability of the individual indices compared to the correlation between them. Otherwise said, the more two things are the same thing, the more likely that subtracting one from the other leaves measurement error rather than construct variance.

Because of the reliance of difference scores in the dot-probe task, Rodebaugh et al. (2016) challenged whether attention bias toward threat exists or whether it is stable across time for those with anxiety.

23.3.4.3.2 Reliability paradox

Another challenge with performance-based assessments of cognition is known as the reliability paradox (Hedge et al., 2018). Many basic cognitive paradigms, such as the Flanker task, were designed for detecting normative cognitive effects. However, a downside of that is that not all of them are good for assessing individual differences. That is, their scores are not reliable for a particular person. Low reliability precludes making strong inferences and decisions about individuals and calls into question the validity of inferences regarding individual differences, or people's change, in scores on those tasks.

The *reliability paradox* is that despite some robust cognitive tasks showing well-established experimental effects, many of these tasks do not produce reliable individual differences, including the Flanker task, Stroop task, and stop-signal task, etc. Experimental effects become well-established, and therefore those tasks become widely used, when between-subject variability is low. However, low between-subject variability leads to low reliability of individual differences. The stability coefficient, i.e., test–retest reliability, an index of reliability of individual differences relies on a Pearson correlation. As described in Section 3.5.1.1.1, correlation requires variability: restricted range leads to weaker associations. When a measure has low between-subject variability, it prevents us from detecting consistent rank ordering of people across time. That is, the very reason such tasks produce robust and easily replicable experimental effects due to low between-person variability makes their use as correlational tools problematic. Moreover, the poor test–retest reliability of many performance-based assessments is exacerbated by the use of difference scores.

The implications of the reliability paradox are that many well-established approaches in experimental, cognitive, and neuropsychology may not translate well to the study of individual differences, even though the measures can be useful for making group-level inferences. It is important to know the reliability of your measures, especially when dealing with issues of trying to understand where a particular person stands on the construct relative to other people.

Unreliability and measurement error are threats to science and knowledge. Unreliability leads to false inferences and failures to replicate findings. As described in Section 4.6, and formalized with the attenuation formula (Equation (4.2)), associations with other variables are weakened to the extent that measurement error exists. If you know the degree of unreliability, you can account for it using the disattenuation formula (Equation (4.3)), to get more accurate estimates of the true associations with other variables.

It is important to test the reliability of your measures and report the reliability in papers. Continually work to improve the reliability of your measures. Ways to improve the reliability of measures are described in Section 3.14. Another way to improve reliability of scores is to aggregate multiple measures using a multimethod approach in structural equation modeling.

23.3.5 Cognitive Neuroscience Approaches

Another branch of cognitive science approaches includes cognitive neuroscience approaches. For example, cognitive neuroscience approaches connect cognitive processes to measures of brain functioning, such as electroencephalography (EEG) or functional magnetic resonance imaging (fMRI). An example of linking cognitive processes to measures of brain functioning might be examining people's digit span in relation to fMRI measures. Cognitive neuroscience techniques are discussed in Chapter 19. Cognitive neuroscience is a high priority of the National Institute of Mental Health with their emphasis on the Research Domain Criteria (RDoC). RDoC seeks to assess the underlying substrates of illness across multiple levels of analysis and the neurodevelopmental trajectories rather than just behavioral symptoms, which are heterogeneous.

23.4 Conclusion

Multiple aspects of cognition can be assessed, including cognitive products, processes, and structures or organization. The general approaches to assessing cognition include endorsement methods and production methods. Cognitive assessments include self-report, think-aloud approaches, random thought sampling, performance-based measures, cognitive modeling, and cognitive neuroscience approaches. One challenge related to the use of performance-based assessment of cognition is that many such tasks involve difference scores, which tend to be lower in reliability than each of the indices that compose it. Another challenge with performance-based assessments of cognition is known as the reliability paradox that despite some robust cognitive tasks showing well-established experimental effects, many of these tasks do not produce reliable individual differences due to low between-subject variability and the use of difference scores.

23.5 Suggested Readings

Dunkley et al. (2019); Treat et al. (2007)

24

Cultural and Individual Diversity

Like ethics, considerations of cultural and individual diversity are relevant to all of our domains as psychologists, including (but not limited to) research, teaching, assessment, intervention, and supervision. Diverse samples provide stronger tests of theories and better generalizability of findings (external validity). In assessment, we need measures that provide us with the best information, and that are reliable and valid for all people we use them with. Diversity is a broad concept, and it spans many dimensions of differences among people.

24.1 Terminology

24.1.1 Diversity, Equity, and Inclusion

24.1.1.1 Diversity

Diversity refers to all aspects of differences between people. Diversity is a characteristic of a group, not a characteristic of an individual. Thus, a person is not diverse. There are many aspects of human difference, including but not limited to race, ethnicity, creed, color, sex, gender, gender identity, sexual orientation, socioeconomic status, language, culture, national origin, religion/spirituality, age, (dis)ability, military/veteran status, personality, political perspective, and associational preferences.

Having a diverse group (e.g., of participants, clients, patients, etc.) is insufficient. It is also important to make sure that we take steps for all groups to feel included (inclusion) and to thrive (equity).

24.1.1.2 Equity

Equity refers to fair and just practices and policies that ensure everyone can thrive. Equity is different from equality. *Equality* involves treating everyone equally (i.e., treating everyone the same). However, due to structural inequities—historic and current (e.g., structural racism and patriarchy)—some people are disadvantaged and marginalized more so than others. Structural racism refers to "the normalization and legitimization of an array of dynamics—historical, cultural, institutional, and interpersonal—that routinely advantage non-Latinx White persons while producing cumulative and chronic adverse outcomes for Black and other people with minoritized identities in housing, education, employment, health care, criminal justice, and psychology." (Byrd et al., 2021, p. 279). Patriarchal societies reflect society's long history of wage gaps, gender discrimination, violence against women, etc. Treating people equally (equality) does not allow everyone to thrive given these different experiences and unequal access to opportunities. Thus, equity seeks to help everyone thrive, including those who are marginalized with fewer access to opportunities.

24.1.1.3 Inclusion

Inclusion refers to providing a community where all members are and feel respected, have a sense of belonging, and are able to participate and achieve their potential.

24.1.2 Aspects of Difference

There are many aspects of difference. However, identifying labels to capture these differences can be challenging. "Asian" is an overly broad term. There are more than 4 billion people from Asian countries, and considerable heterogeneity. "Hispanic" is based on language (i.e., a person from a Spanish speaking country), whereas "Latino/a/x" and "African American" are based on geography (i.e., a person from a Latin American country). Traditional classifications of race/ethnicity by the National Institutes of Health miss groups that may be important to distinguish, including Arab, Middle Eastern, or North African (AMENA) populations.

Labels by the 2020 U.S. Census attempt to be more precise than traditional classifications of race and ethnicity by the National Institutes of Health. For the classification of "Hispanic, Latino, or Spanish origin" in the 2020 U.S. Census, see Figure 24.1. Notice how the question distinguishes between identities of people from (or whose ancestors were from) various countries, including Mexico, Puerto Rico, Cuba, etc.

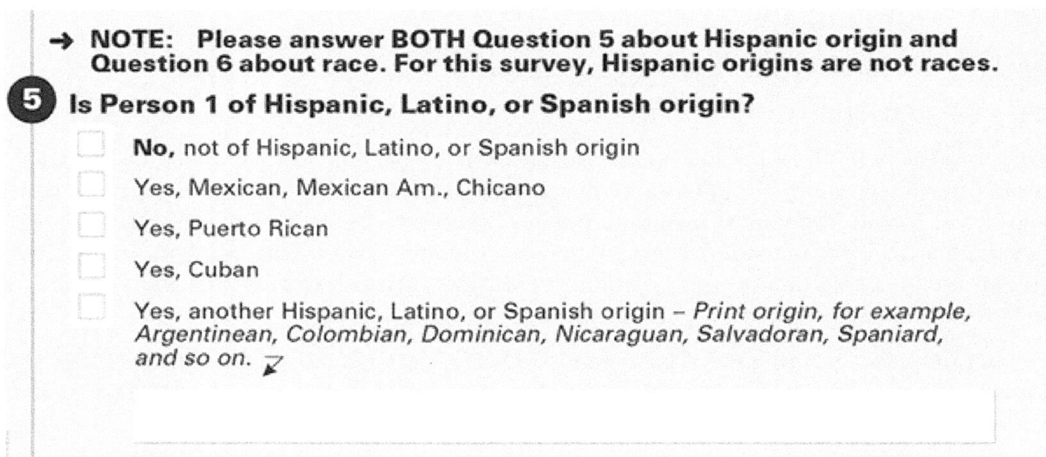
→ **NOTE: Please answer BOTH Question 5 about Hispanic origin and Question 6 about race. For this survey, Hispanic origins are not races.**

5 Is Person 1 of Hispanic, Latino, or Spanish origin?

- ☐ **No,** not of Hispanic, Latino, or Spanish origin
- ☐ Yes, Mexican, Mexican Am., Chicano
- ☐ Yes, Puerto Rican
- ☐ Yes, Cuban
- ☐ Yes, another Hispanic, Latino, or Spanish origin – *Print origin, for example, Argentinean, Colombian, Dominican, Nicaraguan, Salvadoran, Spaniard, and so on.*

FIGURE 24.1 Question Asking About One's Hispanic Origin in the 2020 U.S. Census. (Figure reprinted from the American Community Survey (2020): https://censusreporter.org/topics/race-hispanic/ [archived at https://perma.cc/LRW6-4JAJ])

For the classification of "Race" in the 2020 U.S. Census, see Figure 24.2. Notice how the question distinguishes between identities of people from (or whose ancestors were from) various countries, including India, China, Philippines, etc.

Society treats people differently based on factors that they are born into and are outside of their control, including their race and their family's socioeconomic status. Socioeconomic status refers to the social standing or class of an individual, and it is often assessed as a combination of education, income, occupation, access to resources, privilege, power, and control (Suzuki et al., 2013). There is also growing attention to neighborhood- and community-level factors associated with deprivation.

6 What is Person 1's race? *Mark (X) one or more boxes.*

- ☐ White
- ☐ Black or African Am.
- ☐ American Indian or Alaska Native — *Print name of enrolled or principal tribe.*
- ☐ Asian Indian
- ☐ Chinese
- ☐ Filipino
- ☐ Other Asian – *Print race, for example, Hmong, Laotian, Thai, Pakistani, Cambodian, and so on.*
- ☐ Japanese
- ☐ Korean
- ☐ Vietnamese
- ☐ Native Hawaiian
- ☐ Guamanian or Chamorro
- ☐ Samoan
- ☐ Other Pacific Islander – *Print race, for example, Fijian, Tongan, and so on.*
- ☐ Some other race – *Print race.*

FIGURE 24.2 Question Asking About One's Race in the 2020 U.S. Census. (Figure reprinted from the American Community Survey (2020): https://censusreporter.org/topics/race-hispanic/ [archived at https://perma.cc/LRW6-4JAJ])

There are also many other important aspects of difference to assess when thinking about individual differences in behavior. For instance, one important aspect of difference is family structure. Family structure includes lots of components, such as whether the parent is a single parent or whether there are two parents, whether the parents are working parents or whether the family has a stay-at-home parent, and whether there are other family members (e.g., grandparents) in the household.

Another important aspect of diversity includes one's sex, gender identity, and gender expression. Sex is the person's gender that was assigned at birth, and includes male, female, and intersex. Gender identity is how one self-identifies in terms of their gender. Gender identity is a spectrum in terms of the degree to which a person identifies as a female/woman/girl, a male/man/boy, or other genders, in terms of personality, likes/dislikes, jobs/hobbies, and roles and expectations. The person's gender identity may be non-binary or genderqueer if they do not identify as a man or woman (e.g., genderfluid). When the person's sex assigned at birth and their gender identity are aligned, the person is cis-gender. When the person's sex assigned at birth and their gender identity are not aligned, the person is transgender. Gender expression deals with how the person's gender is expressed to others, including their appearance.

Another dimension of diversity is whether someone is from a rural versus urban area. People from rural areas may have less access to resources. Another aspect of diversity is refugee or immigrant status. Refugee and immigrant groups may have less access to resources and may have language barriers, in addition to difficulty finding work, and fear of deportation.

It is also important to consider diversity in terms of sexual orientation and sexual behaviors. There is a distinction between one's sexual orientation (e.g., lesbian, gay, bisexual, heterosexual, pansexual, asexual)—that is, who one is sexually or romantically attracted to—versus whom one has sex with (i.e., sexual behavior). There are also differences in terms of the degree of people's sexual risk taking and sexual aggression.

Ability and disability are other important facets of diversity, including learning disabilities. Additionally, there are important brain-related differences that lead people to interact and experience the world in different ways, as reflected in the term, neurodiversity. Neurodiversity can include differences related to autism and other conditions such as attention-deficit hyperactivity disorder.

Age is another important dimension of diversity. Consider the issue of heterotypic continuity. For example, externalizing problems look different at different ages and should be assessed in different ways with different measures at different ages (F. R. Chen & Jaffee, 2015; J. L. Miller et al., 2009; Moffitt, 1993; Patterson, 1993; Petersen et al., 2015; Petersen & LeBeau, 2022; Wakschlag et al., 2010).

Another important aspect of diversity is culture, which includes belief systems, value orientations, psychological processes, worldview, learned and transmitted beliefs, and practices (Suzuki et al., 2013). A person's culture has many facets, including but not limited to experiences related to geographic boundaries, language, religious belief, social class, gender, sexual orientation, and ability status (Suzuki et al., 2013). However, culture and one's related identities are dynamic and changing (Suzuki et al., 2013), which makes them challenging to assess. Culture tends to be ignored in psychological research relative to other facets of diversity, but culture is arguably the most important in terms of influencing behavior. Additional dimensions of difference include religion and spirituality.

Another aspect of diversity is intersectionality, the intersecting of multiple identities. Intersectionality deals with how the combination of various identities can combine to influence behavior and bias.

There are many other important aspects of difference, too. This was not an exhaustive list!

24.2 Assessing Cultural and Individual Diversity: Multicultural Assessment Frameworks

A review of frameworks for multicultural assessment is provided by L. M. Edwards et al. (2017).

24.2.1 The ADDRESSING Model

The *ADDRESSING* model (Hays, 2016) provides a framework to consider some of the commonly examined differences between people within a clinical context. ADDRESSING is an acronym that stands for:

- **A**ge and generational differences
- **D**evelopmental or other **D**isability
- **R**eligion and spiritual orientation
- **E**thnic and racial identity

- **S**ocioeconomic status
- **S**exual orientation
- **I**ndigenous heritage
- **N**ational origin
- **G**ender

These are important aspects of differences between people that can be helpful to understand when working with a client and how they self-identify. For instance, the therapist could ask the client how they self-identify in each of these domains and how their identity is meaningful to them. In addition to the aspects of diversity identified in ADDRESSING, there are other aspects of diversity and difference that may be worth considering, including but not limited to personality, culture, and political beliefs.

24.2.2 DSM-5 Cultural Formulation Interview

The Diagnostic and Statistical Manual of Mental Disorders (DSM) provides a framework for clinicians to organize cultural information about a client using the Cultural Formulation Interview (Lewis-Fernández et al., 2014). The Cultural Formulation Interview is a semi-structured interview and is available here: https://www.psychiatry.org/File%20Library/Psychiatrists/Practice/DSM/APA_DSM5_Cultural-Formulation-Interview.pdf (archived at https://perma.cc/3EWR-LGEN).

24.2.3 Multicultural Assessment Procedure

The Multicultural Assessment Procedure was developed by Ridley et al. (1998). The framework includes four phases:

1. Gather clinical data, including cultural data, through history taking and multiple methods for the purpose of formulating a case conceptualization
2. Interpret clinical and cultural data to formulate a hypothesis, while keeping in mind to:
   - differentiate the cultural data as being either idiosyncratic (i.e., unique to the individual client and would not necessarily be expected of other members of the client's culture) or culture-specific
   - consider base rates
   - differentiate dispositional from environmental stressors
   - differentiate clinically significant data from data that are not clinically significant
3. Incorporate cultural data with other clinical information to test the hypotheses by ruling out medical explanations and using appropriate assessments and testing
4. Arrive at a sound assessment decision (case conceptualization)

The procedure also includes debiasing strategies to minimize the likelihood of clinical judgment errors. Ridley et al. (2001) expanded on this framework in consideration of ethical issues in multicultural assessment.

24.2.4 Multicultural Assessment–Intervention Process

The Multicultural Assessment–Intervention Process was developed by R. H. Dana (1998). The process provides a flowchart for clinicians to conduct assessment by asking relevant questions about cultural orientation, type of assessment instrument (e.g., etic or emic), cultural formulation for diagnosis, and intervention approach (e.g., universal, culture-general, culture-specific, identity-specific, etc.). *Etic* assessments are culture-general, whereas *emic* assessments are culture-specific.

24.3 Assessments with Ethnic, Linguistic, and Culturally Diverse Populations

24.3.1 Methodological and Conceptual Challenges in Research

Methodological and conceptual challenges for conducting research with ethnic minorities are described by Okazaki & Sue (1995). Guidelines for conducting research with diverse groups are described by Burlew et al. (2019).

24.3.1.1 Use of Terms: Race, Ethnicity, Culture

Use of terminology with respect to race, ethnicity, and culture is a key challenge in assessment of diverse samples. Many people refer to race, ethnicity, and culture interchangeably, which reflects conceptual confusion. There is no definition of race, ethnicity, and culture that is universally agreed on (Okazaki & Sue, 1995). As described by Okazaki & Sue (1995), "the use of the term 'race' appears to imply biological factors, as races are typically defined by observable physiognomic features such as skin color, hair type and color, eye color, stature, facial features, and so forth" (p. 367). By contrast, ethnicity (ethnic status) has been defined as "an easily identifiable characteristic that implies a common cultural history with others possessing the same characteristic" (Eaton, 1980, p. 160). Ethnic identifiers for evaluating whether people share a "common cultural history" include racial, national, tribal, religious, linguistic, or cultural origin or background. Thus, race and ethnicity, though conceptually distinct, are related as race can be an ethnic identifier.

Researchers have argued that race designations are arbitrary (Helms et al., 2005), that race is a social, cultural, and/or political construct rather than a biological construct (Sternberg et al., 2005; Yudell et al., 2016), that race has no genetic basis (Yudell et al., 2016), that within-race differences are greater than between-race differences (Zuckerman, 1990), and that racial categories lack conceptual meaning (Helms et al., 2005). According to the American Anthropological Association (1998, p. 712), "physical variations in the human species have no meaning except the social ones that humans put on them". However, even though race does not appear to have a genetic or biological basis and therefore appears to be a social construct rather than a biological construct, racism as a social problem is real and is a major issue (Smedley & Smedley, 2005). People are born into different social reactions based on their race. Thus, race is important to consider from a perspective of racialized experiences and discrimination even if the racial categories do not represent underlying biological differences.

In terms of determining what to assess and analyze, it is important for the researcher to determine whether they are interested in evaluating race as a biological variable, ethnicity as a demographic variable, or an aspect of cultural experience as a psychological variable (Okazaki & Sue, 1995). Researchers often use race and/or ethnicity as proxy variables for psychological variables such as cultural values, self-concept, minority status, etc. However, race and ethnicity are distal to the variables that may be of most psychological interest. Some people identify their primary culture as being different from their self-identified ethnicity.

It is thus important to assess the psychological processes of interest, rather than merely relying on racial or ethnic categories as proxies.

Culture refers to a psychological variable: i.e., the social context. Researchers often group people together based on race or ethnicity with the implicit assumption that they share some cultural experience. According to Okazaki and Sue (1995), assumptions underlying the use of race or ethnicity in a study should be made explicit. Research should directly assess the underlying psychological variables associated with culture, such as different spiritual practices, that are hypothesized to produce the racial/ethnic/cultural differences. That is, it is generally best not to rely solely on race or ethnicity, which are imprecise, to classify people unless the goal is to classify people based on racialized reactions and experiences. Thus, the researcher can classify people according to race/ethnicity but can also examine the more proximal cultural variables that are thought to drive group-related differences.

24.3.1.2 Whether to Examine Individual Differences or Group Characteristics

One question the researcher should consider is whether they are interested in understanding individual differences or group characteristics. Both can be valuable and important questions to examine. However, researchers should not underestimate within-group heterogeneity (Okazaki & Sue, 1995). The greater the within-group heterogeneity, the less accurate predictions tend to be. Moreover, inferences at the group-level cannot necessarily be applied to the individual level; the confounding of an individual with the individual's culture leads to stereotyping (Okazaki & Sue, 1995), which should be avoided.

24.3.1.3 Selecting Participants

One question is which groups to include in the research design and in what proportion. For group-related comparisons, the researcher would need a large enough sample size for every group examined to have adequate power to identify group-related differences. If the researcher is interested in studying a particular group, a question is whether to use a comparison group. A comparison group can provide a basis of comparison to better interpret the findings in the group of interest. However, inclusion of a comparison group can add time, cost, and as a result may lead to achieving a smaller sample in the group of interest. Moreover, the group comparison approach has been criticized for reinforcing racial stereotypes, reinforcing Whites as the standard group and non-White behavior as deviant, and overlooking within-group variation (Okazaki & Sue, 1995). Thus, decisions about which groups to include, in what proportion, and whether to include a comparison group should be guided by the questions and purpose of the study. Practical considerations can come into play, and having a comparison group should not be considered the necessary default for all studies. Moreover, White groups should not be considered the default.

24.3.1.4 Ensuring Fair Group Comparisons

Another issue is how to achieve fair group comparisons. One approach is to match groups by selecting participants a priori to be similar on relevant, secondary characteristics such as demographic characteristics (e.g., age, sex, socioeconomic status) or other abilities (e.g., intelligence). The goal of matching is for participants to be as similar as possible in the relevant characteristics apart from their group classification. However, there are challenges to matching groups on all relevant characteristics. Another approach is to control for these secondary characteristics post hoc in the statistical analysis. Which variables to include as control variables is an important question that depends on the goal. A key question is which variables to match participants on. However, there is not an agreed-upon list of matching variables. Generally, researchers recommend controlling for social and demographic characteristics such as educational attainment, income level, and language fluency, when group-related differences exist on those variables and the researcher believes that such differences may moderate the associations of interest (Okazaki & Sue, 1995). When comparing Black and White participants, it is important to control for group differences in socioeconomic status, especially in the U.S.

In addition to main effects of group status, it may also be important to consider *interaction* effects of group status, consistent with an intersectionality approach. However, power to detect interactions tends to be weaker than power to detect main effects, both because of smaller effect sizes (https://statmodeling.stat.columbia.edu/2018/03/15/need-16-times-sample-size-estimate-interaction-estimate-main-effect, archived at https://perma.cc/E3KA-SGB7) and because of smaller sample sizes of the intersecting groups.

24.3.1.5 Sampling

Researchers face important questions with how to identify, sample, and recruit ethnic minority samples. Groups, such as ethnic groups, may be classified at a broad level (e.g., Latinx or Hispanic) or at a more specific level (e.g., Puerto Rican, Mexican American, etc.); however, these approaches do not need to be mutually exclusive. Researchers must also determine how to classify people of mixed racial or ethnic backgrounds. It is also important to note that it is an incorrect assumption that once people are identified as belonging to a particular ethnic-cultural group, that they share a common understanding of their own ethnicity or culture and identify with the ethnic-cultural group (Okazaki & Sue, 1995).

There are challenges of recruiting a sizeable sample size with specific ethnic-cultural groups (e.g., Japanese Americans). This is partly a challenge of small overall population size (e.g., American Indians). This is also partly a challenge of difficult-to-reach populations who are distrustful of science and researchers. Research has exploited under-privileged populations (e.g., the Tuskegee syphilis study in Black men), which has led to changes in the consent process to ensure that participation is voluntary. There may also be selection effects, such that the people who are willing to participate in research may differ in important ways from those less willing to participate in research, which is a challenge to generalizability. To address sample size challenges, researchers often combine data from multiple ethnic-cultural groups with some common origin. For instance, researchers might combine Chinese Americans, Japanese Americans, and Korean Americans into one group. Or, researchers might combine people from multiple tribal groups among American Indians. However, broadening the ethnic grouping increases the heterogeneity of the groups, so the researcher must decide which are the sources of variability that can and cannot be overlooked (Okazaki & Sue, 1995).

Much of the literature in general and on diversity, in particular, is from research on college students. There are limitations of conducting research on college students. College students are not representative of the broader population. Research using college students underestimates the population heterogeneity in terms of demographic and psychosocial diversity.

One goal of research is to learn findings that apply to the broader population, with the goal of having a representative sample, where the mean of the sample is approximately the same as the mean of the population. However, having a population-representative sample is not as useful for comparing differences between groups. To do this, we would need large samples of each group—e.g., equally weighted samples. Most research is on participants from WEIRD countries (Henrich et al., 2010): Western, educated, industrialized, rich, and democratic (WEIRD) societies. This further limits the potential generalizability of findings to different cultures.

Provide a thorough description of the sample and sampling methodology used. For instance, it can be helpful to describe participants on additional dimensions to race and ethnicity, including generational status, acculturation, self-identification, ethnic and cultural composition of the neighborhoods or communities, etc. (Okazaki & Sue, 1995). Acculturation deals with the change that individuals undergo due to contact with members of different cultures, and it includes strategies such as assimilation, separation, marginalization, and integration (Suzuki et al., 2013).

24.3.1.6 Establishing Equivalence of Measures Across Groups

Five key areas need to be empirically evaluated in using or adapting instruments across cultures or groups to reduce or eliminate cultural bias (Hunsley & Mash, 2007):

- Conceptual equivalence
- Linguistic (or translation) equivalence
- Psychological equivalence of the items
- Functional equivalence
- Metric and scalar equivalence (i.e., measurement invariance)

Conceptual equivalence refers to establishing that the construct has the same meaning across groups. Linguistic (or translation) equivalence refers to the measure having the same linguistic meaning in each language to which it has been translated. Best practices for establishing translation equivalence include having experts translate and back-translate the measure, comparing both the original and back-translated versions, and revising the translation accordingly (Okazaki & Sue, 1995). Psychological equivalence of the items deals with establishing that the psychological effect each item has for each group or in the different versions.

Functional equivalence deals with establishing similar predictive and concurrent criterion-related validity to prevent test bias (i.e., similar regression intercepts and slopes between measure and criterion). Functional equivalence can be difficult to establish when both the test and the external criteria of interest are both rooted in the same dominant universalist cultural epistemology or worldview; instead, it may be advantageous to validate tests against external criteria that are grounded in the nondominant group's culture (Suzuki et al., 2013).

Metric and scalar equivalence (i.e., measurement invariance) deal with establishing that the construct is measured on the same metric across groups, that is, a particular score reflects the same level on the construct for people in each group. Metric equivalence/invariance deals with establishing that items' discrimination parameters (or factor loadings) are the same across groups. Scalar equivalence/invariance deals with establishing that both items' discrimination parameters (or factor loadings) and difficulty parameters (or intercepts) are the same across groups.

24.3.1.7 Methods of Assessment

It is debatable whether some assessment methods may be more likely to result in cultural or ethnic bias compared to other assessment methods (Okazaki & Sue, 1995). Certain types of assessment techniques might be more likely to bias or obscure differences between cultural groups. This especially depends on who is doing the observing and their own beliefs. There may be selection biases regarding the types of people who are willing to participate in in-depth studies that involve observational or psychophysiological assessment. It may be worth considering supplementing quantitative measurement approaches with qualitative measurement approaches, such as interviews and life histories, which may be better able to capture cultural factors. In general, it is advantageous to assess people using multiple measures and methods to establish convergent validity of cultural constructs (Okazaki & Sue, 1995).

24.3.1.8 Interpretation of Data

Another challenge deals with how to interpret data from group comparison designs. Historically, group differences in scores were most commonly interpreted from a deficit-based narrative rather than a strengths-based narrative (Byrd et al., 2021).

24.3.2 APA Guidelines

There are many disparities in psychological services for under-served populations, including health disparities, diagnostic disparities, and disparities in the use and availability of psychological services (Rivera Mindt et al., 2010). To help address these disparities, the American Psychological Association (APA) Office of Ethnic Minority Affairs published guidelines for providers of psychological services to ethnic, linguistic, and culturally diverse populations (American Psychological Association Office of Ethnic Minority Affairs, 1993). Their guidelines included suggestions such as:

- Whenever possible, provide information in writing along with oral explanations.
- Whenever possible, provide the information and interact in the language that is understandable to the client. If that is not feasible, make an appropriate referral. If this is not possible, provide a translator with cultural knowledge and an appropriate professional background. When no translator is available, then use a trained paraprofessional from the client's culture as a translator.
- If you do not possess knowledge and training about an ethnic group, seek consultation with, and/or make referrals to, appropriate experts as necessary.
- Consider the validity of a given instrument or procedure and interpret the resulting data, while keeping in mind the cultural and linguistic characteristics of the client.
- Be aware of the test's reference population and possible limitations of using the instrument with other populations.
- Seek to help clients determine whether a "problem" stems from racism or bias in others so that the client does not inappropriately personalize problems.

The APA has also published guidelines for working with particular groups, including:

- Groups based on race and ethnicity (https://www.apa.org/about/policy/guidelines-race-ethnicity.pdf, archived at https://perma.cc/4LM9-X6JN)
- People with low income (https://www.apa.org/about/policy/guidelines-low-income.pdf, archived at https://perma.cc/PZQ5-8YFG)
- People with disabilities (https://www.apa.org/pi/disability/resources/assessment-disabilities, archived at https://perma.cc/5YZ8-FNJT; PDF: https://perma.cc/KYY4-CQFQ)
- People who are transgender or gender nonconforming (https://www.apa.org/practice/guidelines/transgender.pdf, archived at https://perma.cc/E9VH-QG3W)
- Sexual minorities (https://www.apa.org/about/policy/psychological-sexual-minority-persons.pdf, archived at https://perma.cc/4BJD-QZCF)
- Girls and women (https://www.apa.org/about/policy/psychological-practice-girls-women.pdf, archived at https://perma.cc/AYA4-KB5W)
- Boys and men (https://www.apa.org/about/policy/boys-men-practice-guidelines.pdf, archived at https://perma.cc/6HWK-W9R6)
- Older adults (https://www.apa.org/practice/guidelines/guidelines-psychological-practice-older-adults.pdf, archived at https://perma.cc/EQ95-Y78Y)

24.3.3 Seek Training and Consultation

Research has shown that relatively few practitioners receive extensive training in multicultural assessment and few use frameworks for multicultural assessment (Brickman et al., 2006; L. M. Edwards et al., 2017). Researchers have encouraged increasing multicultural education, training, awareness, and knowledge, increasing multicultural psychological research, and increasing the provision of culturally competent psychological services to ethnic minorities (Rivera Mindt et al., 2010). It can also be worthwhile to consult with informal support systems, including churches, ethnic clubs, family associations, and community leaders (Leong & Kalibatseva, 2016).

24.3.4 Develop Awareness of Cultural Differences

One goal should be to develop cultural competence with the groups, communities, and individuals with which one works or interacts. It can be helpful to be aware of cultural differences, including cultural differences in communication style and use of language (Leong & Kalibatseva, 2016).

24.3.5 Show Cultural Humility

Another goal should be to show cultural humility. Tervalon & Murray-Garcia (1998) describe three key aspects of cultural humility: (1) a life-long commitment to self-evaluation and self-critique, (2) fixing power imbalances, and (3) developing mutually beneficial and nonpaternalistic partnerships with communities who advocate for others. For instance, it is important to be aware of one's biases and stereotypical beliefs. Cultural humility involves treating the client as the expert on their experience. Therefore, cultural humility involves collaboration between the clinician and client, because each brings important knowledge. The client brings their knowledge of their situation, and their preferences. The clinician brings their scientific knowledge about strengths and difficulties, and about behavior change.

24.3.6 Do Not Assume or Stereotype

It is important to consider cultural factors; at the same time, groups are not monolithic and every person is unique. Do not assume about someone based on their demographics, which is stereotyping. Just because a person comes from a particular group does not mean the person shares all beliefs, behaviors, etc. with the group (Okazaki & Sue, 1995). Thus, it is important to be aware of within-group differences, as well (Leong & Kalibatseva, 2016; Okazaki & Sue, 1995), which are often as large or larger than between-group differences (Zuckerman, 1990). Show genuine interest and curiosity to get to know a person as an individual.

24.3.7 Ensure Adequate Representation of Under-Represented Groups in Research

There are important issues of generalizability of research findings. Participant samples historically have been largely White and middle or upper middle class. This reduces the potential generalizability of findings, and limits effectiveness of treatments to under-represented populations, many of whom have experienced discrimination and social disadvantage. Many groups, including people who are Black or Latinx, and gender and sexual minorities have not been adequately represented in research studies. As a result, the knowledge gained from unrepresentative studies may not generalize to other under-represented groups. Science plays an important role in advancing knowledge that can lead to the development of new treatments. However, groups who are under-represented in research are less likely to benefit from the new treatments because the knowledge upon which the treatments were developed and tested may not generalize to the under-represented groups. Moreover, the lack of inclusion of under-represented groups in studies leads to inappropriate normative data. Thus, it is crucial to have better representation of historically marginalized and minoritized groups in science, including people who are Black or Latinx, and gender and sexual minorities.

People from Finland and Sweden are often studied to examine health-related questions. Because they have a socialized health care system, the government keeps medical records on all citizens, so researchers can examine millions of participants, and can study rare conditions and behaviors with a low base rate, like suicide (Lysell et al., 2018). However, there are questions of generalizability from the Scandinavian population and health care system to those of other countries, including the United States. One could hypothetically use propensity score matching for matching their sample to other populations, but one cannot really do that because they have too many empty cells for propensity score matching due to too few people of various under-represented racial/ethnic groups.

24.3.8 Use Appropriate Measurement

24.3.8.1 Do Not Use Offensive Content or Procedures

It is important to use stimuli that are valid for the populations being tested. It is important to avoid using content or procedures that are culturally or racially insensitive, or that are racist, sexist, heteronormative, and/or ableist (Byrd et al., 2021). When developing assessments, it may be important to evaluate stimuli in focus groups to ensure they are not offensive.

One of the most widely used standardized assessments in psychological assessment is the Boston Naming Test, a measure of visual confrontation naming that is used to assess cognitive impairment, aphasia, and dementia. The Boston Naming Test includes a noose as one of the items. Historically, lynchings with a noose were used in the United States as a form of racial terror against Black people. Thus, the use of a noose as an item in the Boston Naming Test is racially insensitive and inappropriate for use because it is deeply offensive and has a harmful nature. It can have a strong negative impact on Black respondents in terms of distress, performance disparities, and health disparities (Byrd et al., 2021).

Culturally offensive stimuli can lead to stereotype threat and compromise the validity of the assessment. Stereotype threat occurs when people are or feel at risk of conforming themselves to stereotypes about their social group, thus leading them to show poorer performance in ways that are consistent with the stereotype. Moreover, the use of offensive procedures likely contributes to greater distrust of the scientific and medical fields among under-served communities, which acts as a barrier to health care and to health disparities. Thus, removing and replacing offensive stimuli may be necessary from a moral and ethical perspective to do no harm and to ensure valid assessment, even if it risks modifying the standardized procedure from which the norms were developed (Byrd et al., 2021). When deviating from standardized procedures, it is important to describe such deviations in resulting papers or reports.

24.3.8.2 Use Culturally Valid Measures

Most measures originated from Western societies (Suzuki et al., 2013) and have been validated only among non-Latinx, English-speaking Whites (Manly, 2005). It is important to use measures that have been validated for the populations with whom they will be used. Many measures have been used for different populations than the populations with which the instruments were developed and validated, such as with immigrants, refugees, or when exporting measures to different countries or cultural contexts. Exporting measures for use with people from different cultures assumes universality (i.e., cross-cultural validity). More work should examine adaptation and validation of measures for other cultures, countries, languages, etc. (Leong & Kalibatseva, 2016). However, some measures may not be able to be applied validly across cultures. Using valid measures for the target population may in some cases mean using culturally specific (etic) instruments rather than universal (emic) instruments. If using measures whose validity and measurement equivalence has not been established, it is important to interpret results with caution and to provide disclaimers in any resulting papers or reports (Leong & Kalibatseva, 2016).

As described in Section 4.3.1.16, it is also important for measures to have cultural validity, which refers to "the effectiveness of a measure or the accuracy of a clinical diagnosis to address the existence and importance of essential cultural factors." (Leong & Kalibatseva, 2016, p. 58). Essential cultural factors may include values, beliefs, experiences, communication patterns, and approaches to knowledge (epistemologies).

Threats to cultural validity of assessments includes: pathoplasticity of psychological disorders, bias in clinical judgment, language capability of the client, biased measures, or inappropriate use or interpretation of measures (Leong & Kalibatseva, 2016).

24.3.8.3 Use Linguistically Appropriate Assessment

It is important to use assessment approaches that are linguistically appropriate for the examinee (Leong & Kalibatseva, 2016). First, the measure should be in a language that is understood by the examinee. Second, the measure should be consistent with the examinee's language ability. Sometimes interpreters or translators may be necessary. However, use of interpreters has been shown to lead to underestimations of patients' emotion suffering and despair (Leong & Kalibatseva, 2016). In addition, clients and therapists can attach different meanings to the same words. It is thus important not to assume that you know what the client means by various terms and not to assume that the client knows what you mean by various terms.

24.3.8.4 Use Follow-Up as Necessary

As described by Suzuki et al. (2013), it may be necessary to use follow-up procedures to clarify people's responses to items or to test the limits by readministering items with additional supports (e.g., modifying instructions to involve more or fewer cues, adjusting the pace of information presented, adjusting memory demands, changing the response format) (Sattler & Hoge, 2006). When deviating from standardized procedures, it is important to describe such deviations in resulting papers or reports.

24.3.8.5 Examine and Correct for Test Bias

As described in Chapter 15, there are two types of test bias: predictive test bias and test structure bias. It is important to evaluate the possibility of both when using assessments across groups.

It is important to establish measurement invariance across groups to ensure that scores have the same meaning for each group (Burlew et al., 2019). If measures are non-invariant, the means (i.e., level) and or associations between constructs could appear to (artifactually) differ across groups, when in reality they do not (F. F. Chen, 2008). Measurement invariance can be examined in terms of item intercepts, item factor loadings, and item residuals. Establishing measurement invariance of just intercepts or factor loadings (or vice versa) is not sufficient to establish measurement invariance because tests can show strong bias in one dimension (e.g., intercepts) even if the test does not show bias in other dimensions (e.g., factor loadings) (Wicherts & Dolan, 2010). Approaches for evaluating measurement invariance across groups are described by Han et al. (2019). To help minimize the potential for test bias, reseachers are encouraged to develop the scales simultaneously across the different groups or cultures (Fernández & Abe, 2018).

It is also important to determine whether the measure's scores show similar relations to meaningful external criteria (Burlew et al., 2019).

Fernández & Abe (2018) provide strategies to address cross-cultural bias, such as excluding words or concepts that are specific to one language or culture. Use of North American neuropsychological tests in other countries has shown to lead to considerable false positives, and the extent of misdiagnosis differs by country (Daugherty et al., 2017).

It is important to examine factors that moderate the validity of assessment, e.g., groups for whom the assessment is biased. Ways to investigate and detect bias are described in Section 15.2. The number of potential moderating variables is so large, that it is not realistic to develop an assessment base that encompasses all of these factors and their interactions. Evidence should be used regarding which factors seem to matter for a given assessment purpose—that is, the factors that have a medium-to-large effect size. It is valuable to examine the effect size of moderators; if the effects are small, it might not be sufficient to scrap the instrument for the population. Gender and cultural differences have shown a number of statistically significant effects for a number of different assessment purposes, but many of the observed effects are quite small and likely trivial, and they do not present compelling reasons to change the assessment (Youngstrom & Van Meter, 2016). Nevertheless, if you do find evidence of bias, it is important to correct for it. Ways to correct for bias using score adjustment and other approaches are discussed in Section 15.5.

24.3.9 Consider Pathoplasticity of Constructs

Constructs can manifest differently across cultures. Pathoplasticity of mental disorders refers to the variability in symptoms, course, outcome, and distribution of mental disorders among various cultural groups (Leong & Kalibatseva, 2016). Some syndromes are considered culture-bound—that is, they exist in some cultures but not in other cultures. Hwabyung is a Korean culture-bound syndrome in which suppressed negative emotions manifest themselves in bodily ways such as chest pains and difficulty breathing. In addition, features associated with a disorder, including the content, severity, or frequency of symptoms, may vary across cultures.

For instance, Asian Americans tend to report a greater degree of psychological disturbance than Whites, which could be due to several reasons (Leong & Kalibatseva, 2016). It is possible that Asian Americans (a) show higher rates of mental health problems than other groups, (b) under-utilize mental health services, and/or (c) are more likely than other groups to be misdiagnosed due to miscommunication, use of invalid instruments for Asian Americans, and/or lack of cultural knowledge on the part of therapists. In addition, how clients act in a diagnostic interview may depend on cultural factors, and it thus may be important to sample the clients more broadly than a diagnostic interview (Leong & Kalibatseva, 2016).

For a case example of pathoplasticity, there is a disorder among the traditional Navajo called "Moth Madness" (American Psychological Association Office of Ethnic Minority Affairs, 1993). Symptoms of Moth Madness include seizure-like behaviors. This disorder is believed by the Navajo to be the supernatural result of incestuous thoughts or behaviors. Both differential diagnosis and intervention should take into consideration the traditional values of Moth Madness.

24.3.10 Formulate a Culturally Informed Case Conceptualization

It can be helpful to discuss your diagnosis and case conceptualization with the client. For instance, you may learn that some behaviors are normative in their culture and may not be distressing or concerning to them. It can thus be helpful to consider client preferences in terms of what to address and how to address it, while adhering to evidence-based approaches.

24.3.11 Bias in Clinical Judgment

As reviewed by Garb (1997), there is evidence of race bias, social class bias, and gender bias in clinical judgment. Race bias, social class bias, and gender bias in clinical judgment occurs when the accuracy of judgments varies as a function of client race, social class, or gender. That is, clinical judgment bias occurs when the accuracy of judgments varies as function of other variables (e.g., race, social class, gender). Bias is not when the *judgments* themselves vary as a function of other factors, but when the *accuracy* of those judgments varies. Examining how judgments differ across groups does not control for differences in clinical severity between the groups. If a clinician rates more people in one group as having a disorder than another group, this is not necessarily evidence of bias because the true prevalence of the condition could differ across groups. Thus, it is important to compare groups with similar levels of symptomatology or to control for level of symptomatology. If clinical judgments are more accurate for White clients than Black clients, we would say that race bias exists.

Accuracy of judgments could vary by the client's race, social class, or gender for several reasons (Garb, 1997). One way in which judgments could be biased is if the diagnostic criteria are biased—for instance, if the diagnoses are more valid for one group (e.g., White clients) than for another group (e.g., Black clients). Another reason that accuracy of judgments could vary as a function of client race, social class, or gender is if the judgments are made based on a biased instrument. Another way that accuracy of judgments could vary as a function of client race, social class, or gender is related to confirmation bias or biases introduced during the usage of a measure. This could occur, for instance if clinicians do not consider alternative hypotheses, and based on their hypotheses, they choose the data to collect that support their hypotheses rather than collecting data that could refute their hypotheses. Bias could also occur in the way that data are integrated from multiple measures or methods. Another form of bias could arise from how test results are used, in terms of inequitable social consequences (Suzuki et al., 2013).

Many studies do not find bias in clinical judgments as a function of race, social class, or gender, but some studies do find evidence of bias (Garb, 1997).

24.3.11.1 Race Bias

One pattern of race bias is that Black and Latinx patients with a psychotic affective disorder are more likely than White patients to be misdiagnosed as having schizophrenia (Garb, 1997). That is, Black and Latinx patients are less likely than White patients to be diagnosed with psychotic affective disorder (with the same symptoms) and are more likely to be diagnosed as having schizophrenia, even when the measures do not indicate that a diagnosis of schizophrenia is justified. Another pattern of race bias is that the risk of violence is overestimated for Black patients but not for White patients (Garb, 1997). In addition, cases of child abuse are more likely to be reported when children are White than when they are Black (even when comparing similar behavior) (Garb, 1997). Race bias has also been observed with respect to antipsychotic medication. Antipsychotic medications are more often prescribed for Black patients than for other patients even for similar levels of psychosis (Garb, 1997). Moreover, affective symptoms in patients who are severely ill are more often under-treated for Black or Latinx patients than for White patients (Garb, 1997).

24.3.11.2 Social Class Bias

One pattern of social class bias is that child abuse is more likely to be reported if a child is from a lower-class background rather than a middle- or upper-class background (even when comparing similar behavior) (Garb, 1997). In addition, middle-class children are more likely to be referred to special education programs compared to lower-class children (Garb, 1997). There is also social class bias in clinicians' decisions about psychotherapy. Referrals for psychotherapy are more often made for middle-class clients than for lower-class clients (Garb, 1997). Clinicians are more likely to recommend psychotherapy and expect a client to do well in psychotherapy when the client is from a middle- or upper-class background compared to when the client is from a lower-class background, leading to a tendency for clinicians to refer clients to different types of treatments based on the client's social class (Garb, 1997). Specifically, lower-class clients are more likely to be referred for supportive psychotherapy, whereas middle-class clients are more likely to be referred for insight-oriented psychotherapy.

24.3.11.3 Gender Bias

One pattern of gender bias is that women are more likely than men to be diagnosed with a histrionic personality disorder, whereas men are more likely than women to be diagnosed with antisocial personality disorder, even when female and male clients do not differ in symptomatology (Garb, 1997). Another pattern is that clinicians tend to overestimate likelihood of violent behavior for male clients and underestimate likelihood of violent behavior for female clients (Garb, 1997; McNiel & Binder, 1995). Although males tend to show more violence than females, studies have shown that false positives tend to be more common for male patients than female patients, whereas false negatives tend to be more common for female patients than male patients (McNiel & Binder, 1995).

In terms of autism, some conceptualizations of autism consider it to be a manifestation of "extreme male brain" (Baron-Cohen, 2002, 2010; Greenberg et al., 2018). Girls diagnosed with autism tend to be more severely affected than boys diagnosed with autism. People are less likely to notice autism in girls. This could possibly be due to girls with autism having fewer restricted interests and lower levels of repetitive behavior compared to boys. Research has tried to develop assessments to equate boys and girls, but girls and boys appear to be unequal in their underlying autism process—that is, boys and girls appear to show sex-specific autism phenotypes (Frazier et al., 2014).

24.3.11.4 Recommendations for Reducing Bias in Clinical Judgment

Garb (1997) makes several recommendations for reducing bias in clinical judgment, including:

- Be aware of biases that have been reported in the clinical judgment literature.
- Use standardized and structured assessment approaches and attend strictly to diagnostic criteria when making diagnoses.
- Use actuarial approaches and statistical prediction rules.

24.3.12 Use Appropriate Normative Data

When group-referenced judgments will be used, it is important to consider what the appropriate norm is. The question of whether separate norms should be used for various racial/ethnic minority groups is of considerable controversy (Burlew et al., 2019). Pros and cons of using group-specific norms are discussed in Section 15.5.2.2.2 and reviewed by Manly (2005). The question about which norms to use is complex, and psychologists should evaluate the cost and benefit of each norm, and use the norm with the greatest benefit and the least cost for the client (Manly & Echemendia, 2007). Burlew et al. (2019) recommend limiting the use of measures that require the use of norms to interpret, and to note in the limitations of a paper or report if a norm based on one group is used to evaluate a person from a different group.

24.3.13 Contextualize Group-Related Differences

When conducting research and identifying different scores between groups, it is important to be cautious not to assume that differences in the scores between groups are caused by the group membership. That is, correlation does not necessarily mean causation! For instance, if the researcher identifies higher rates of suicide in transgender than cisgender individuals (as has been observed, Toomey et al., 2018), it is important not to automatically assume the higher suicide rate is *because of* the person's transgender status, per se. Rather, there are likely many aspects of discrimination and victimization that transgender individuals experience that, unfortunately, may increase their suicide rate relative to cisgender individuals.

It is important to contextualize test score differences between groups within sociocultural and historical inequities rather than interpreting group-related differences in tests scores from a deficit-based narrative (Byrd et al., 2021). It is important to avoid interpretive bias and to pay attention not to over- or under-pathologize (Okazaki & Sue, 1995). Over-pathologizing can lead to stigmatization and institutionalization. Underestimating psychopathology can deprive patients of treatments or services that they would benefit from. For instance, one should be aware of the danger of underestimating psychopathology for clients from different cultures (from that of the therapist) through over-attributing bizarre behavior or thought patterns to the client's culture (Okazaki & Sue, 1995).

24.3.14 Dissemination and Implementation

Dissemination and implementation deals not just with finding differences between groups, but what to do about these differences. Aspirationally, we would successfully be able to custom-tailor treatments to individuals based on their individual characteristics. The goal is to identify the best treatment for each group, or ideally, each individual.

24.3.15 Use Inclusive and Bias-Free Language

It is important to use bias-free language, as discussed in the publication manual of the American Psychological Association [APA; American Psychological Association (2020)]. Guidelines for bias-free language include the following:

1. Describe at the appropriate level of specificity
   a. Focus on relevant characteristics
   b. Acknowledge relevant differences that exist
   c. Be appropriately specific
2. Be sensitive to labels

a. Acknowledge people's humanity
b. Provide operational definitions and labels
c. Avoid false hierarchies

When writing reports, manuscripts, or in conversation, it can be helpful to use inclusive and person-first language. The aim of people-first language is to reduce stigma because it treats everyone as a human first. People-first language puts the person before the disability and describes the difficulties a person has rather than who a person is. For instance, say "a child with intellectual disability" instead of "an intellectually disabled child". That said, some individuals may prefer identity-first labels (e.g., autistic person) rather than person-first labels for their own identities. Thus, it is important to use the labels preferred by the particular client. The APA guidelines for inclusive language are located here: https://www.apa.org/about/apa/equity-diversity-inclusion/language-guide.pdf (archived at https://perma.cc/82QH-ED96).

24.4 Conclusion

Diverse samples provide stronger tests of theories and better generalizability of findings (external validity). We need measures that are reliable and valid for all people we use them with. There are various multicultural frameworks to assessment. Guidelines for assessment of diverse populations are discussed. Recommendations include developing and using appropriate and valid measures for the target population(s), ensuring fair group comparisons, seeking training and consultation, developing awareness of cultural differences, showing cultural humility, avoiding assuming or stereotyping, ensuring adequate representation of under-represented minorities, considering pathoplasticity of constructs, formulating a culturally informed case conceptualization, using appropriate normative data, contextualizing group-related differences, and using inclusive language.

24.5 Suggested Readings

Burlew et al. (2019); Byrd et al. (2021); Okazaki & Sue (1995)

References

Achenbach, T. M. (2001). What are norms and why do we need valid ones? *Clinical Psychology: Science and Practice*, *8*(4), 446–450. https://doi.org/10.1093/clipsy.8.4.446

Ackerman, P. L. (2013). Assessment of intellectual functioning in adults. In K. F. Geisinger, J. F. Carlson, J.-I. C. Hansen, N. R. Kuncel, S. P. Reise, & M. C. Rodriguez (Eds.), *APA handbook of testing and assessment in psychology, Vol 2: Testing and assessment in clinical and counseling psychology* (pp. 119–132). American Psychological Association.

Ægisdóttir, S., White, M. J., Spengler, P. M., Maugherman, A. S., Anderson, L. A., Cook, R. S., Nichols, C. N., Lampropoulos, G. K., Walker, B. S., Cohen, G., & Rush, J. D. (2006). The meta-analysis of clinical judgment project: Fifty-six years of accumulated research on clinical versus statistical prediction. *The Counseling Psychologist*, *34*(3), 341–382. https://doi.org/10.1177/0011000005285875

Aguinis, H., Culpepper, S. A., & Pierce, C. A. (2010). Revival of test bias research in preemployment testing. *Journal of Applied Psychology*, *95*(4), 648–680. https://doi.org/10.1037/a0018714

American Educational Research Association, American Psychological Association, & National Council on Measurement in Education. (2014). *Standards for educational and psychological testing*. American Educational Research Association.

American Psychological Association. (2017). *Ethical principles of psychologists and code of conduct*.

American Psychological Association. (2020). *Publication manual of the American Psychological Association* (7th ed.).

American Psychological Association Office of Ethnic Minority Affairs. (1993). Guidelines for providers of psychological services to ethnic, linguistic, and culturally diverse populations. *American Psychologist*, *48*(1), 45–48. https://doi.org/10.1037/0003-066X.48.1.45

Antony, M. M., & Rowa, K. (2005). Evidence-based assessment of anxiety disorders in adults. *Psychological Assessment*, *17*(3), 256–266. https://doi.org/10.1037/1040-3590.17.3.256

Arnett, A., Pennington, B., Willcutt, E., Dmitrieva, J., Byrne, B., Samuelsson, S., & Olson, R. (2012). A cross-lagged model of the development of ADHD inattention symptoms and rapid naming speed. *Journal of Abnormal Child Psychology*, *40*(8), 1313–1326. https://doi.org/10.1007/s10802-012-9644-5

Arvey, R. D., Bouchard, T. J., Carroll, J. B., Cattell, R. B., Cohen, D. B., Dawis, R. V., Detterman, D. K., Dunnette, M., Eysenck, H., Feldman, J. M., Fleishman, E. A., Gilmore, G. C., Gordon, R. A., Gottfredson, L. S., Greene, R. L., Haier, R. J., Hardin, G., Hogan, R., Horn, J. M., . . . Willerman, L. (1994). Mainstream science on intelligence. *Wall Street Journal*, *13*(1), 18–25.

Atanasov, P., Witkowski, J., Ungar, L., Mellers, B., & Tetlock, P. (2020). Small steps to accuracy: Incremental belief updaters are better forecasters. *Organizational Behavior and Human Decision Processes*, *160*, 19–35. https://doi.org/10.1016/j.obhdp.2020.02.001

Austin, P. C., & Steyerberg, E. W. (2014). Graphical assessment of internal and external calibration of logistic regression models by using loess smoothers. *Statistics in Medicine*, *33*(3), 517–535. https://doi.org/10.1002/sim.5941

Avugos, S., Köppen, J., Czienskowski, U., Raab, M., & Bar-Eli, M. (2013). The "hot hand" reconsidered: A meta-analytic approach. *Psychology of Sport and Exercise*, *14*(1), 21–27. https://doi.org/10.1016/j.psychsport.2012.07.005

Baird, C., & Wagner, D. (2000). The relative validity of actuarial- and consensus-based risk assessment systems. *Children and Youth Services Review*, *22*(11), 839–871. https://doi.org/10.1016/S0190-7409(00)00122-5

Bakeman, R., & Goodman, S. H. (2020). Interobserver reliability in clinical research: Current issues and discussion of how to establish best practices. *Journal of Abnormal Psychology*, *129*(1), 5–13. https://doi.org/10.1037/abn0000487

Baker, F. B., & Kim, S.-H. (2017). *The basics of item response theory using R*. Springer.

Ballesteros-Pérez, P., González-Cruz, M. C., & Mora-Melià, D. (2018). Explaining the Bayes' theorem graphically. *Proceedings of the International Technology, Education and Development Conference*.

Baltes, P. B. (1968). Longitudinal and cross-sectional sequences in the study of age and generation effects. *Human Development*, *11*(3), 145–171. http://www.jstor.org/stable/26761719

Bandalos, D. L. (2018). *Measurement theory and applications for the social sciences*. Guilford Publications.

Bar-Eli, M., Avugos, S., & Raab, M. (2006). Twenty years of "hot hand" research: Review and critique. *Psychology of Sport and Exercise*, *7*(6), 525–553. https://doi.org/10.1016/j.psychsport.2006.03.001

Baron-Cohen, S. (2002). The extreme male brain theory of autism. *Trends in Cognitive Sciences*, *6*(6), 248–254. https://doi.org/10.1016/S1364-6613(02)01904-6

Baron-Cohen, S. (2010). Empathizing, systemizing, and the extreme male brain theory of autism. In I. Savic (Ed.), *Progress in brain research* (Vol. 186, pp. 167–175). Elsevier.

Barrash, J., Stillman, A., Anderson, S. W., Uc, E. Y., Dawson, J. D., & Rizzo, M. (2010). Prediction of driving ability with neuropsychological tests: Demographic adjustments diminish accuracy. *Journal of the International Neuropsychological Society*, *16*(4), 679–686. https://doi.org/10.1017/S1355617710000470

Bates, D., Maechler, M., Bolker, B., & Walker, S. (2022). *lme4: Linear mixed-effects models using Eigen and S4*. https://github.com/lme4/lme4/

Bauer, D. J., Belzak, W. C. M., & Cole, V. T. (2020). Simplifying the assessment of measurement invariance over multiple background variables: Using regularized moderated nonlinear factor analysis to detect differential item functioning. *Structural Equation Modeling: A Multidisciplinary Journal*, *27*(1), 43–55. https://doi.org/10.1080/10705511.2019.1642754

Beltz, A. M., Wright, A. G. C., Sprague, B. N., & Molenaar, P. C. M. (2016). Bridging the nomothetic and idiographic approaches to the analysis of clinical data. *Assessment*, *23*(4), 447–458. https://doi.org/10.1177/1073191116648209

Belzak, W. C. M., & Bauer, D. J. (2020). Improving the assessment of measurement invariance: Using regularization to select anchor items and identify differential item functioning. *Psychological Methods*, *25*(6), 673–690. https://doi.org/10.1037/met0000253

Benjamin, L. T. (2005). A history of clinical psychology as a profession in America (and a glimpse of its future). *Annual Review of Clinical Psychology*, *1*, 1–30. https://doi.org/10.1146/annurev.clinpsy.1.102803.143758

Bennett, C. M., Miller, M. B., & Wolford, G. L. (2009). Neural correlates of interspecies perspective taking in the post-mortem Atlantic Salmon: An argument for multiple comparisons correction. *NeuroImage*, *47*, S125. https://doi.org/10.1016/S1053-8119(09)71202-9

Bennett, C. M., Miller, M. B., & Wolford, G. L. (2010). Neural correlates of interspecies perspective taking in the post-mortem Atlantic Salmon: An argument for multiple comparisons correction. *Journal of Serendipitous and Unexpected Results*, *1*, 1–5. https://teenspecies.github.io/pdfs/NeuralCorrelates.pdf

Benning, S. D., Bachrach, R. L., Smith, E. A., Freeman, A. J., & Wright, A. G. C. (2019). The registration continuum in clinical science: A guide toward transparent practices. *Journal of Abnormal Psychology*, *128*(6), 528–540. https://doi.org/10.1037/abn0000451

Bensch, D., Maaß, U., Greiff, S., Horstmann, K. T., & Ziegler, M. (2019). The nature of faking: A homogeneous and predictable construct? *Psychological Assessment*, *31*(4), 532–544. https://doi.org/10.1037/pas0000619

Berry, D., & Willoughby, M. T. (2017). On the practical interpretability of cross-lagged panel models: Rethinking a developmental workhorse. *Child Development*, *88*(4), 1186–1206. https://doi.org/10.1111/cdev.12660

Bersoff, D. N., DeMatteo, D., & Foster, E. E. (2012). Assessment and testing. In S. J. Knapp (Ed.), *APA handbook of ethics in psychology, Vol 2: Practice, teaching, and research* (pp. 45–74). American Psychological Association.

Bickel, J. E., & Kim, S. D. (2008). Verification of The Weather Channel probability of precipitation forecasts. *Monthly Weather Review*, *136*(12), 4867–4881. https://doi.org/10.1175/2008MWR2547.1

Bland, J. M., & Altman, D. G. (1986). Statistical methods for assessing agreement between two methods of clinical measurement. *The Lancet*, *327*(8476), 307–310. https://doi.org/10.1016/S0140-6736(86)90837-8

Bland, J. M., & Altman, D. G. (1999). Measuring agreement in method comparison studies. *Statistical Methods in Medical Research*, *8*(2), 135–160. https://doi.org/10.1177/096228029900800204

Blashfield, R. K., Keeley, J. W., Flanagan, E. H., & Miles, S. R. (2014). The cycle of classification: DSM-I through DSM-5. *Annual Review of Clinical Psychology*, *10*(1), 25–51. https://doi.org/10.1146/annurev-clinpsy-032813-153639

Blumberg, M. S. (2013). Homology, correspondence, and continuity across development: The case of sleep. *Developmental Psychobiology*, *55*(1), 92–100. https://doi.org/10.1002/dev.21024

Bocskocsky, A., Ezekowitz, J., & Stein, C. (2014). The hot hand: A new approach to an old "fallacy." *MIT Sloan Sports Analytics Conference.*

Bolger, F., & Önkal-Atay, D. (2004). The effects of feedback on judgmental interval predictions. *International Journal of Forecasting*, *20*(1), 29–39. https://doi.org/10.1016/S0169-2070(03)00009-8

Bollen, K. A. (1989). *Structural equations with latent variables*. John Wiley & Sons.

Bollen, K. A. (2002). Latent variables in psychology and the social sciences. *Annual Review of Psychology*, *53*(1), 605–634. https://doi.org/10.1146/annurev.psych.53.100901.135239

Bollen, K. A., & Bauldry, S. (2011). Three Cs in measurement models: Causal indicators, composite indicators, and covariates. *Psychological Methods*, *16*(3), 265–284. https://doi.org/10.1037/a0024448

Bollen, K. A., & Diamantopoulos, A. (2017). In defense of causal-formative indicators: A minority report. *Psychological Methods*, *22*(3), 581–596. https://doi.org/10.1037/met0000056

Bollen, K. A., & Lennox, R. D. (1991). Conventional wisdom on measurement: A structural equation perspective. *Psychological Bulletin*, *110*(2), 305–314. https://doi.org/10.1037/0033-2909.110.2.305

Boring, E. G. (1923). Intelligence as the tests test it. *New Republic*, *36*, 35–37.

Bornstein, R. F. (2011). Toward a process-focused model of test score validity: Improving psychological assessment in science and practice. *Psychological Assessment*, *23*(2), 532–544. https://doi.org/10.1037/a0022402

Borsboom, D. (2003). *Conceptual issues in psychological measurement*. Universiteit van Amsterdam.

Box, G. E. P. (1979). Robustness in the strategy of scientific model building. In R. L. Launer & G. N. Wilkinson (Eds.), *Robustness in statistics.* Academic Press.

Brennan, R. L. (1992). Generalizability theory. *Educational Measurement: Issues and Practice, 11*(4), 27–34. https://doi.org/10.1111/j.1745-3992.1992.tb00260.x

Brennan, R. L. (2001). *Generalizability theory.* Springer New York. https://books.google.com/books?id=nbHbBwAAQBAJ

Brickman, A. M., Cabo, R., & Manly, J. J. (2006). Ethical issues in cross-cultural neuropsychology. *Applied Neuropsychology, 13*(2), 91–100. https://doi.org/10.1207/s15324826an1302_4

Brown, R. T., Reynolds, C. R., & Whitaker, J. S. (1999). Bias in mental testing since bias in mental testing. *School Psychology Quarterly, 14*(3), 208–238. https://doi.org/10.1037/h0089007

Buchanan, T. (2002). Online assessment: Desirable or dangerous? *Professional Psychology: Research and Practice, 33*(2), 148–154. https://doi.org/10.1037/0735-7028.33.2.148

Burchett, D., & Ben-Porath, Y. S. (2019). Methodological considerations for developing and evaluating response bias indicators. *Psychological Assessment, 31*(12), 1497–1511. https://doi.org/10.1037/pas0000680

Burisch, M. (1984). Approaches to personality inventory construction: A comparison of merits. *American Psychologist, 39,* 214–227. https://doi.org/10.1037/0003-066X.39.3.214

Bürkner, P.-C. (2021). Bayesian item response modeling in R with brms and Stan. *Journal of Statistical Software, 100*(5), 1–54. https://doi.org/10.18637/jss.v100.i05

Burlew, A. K., Peteet, B. J., McCuistian, C., & Miller-Roenigk, B. D. (2019). Best practices for researching diverse groups. *American Journal of Orthopsychiatry, 89*(3), 354–368. https://doi.org/10.1037/ort0000350

Buros Center for Testing. (2021). *The twenty-first mental measurements yearbook.* Buros Center for Testing.

Busemeyer, J. R., & Stout, J. C. (2002). A contribution of cognitive decision models to clinical assessment: Decomposing performance on the Bechara gambling task. *Psychological Assessment, 14*(3), 253–262. https://doi.org/10.1037/1040-3590.14.3.253

Button, K. S., Ioannidis, J. P. A., Mokrysz, C., Nosek, B. A., Flint, J., Robinson, E. S. J., & Munafo, M. R. (2013a). Confidence and precision increase with high statistical power. *Nature Reviews Neuroscience, 14*(8), 585–585. https://doi.org/10.1038/nrn3475-c4

Button, K. S., Ioannidis, J. P. A., Mokrysz, C., Nosek, B. A., Flint, J., Robinson, E. S. J., & Munafo, M. R. (2013b). Power failure: Why small sample size undermines the reliability of neuroscience. *Nature Reviews Neuroscience, 14*(5), 365–376. https://doi.org/10.1038/nrn3475

Byrd, D. A., Rivera Mindt, M. M., Clark, U. S., Clarke, Y., Thames, A. D., Gammada, E. Z., & Manly, J. J. (2021). Creating an antiracist psychology by addressing professional complicity in psychological assessment. *Psychological Assessment, 33*(3), 279–285. https://doi.org/10.1037/pas0000993

Calamia, M. (2019). Practical considerations for evaluating reliability in ambulatory assessment studies. *Psychological Assessment, 31*(3), 285–291. https://doi.org/10.1037/pas0000599

Camilli, G. (2013). Ongoing issues in test fairness. *Educational Research and Evaluation, 19*(2–3), 104–120. https://doi.org/10.1080/13803611.2013.767602

Campbell, D. T., & Fiske, D. W. (1959). Convergent and discriminant validation by the multitrait-multimethod matrix. *Psychological Bulletin, 56*(2), 81–105. https://doi.org/10.1037/h0046016

Campbell, L., Vasquez, M., Behnke, S., & Kinscherff, R. (2010). *APA ethics code commentary and case illustrations* (pp. v, 392–v, 392). American Psychological Association.

Carlson, S. M., & Zelazo, P. D. (2014). *Minnesota executive function scale. Test manual.* Reflection Sciences, LLC.

Carpenter, R. W., Wycoff, A. M., & Trull, T. J. (2016). Ambulatory assessment: New adventures in characterizing dynamic processes. *Assessment*, *23*(4), 414–424. https://doi.org/10.1177/1073191116632341

Cashel, M. L. (2002). Child and adolescent psychological assessment: Current clinical practices and the impact of managed care. *Professional Psychology: Research and Practice*, *33*(5), 446–453. https://doi.org/10.1037/0735-7028.33.5.446

Caspi, A., Houts, R. M., Ambler, A., Danese, A., Elliott, M. L., Hariri, A., Harrington, H., Hogan, S., Poulton, R., Ramrakha, S., Rasmussen, L. J. H., Reuben, A., Richmond-Rakerd, L., Sugden, K., Wertz, J., Williams, B. S., & Moffitt, T. E. (2020). Longitudinal assessment of mental health disorders and comorbidities across 4 decades among participants in the Dunedin Birth Cohort Study. *JAMA Network Open*, *3*(4), e203221–e203221. https://doi.org/10.1001/jamanetworkopen.2020.3221

Caspi, A., Houts, R. M., Belsky, D. W., Goldman-Mellor, S. J., Harrington, H., Israel, S., Meier, M. H., Ramrakha, S., Shalev, I., Poulton, R., & Moffitt, T. E. (2014). The p factor: One general psychopathology factor in the structure of psychiatric disorders? *Clinical Psychological Science*, *2*(2), 119–137. https://doi.org/10.1177/2167702613497473

Caspi, A., & Shiner, R. L. (2006). Personality development. In N. Eisenberg, W. Damon, & R. M. Lerner (Eds.), *Handbook of child psychology* (6th ed., Vol. 3, pp. 300–365). John Wiley & Sons, Inc.

Chalmers, P. (2020). *mirt: Multidimensional item response theory.* https://CRAN.R-project.org/package=mirt

Chalmers, P. (2021). *mirtCAT: Computerized adaptive testing with multidimensional item response theory.* https://CRAN.R-project.org/package=mirtCAT

Chandler, J., Sisso, I., & Shapiro, D. (2020). Participant carelessness and fraud: Consequences for clinical research and potential solutions. *Journal of Abnormal Psychology*, *129*(1), 49–55. https://doi.org/10.1037/abn0000479

Charba, J. P., & Klein, W. H. (1980). Skill in precipitation forecasting in the National Weather Service. *Bulletin of the American Meteorological Society*, *61*(12), 1546–1555. https://doi.org/10.1175/1520-0477(1980)061%3C1546:SIPFIT%3E2.0.CO;2

Chen, F. F. (2007). Sensitivity of goodness of fit indexes to lack of measurement invariance. *Structural Equation Modeling: A Multidisciplinary Journal*, *14*(3), 464–504. https://doi.org/10.1080/10705510701301834

Chen, F. F. (2008). What happens if we compare chopsticks with forks? The impact of making inappropriate comparisons in cross-cultural research. *Journal of Personality and Social Psychology*, *95*(5), 1005–1018. https://doi.org/10.1037/a0013193

Chen, F. R., & Jaffee, S. R. (2015). The heterogeneity in the development of homotypic and heterotypic antisocial behavior. *Journal of Developmental and Life-Course Criminology*, *1*(3), 269–288. https://doi.org/10.1007/s40865-015-0012-3

Chen, Y., Prudêncio, R. B. C., Diethe, T., & Flach, P. (2019). β3-IRT: A new item response model and its applications. *arXiv:1903.04016.* https://arxiv.org/abs/1903.04016

Cheng, Y., Shao, C., & Lathrop, Q. N. (2016). The mediated MIMIC model for understanding the underlying mechanism of DIF. *Educational and Psychological Measurement*, *76*(1), 43–63. https://doi.org/10.1177/0013164415576187

Cheung, G. W., & Rensvold, R. B. (2002). Evaluating goodness-of-fit indexes for testing measurement invariance. *Structural Equation Modeling: A Multidisciplinary Journal*, *9*(2), 233–255. https://doi.org/10.1207/s15328007sem0902_5

Childs, D. Z., Hindle, B. J., & Warren, P. H. (2021). *APS 240: Data analysis and statistics with R.* https://dzchilds.github.io/stats-for-bio/

Choca, J. P., & Rossini, E. D. (2018). *Assessment using the Rorschach inkblot test.* American Psychological Association.

Cicchetti, D., & Rogosch, F. A. (2002). A developmental psychopathology perspective on adolescence. *Journal of Consulting and Clinical Psychology, 70*(1), 6–20. https://doi.org/10.1037/0022-006X.70.1.6

Civelek, M. E. (2018). *Essentials of structural equation modeling.* Zea E-Books.

Clark, L. A., & Watson, D. (1995). Constructing validity: Basic issues in objective scale development. *Psychological Assessment, 7*, 309–319. https://doi.org/10.1037/1040-3590.7.3.309

Clark, L. A., & Watson, D. (2019). Constructing validity: New developments in creating objective measuring instruments. *Psychological Assessment, 31*(12), 1412–1427. https://doi.org/10.1037/pas0000626

Clark, M. J., & Grandy, J. (1984). *Sex differences in the academic performance of Scholastic Aptitude Test takers: College board report no. 84-8.* College Board Publications.

Clark, S. J., & Desharnais, R. A. (1998). Honest answers to embarrassing questions: Detecting cheating in the randomized response model. *Psychological Methods, 3*(2), 160–168. https://doi.org/10.1037/1082-989X.3.2.160

Cole, N. S. (1981). Bias in testing. *American Psychologist, 36*(10), 1067–1077. https://doi.org/10.1037/0003-066X.36.10.1067

Cole, V., Gottfredson, N., & Giordano, M. (2018). *aMNLFA: Automated fitting of moderated nonlinear factor analysis through the Mplus program.* https://CRAN.R-project.org/package=aMNLFA

Committee on the General Aptitude Test Battery, Commission on Behavioral and Social Sciences and Education, & National Research Council. (1989). *Fairness in employment testing: Validity generalization, minority issues, and the general aptitude test battery.* National Academies Press.

Conradt, E., Crowell, S. E., & Cicchetti, D. (2021). Using development and psychopathology principles to inform the research domain criteria (RDoC) framework. *Development and Psychopathology, 33*(5), 1521–1525. https://doi.org/10.1017/S0954579421000985

Cooper, L. D., & Balsis, S. (2009). When less is more: How fewer diagnostic criteria can indicate greater severity. *Psychological Assessment, 21*(3), 285–293. https://doi.org/10.1037/a0016698

Cortina, J. M. (1993). What is coefficient alpha? An examination of theory and applications. *Journal of Applied Psychology, 78*, 98–104. https://doi.org/10.1037/0021-9010.78.1.98

Costa Jr., P. T., McCrae, R. R., & Löckenhoff, C. E. (2019). Personality across the life span. *Annual Review of Psychology, 70*(1), 423–448. https://doi.org/10.1146/annurev-psych-010418-103244

Counsell, A., Cribbie, R. A., & Flora, D. B. (2020). Evaluating equivalence testing methods for measurement invariance. *Multivariate Behavioral Research, 55*(2), 312–328. https://doi.org/10.1080/00273171.2019.1633617

Cronbach, L. J., & Meehl, P. E. (1955). Construct validity in psychological tests. *Psychological Bulletin, 52*(4), 281–302. https://doi.org/10.1037/h0040957

Curran, P. J., Howard, A. L., Bainter, S. A., Lane, S. T., & McGinley, J. S. (2014). The separation of between-person and within-person components of individual change over time: A latent curve model with structured residuals. *Journal of Consulting and Clinical Psychology, 82*, 8–94. https://doi.org/10.1037/a0035297

Dana, J., & Thomas, R. (2006). In defense of clinical judgment . . . and mechanical prediction. *Journal of Behavioral Decision Making, 19*(5), 413–428. https://doi.org/10.1002/bdm.537

Dana, R. H. (1998). Multicultural assessment of personality and psychopathology in the United States: Still art, not yet science, and controversial. *European Journal of Psychological Assessment, 14*(1), 62–70. https://doi.org/10.1027/1015-5759.14.1.62

Daugherty, J. C., Puente, A. E., Fasfous, A. F., Hidalgo-Ruzzante, N., & Pérez-Garcia, M. (2017). Diagnostic mistakes of culturally diverse individuals when using North American neuropsychological tests. *Applied Neuropsychology: Adult, 24*(1), 16–22. https://doi.org/10.1080/23279095.2015.1036992

Davison, G. C., Vogel, R. S., & Coffman, S. G. (1997). Think-aloud approaches to cognitive assessment and the articulated thoughts in simulated situations paradigm. *Journal of Consulting and Clinical Psychology, 65*(6), 950–958. https://doi.org/10.1037/0022-006X.65.6.950

Dawes, R. M. (1986). Representative thinking in clinical judgment. *Clinical Psychology Review, 6*, 425–441. https://doi.org/10.1016/0272-7358(86)90030-9

Dawes, R. M., Faust, D., & Meehl, P. E. (1989). Clinical versus actuarial judgment. *Science, 243*(4899), 1668–1674. https://doi.org/10.1126/science.2648573

Diamantopoulos, A., Riefler, P., & Roth, K. P. (2008). Advancing formative measurement models. *Journal of Business Research, 61*(12), 1203–1218. https://doi.org/10.1016/j.jbusres.2008.01.009

Dien, J. (2012). Applying principal components analysis to event-related potentials: A tutorial. *Developmental Neuropsychology, 37*(6), 497–517. https://doi.org/10.1080/87565641.2012.697503

Dinno, A. (2014). *Gently clarifying the application of Horn's parallel analysis to principal component analysis versus factor analysis.* http://archives.pdx.edu/ds/psu/10527

Dombrowski, S. C., McGill, R. J., & Morgan, G. B. (2021). Monte Carlo modeling of contemporary intelligence test (IQ) factor structure: Implications for IQ assessment, interpretation, and theory. *Assessment, 28*(3), 977–993. https://doi.org/10.1177/1073191119869828

Dorans, N. J. (2017). Contributions to the quantitative assessment of item, test, and score fairness. In R. E. Bennett & M. von Davier (Eds.), *Advancing human assessment* (pp. 201–230). Springer, Cham.

Dubois, J., & Adolphs, R. (2016). Building a science of individual differences from fMRI. *Trends in Cognitive Sciences, 20*(6), 425–443. https://doi.org/10.1016/j.tics.2016.03.014

Dueber, D. (2019). *dmacs: Measurement nonequivalence effect size calculator.* https://github.com/ddueber/dmacs

Duncan, G. J., Engel, M., Claessens, A., & Dowsett, C. J. (2014). Replication and robustness in developmental research. *Developmental Psychology, 50*(11), 2417–2425. https://doi.org/10.1037/a0037996

Dunkley, D. M., Segal, Z. V., & Blankstein, K. R. (2019). Cognitive assessment: Issues and methods. In K. S. Dobson & D. J. A. Dozois (Eds.), *Handbook of cognitive-behavioral therapies* (4th ed., pp. 85–119). Guilford Press.

Dunn, T. J., Baguley, T., & Brunsden, V. (2014). From alpha to omega: A practical solution to the pervasive problem of internal consistency estimation. *British Journal of Psychology, 105*(3), 399–412. https://doi.org/10.1111/bjop.12046

Dunning, D., Heath, C., & Suls, J. M. (2004). Flawed self-assessment: Implications for health, education, and the workplace. *Psychological Science in the Public Interest, 5*, 69–106. https://doi.org/10.1111/j.1529-1006.2004.00018.x

Durbin, C. E., Wilson, S., & MacDonald, I., Angus W. (2022). Integrating development into the research domain criteria (RDoC) framework: Introduction to the special section. *Journal of Psychopathology and Clinical Science, 131*(6), 535–541. https://doi.org/10.1037/abn0000767

Eaton, W. W. (1980). *The sociology of mental disorders.* Praeger.

Eddy, D. M. (1982). Probabilistic reasoning in clinical medicine: Problems and opportunities. In D. Kahneman, P. Slovic, & A. Tversky (Eds.), *Judgment under uncertainty: Heuristics and biases* (pp. 249–267). Cambridge University Press.

Edwards, J. R. (2011). The fallacy of formative measurement. *Organizational Research Methods, 14*(2), 370–388. https://doi.org/10.1177/1094428110378369

Edwards, J. R., & Bagozzi, R. P. (2000). On the nature and direction of relationships between constructs and measures. *Psychological Methods, 5*(2), 155–174. https://doi.org/10.1037/1082-989X.5.2.155

Edwards, L. M., Burkard, A. W., Adams, H. A., & Newcomb, S. A. (2017). A mixed-method study of psychologists' use of multicultural assessment. *Professional Psychology: Research and Practice, 48*(2), 131–138. https://doi.org/10.1037/pro0000095

Ellard, K. K., Fairholme, C. P., Boisseau, C. L., Farchione, T. J., & Barlow, D. H. (2010). Unified protocol for the transdiagnostic treatment of emotional disorders: Protocol development and initial outcome data. *Cognitive and Behavioral Practice, 17*(1), 88–101. https://doi.org/10.1016/j.cbpra.2009.06.002

Embretson, S. E. (1996). The new rules of measurement. *Psychological Assessment, 8*, 341–349. https://doi.org/10.1037/1040-3590.8.4.341

Embretson, S. E., & Reise, S. P. (2000). *Item response theory for psychologists* (Vol. 4). Lawrence Erlbaum Associates.

Evans, S. C., & Shaughnessy, S. (in press). Emotion regulation as central to psychopathology across childhood and adolescence: A commentary on Nobakht et al. (2023). *Journal of Child Psychology and Psychiatry*. https://doi.org/https://doi.org/10.1111/jcpp.13910

Executive Board of the American Anthropological Association. (1998). AAA statement on race. *American Anthropologist, 100*(3), 712–713. https://doi.org/10.1525/aa.1998.100.3.712

Exner, J. E. (1974). *The Rorschach: A comprehensive system*. John Wiley & Sons.

Exner, J. E., & Erdberg, S. P. (2005). *The Rorschach, a comprehensive system: Advanced interpretation* (3rd ed., Vol. 2). John Wiley & Sons, Inc.

Falotico, R., & Quatto, P. (2010). On avoiding paradoxes in assessing inter-rater agreement. *Italian Journal of Applied Statistics, 22*, 151–160.

Faraone, S. V., & Tsuang, M. T. (1994). Measuring diagnostic accuracy in the absence of a "gold standard." *American Journal of Psychiatry, 151*, 650–657. https://doi.org/10.1176/ajp.151.5.650

Farrington, D. P., & Loeber, R. (1989). Relative improvement over chance (RIOC) and phi as measures of predictive efficiency and strength of association in 2×2 tables. *Journal of Quantitative Criminology, 5*(3), 201–213. https://doi.org/10.1007/BF01062737

Farris, C., Treat, T. A., Viken, R. J., & McFall, R. M. (2008). Perceptual mechanisms that characterize gender differences in decoding women's sexual intent. *Psychological Science, 19*(4), 348–354. https://doi.org/10.1111/j.1467-9280.2008.02092.x

Farris, C., Viken, R. J., Treat, T. A., & McFall, R. M. (2006). Heterosocial perceptual organization: Application of the choice model to sexual coercion. *Psychological Science (0956-7976), 17*(10), 869–875. https://doi.org/10.1111/j.1467-9280.2006.01796.x

Fernández, A. L., & Abe, J. (2018). Bias in cross-cultural neuropsychological testing: Problems and possible solutions. *Culture and Brain, 6*(1), 1–35. https://doi.org/10.1007/s40167-017-0050-2

Fiske, D. W., & Campbell, D. T. (1992). Citations do not solve problems. *Psychological Bulletin, 112*(3), 393–395. https://doi.org/10.1037/0033-2909.112.3.393

Fletcher, R. R., Nakeshimana, A., & Olubeko, O. (2021). Addressing fairness, bias, and appropriate use of artificial intelligence and machine learning in global health. *Frontiers in Artificial Intelligence, 3*(116). https://doi.org/10.3389/frai.2020.561802

Flora, D. B. (2020). Your coefficient alpha is probably wrong, but which coefficient omega is right? A tutorial on using R to obtain better reliability estimates. *Advances in Methods and Practices in Psychological Science, 3*(4), 484–501. https://doi.org/10.1177/2515245920951747

Floyd, F. J., & Widaman, K. F. (1995). Factor analysis in the development and refinement of clinical assessment instruments. *Psychological Assessment*, *7*, 286–299. https://doi.org/10.1037/1040-3590.7.3.286

Fontaine, N. M. G., & Petersen, I. T. (2017). Developmental trajectories of psychopathology: An overview of approaches and applications. In L. Centifanti & D. Williams (Eds.), *The wiley handbook of developmental psychopathology* (pp. 5–28). Wiley-Blackwell.

Forbey, J. D., & Ben-Porath, Y. S. (2007). Computerized adaptive personality testing: A review and illustration with the MMPI-2 computerized adaptive version. *Psychological Assessment*, *19*(1), 14–24. https://doi.org/10.1037/1040-3590.19.1.14

Fornell, C., & Larcker, D. F. (1981). Evaluating structural equation models with unobservable variables and measurement error. *Journal of Marketing Research*, *18*(1), 39–50. https://doi.org/10.2307/3151312

Fox, J., Weisberg, S., & Price, B. (2022). *Car: Companion to applied regression*. https://CRAN.R-project.org/package=car

Frank, L. K. (1939). Projective methods for the study of personality. *Journal of Psychology*, *8*, 389–413. https://doi.org/10.1080/00223980.1939.9917671

Frazier, T. W., Georgiades, S., Bishop, S. L., & Hardan, A. Y. (2014). Behavioral and cognitive characteristics of females and males with autism in the simons simplex collection. *Journal of the American Academy of Child & Adolescent Psychiatry*, *53*(3), 329–340.e3. https://doi.org/10.1016/j.jaac.2013.12.004

Freese, J., & Peterson, D. (2017). Replication in social science. *Annual Review of Sociology*.

Freud, S. (1911). Psycho-analytic notes on an autobiographical account of a case of paranoia (dementia paranoides). In J. Strachey (Ed.), *The standard edition of the complete psychological works of Sigmund Freud: The case of Schreber, papers on technique and other works, Vol. 12 (1911–1913)* (pp. 1–82).

Fried, E. I. (2022). Studying mental health problems as systems, not syndromes. *Current Directions in Psychological Science*, *31*(6), 500–508. https://doi.org/10.1177/09637214221114089

Furr, R. M. (2017). *Psychometrics: An introduction*. SAGE publications.

Furr, R. M., & Heuckeroth, S. (2019). The "quantifying construct validity" procedure: Its role, value, interpretations, and computation. *Assessment*, *26*(4), 555–566. https://doi.org/10.1177/1073191118820638

Galatzer-Levy, I. R., & Bryant, R. A. (2013). 636,120 ways to have posttraumatic stress disorder. *Perspectives on Psychological Science*, *8*(6), 651–662. https://doi.org/10.1177/1745691613504115

Gambrill, E. (2014). The diagnostic and statistical manual of mental disorders as a major form of dehumanization in the modern world. *Research on Social Work Practice*, *24*(1), 13–36. https://doi.org/10.1177/1049731513499411

Gandrud, C. (2020). *Reproducible research with R and R studio* (3rd ed.). CRC Press. https://www.routledge.com/Reproducible-Research-with-R-and-RStudio/Gandrud/p/book/9780367143985

Garb, H. N. (1997). Race bias, social class bias, and gender bias in clinical judgment. *Clinical Psychology: Science and Practice*, *4*(2), 99–120. https://doi.org/10.1111/j.1468-2850.1997.tb00104.x

Garb, H. N. (2005). Clinical judgment and decision making. *Annual Review of Clinical Psychology*, *1*, 67–89. https://doi.org/10.1146/annurev.clinpsy.1.102803.143810

Garb, H. N. (2007). Computer-administered interviews and rating scales. *Psychological Assessment*, *19*(1), 4–13. https://doi.org/10.1037/1040-3590.19.1.4

Garb, H. N., & Wood, J. M. (2019). Methodological advances in statistical prediction. *Psychological Assessment*, *31*(12), 1456–1466. https://doi.org/10.1037/pas0000673

Garb, H. N., Wood, J. M., Lilienfeld, S. O., & Nezworski, M. T. (2005). Roots of the Rorschach controversy. *Clinical Psychology Review*, *25*(1), 97–118. https://doi.org/10.1016/j.cpr.2004.09.002

Garber, J., & Weersing, V. R. (2010). Comorbidity of anxiety and depression in youth: Implications for treatment and prevention. *Clinical Psychology: Science and Practice*, *17*(4), 293–306. https://doi.org/10.1111/j.1468-2850.2010.01221.x

Gelman, A., & Loken, E. (2013). The garden of forking paths: Why multiple comparisons can be a problem, even when there is no "fishing expedition" or "p-hacking" and the research hypothesis was posited ahead of time. *Department of Statistics, Columbia University.*

Gibbons, R. D., Weiss, D. J., Frank, E., & Kupfer, D. (2016). Computerized adaptive diagnosis and testing of mental health disorders. *Annual Review of Clinical Psychology*, *12*(1), 83–104. https://doi.org/10.1146/annurev-clinpsy-021815-093634

Gilovich, T., Vallone, R., & Tversky, A. (1985). The hot hand in basketball: On the misperception of random sequences. *Cognitive Psychology*, *17*(3), 295–314. https://doi.org/10.1016/0010-0285(85)90010-6

Gipps, C., & Stobart, G. (2009). Fairness in assessment. In C. Wyatt-Smith & J. J. Cumming (Eds.), *Educational assessment in the 21st century: Connecting theory and practice* (pp. 105–118). Springer Netherlands. https://doi.org/10.1007/978-1-4020-9964-9_6

Girard, J. M., & Cohn, J. F. (2016). A primer on observational measurement. *Assessment*, *23*(4), 404–413. https://doi.org/10.1177/1073191116635807

Gneiting, T., & Walz, E.-M. (2021). Receiver operating characteristic (ROC) movies, universal ROC (UROC) curves, and coefficient of predictive ability (CPA). *Machine Learning*. https://doi.org/10.1007/s10994-021-06114-3

Gonzalez, O., & Pelham, W. E. (2021). When does differential item functioning matter for screening? A method for empirical evaluation. *Assessment*, *28*(2), 446–456. https://doi.org/10.1177/1073191120913618

Goodwin, L. D., & Leech, N. L. (2006). Understanding correlation: Factors that affect the size of r. *The Journal of Experimental Education*, *74*(3), 249–266. https://doi.org/10.3200/JEXE.74.3.249-266

Gottfredson, L. S. (1994). The science and politics of race-norming. *American Psychologist*, *49*(11), 955–963. https://doi.org/10.1037/0003-066X.49.11.955

Gottfredson, L. S. (1997). Mainstream science on intelligence: An editorial with 52 signatories, history, and bibliography. *Intelligence*, *24*(1), 13–23.

Gottfredson, N. C., Cole, V. T., Giordano, M. L., Bauer, D. J., Hussong, A. M., & Ennett, S. T. (2019). Simplifying the implementation of modern scale scoring methods with an automated R package: Automated moderated nonlinear factor analysis (aMNLFA). *Addictive Behaviors*, *94*, 65–73. https://doi.org/10.1016/j.addbeh.2018.10.031

Graham, J. M. (2006). Congeneric and (essentially) tau-equivalent estimates of score reliability: What they are and how to use them. *Educational and Psychological Measurement*, *66*(6), 930–944. https://doi.org/10.1177/0013164406288165

Graham, J. R., Veltri, C. O. C., & Lee, T. T. C. (2022). *MMPI instruments: Assessing personality and psychopathology* (6th ed.). Oxford University Press.

Granziol, U., Brancaccio, A., Pizziconi, G., Spangaro, M., Gentili, F., Bosia, M., Gregori, E., Luperini, C., Pavan, C., Santarelli, V., Cavallaro, R., Cremonese, C., Favaro, A., Rossi, A., Vidotto, G., & Spoto, A. (2022). On the implementation of computerized adaptive observations for psychological assessment. *Assessment*, *29*(2), 225–241. https://doi.org/10.1177/1073191120960215

Green, S. B., & Yang, Y. (2015). Evaluation of dimensionality in the assessment of internal consistency reliability: Coefficient alpha and omega coefficients. *Educational Measurement: Issues and Practice*, *34*(4), 14–20. https://doi.org/10.1111/emip.12100

Greenberg, D. M., Warrier, V., Allison, C., & Baron-Cohen, S. (2018). Testing the empathizing–systemizing theory of sex differences and the extreme male brain theory of autism in half a million people. *Proceedings of the National Academy of Sciences*, *115*(48), 12152–12157. https://doi.org/10.1073/pnas.1811032115

Grove, W. M., & Meehl, P. E. (1996). Comparative efficiency of informal (subjective, impressionistic) and formal (mechanical, algorithmic) prediction procedures: The clinical–statistical controversy. *Psychology, Public Policy, and Law*, *2*(2), 293–323. https://doi.org/10.1037/1076-8971.2.2.293

Grove, W. M., Zald, D. H., Lebow, B. S., Snitz, B. E., & Nelson, C. (2000). Clinical versus mechanical prediction: A meta-analysis. *Psychological Assessment*, *12*(1), 19–30. https://doi.org/10.1037/1040-3590.12.1.19

Gunn, H. J., Grimm, K. J., & Edwards, M. C. (2020). Evaluation of six effect size measures of measurement non-invariance for continuous outcomes. *Structural Equation Modeling: A Multidisciplinary Journal*, *27*(4), 503–514. https://doi.org/10.1080/10705511.2019.1689507

Gwet, K. L. (2008). Computing inter-rater reliability and its variance in the presence of high agreement. *British Journal of Mathematical and Statistical Psychology*, *61*(1), 29–48. https://doi.org/10.1348/000711006X126600

Gwet, K. L. (2021a). *Handbook of inter-rater reliability: The definitive guide to measuring the extent of agreement among raters, Vol. 1: Analysis of categorical ratings* (5th ed.). AgreeStat Analytics.

Gwet, K. L. (2021b). *Handbook of inter-rater reliability: The definitive guide to measuring the extent of agreement among raters, Vol. 2: Analysis of quantitative ratings* (5th ed.). AgreeStat Analytics.

Hagquist, C. (2019). Explaining differential item functioning focusing on the crucial role of external information – an example from the measurement of adolescent mental health. *BMC Medical Research Methodology*, *19*(1), 185. https://doi.org/10.1186/s12874-019-0828-3

Hagquist, C., & Andrich, D. (2017). Recent advances in analysis of differential item functioning in health research using the Rasch model. *Health and Quality of Life Outcomes*, *15*(1), 181. https://doi.org/10.1186/s12955-017-0755-0

Hall, G. C. N., Bansal, A., & Lopez, I. R. (1999). Ethnicity and psychopathology: A meta-analytic review of 31 years of comparative MMPI/MMPI-2 research. *Psychological Assessment*, *11*(2), 186–197. https://doi.org/10.1037/1040-3590.11.2.186

Hamaker, E. L., Kuiper, R. M., & Grasman, R. P. P. P. (2015). A critique of the cross-lagged panel model. *Psychological Methods*, *20*(1), 102–116. https://doi.org/10.1037/a0038889

Han, K., Colarelli, S. M., & Weed, N. C. (2019). Methodological and statistical advances in the consideration of cultural diversity in assessment: A critical review of group classification and measurement invariance testing. *Psychological Assessment*, *31*(12), 1481–1496. https://doi.org/10.1037/pas0000731

Hardin, A. M., Chang, J. C.-J., Fuller, M. A., & Torkzadeh, G. (2011). Formative measurement and academic research: In search of measurement theory. *Educational and Psychological Measurement*, *71*(2), 281–305. https://doi.org/10.1177/0013164410370208

Harrell, F. (2015). *Regression modeling strategies: With applications to linear models, logistic and ordinal regression, and survival analysis*. Springer.

Harrell, Jr., F. E. (2021). *rms: Regression modeling strategies*. https://CRAN.R-project.org/package=rms

Hayes, A. F., & Coutts, J. J. (2020). Use omega rather than cronbach's alpha for estimating reliability. but.... *Communication Methods and Measures*, *14*(1), 1–24. https://doi.org/10.1080/19312458.2020.1718629

Hayes, S. C., Nelson, R. O., & Jarrett, R. B. (1987). The treatment utility of assessment: A functional approach to evaluating assessment quality. *American Psychologist*, *42*, 963–974. https://doi.org/10.1037/0003-066X.42.11.963

Haynes, S. N. (2001). Clinical applications of analogue behavioral observation: Dimensions of psychometric evaluation. *Psychological Assessment*, *13*(1), 73–85. https://doi.org/10.1037/1040-3590.13.1.73

Haynes, S. N., & Yoshioka, D. T. (2007). Clinical assessment applications of ambulatory biosensors. *Psychological Assessment*, *19*(1), 44–57. https://doi.org/10.1037/1040-3590.19.1.44

Hays, P. A. (2016). *Addressing cultural complexities in practice: Assessment, diagnosis, and therapy*. American Psychological Association.

Hedge, C., Powell, G., & Sumner, P. (2018). The reliability paradox: Why robust cognitive tasks do not produce reliable individual differences. *Behavior Research Methods*, *50*(3), 1166–1186. https://doi.org/10.3758/s13428-017-0935-1

Helms, J. E. (2006). Fairness is not validity or cultural bias in racial-group assessment: A quantitative perspective. *American Psychologist*, *61*(8), 845–859. https://doi.org/10.1037/0003-066X.61.8.845

Helms, J. E., Jernigan, M., & Mascher, J. (2005). The meaning of race in psychology and how to change it: A methodological perspective. *American Psychologist*, *60*(1), 27–36. https://doi.org/10.1037/0003-066X.60.1.27

Henrich, J., Heine, S. J., & Norenzayan, A. (2010). Most people are not WEIRD. *Nature*, *466*(7302), 29–29. https://doi.org/10.1038/466029a

Henseler, J., Ringle, C. M., & Sarstedt, M. (2015). A new criterion for assessing discriminant validity in variance-based structural equation modeling. *Journal of the Academy of Marketing Science*, *43*(1), 115–135. https://doi.org/10.1007/s11747-014-0403-8

Hertzog, C., & Nesselroade, J. R. (2003). Assessing psychological change in adulthood: An overview of methodological issues. *Psychology and Aging*, *18*(4), 639–657. https://doi.org/10.1037/0882-7974.18.4.639

Himmelstein, P. H., Woods, W. C., & Wright, A. G. C. (2019). A comparison of signal- and event-contingent ambulatory assessment of interpersonal behavior and affect in social situations. *Psychological Assessment*, *31*(7), 952–960. https://doi.org/10.1037/pas0000718

Hinshaw, S. P., & Nigg, J. T. (1999). Behavior rating scales in the assessment of disruptive behavior problems in childhood. In D. Shaffer, C. P. Lucas, & J. E. Richters (Eds.), *Diagnostic assessment in child and adolescent psychopathology*. (pp. 91–126). The Guilford Press.

Hoch, S. J. (1985). Counterfactual reasoning and accuracy in predicting personal events. *Journal of Experimental Psychology: Learning, Memory, and Cognition*, *11*(4), 719–731. https://doi.org/10.1037/0278-7393.11.1-4.719

Holmlund, T. B., Foltz, P. W., Cohen, A. S., Johansen, H. D., Sigurdsen, R., Fugelli, P., Bergsager, D., Cheng, J., Bernstein, J., Rosenfeld, E., & Elvevåg, B. (2019). Moving psychological assessment out of the controlled laboratory setting: Practical challenges. *Psychological Assessment*, *31*(3), 292–303. https://doi.org/10.1037/pas0000647

Hough, S. E. (2016). *Predicting the unpredictable: The tumultuous science of earthquake prediction*. Princeton University Press.

Howell, R. D., Breivik, E., & Wilcox, J. B. (2007). Reconsidering formative measurement. *Psychological Methods*, *12*(2), 205–218. https://doi.org/10.1037/1082-989X.12.2.205

Huebner, A., & Lucht, M. (2019). Generalizability theory in R. *Practical Assessment, Research & Evaluation*, *24*(5), 2. https://doi.org/10.7275/5065-gc10

Hunsley, J., Lee, C. M., Wood, J. M., & Taylor, W. (2015). Controversial and questionable assessment techniques. In S. O. Lilienfeld, S. J. Lynn, & J. M. Lohr (Eds.), *Science and pseudoscience in clinical psychology* (2nd ed., pp. 42–82). The Guilford Press.

Hunsley, J., & Mash, E. J. (2007). Evidence-based assessment. *Annual Review of Clinical Psychology, 3*, 29–51. https://doi.org/10.1146/annurev.clinpsy.3.022806.091419

Hurlburt, R. T. (1997). Randomly sampling thinking in the natural environment. *Journal of Consulting and Clinical Psychology, 65*(6), 941–949. https://doi.org/10.1037/0022-006X.65.6.941

Hussong, A. M., Bauer, D. J., Giordano, M. L., & Curran, P. J. (2020). Harmonizing altered measures in integrative data analysis: A methods analogue study. *Behavior Research Methods.* https://doi.org/10.3758/s13428-020-01472-7

Hussong, A. M., Curran, P. J., & Bauer, D. J. (2013). Integrative data analysis in clinical psychology research. *Annual Review of Clinical Psychology, 9*(1), 61–89. https://doi.org/10.1146/annurev-clinpsy-050212-185522

Hyndman, R. J., & Athanasopoulos, G. (2018). *Forecasting: Principles and practice* (2nd ed.). OTexts.

Jensen, A. R. (1980). Précis of bias in mental testing. *Behavioral and Brain Sciences, 3*(3), 325–333. https://doi.org/10.1017/S0140525X00005161

Jiang, Z. (2018). Using the linear mixed-effect model framework to estimate generalizability variance components in R. *Methodology, 14*(3), 133–142. https://doi.org/10.1027/1614-2241/a000149

John, L. K., Loewenstein, G., & Prelec, D. (2012). Measuring the prevalence of questionable research practices with incentives for truth telling. *Psychological Science, 23*(5), 524–532. https://doi.org/10.1177/0956797611430953

Johnson, J. E. V., & Bruce, A. C. (2001). Calibration of subjective probability judgments in a naturalistic setting. *Organizational Behavior and Human Decision Processes, 85*(2), 265–290. https://doi.org/10.1006/obhd.2000.2949

Jonson, J. L., & Geisinger, K. F. (2022). *Fairness in educational and psychological testing: Examining theoretical, research, practice, and policy implications of the 2014 standards.* American Educational Research Association,.

Jorgensen, T. D., Kite, B. A., Chen, P.-Y., & Short, S. D. (2018). Permutation randomization methods for testing measurement equivalence and detecting differential item functioning in multiple-group confirmatory factor analysis. *Psychological Methods, 23*(4), 708–728. https://doi.org/10.1037/met0000152

Jorgensen, T. D., Pornprasertmanit, S., Schoemann, A. M., & Rosseel, Y. (2021). *semTools: Useful tools for structural equation modeling.* https://github.com/simsem/semTools/wiki

Kazdin, A. E. (1995). Preparing and evaluating research reports. *Psychological Assessment, 7*(3), 228–237. https://doi.org/10.1037/1040-3590.7.3.228

Kelley, K. (2020). *MBESS: The MBESS R package.* http://nd.edu/~kkelley/site/MBESS.html

Kelley, K., & Pornprasertmanit, S. (2016). Confidence intervals for population reliability coefficients: Evaluation of methods, recommendations, and software for composite measures. *Psychological Methods, 21*(1), 69–92. https://doi.org/10.1037/a0040086

Keren, G. (1987). Facing uncertainty in the game of bridge: A calibration study. *Organizational Behavior and Human Decision Processes, 39*(1), 98–114. https://doi.org/10.1016/0749-5978(87)90047-1

Kessler, R. C., Bossarte, R. M., Luedtke, A., Zaslavsky, A. M., & Zubizarreta, J. R. (2020). Suicide prediction models: A critical review of recent research with recommendations for the way forward. *Molecular Psychiatry, 25*(1), 168–179. https://doi.org/10.1038/s41380-019-0531-0

Kievit, R. A., Brandmaier, A. M., Ziegler, G., Harmelen, A.-L. van, Mooij, S. M. M. de, Moutoussis, M., Goodyer, I., Bullmore, E., Jones, P. B., Fonagy, P., Lindenberger, U., & Dolan, R. J. (2018). Developmental cognitive neuroscience using latent change score models: A tutorial and applications. *Developmental Cognitive Neuroscience*, *33*, 99–117. https://doi.org/10.1016/j.dcn.2017.11.007

Kievit, R., Frankenhuis, W., Waldorp, L., & Borsboom, D. (2013). Simpson's paradox in psychological science: A practical guide. *Frontiers in Psychology*, *4*(513). https://doi.org/10.3389/fpsyg.2013.00513

Klein, D. F., & Cleary, T. A. (1969). Platonic true scores: Further comment. *Psychological Bulletin*, *71*(4), 278–280. https://doi.org/10.1037/h0026852

Kline, R. B. (2023). *Principles and practice of structural equation modeling* (5th ed.). Guilford Publications.

Koehler, D. J., Brenner, L., & Griffin, D. (2002). The calibration of expert judgment: Heuristics and biases beyond the laboratory. In T. Gilovich, D. Griffin, & D. Kahneman (Eds.), *Heuristics and biases: The psychology of intuitive judgment*. Cambridge University Press.

Koriat, A., Lichtenstein, S., & Fischhoff, B. (1980). Reasons for confidence. *Journal of Experimental Psychology: Human Learning and Memory*, *6*(2), 107–118. https://doi.org/10.1037/0278-7393.6.2.107

Korotitsch, W. J., & Nelson-Gray, R. O. (1999). An overview of self-monitoring research in assessment and treatment. *Psychological Assessment*, *11*(4), 415–425. https://doi.org/10.1037/1040-3590.11.4.415

Kotov, R., Krueger, R. F., Watson, D., Achenbach, T. M., Althoff, R. R., Bagby, R. M., Brown, T. A., Carpenter, W. T., Caspi, A., Clark, L. A., Eaton, N. R., Forbes, M. K., Forbush, K. T., Goldberg, D., Hasin, D., Hyman, S. E., Ivanova, M. Y., Lynam, D. R., Markon, K., … Zimmerman, M. (2017). The hierarchical taxonomy of psychopathology (HiTOP): A dimensional alternative to traditional nosologies. *Journal of Abnormal Psychology*, *126*(4), 454–477. https://doi.org/10.1037/abn0000258

Kotov, R., Krueger, R. F., Watson, D., Cicero, D. C., Conway, C. C., DeYoung, C. G., Eaton, N. R., Forbes, M. K., Hallquist, M. N., Latzman, R. D., Mullins-Sweatt, S. N., Ruggero, C. J., Simms, L. J., Waldman, I. D., Waszczuk, M. A., & Wright, A. G. C. (2021). The hierarchical taxonomy of psychopathology (HiTOP): A quantitative nosology based on consensus of evidence. *Annual Review of Clinical Psychology*, *17*(1), 83–108. https://doi.org/10.1146/annurev-clinpsy-081219-093304

Kozak, M. J., & Cuthbert, B. N. (2016). The NIMH research domain criteria initiative: Background, issues, and pragmatics. *Psychophysiology*, *53*(3), 286–297. https://doi.org/10.1111/psyp.12518

Kraemer, H., Yesavage, J., Taylor, J., & Kupfer, D. (2000). How can we learn about developmental processes from cross-sectional studies, or can we? *American Journal of Psychiatry*, *157*(2), 163–171. https://doi.org/10.1176/APPI.AJP.157.2.163

Kriegman, L. S., & Kriegman, G. (1965). The PaTE report: A new psychodynamic and therapeutic evaluative procedure. *The Psychiatric Quarterly*, *39*(1), 646–674. https://doi.org/10.1007/BF01569493

Krosnick, J. A. (1999). Survey research. *Annual Review of Psychology*, *50*, 537–567. https://doi.org/10.1146/annurev.psych.50.1.537

Krueger, R. F., Nichol, P. E., Hicks, B. M., Markon, K. E., Patrick, C. J., lacono, W. G., & McGue, M. (2004). Using latent trait modeling to conceptualize an alcohol problems continuum. *Psychological Assessment*, *16*(2), 107–119. https://doi.org/10.1037/1040-3590.16.2.107

Kuhn, M. (2022). *caret: Classification and regression training*. https://github.com/topepo/caret/

Kuncel, N. R., & Hezlett, S. A. (2010). Fact and fiction in cognitive ability testing for admissions and hiring decisions. *Current Directions in Psychological Science*, *19*(6), 339–345. https://doi.org/10.1177/0963721410389459

Kundu, S., Aulchenko, Y. S., & Janssens, A. C. J. W. (2020). *PredictABEL: Assessment of risk prediction models*. https://CRAN.R-project.org/package=PredictABEL

Lai, M. H. C. (2021). Adjusting for measurement noninvariance with alignment in growth modeling. *Multivariate Behavioral Research*, 1–18. https://doi.org/10.1080/00273171.2021.1941730

Larson, M. J., & Carbine, K. A. (2017). Sample size calculations in human electrophysiology (EEG and ERP) studies: A systematic review and recommendations for increased rigor. *International Journal of Psychophysiology*, *111*, 33–41. https://doi.org/10.1016/j.ijpsycho.2016.06.015

Lee, K., Bull, R., & Ho, R. M. H. (2013). Developmental changes in executive functioning. *Child Development*, *84*(6), 1933–1953. https://doi.org/10.1111/cdev.12096

Lee Meeuw Kjoe, P. R., Agelink van Rentergem, J. A., Vermeulen, I. E., & Schagen, S. B. (2021). How to correct for computer experience in online cognitive testing? *Assessment*, *28*(5), 1247–1255. https://doi.org/10.1177/1073191120911098

Lek, K. M., & Van De Schoot, R. (2018). A comparison of the single, conditional and person-specific standard error of measurement: What do they measure and when to use them? *Frontiers in Applied Mathematics and Statistics*, *4*(40). https://doi.org/10.3389/fams.2018.00040

Lele, S. R., Keim, J. L., & Solymos, P. (2019). *ResourceSelection: Resource selection (probability) functions for use-availability data*. https://github.com/psolymos/ResourceSelection

Leong, F. T. L., & Kalibatseva, Z. (2016). Threats to cultural validity in clinical diagnosis and assessment: Illustrated with the case of Asian Americans. In N. Zane, G. Bernal, & F. T. L. Leong (Eds.), *Evidence-based psychological practice with ethnic minorities: Culturally informed research and clinical strategies* (pp. 57–74). American Psychological Association.

Lewis-Fernández, R., Aggarwal, N. K., Bäärnhielm, S., Rohlof, H., Kirmayer, L. J., Weiss, M. G., Jadhav, S., Hinton, L., Alarcón, R. D., Bhugra, D., Groen, S., Dijk, R. van, Qureshi, A., Collazos, F., Rousseau, C., Caballero, L., Ramos, M., & Lu, F. (2014). Culture and psychiatric evaluation: Operationalizing cultural formulation for DSM-5. *Psychiatry: Interpersonal and Biological Processes*, *77*(2), 130–154. https://doi.org/10.1521/psyc.2014.77.2.130

Lilienfeld, S. O. (2007). Psychological treatments that cause harm. *Perspectives on Psychological Science*, *2*(1), 53–70. https://doi.org/10.1111/j.1745-6916.2007.00029.x

Lilienfeld, S. O. (2017). Psychology's replication crisis and the grant culture: Righting the ship. *Perspectives on Psychological Science*, *12*(4), 660–664. https://doi.org/10.1177/1745691616687745

Lilienfeld, S. O., Sauvigne, K., Lynn, S. J., Latzman, R. D., Cautin, R., & Waldman, I. D. (2015). Fifty psychological and psychiatric terms to avoid: A list of inaccurate, misleading, misused, ambiguous, and logically confused words and phrases. *Frontiers in Psychology*, *6*. https://doi.org/10.3389/fpsyg.2015.01100

Lilienfeld, S. O., Wood, J. M., & Garb, H. N. (2000). The scientific status of projective techniques. *Psychological Science in the Public Interest*, *1*, 27–66. https://doi.org/10.1111/1529-1006.002

Lindhiem, O., Petersen, I. T., Mentch, L. K., & Youngstrom, E. A. (2020). The importance of calibration in clinical psychology. *Assessment*, *27*(4), 840–854. https://doi.org/10.1177/1073191117752055

Lindzey, G. (1952). Thematic apperception test: Interpretive assumptions and related empirical evidence. *Psychological Bulletin*, *49*, 1–25. https://doi.org/10.1037/h0062363

Little, T. D. (2013). *Longitudinal structural equation modeling.* The Guilford Press.

Little, T. D., Preacher, K. J., Selig, J. P., & Card, N. A. (2007). New developments in latent variable panel analyses of longitudinal data. *International Journal of Behavioral Development, 31*(4), 357–365. https://doi.org/10.1177/0165025407077757

Little, T. D., Slegers, D. W., & Card, N. A. (2006). A non-arbitrary method of identifying and scaling latent variables in SEM and MACS models. *Structural Equation Modeling, 13*(1), 59–72. https://doi.org/10.1207/s15328007sem1301_3

Liu, Y., Millsap, R. E., West, S. G., Tein, J.-Y., Tanaka, R., & Grimm, K. J. (2017). Testing measurement invariance in longitudinal data with ordered-categorical measures. *Psychological Methods, 22*(3), 486–506. https://doi.org/10.1037/met0000075

Lobbestael, J., Leurgans, M., & Arntz, A. (2011). Inter-rater reliability of the Structured Clinical Interview for DSM-IV Axis I Disorders (SCID I) and Axis II Disorders (SCID II). *Clinical Psychology & Psychotherapy, 18*(1), 75–79. https://doi.org/10.1002/cpp.693

Loevinger, J. (1957). Objective tests as instruments of psychological theory. *Psychological Reports, 3*(3), 635–694. https://doi.org/10.2466/pr0.1957.3.3.635

Loken, E., & Gelman, A. (2017). Measurement error and the replication crisis. *Science, 355*(6325), 584–585. https://doi.org/10.1126/science.aal3618

Lubke, G. H., McArtor, D. B., Boomsma, D. I., & Bartels, M. (2018). Genetic and environmental contributions to the development of childhood aggression. *Developmental Psychology, 54*(1), 39–50. https://doi.org/10.1037/dev0000403

Lüdecke, D., Ben-Shachar, M. S., Patil, I., Waggoner, P., & Makowski, D. (2021). performance: An R package for assessment, comparison and testing of statistical models. *Journal of Open Source Software, 6*(60), 3139. https://doi.org/10.21105/joss.03139

Lupien, S. J., Sasseville, M., François, N., Giguère, C. E., Boissonneault, J., Plusquellec, P., Godbout, R., Xiong, L., Potvin, S., Kouassi, E., & Lesage, A. (2017). The DSM5/RDoC debate on the future of mental health research: Implication for studies on human stress and presentation of the signature bank. *Stress, 20*(1), 2–18. https://doi.org/10.1080/10253890.2017.1286324

Lutz, W., Schwartz, B., & Delgadillo, J. (2022). Measurement-based and data-informed psychological therapy. *Annual Review of Clinical Psychology, 18*(1), 71–98. https://doi.org/10.1146/annurev-clinpsy-071720-014821

Lysell, H., Dahlin, M., Viktorin, A., Ljungberg, E., D'Onofrio, B. M., Dickman, P., & Runeson, B. (2018). Maternal suicide – register based study of all suicides occurring after delivery in sweden 1974–2009. *PLOS ONE, 13*(1), e0190133. https://doi.org/10.1371/journal.pone.0190133

MacCallum, R. C., & Austin, J. T. (2000). Applications of structural equation modeling in psychological research. *Annual Review of Psychology, 51*(1), 201–226. https://doi.org/10.1146/annurev.psych.51.1.201

Magis, D. (2013). A note on the item information function of the four-parameter logistic model. *Applied Psychological Measurement, 37*(4), 304–315. https://doi.org/10.1177/0146621613475471

Makridakis, S., Hogarth, R. M., & Gaba, A. (2009). Forecasting and uncertainty in the economic and business world. *International Journal of Forecasting, 25*(4), 794–812. https://doi.org/10.1016/j.ijforecast.2009.05.012

Manly, J. J. (2005). Advantages and disadvantages of separate norms for African Americans. *The Clinical Neuropsychologist, 19*(2), 270–275. https://doi.org/10.1080/13854040590945346

Manly, J. J., & Echemendia, R. J. (2007). Race-specific norms: Using the model of hypertension to understand issues of race, culture, and education in neuropsychology. *Archives of Clinical Neuropsychology, 22*(3), 319–325. https://doi.org/10.1016/j.acn.2007.01.006

Markon, K. E. (2019). Bifactor and hierarchical models: Specification, inference, and interpretation. *Annual Review of Clinical Psychology, 15*(1), 51–69. https://doi.org/10.1146/annurev-clinpsy-050718-095522

Markon, K. E., Chmielewski, M., & Miller, C. J. (2011). The reliability and validity of discrete and continuous measures of psychopathology: A quantitative review. *Psychological Bulletin, 137*(5), 856–879. https://doi.org/10.1037/a0023678

Markus, K. A. (2018). Three conceptual impediments to developing scale theory for formative scales. *Methodology, 14*(4), 156–164. https://doi.org/10.1027/1614-2241/a000154

Marsh, H. W., Morin, A. J. S., Parker, P. D., & Kaur, G. (2014). Exploratory structural equation modeling: An integration of the best features of exploratory and confirmatory factor analysis. *Annual Review of Clinical Psychology, 10*(1), 85–110. https://doi.org/10.1146/annurev-clinpsy-032813-153700

Masche, J. G., & Dulmen, M. H. M. van. (2004). Advances in disentangling age, cohort, and time effects: No quadrature of the circle, but a help. *Developmental Review, 24*(3), 322–342. https://doi.org/10.1016/j.dr.2004.04.002

Matthews, M., Abdullah, S., Murnane, E., Voida, S., Choudhury, T., Gay, G., & Frank, E. (2016). Development and evaluation of a smartphone-based measure of social rhythms for bipolar disorder. *Assessment, 23*(4), 472–483. https://doi.org/10.1177/1073191116656794

McArdle, J. J., & Grimm, K. J. (2011). An empirical example of change analysis by linking longitudinal item response data from multiple tests. In A. A. von Davier (Ed.), *Statistical models for test equating, scaling, and linking* (pp. 71–88). Springer Science & Business Media.

McArdle, J. J., Grimm, K. J., Hamagami, F., Bowles, R. P., & Meredith, W. (2009). Modeling life-span growth curves of cognition using longitudinal data with multiple samples and changing scales of measurement. *Psychological Methods, 14*(2), 126–149. https://doi.org/10.1037/a0015857

McClelland, D. C. (1973). Testing for competence rather than for "intelligence." *American Psychologist, 28*, 1–14. https://doi.org/10.1037/h0034092

McClelland, D. C. (1994). The knowledge-testing-educational complex strikes back. *American Psychologist, 49*(1), 66–69. https://doi.org/10.1037/0003-066X.49.1.66

McFall, R. M. (1991). Manifesto for a science of clinical psychology. *The Clinical Psychologist, 44*(6), 75–91.

McFall, R. M. (2000). Elaborate reflections on a simple manifesto. *Applied & Preventive Psychology, 9*(1), 5–21. https://doi.org/10.1016/s0962-1849(05)80035-6

McNally, R. J. (2021). Network analysis of psychopathology: Controversies and challenges. *Annual Review of Clinical Psychology, 17*(1), 31–53. https://doi.org/10.1146/annurev-clinpsy-081219-092850

McNeish, D. (2018). Thanks coefficient alpha, we'll take it from here. *Psychological Methods, 23*(3), 412–433. https://doi.org/10.1037/met0000144

McNeish, D., & Wolf, M. G. (2023). Dynamic fit index cutoffs for confirmatory factor analysis models. *Psychological Methods, 28*(1), 61–88. https://doi.org/10.1037/met0000425

McNiel, D. E., & Binder, R. L. (1995). Correlates of accuracy in the assessment of psychiatric inpatients' risk of violence. *American Journal of Psychiatry, 152*(6), 901–906. https://doi.org/10.1176/ajp.152.6.901

Meade, A. W. (2010). A taxonomy of effect size measures for the differential functioning of items and scales. *Journal of Applied Psychology, 95*(4), 728–743. https://doi.org/10.1037/a0018966

Meehl, P. E. (1957). When shall we use our heads instead of the formula? *Journal of Counseling Psychology, 4*(4), 268–273. https://doi.org/10.1037/h0047554

Meehl, P. E. (1978). Theoretical risks and tabular asterisks: Sir Karl, Sir Ronald, and the slow progress of soft psychology. *Journal of Consulting and Clinical Psychology*, *46*(4), 806–834. https://doi.org/10.1037/0022-006x.46.4.806

Meehl, P. E. (1986). Causes and effects of my disturbing little book. *Journal of Personality Assessment*, *50*(3), 370–375. https://doi.org/10.1207/s15327752jpa5003_6

Meehl, P. E., & Rosen, A. (1955). Antecedent probability and the efficiency of psychometric signs, patterns, or cutting scores. *Psychological Bulletin*, *52*(3), 194–216. https://doi.org/10.1037/h0048070

Melikyan, Z. A., Agranovich, A. V., & Puente, A. E. (2019). Fairness in psychological testing. In G. Goldstein, D. N. Allen, & J. DeLuca (Eds.), *Handbook of psychological assessment (fourth edition)* (pp. 551–572). Academic Press. https://doi.org/10.1016/B978-0-12-802203-0.00018-3

Meyer, G. J., Erard, R. E., Erdberg, P., Mihura, J. L., & Viglione, D. J. (2011). *Rorschach Performance Assessment System: Administration, coding, interpretation, and technical manual.* Rorschach Performance Asesseement Systems LLC.

Miller, G. A., Elbert, T., Sutton, B. P., & Heller, W. (2007). Innovative clinical assessment technologies: Challenges and opportunities in neuroimaging. *Psychological Assessment*, *19*(1), 58–73. https://doi.org/10.1037/1040-3590.19.1.58

Miller, G. A., Rockstroh, B. S., Hamilton, H. K., & Yee, C. M. (2016). Psychophysiology as a core strategy in RDoC. *Psychophysiology*, *53*(3), 410–414. https://doi.org/10.1111/psyp.12581

Miller, J. B., & Sanjurjo, A. (2014). A cold shower for the hot hand fallacy. *Innocenzo Gasparini Institute for Economic Research.* https://repec.unibocconi.it/igier/igi/wp/2014/518.pdf

Miller, J. L., Vaillancourt, T., & Boyle, M. H. (2009). Examining the heterotypic continuity of aggression using teacher reports: Results from a national Canadian study. *Social Development*, *18*(1), 164–180. https://doi.org/10.1111/j.1467-9507.2008.00480.x

Millsap, R. E. (2011). *Statistical approaches to measurement invariance.* Taylor & Francis.

Moeller, J. (2015). A word on standardization in longitudinal studies: don't. *Frontiers in Psychology*, *6*(1389), 1–4. https://doi.org/10.3389/fpsyg.2015.01389

Moffitt, T. E. (1993). Adolescence-limited and life-course-persistent antisocial behavior: A developmental taxonomy. *Psychological Review*, *100*(4), 674–701. https://doi.org/10.1037/0033-295X.100.4.674

Moffitt, T. E. (2006a). A review of research on the taxonomy of life-course persistent versus adolescence-limited antisocial behavior. *Taking Stock: The Status of Criminological Theory*, *15*, 277–312.

Moffitt, T. E. (2006b). Life-course-persistent versus adolescence-limited antisocial behavior. In D. C. D. J. Cohen (Ed.), *Developmental psychopathology, vol 3: Risk, disorder, and adaptation (2nd ed.)* (pp. 570–598). John Wiley & Sons Inc.

Moore, C. T. (2016). *gtheory: Apply generalizability theory with R.* http://EvaluationDashboard.com

Morgan, C. D., & Murray, H. A. (1935). A method for investigating fantasies: The thematic apperception test. *Archives of Neurology & Psychiatry*, *34*(2), 289–306. https://doi.org/10.1001/archneurpsyc.1935.02250200049005

Morley, S. K., Brito, T. V., & Welling, D. T. (2018). Measures of model performance based on the log accuracy ratio. *Space Weather*, *16*(1), 69–88. https://doi.org/10.1002/2017SW001669

Mullins-Sweatt, S. N., & Widiger, T. A. (2009). Clinical utility and DSM-V. *Psychological Assessment*, *21*(3), 302–312. https://doi.org/10.1037/a0016607

Murphy, A. H., & Winkler, R. L. (1984). Probability forecasting in meterology. *Journal of the American Statistical Association*, *79*(387), 489–500. https://doi.org/10.2307/2288395

Muthén, L. K., & Muthén, B. O. (2019). *Mplus version 8.4*. Muthén & Muthén.

Nagy, T. F. (2011). *Essential ethics for psychologists: A primer for understanding and mastering core issues* (pp. x, 252–x, 252). American Psychological Association.

Nelson-Gray, R. O. (2003). Treatment utility of psychological assessment. *Psychological Assessment, 15*(4), 521–531. https://doi.org/10.1037/1040-3590.15.4.521

Nisbett, R. E., & Wilson, T. D. (1977). Telling more than we can know: Verbal reports on mental processes. *Psychological Review, 84*(3), 231–259. https://doi.org/10.1037/0033-295x.84.3.231

Nunnally, J. C., & Bernstein, I. H. (1994). *Psychometric theory* (3rd ed.). McGraw-Hill.

Nye, C. D., Bradburn, J., Olenick, J., Bialko, C., & Drasgow, F. (2019). How big are my effects? Examining the magnitude of effect sizes in studies of measurement equivalence. *Organizational Research Methods, 22*(3), 678–709. https://doi.org/10.1177/1094428118761122

Okazaki, S., & Sue, S. (1995). Methodological issues in assessment research with ethnic minorities. *Psychological Assessment, 7*(3), 367–375. https://doi.org/10.1037/1040-3590.7.3.367

Open Science Collaboration. (2015). Estimating the reproducibility of psychological science. *Science, 349*(6251). https://doi.org/10.1126/science.aac4716

Orth, U., Clark, D. A., Donnellan, M. B., & Robins, R. W. (2021). Testing prospective effects in longitudinal research: Comparing seven competing cross-lagged models. *Journal of Personality and Social Psychology, 120*(4), 1013–1034. https://doi.org/10.1037/pspp0000358

Oskamp, S. (1965). Overconfidence in case-study judgments. *Journal of Consulting Psychology, 29*(3), 261–265. https://doi.org/10.1037/h0022125

Patrick, C. J., Iacono, W. G., & Venables, N. C. (2019). Incorporating neurophysiological measures into clinical assessments: Fundamental challenges and a strategy for addressing them. *Psychological Assessment, 31*(7), 952–960. https://doi.org/10.1037/pas0000713

Patterson, G. R. (1993). Orderly change in a stable world: The antisocial trait as a chimera. *Journal of Consulting and Clinical Psychology, 61*(6), 911–919. https://doi.org/10.1037/0022-006X.61.6.911

Paulus, J. K., & Kent, D. M. (2020). Predictably unequal: Understanding and addressing concerns that algorithmic clinical prediction may increase health disparities. *Npj Digital Medicine, 3*(1), 99. https://doi.org/10.1038/s41746-020-0304-9

Pearl, J. (2013). Linear models: A useful "microscope" for causal analysis. *Journal of Causal Inference, 1*(1), 155–170. https://doi.org/10.1515/jci-2013-0003

Peters, G.-J. (2014). The alpha and the omega of scale reliability and validity: Why and how to abandon Cronbach's alpha and the route towards more comprehensive assessment of scale quality. *European Health Psychologist, 16*(2), 56–69.

Petersen, I. T. (2024). *petersenlab: Package of R functions for the Petersen Lab*. https://doi.org/10.5281/zenodo.7602890

Petersen, I. T., Apfelbaum, K. S., & McMurray, B. (in press). Adapting open science and pre-registration to longitudinal research. *Infant and Child Development*. https://doi.org/10.1002/icd.2315

Petersen, I. T., Bates, J. E., D'Onofrio, B. M., Coyne, C. A., Lansford, J. E., Dodge, K. A., Pettit, G. S., & Van Hulle, C. A. (2013). Language ability predicts the development of behavior problems in children. *Journal of Abnormal Psychology, 122*(2), 542–557. https://doi.org/10.1037/a0031963

Petersen, I. T., Bates, J. E., Dodge, K. A., Lansford, J. E., & Pettit, G. S. (2015). Describing and predicting developmental profiles of externalizing problems from childhood to adulthood. *Development and Psychopathology, 27*(3), 791–818. https://doi.org/10.1017/S0954579414000789

Petersen, I. T., Bates, J. E., McQuillan, M. E., Hoyniak, C. P., Staples, A. D., Rudasill, K. M., Molfese, D. L., & Molfese, V. J. (2021). Heterotypic continuity of inhibitory control in early childhood: Evidence from four widely used measures. *Developmental Psychology, 57*(11), 1755–1771. https://doi.org/10.1037/dev0001025

Petersen, I. T., Choe, D. E., & LeBeau, B. (2020). Studying a moving target in development: The challenge and opportunity of heterotypic continuity. *Developmental Review, 58*, 100935. https://doi.org/10.1016/j.dr.2020.100935

Petersen, I. T., Hoyniak, C. P., McQuillan, M. E., Bates, J. E., & Staples, A. D. (2016). Measuring the development of inhibitory control: The challenge of heterotypic continuity. *Developmental Review, 40*, 25–71. https://doi.org/10.1016/j.dr.2016.02.001

Petersen, I. T., & LeBeau, B. (2021). Language ability in the development of externalizing behavior problems in childhood. *Journal of Educational Psychology, 113*(1), 68–85. https://doi.org/10.1037/edu0000461

Petersen, I. T., & LeBeau, B. (2022). Creating a developmental scale to chart the development of psychopathology with different informants and measures across time. *Journal of Psychopathology and Clinical Science, 131*(6), 611–625. https://doi.org/10.1037/abn0000649

Petersen, I. T., LeBeau, B., & Choe, D. E. (2021). Creating a developmental scale to account for heterotypic continuity in development: A simulation study. *Child Development, 92*(1), e1–e19. https://doi.org/10.1111/cdev.13433

Petersen, I. T., Lindhiem, O., LeBeau, B., Bates, J. E., Pettit, G. S., Lansford, J. E., & Dodge, K. A. (2018). Development of internalizing problems from adolescence to emerging adulthood: Accounting for heterotypic continuity with vertical scaling. *Developmental Psychology, 54*(3), 586–599. https://doi.org/10.1037/dev0000449

Petscher, Y., Justice, L. M., & Hogan, T. (2018). Modeling the early language trajectory of language development when the measures change and its relation to poor reading comprehension. *Child Development, 89*(6), 2136–2156. https://doi.org/10.1111/cdev.12880

Piasecki, T. M., Hufford, M. R., Solhan, M., & Trull, T. J. (2007). Assessing clients in their natural environments with electronic diaries: Rationale, benefits, limitations, and barriers. *Psychological Assessment, 19*(1), 25–43. https://doi.org/10.1037/1040-3590.19.1.25

Podsakoff, P. M., MacKenzie, S. B., & Podsakoff, N. P. (2012). Sources of method bias in social science research and recommendations on how to control it. *Annual Review of Psychology, 63*(1), 539–569. https://doi.org/10.1146/annurev-psych-120710-100452

Putnam, S. P., Rothbart, M. K., & Gartstein, M. A. (2008). Homotypic and heterotypic continuity of fine-grained temperament during infancy, toddlerhood, and early childhood. *Infant & Child Development, 17*(4), 387–405. https://doi.org/10.1002/ICD.582

Putnick, D. L., & Bornstein, M. H. (2016). Measurement invariance conventions and reporting: The state of the art and future directions for psychological research. *Developmental Review, 41*, 71–90. https://doi.org/10.1016/j.dr.2016.06.004

R Core Team. (2022). *R: A language and environment for statistical computing.* R Foundation for Statistical Computing. https://www.R-project.org/

Raiche, G., & Magis, D. (2020). *nFactors: Parallel analysis and other non graphical solutions to the Cattell scree test.* https://CRAN.R-project.org/package=nFactors

Raugh, I. M., Chapman, H. C., Bartolomeo, L. A., Gonzalez, C., & Strauss, G. P. (2019). A comprehensive review of psychophysiological applications for ecological momentary assessment in psychiatric populations. *Psychological Assessment, 31*(3), 304–317. https://doi.org/10.1037/pas0000651

Raykov, T. (2001). *Bias of coefficient α for fixed congeneric measures with correlated errors.* *25*(1), 69–76. https://doi.org/10.1177/01466216010251005

Raykov, T., & Marcoulides, G. A. (2019). Thanks coefficient alpha, we still need you! *Educational and Psychological Measurement, 79*(1), 200–210. https://doi.org/10.1177/0013164417725127

Raykov, T., Marcoulides, G. A., Harrison, M., & Zhang, M. (2020). On the dependability of a popular procedure for studying measurement invariance: A cause for concern? *Structural Equation Modeling: A Multidisciplinary Journal, 27*(4), 649–656. https://doi.org/10.1080/10705511.2019.1610409

Reise, S. P., & Waller, N. G. (2009). Item response theory and clinical measurement. *Annual Review of Clinical Psychology, 5*(1), 27–48. https://doi.org/10.1146/annurev.clinpsy.032408.153553

Revelle, W. (2022). *psych: Procedures for psychological, psychometric, and personality research.* https://personality-project.org/r/psych/

Revelle, W., & Condon, D. M. (2019). Reliability from α to ω: A tutorial. *Psychological Assessment, 31*(12), 1395–1411. https://doi.org/10.1037/pas0000754

Revelle, W., & Rocklin, T. (1979). Very simple structure: An alternative procedure for estimating the optimal number of interpretable factors. *Multivariate Behavioral Research, 14*(4), 403–414. https://doi.org/10.1207/s15327906mbr1404_2

Reynolds, C. R., Altmann, R. A., & Allen, D. N. (2021). The problem of bias in psychological assessment. In C. R. Reynolds, R. A. Altmann, & D. N. Allen (Eds.), *Mastering modern psychological testing: Theory and methods* (pp. 573–613). Springer International Publishing. https://doi.org/10.1007/978-3-030-59455-8_15

Reynolds, C. R., & Suzuki, L. A. (2012). Bias in psychological assessment: An empirical review and recommendations. In I. B. Weiner, J. R. Graham, & J. A. Naglieri (Eds.), *Handbook of psychology, Vol. 10: Assessment psychology, Part 1: Assessment issues* (2nd ed., pp. 82–113).

Rice, M. E., Harris, G. T., & Lang, C. (2013). Validation of and revision to the VRAG and SORAG: The Violence Risk Appraisal Guide—Revised (VRAG-R). *Psychological Assessment, 25*(3), 951–965. https://doi.org/10.1037/a0032878

Ridley, C. R., Hill, C. L., & Wiese, D. L. (2001). Ethics in multicultural assessment a model of reasoned application. In D. L. Wiese (Ed.), *Handbook of multicultural assessment: Clinical, psychological, and educational applications* (p. 29).

Ridley, C. R., Li, L. C., & Hill, C. L. (1998). Multicultural assessment: Reexamination, reconceptualization, and practical application. *The Counseling Psychologist, 26*(6), 827–910. https://doi.org/10.1177/0011000098266001

Rigdon, E. E. (2010). Polychoric correlation coefficient. In N. J. Salkind (Ed.), *Encyclopedia of research design.* SAGE Publications. https://doi.org/10.4135/9781412961288

Rivera Mindt, M., Byrd, D., Saez, P., & Manly, J. (2010). Increasing culturally competent neuropsychological services for ethnic minority populations: A call to action. *The Clinical Neuropsychologist, 24*(3), 429–453. https://doi.org/10.1080/13854040903058960

Roberts, A. C., Yeap, Y. W., Seah, H. S., Chan, E., Soh, C.-K., & Christopoulos, G. I. (2019). Assessing the suitability of virtual reality for psychological testing. *Psychological Assessment, 31*(3), 318–328. https://doi.org/10.1037/pas0000663

Robin, X., Turck, N., Hainard, A., Tiberti, N., Lisacek, F., Sanchez, J.-C., & Müller, M. (2021). *pROC: Display and analyze ROC curves.* http://expasy.org/tools/pROC/

Robitzsch, A. (2019). *mnlfa: Moderated nonlinear factor analysis.* https://CRAN.R-project.org/package=mnlfa

Rodebaugh, T. L., Scullin, R. B., Langer, J. K., Dixon, D. J., Huppert, J. D., Bernstein, A., Zvielli, A., & Lenze, E. J. (2016). Unreliability as a threat to understanding psychopathology: The cautionary tale of attentional bias. *Journal of Abnormal Psychology, 125*(6), 840–851. https://doi.org/10.1037/abn0000184

Roemer, E., Schuberth, F., & Henseler, J. (2021). HTMT2–an improved criterion for assessing discriminant validity in structural equation modeling. *Industrial Management & Data Systems*, *121*(12), 2637–2650. https://doi.org/10.1108/IMDS-02-2021-0082

Rönkkö, M., & Cho, E. (2020). An updated guideline for assessing discriminant validity. *Organizational Research Methods*, 1094428120968614. https://doi.org/10.1177/1094428120968614

Rosseel, Y., Jorgensen, T. D., & Rockwood, N. (2022). *lavaan: Latent variable analysis*. https://lavaan.ugent.be

Royal, K. (2016). "Face validity" is not a legitimate type of validity evidence! *The American Journal of Surgery*, *212*(5), 1026–1027. https://doi.org/10.1016/j.amjsurg.2016.02.018

Ruiz, M. A., Drake, E. B., Glass, A., Marcotte, D., & Gorp, W. G. van. (2002). Trying to beat the system: Misuse of the internet to assist in avoiding the detection of psychological symptom dissimulation. *Professional Psychology: Research and Practice*, *33*(3), 294–299. https://doi.org/10.1037/0735-7028.33.3.294

Ruscio, J., & Roche, B. (2012). Determining the number of factors to retain in an exploratory factor analysis using comparison data of known factorial structure. *Psychological Assessment*, *24*(2), 282–292. https://doi.org/10.1037/a0025697

Rush, A. J., First, M. B., & Blacker, D. (2009). *Handbook of psychiatric measures*. American Psychiatric Publishing.

Rushton, J. P., Brainerd, C. J., & Pressley, M. (1983). Behavioral development and construct validity: The principle of aggregation. *Psychological Bulletin*, *94*(1), 18–38. https://doi.org/10.1037/0033-2909.94.1.18

Russo, J. E., & Schoemaker, P. J. (1992). Managing overconfidence. *Sloan Management Review*, *33*(2), 7.

Sackett, P. R., Borneman, M. J., & Connelly, B. S. (2008). High stakes testing in higher education and employment: Appraising the evidence for validity and fairness. *American Psychologist*, *63*, 215–227. https://doi.org/10.1037/0003-066X.63.4.215

Sackett, P. R., Schmitt, N., Ellingson, J. E., & Kabin, M. B. (2001). High-stakes testing in employment, credentialing, and higher education. *American Psychologist*, *56*, 301–318. https://doi.org/10.1037/0003-066X.56.4.302

Sackett, P. R., & Wilk, S. L. (1994). Within-group norming and other forms of score adjustment in preemployment testing. *American Psychologist*, *49*(11), 929–954. https://doi.org/10.1037/0003-066X.49.11.929

Sattler, J. M., & Hoge, R. D. (2006). *Assessment of children: Behavioral, social, and clinical foundations* (5th ed.). Jerome M. Sattler, Publisher, Inc.

Schaefer, J. D., Caspi, A., Belsky, D. W., Harrington, H., Houts, R., Horwood, L. J., Hussong, A., Ramrakha, S., Poulton, R., & Moffitt, T. E. (2017). Enduring mental health: Prevalence and prediction. *Journal of Abnormal Psychology*, *126*(2), 212–224. https://doi.org/10.1037/abn0000232

Schaie, K. W. (1965). A general model for the study of developmental problems. *Psychological Bulletin*, *64*(2), 92–107. https://doi.org/10.1037/h0022371

Schaie, K. W. (2005). *Developmental influences on adult intelligence: The Seattle longitudinal study*. Oxford University Press.

Schaie, K. W., & Baltes, P. B. (1975). On sequential strategies in developmental research. *Human Development*, *18*(5), 384–390. https://doi.org/10.1159/000271498

Schmidt, F. L., & Hunter, J. E. (1981). Employment testing: Old theories and new research findings. *American Psychologist*, *36*(10), 1128–1137. https://doi.org/10.1037/0003-066X.36.10.1128

Schmidt, F. L., & Hunter, J. E. (1996). Measurement error in psychological research: Lessons from 26 research scenarios. *Psychological Methods*, *1*(2), 199–223. https://doi.org/10.1037/1082-989X.1.2.199

Schneider, W. J. (2021). *simstandard: Generate standardized data.* https://github.com/wjschne/simstandard

Schuberth, F. (2023). The Henseler-Ogasawara specification of composites in structural equation modeling: A tutorial. *Psychological Methods, 28*(4), 843–859. https://doi.org/10.1037/met0000432

Schulenberg, J. E., & Maslowsky, J. (2009). Taking substance use and development seriously: Developmentally distal and proximal influences on adolescence drug use. *Monographs of the Society for Research in Child Development, 74*(3), 121–130. https://doi.org/10.1111/j.1540-5834.2009.00544.x

Sechrest, L. (1963). Incremental validity: A recommendation. *Educational and Psychological Measurement, 23*, 153–158. https://doi.org/10.1177/001316446302300113

Sechrest, L., Stickle, T. R., & Stewart, M. (1998). The role of assessment in clinical psychology. In A. Bellack, M. Hersen, & C. R. Reynolds (Eds.), *Comprehensive clinical psychology, Vol. 4: Assessment.* Pergamon.

Sellbom, M. (2019). The MMPI-2-restructured form (MMPI-2-RF): Assessment of personality and psychopathology in the twenty-first century. *Annual Review of Clinical Psychology, 15*(1), 149–177. https://doi.org/10.1146/annurev-clinpsy-050718-095701

Sellbom, M., & Tellegen, A. (2019). Factor analysis in psychological assessment research: Common pitfalls and recommendations. *Psychological Assessment, 31*(12), 1428–1441. https://doi.org/10.1037/pas0000623

Sharp, K. L., Williams, A. J., Rhyner, K. T., & Ilardi, S. S. (2013). The clinical interview. In K. F. Geisinger, J. F. Carlson, J.-I. C. Hansen, N. R. Kuncel, S. P. Reise, & M. C. Rodriguez (Eds.), *APA handbook of testing and assessment in psychology, Vol. 2: Testing and assessment in clinical and counseling psychology* (pp. 103–117). American Psychological Association.

Shavelson, R. J., Webb, N. M., & Rawley, R. L. (1989). Generalizability theory. *American Psychologist, 44*, 922–932. https://doi.org/10.1037/0003-066X.44.6.922

Shrout, P. E., & Rodgers, J. L. (2018). Psychology, science, and knowledge construction: Broadening perspectives from the replication crisis. *Annual Review of Psychology, 69*(1), 487–510. https://doi.org/10.1146/annurev-psych-122216-011845

Sijtsma, K. (2008). On the use, the misuse, and the very limited usefulness of cronbach's alpha. *Psychometrika, 74*(1), 107. https://doi.org/10.1007/s11336-008-9101-0

Silver, N. (2012). *The signal and the noise: Why so many predictions fail–but some don't.* Penguin.

Silverberg, N. D., & Millis, S. R. (2009). Impairment versus deficiency in neuropsychological assessment: Implications for ecological validity. *Journal of the International Neuropsychological Society, 15*(1), 94–102. https://doi.org/10.1017/S1355617708090139

Simms, L. J., Zelazny, K., Williams, T. F., & Bernstein, L. (2019). Does the number of response options matter? Psychometric perspectives using personality questionnaire data. *Psychological Assessment, 31*(4), 557–566. https://doi.org/10.1037/pas0000648

Skala, D. (2008). Overconfidence in psychology and finance–an interdisciplinary literature review. *Bank i Kredyt, 4*, 33–50.

Slack, M. K., & Draugalis, J., Jolaine R. (2001). Establishing the internal and external validity of experimental studies. *American Journal of Health-System Pharmacy, 58*(22), 2173–2181. https://doi.org/10.1093/ajhp/58.22.2173

Smedley, A., & Smedley, B. D. (2005). Race as biology is fiction, racism as a social problem is real: Anthropological and historical perspectives on the social construction of race. *American Psychologist, 60*(1), 16–26. https://doi.org/10.1037/0003-066X.60.1.16

Smith, G. T., Atkinson, E. A., Davis, H. A., Riley, E. N., & Oltmanns, J. R. (2020). The general factor of psychopathology. *Annual Review of Clinical Psychology, 16*(1), 75–98. https://doi.org/10.1146/annurev-clinpsy-071119-115848

Smith, G. T., McCarthy, D. M., & Anderson, K. G. (2000). On the sins of short-form development. *Psychological Assessment*, *12*(1), 102–111. https://doi.org/10.1037/1040-3590.12.1.102

Sobell, L. C., & Sobell, M. B. (2008). Timeline followback (TLFB). In A. J. Rush Jr., M. B. First, & D. Blacker (Eds.), *Handbook of psychiatric measures* (2nd ed., pp. 466–468). American Psychiatric Publishing.

Sommers-Flanagan, J., & Sommers-Flanagan, R. (2016). *Clinical interviewing.* Wiley.

Somoza, E., Soutullo-Esperon, L., & Mossman, D. (1989). Evaluation and optimization of diagnostic tests using receiver operating characteristic analysis and information theory. *International Journal of Bio-Medical Computing*, *24*(3), 153–189. https://doi.org/10.1016/0020-7101(89)90029-9

Stanislaw, H., & Todorov, N. (1999). Calculation of signal detection theory measures. *Behavior Research Methods, Instruments, & Computers*, *31*(1), 137–149. https://doi.org/10.3758/bf03207704

Stanton, K., McDonnell, C. G., Hayden, E. P., & Watson, D. (2020). Transdiagnostic approaches to psychopathology measurement: Recommendations for measure selection, data analysis, and participant recruitment. *Journal of Abnormal Psychology*, *129*(1), 21–28. https://doi.org/10.1037/abn0000464

Staples, A. D., Bates, J. E., Petersen, I. T., McQuillan, M. E., & Hoyniak, C. (2019). Measuring sleep in young children and their mothers: Identifying actigraphic sleep composites. *International Journal of Behavioral Development*, *43*(3), 278–285. https://doi.org/10.1177/0165025419830236

Sternberg, R. J., Grigorenko, E. L., & Kidd, K. K. (2005). Intelligence, race, and genetics. *American Psychologist*, *60*(1), 46–59. https://doi.org/10.1037/0003-066x.60.1.46

Stevens, R. J., & Poppe, K. K. (2020). Validation of clinical prediction models: What does the "calibration slope" really measure? *Journal of Clinical Epidemiology*, *118*, 93–99. https://doi.org/10.1016/j.jclinepi.2019.09.016

Steyerberg, E. W., & Vergouwe, Y. (2014). Towards better clinical prediction models: Seven steps for development and an ABCD for validation. *European Heart Journal*, *35*(29), 1925–1931. https://doi.org/10.1093/eurheartj/ehu207

Steyerberg, E. W., Vickers, A. J., Cook, N. R., Gerds, T., Gonen, M., Obuchowski, N., Pencina, M. J., & Kattan, M. W. (2010). Assessing the performance of prediction models: A framework for traditional and novel measures. *Epidemiology*, *21*(1), 128–138. https://doi.org/10.1097/EDE.0b013e3181c30fb2

Strauss, M. E., & Smith, G. T. (2009). Construct validity: Advances in theory and methodology. *Annual Review of Clinical Psychology*, *5*(1), 1–25. https://doi.org/10.1146/annurev.clinpsy.032408.153639

Sullivan, H. S. (1970). *The psychiatric interview.* Norton.

Summerfeldt, L. J., Kloosterman, P. H., & Antony, M. M. (2010). Structured and semistructured diagnostic interviews. In M. M. Antony & D. H. Barlow (Eds.), *Handbook of assessment and treatment planning for psychological disorders* (2nd ed., pp. 95–137). Guilford Press.

Suzuki, L. A., Onoue, M. A., & Hill, J. S. (2013). Clinical assessment: A multicultural perspective. In K. F. Geisinger, J. F. Carlson, J.-I. C. Hansen, N. R. Kuncel, S. P. Reise, & M. C. Rodriguez (Eds.), *APA handbook of testing and assessment in psychology, Vol. 2: Testing and assessment in clinical and counseling psychology* (pp. 193–212). American Psychological Association.

Swets, J. A., Dawes, R. M., & Monahan, J. (2000). Psychological science can improve diagnostic decisions. *Psychological Science in the Public Interest*, *1*, 1–26. https://doi.org/10.1111/1529-1006.001

Tackett, J. L., Brandes, C. M., King, K. M., & Markon, K. E. (2019). Psychology's replication crisis and clinical psychological science. *Annual Review of Clinical Psychology, 15*(1), 579–604. https://doi.org/10.1146/annurev-clinpsy-050718-095710

Tackett, J. L., Brandes, C. M., & Reardon, K. W. (2019). Leveraging the open science framework in clinical psychological assessment research. *Psychological Assessment, 31*(12), 1386–1394. https://doi.org/10.1037/pas0000583

Tackett, J. L., Lang, J. W. B., Markon, K. E., & Herzhoff, K. (2019). A correlated traits, correlated methods model for thin-slice child personality assessment. *Psychological Assessment, 31*(4), 545–556. https://doi.org/10.1037/pas0000635

Tervalon, M., & Murray-Garcia, J. (1998). Cultural humility versus cultural competence: A critical distinction in defining physician training outcomes in multicultural education. *Journal of Health Care for the Poor and Underserved, 9*(2), 117–125.

Tetlock, P. E. (2017). *Expert political judgment: How good is it? How can we know? - New edition.* Princeton University Press.

Textor, J., van der Zander, B., & Ankan, A. (2021). *dagitty: Graphical analysis of structural causal models.* https://CRAN.R-project.org/package=dagitty

Thomas, M. L. (2019). Advances in applications of item response theory to clinical assessment. *Psychological Assessment, 31*(12), 1442–1455. https://doi.org/10.1037/pas0000597

Thorndike, R. L. (1971). Concepts of culture-fairness. *Journal of Educational Measurement, 8*(2), 63–70. https://doi.org/10.1111/j.1745-3984.1971.tb00907.x

Tiego, J., Martin, E. A., DeYoung, C. G., Hagan, K., Cooper, S. E., Pasion, R., Satchell, L., Shackman, A. J., Bellgrove, M. A., Fornito, A., Abend, R., Goulter, N., Eaton, N. R., Kaczkurkin, A. N., & Nusslock, R. (2023). Precision behavioral phenotyping as a strategy for uncovering the biological correlates of psychopathology. *Nature Mental Health, 1*, 304–315. https://doi.org/10.1038/s44220-023-00057-5

Tofallis, C. (2015). A better measure of relative prediction accuracy for model selection and model estimation. *Journal of the Operational Research Society, 66*(8), 1352–1362. https://doi.org/10.1057/jors.2014.103

Tong, Y., & Kolen, M. J. (2007). Comparisons of methodologies and results in vertical scaling for educational achievement tests. *Applied Measurement in Education, 20*(2), 227–253. https://doi.org/10.1080/08957340701301207

Toomey, R. B., Syvertsen, A. K., & Shramko, M. (2018). Transgender adolescent suicide behavior. *Pediatrics, 142*(4). https://doi.org/10.1542/peds.2017-4218

Trafimow, D. (2015). A defense against the alleged unreliability of difference scores. *Cogent Mathematics, 2*(1), 1064626. https://doi.org/10.1080/23311835.2015.1064626

Treat, T. A., McFall, R. M., Viken, R. J., Kruschke, J. K., Nosofsky, R. M., & Wang, S. S. (2007). Clinical cognitive science: Applying quantitative models of cognitive processing to examine cognitive aspects of psychopathology. In R. W. J. Neufeld (Ed.), *Advances in clinical cognitive science: Formal modeling of processes and symptoms* (pp. 179–205). American Psychological Association.

Treat, T. A., & Viken, R. J. (2023). Measuring test performance with signal detection theory techniques. In H. Cooper, M. N. Coutanche, L. M. McMullen, A. T. Panter, D. Rindskopf, & K. J. Sher (Eds.), *APA handbook of research methods in psychology: Foundations, planning, measures, and psychometrics* (2nd ed., Vol. 1, pp. 837–858). American Psychological Association.

Treiblmaier, H., Bentler, P. M., & Mair, P. (2011). Formative constructs implemented via common factors. *Structural Equation Modeling: A Multidisciplinary Journal, 18*(1), 1–17. https://doi.org/10.1080/10705511.2011.532693

Trull, T. J., & Ebner-Priemer, U. W. (2020). Ambulatory assessment in psychopathology research: A review of recommended reporting guidelines and current practices. *Journal of Abnormal Psychology, 129*(1), 56–63. https://doi.org/10.1037/abn0000473

Tversky, A., & Kahneman, D. (1974). Judgment under uncertainty: Heuristics and biases. *Science*, *185*(4157), 1124–1131. https://doi.org/10.1126/science.185.4157.1124

Ursenbach, J., O'Connell, M. E., Neiser, J., Tierney, M. C., Morgan, D., Kosteniuk, J., & Spiteri, R. J. (2019). Scoring algorithms for a computer-based cognitive screening tool: An illustrative example of overfitting machine learning approaches and the impact on estimates of classification accuracy. *Psychological Assessment*, *31*(11), 1377–1382. https://doi.org/10.1037/pas0000764

Van De Schoot, R., Kluytmans, A., Tummers, L., Lugtig, P., Hox, J., & Muthen, B. (2013). Facing off with scylla and charybdis: A comparison of scalar, partial, and the novel possibility of approximate measurement invariance. *Frontiers in Psychology*, *4*(770). https://doi.org/10.3389/fpsyg.2013.00770

Van De Schoot, R., Schmidt, P., De Beuckelaer, A., Lek, K., & Zondervan-Zwijnenburg, M. (2015). Editorial: Measurement invariance. *Frontiers in Psychology*, *6*(1064). https://doi.org/10.3389/fpsyg.2015.01064

van der Nest, G., Lima Passos, V., Candel, M. J. J. M., & van Breukelen, G. J. P. (2020). An overview of mixture modelling for latent evolutions in longitudinal data: Modelling approaches, fit statistics and software. *Advances in Life Course Research*, *43*, 100323. https://doi.org/10.1016/j.alcr.2019.100323

Vaz, S., Falkmer, T., Passmore, A. E., Parsons, R., & Andreou, P. (2013). The case for using the repeatability coefficient when calculating test–retest reliability. *PLOS ONE*, *8*(9), e73990. https://doi.org/10.1371/journal.pone.0073990

Vispoel, W. P., Hong, H., & Lee, H. (2023). Benefits of doing generalizability theory analyses within structural equation modeling frameworks: Illustrations using the Rosenberg self-esteem scale. *Structural Equation Modeling: A Multidisciplinary Journal*, 1–17. https://doi.org/10.1080/10705511.2023.2187734

Vispoel, W. P., Lee, H., Xu, G., & Hong, H. (2022). Integrating bifactor models into a generalizability theory based structural equation modeling framework. *The Journal of Experimental Education*, 1–21. https://doi.org/10.1080/00220973.2022.2092833

Vispoel, W. P., Morris, C. A., & Kilinc, M. (2018). Applications of generalizability theory and their relations to classical test theory and structural equation modeling. *Psychological Methods*, *23*(1), 1–26. https://doi.org/10.1037/met0000107

Vispoel, W. P., Morris, C. A., & Kilinc, M. (2019). Using generalizability theory with continuous latent response variables. *Psychological Methods*, *24*(2), 153–178. https://doi.org/10.1037/met0000177

Voorhees, C. M., Brady, M. K., Calantone, R., & Ramirez, E. (2016). Discriminant validity testing in marketing: An analysis, causes for concern, and proposed remedies. *Journal of the Academy of Marketing Science*, *44*(1), 119–134. https://doi.org/10.1007/s11747-015-0455-4

Wakschlag, L. S., Tolan, P. H., & Leventhal, B. L. (2010). Research review: "Ain't misbehavin": Towards a developmentally-specified nosology for preschool disruptive behavior. *Journal of Child Psychology and Psychiatry*, *51*(1), 3–22. https://doi.org/10.1111/j.1469-7610.2009.02184.x

Wang, S., Jiao, H., & Zhang, L. (2013). Validation of longitudinal achievement constructs of vertically scaled computerised adaptive tests: A multiple-indicator, latent-growth modelling approach. *International Journal of Quantitative Research in Education*, *1*(4), 383–407. https://doi.org/10.1504/IJQRE.2013.058307

Wang, T., Merkle, E. C., & Zeileis, A. (2014). Score-based tests of measurement invariance: Use in practice. *Frontiers in Psychology*, *5*. https://doi.org/10.3389/fpsyg.2014.00438

Wang, W.-C., Shih, C.-L., & Yang, C.-C. (2009). The MIMIC method with scale purification for detecting differential item functioning. *Educational and Psychological Measurement*, *69*(5), 713–731. https://doi.org/10.1177/0013164409332228

Watkins, C. E., Campbell, V. L., Nieberding, R., & Hallmark, R. (1995). Contemporary practice of psychological assessment by clinical psychologists. *Professional Psychology: Research and Practice*, *26*(1), 54–60. https://doi.org/10.1037/0735-7028.26.1.54

Weems, C. F. (2008). Developmental trajectories of childhood anxiety: Identifying continuity and change in anxious emotion. *Developmental Review*, *28*(4), 488–502. https://doi.org/10.1016/j.dr.2008.01.001

Wei, T., & Simko, V. (2021). *R package "corrplot": Visualization of a correlation matrix.* https://github.com/taiyun/corrplot

Weintraub, S., Bauer, P. J., Zelazo, P. D., Wallner-Allen, K., Dikmen, S. S., Heaton, R. K., Tulsky, D. S., Slotkin, J., Blitz, D. L., Carlozzi, N. E., Havlik, R. J., Beaumont, J. L., Mungas, D., Manly, J. J., Borosh, B. G., Nowinski, C. J., & Gershon, R. C. (2013). I. NIH toolbox cognition battery (CB): Introduction and pediatric data. *Monographs of the Society for Research in Child Development*, *78*(4), 1–15. https://doi.org/10.1111/mono.12031

Weiss, B., & Garber, J. (2003). Developmental differences in the phenomenology of depression. *Development and Psychopathology*, *15*(2), 403–430. https://doi.org/10.1017/S0954579403000221

Whitbourne, S. K. (2019). *Longitudinal, cross-sectional, and sequential designs in lifespan developmental psychology.* Oxford University Press.

Wicherts, J. M., & Dolan, C. V. (2010). Measurement invariance in confirmatory factor analysis: An illustration using IQ test performance of minorities. *Educational Measurement: Issues and Practice*, *29*(3), 39–47. https://doi.org/10.1111/j.1745-3992.2010.00182.x

Wickham, H. (2021). *tidyverse: Easily install and load the tidyverse.* https://CRAN.R-project.org/package=tidyverse

Wickham, H., Averick, M., Bryan, J., Chang, W., McGowan, L. D., François, R., Grolemund, G., Hayes, A., Henry, L., Hester, J., Kuhn, M., Pedersen, T. L., Miller, E., Bache, S. M., Müller, K., Ooms, J., Robinson, D., Seidel, D. P., Spinu, V., ... Yutani, H. (2019). Welcome to the tidyverse. *Journal of Open Source Software*, *4*(43), 1686. https://doi.org/10.21105/joss.01686

Widiger, T. A. (2002). Personality disorders. In M. M. Antony & D. H. Barlow (Eds.), *Handbook of assessment and treatment planning for psychological disorders* (pp. 453–480). Guilford Publications.

Wiggins, J. S. (1973). *Personality and prediction: Principles of personality assessment.* Addison-Wesley.

Willett, W. (2012). Correction for the effects of measurement error. In W. Willett (Ed.), *Nutritional epidemiology* (3rd ed., pp. 287–304). Oxford University Press.

Williams, A. J., Botanov, Y., Kilshaw, R. E., Wong, R. E., & Sakaluk, J. K. (2021). Potentially harmful therapies: A meta-scientific review of evidential value. *Clinical Psychology: Science and Practice*, *28*(1), 5–18. https://doi.org/10.1111/cpsp.12331

Wood, J. M., Garb, H. N., Lilienfeld, S. O., & Nezworski, M. T. (2002). Clinical assessment. *Annual Review of Psychology*, *53*(1), 519. https://doi.org/10.1146/annurev.psych.53.100901.135136

Wood, J. M., Nezworski, M. T., Garb, H. N., & Lilienfeld, S. O. (2001). Problems with the norms of the Comprehensive System for the Rorschach: Methodological and conceptual considerations. *Clinical Psychology: Science and Practice*, *8*(3), 397–402. https://doi.org/10.1093/clipsy.8.3.397

Wood, J. M., Nezworski, M. T., & Stejskal, W. J. (1996a). The Comprehensive System for the Rorschach: A critical examination. *Psychological Science*, *7*(1), 3–10. https://doi.org/10.1111/j.1467-9280.1996.tb00658.x

Wood, J. M., Nezworski, M. T., & Stejskal, W. J. (1996b). Thinking critically about the Comprehensive System for the Rorschach: A reply to exner. *Psychological Science*, *7*(1), 14–17. https://doi.org/10.1111/j.1467-9280.1996.tb00660.x

Wood, J. M., Teresa, P. M., Garb, H. N., & Lilienfeld, S. O. (2001). The misperception of psychopathology: Problems with the norms of the Comprehensive System for the Rorschach. *Clinical Psychology: Science and Practice*, *8*(3), 350–373. https://doi.org/10.1093/clipsy.8.3.350

Woody, M. L., & Gibb, B. E. (2015). Integrating NIMH Research Domain Criteria (RDoC) into depression research. *Current Opinion in Psychology*, *4*, 6–12. https://doi.org/10.1016/j.copsyc.2015.01.004

Wright, A. G. C., Gates, K. M., Arizmendi, C., Lane, S. T., Woods, W. C., & Edershile, E. A. (2019). Focusing personality assessment on the person: Modeling general, shared, and person specific processes in personality and psychopathology. *Psychological Assessment*, *31*(4), 502–515. https://doi.org/10.1037/pas0000617

Wright, A. G. C., & Woods, W. C. (2020). Personalized models of psychopathology. *Annual Review of Clinical Psychology*, *16*(1), 49–74. https://doi.org/10.1146/annurev-clinpsy-102419-125032

Wright, A. G. C., & Zimmermann, J. (2019). Applied ambulatory assessment: Integrating idiographic and nomothetic principles of measurement. *Psychological Assessment*, *31*(12), 1467–1480. https://doi.org/10.1037/pas0000685

Yang, Y., & Land, K. C. (2013). *Age-period-cohort analysis: New models, methods, and empirical applications*. Taylor & Francis.

Youngstrom, E. A., Halverson, T. F., Youngstrom, J. K., Lindhiem, O., & Findling, R. L. (2018). Evidence-based assessment from simple clinical judgments to statistical learning: Evaluating a range of options using pediatric bipolar disorder as a diagnostic challenge. *Clinical Psychological Science*, *6*(2), 243–265. https://doi.org/10.1177/2167702617741845

Youngstrom, E. A., & Van Meter, A. (2016). Empirically supported assessment of children and adolescents. *Clinical Psychology: Science and Practice*, *23*(4), 327–347. https://doi.org/10.1111/cpsp.12172

Youngstrom, E. A., Van Meter, A., Frazier, T. W., Hunsley, J., Prinstein, M. J., Ong, M.-L., & Youngstrom, J. K. (2017). Evidence-based assessment as an integrative model for applying psychological science to guide the voyage of treatment. *Clinical Psychology: Science and Practice*, *24*(4), 331–363. https://doi.org/10.1111/cpsp.12207

Yu, X., Schuberth, F., & Henseler, J. (2023). Specifying composites in structural equation modeling: A refinement of the Henseler-Ogasawara specification. *Statistical Analysis and Data Mining: The ASA Data Science Journal*, *16*(4), 348–357. https://doi.org/https://doi.org/10.1002/sam.11608

Yudell, M., Roberts, D., DeSalle, R., & Tishkoff, S. (2016). Taking race out of human genetics. *Science*, *351*(6273), 564–565. https://doi.org/10.1126/science.aac4951

Zhang, J., & Mueller, S. T. (2005). A note on ROC analysis and non-parametric estimate of sensitivity. *Psychometrika*, *70*(1), 203–212. https://doi.org/10.1007/s11336-003-1119-8

Zieky, M. J. (2006). Fairness review in assessment. In S. M. Downing & T. M. Haladyna (Eds.), *Handbook of test development* (pp. 359–376). Routledge. https://doi.org/10.4324/9780203874776.ch16

Zieky, M. J. (2013). Fairness review in assessment. In K. F. Geisinger, B. A. Bracken, J. F. Carlson, J.-I. C. Hansen, N. R. Kuncel, S. P. Reise, & M. C. Rodriguez (Eds.), *APA handbook of testing and assessment in psychology, Vol. 1: Test theory and testing and assessment in industrial and organizational psychology* (pp. 293–302). American Psychological Association. https://doi.org/10.1037/14047-017

Zuckerman, M. (1990). Some dubious premises in research and theory on racial differences: Scientific, social, and ethical issues. *American Psychologist*, *45*(12), 1297–1303. https://doi.org/10.1037/0003-066X.45.12.1297

Index

For Product Safety Concerns and Information please contact our EU
representative GPSR@taylorandfrancis.com
Taylor & Francis Verlag GmbH, Kaufingerstraße 24, 80331 München, Germany

www.ingramcontent.com/pod-product-compliance
Ingram Content Group UK Ltd.
Pitfield, Milton Keynes, MK11 3LW, UK
UKHW050056200926
475702UK00019B/2874
* 9 7 8 1 0 3 2 4 1 1 3 4 7 *